Textbook of
Cosmetic Dermatology

Textbook of
Cosmetic Dermatology

SECOND EDITION

Edited by

Robert Baran, MD
Nail Disease Center
42 rue des Serbes
06400 Cannes
France

Howard I Maibach, MD
University of California
Department of Dermatology
Medical Center Way, Surge 110
San Francisco, CA 94143–0989
USA

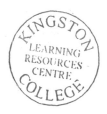

MARTIN DUNITZ

© Martin Dunitz Ltd 1994, 1998

First published in the United Kingdom in
1994 by Martin Dunitz Ltd, 7–9 Pratt Street
London NW1 0AE

Second edition 1998

A CIP catalogue record for this book is available from the British Library

ISBN 1-85317-478-5

Distributed in the United States by:
Blackwell Science Inc.
Commerce Place, 350 Main Street
Malden, MA 02148, USA
Tel: 1–800–215–1000

Distributed in Canada by:
Login Brothers Book Company
324 Salteaux Crescent
Winnipeg, Manitoba, R3J 3T2
Canada
Tel: 204–224–4068

Distributed in Brazil by:
Ernesto Reichmann Distribuidora de Livros, Ltda
Rue Coronel Marques 335, Tatuape 03440–000
São Paulo,
Brazil

Composition by Wearset, Boldon, Tyne and Wear
Printed and bound in Singapore by Kyodo Printing Co (S'pore) Pte Ltd

Contents

Preface ix

Contributors.. xi

Comment: Drugs, cosmetics and cosmeceuticals *Robert Baran, Howard I Maibach* xvii

PART ONE   INFLUENCES ON SKIN PARAMETERS

   1. Climatic influence on cosmetic skin parameters *Mathias Rohr, Karlheinz Schrader* 1
   2. Skin and gender *Ethel Tur, Sarah Brenner*... 17

PART TWO   PHARMACOLOGY OF COSMETIC PRODUCTS

   3. In vitro skin toxicity assays for predicting cosmetic-induced irritancy
      Jeff D Harvell, Howard I Maibach... 33
   4. Perfumes *Walter G Larsen* 41
   5. Regulation *Nicola Loprieno* 49

PART THREE   CUTANEOUS ABSORPTION AND COSMETOLOGY

   6. Cosmetic percutaneous absorption *Ronald C Wester, Howard I Maibach* 75
   7. Percutaneous penetration and diffusion of cosmetic ingredients: Implications for
      safety and efficacy *Jean-Paul L Marty* 85
   8. Transungual drug delivery systems: What's new and relevant?
      Jean-Paul L Marty, Robert Baran 95

PART FOUR   COSMETOLOGY FOR NORMAL SKIN

   9. Ceramides and the skin *Anthony Rawlings, Clive R Harding, Kurt M Schilling*................... 99
  10. Main finished products: Moisturizing and cleansing creams
      Daniel H Maes, Kenneth D Marenus.. 113
  11. Skin care products for normal, dry and greasy skin
      David Black, Stéphane Diridollou, Jean-Michel Lagarde, Yvon Gall 125
  12. Self-tanning products *Daniel H Maes, Kenneth D Marenus*....................................... 151
  13. Masks and astringents/toners *Myra O Barker* 155

PART FIVE   COSMETOLOGY FOR SPECIAL LOCATIONS

  14. Ancillary skin care products *Zoe Diana Draelos* 167
  15. Topical deodorants *Daniel Lambert* 171

16. Hair care *Rodney Dawber* 177

17. Isolated dandruff *Caroline W Cardin* 193

18. Facial and body hair *Rodney Dawber* 201

19. Eye make-up *Anne-Marie Orecchioni* 205

20. Nail varnish formulation *Douglas Schoon* 213

21. Cosmetology for normal nails *Robert Baran, Douglas Schoon* 219

22. Cosmetics for abnormal and pathological nails *Robert Baran, Douglas Schoon* 233

23. Efficacy of moisturizers assessed through bioengineering techniques
Whitney Hannon, Howard I Maibach 245

24. Hand and body lotions *F Anthony Simion, Michael S Starch, Pamela S Witt,
Judith K Woodford, Keith J Edgett* 285

25. Infrared irradiation: Skin effects and protection *Kenneth D Marenus, Daniel H Maes* 309

26. Efficacy of sunscreens *Nicholas J Lowe* 317

27. The vulva *Peter Elsner, Howard I Maibach* 331

PART SIX   COSMETIC TREATMENT OF SPECIAL CONDITIONS

28. Sensitive skin: What is it? *Smita Amin, Patricia Engasser, Howard I Maibach* 343

29. Role of lipids in irritant dermatitis *Anna Di Nardo, Philip W Wertz,
Howard I Maibach* 351

30. Ichthyosis *Rudolf Happle* 359

31. Atopic dermatitis *Georg Rajka* 367

32. Telangiectases *Albert-Adrien Ramelet* 373

33. Hirsutism *Rodney Dawber* 381

34. Pigmentation: Dyschromia *Sumar Kumit Bose, Jean-Paul Ortonne* 391

35. Camouflage cosmetics *Victoria L Rayner* 417

36. Acne *Robert Baran, Martine Chivot, Alan R Shalita* 433

37. Idiopathic hyperhidrosis *Daniel Lambert* 445

38. Aging and photoaging *William M Cunningham* 455

39. Modulation of inflammatory reactions in skin: A new approach to the treatment of
premature aging *Daniel H Maes, Kenneth D Marenus* 469

40. Menopause, skin and cosmetology *Claire Beylot* 487

PART SEVEN   SKIN CARE FOR SPECIAL GROUPS

41. Cosmetics for men *Robert Baran* 495

42. Cosmetic dermatology in children *Danielle Marcoux, John Harper* 505

43. Ethnic cosmetics: Blacks, Hispanics and Orientals
Alessandra Pelosi, Enzo Berardesca, Howard I Maibach 515

PART EIGHT   NON-INVASIVE ASSESSMENT TECHNIQUES IN COSMETOLOGY

44. Measurement of blood flow in the cutaneous microvasculature
Maria Beatriz Lagos, Andreas J Bircher, Howard I Maibach 523

45. Stratum corneum water content and TEWL *Enzo Berardesca, Howard I Maibach* 529

46. Non-invasive techniques for cutaneous investigation *Jean Luc Lévêque* 537

47. The phototrichogram *Monique Courtois* 545
48. Thermal sensory analysis *Gil Yosipovitch* 549

PART NINE   TECHNIQUES IN COSMETOLOGICAL TREATMENT

49. Reduction syringe liposculpturing *Pierre F Fournier* 553
50. Syringe fat transfer *Pierre F Fournier* 569
51. Facial chemical peel *Randall K Roenigk* 585
52. Dermabrasion for rejuvenation and scar revision *Henry H Roenigk Jr* 595
53. Soft-tissue augmentation *C William Hanke, Jenette Michalak* 613
54. Gore-tex and facial rejuvenation *Claude Lassus* 623
55. Hair loss: Surgical treatments *Henry H Roenigk Jr* 633
56. Electrical stimulation of skin (ESS) in skin aging and scars: 13 years'
  experience with electrorhytidopuncture *Liliane Schnitzler, Philippe Simonin* 643
57. Cosmetic cutaneous laser surgery *Timothy J Rosio* 657
58. Cosmetic cryosurgery *Rodney D Sinclair, Christopher Tzermias, Rodney Dawber* 691
59. Cosmetic denervation with botulinum (Botox) toxin *James E Fulton Jr* 701

PART TEN   SIDE-EFFECTS AND SOCIAL ASPECTS OF COSMETOLOGY

60. Adverse cosmetic reactions *Smita Amin, Patricia Engasser, Howard I Maibach* 709
61. Social, psychological and psychiatric aspects of cosmetic use *John A Cotterill* 747

INDEX 755

Preface

The focus in this new edition of *Textbook of Cosmetic Dermatology*, as in the first, is on the scientific aspects of cosmetics and skin care. We tried to fill a gap in the medical literature concerning this field, and the worldwide success of the first edition, coupled with the encouragement of many readers, prompted us to continue along the same lines.

Recent developments in physical and clinical techniques together with the newer surgical approaches are described. There is a pharmacological section – essential for the understanding of cosmetology – and a clinical section that discusses normal skin as well as certain pathological skin conditions. Dermatological surgery has a natural place here.

The chapters from the first edition have been comprehensively revised and updated; many have been completely rewritten. This edition has additional chapters on topics such as climatic influences on cosmetic skin parameters, skin and gender, sensitive skin, modulation of inflammatory reactions in skin, and thermal sensory analysis.

As with the first edition, this book is the fruit of the work of an international team, and each subject has been dealt with by a renowned specialist. It is a textbook aimed at readers who wish to broaden their knowledge, and all those who are interested in cosmetic dermatology – specialists, general practitioners and beauticians – will find the information they require in this book. Those who wish to go deeper into topics in which they have a special interest can do so thanks to numerous references aimed at helping them to advance in their study.

Finally, sincere thanks are due to our Publishers, and especially to their Managing Editor, Alison Campbell.

Robert Baran
Howard I Maibach

Contributors

Smita Amin, MD, FRCPC
Division of Dermatology
Department of Medicine
The Toronto Hospital, Western Division
University of Toronto
Toronto, Ontario M5T 2SB
Canada

Robert Baran, MD
Nail Disease Center
42 rue des Serbes
06400 Cannes
France

Myra O Barker, PhD
Chief Scientific Officer
Mary Kay Holding Corporation
Global Research and Development Group
1430 Regal Row, Suite 340
Dallas, TX 75247–3698
USA

Enzo Berardesca, MD
Clinica Dermatologica
dell'Università di Pavia
Policlinico S. Matteo
27100 Pavia
Italy

Claire Beylot, MD
Professor of Dermatology
University of Bordeaux II
Hôpital du Haut-Lévêque
CHU de Bordeaux
33604 Pessac
France

Andreas J Bircher, MD
Department of Dermatology
University Hospital
Petersgraben
CH-4031 Basel
Switzerland

David Black, PhD
Institut de Recherche Pierre Fabre
Département Recherche et Evaluation
Dermocosmétique
BP 4404
31405 Toulouse
France

Sumit Kumar Bose, MD
Skin Institute and
School of Dermatology
New-Delhi
India

Sarah Brenner, MD
Tel Aviv University
Sackler School of Medicine
Tel Aviv 64239
Israel

Caroline W Cardin, MSc
Procter & Gamble Company
11511 Reed Hartman Highway
Cincinnati, OH 45241–9974
USA

Martine Chivot, MD
288 rue Saint-Jacques
75005 Paris
France

John A Cotterill, MD, FRCP
Lasercare Clinics
1 Park View
Harrogate
North Yorkshire, HG1 5LY
UK

Monique Courtois, MD
Laboratoire L'Oréal
8 Impasse Barbier
92117 Clichy Cedex
France

William M Cunningham, MD
Cu-Tech Inc
International Cutaneous Technologies and
Development
99 Cherry Hill Road
Parsippany, NJ 07054
USA

Rodney Dawber, MA, FRCP
Consultant Dermatologist
Department of Dermatology
Churchill Hospital
Headington
Oxford OX3 7JH
UK

Anna Di Nardo, MD
Clinica Dermatologica
Università Degli Studi di Modena
Policlinico
Largo del Pozzo, 71
41100 Modena
Italy

Stéphane Diridollou, PhD
Institut de Recherche Pierre Fabre
Département Recherche et Evaluation
Dermocosmétique
BP 4404
31405 Toulouse
France

Zoe Diana Draelos, MD
Dermatology Consulting Services
624 Quaker Lane, Suite B-114
High Point, NC 27262
USA

Keith J Edgett
Andrew Jergens Co
2535 Spring Grove Avenue
Cincinnati, OH 45214
USA

Peter Elsner, MD
Department of Dermatology
Friedrich-Schiller-University
Erfurter Strasse 35
D 07743 Jena
Germany

Patricia Engasser, MD
University of California
Department of Dermatology
Medical Center Way, Surge 110
San Francisco, CA 94143–0989
USA

Pierre F Fournier, MD
Aesthetic Plastic Surgery
55 Boulevard de Strasbourg
75010 Paris
France

James E Fulton Jr, MD, PhD
Fulton Skin Institute
1617 Westcliff Drive, Suite 100
Newport Beach, CA 92660
USA

Yvon Gall, MD
Institut de Recherche Pierre Fabre
Département Recherche et Evaluation
Dermocosmétique
BP 4404
31405 Toulouse
France

C William Hanke, MD, FACP
Carmel Medical Center
13450 N Meridion Street, Suite 355
Carmel, IN 46032
USA

Whitney Hannon, MD
University of California
Department of Dermatology
Medical Center Way, Surge 110
San Francisco, CA 94143-0989
USA

Rudolf Happle, MD
Dermatologische Klinik der Universität Marburg
Deutschhausstrasse 9
35033 Marburg
Germany

Clive R Harding, BSc
Department of Cell Biology and Physiology
Unilever Research
Colworth House Laboratory
Sharnbrook
Bedford, MK44 1LQ
UK

John Harper, MD, MRCP
Consultant in Paediatric Dermatology
The Hospital for Sick Children
Great Ormond Street
London WC1N 3JH
UK

Jeff D Harvell, MD
Department of Dermatology
School of Medicine
San Francisco, CA 94143-0989
USA

Jean-Michel Lagarde, MSc
Institut de Recherche Pierre Fabre
Département Recherche et Evaluation
Dermocosmétique
BP 4404
31405 Toulouse
France

Maria Beatriz Lagos, MD
21 Arguilla Street
San Lorenzo Village
Makati City
Philippines 1223

Daniel Lambert, MD
Clinique Dermatologique
Hôpital du Bocage
21034 Dijon Cedex
France

Walter G Larsen, MD
Portland Dermatology Clinic
2250 NW Flanders
Portland, OR 97210
USA

Claude Lassus, MD
Chirurgie Maxillo-Faciale
Plastique Reconstructrice et Esthétique
Palais Négresco
1 rue de Rivoli
06000 Nice
France

Jean Luc Lévêque, PhD
Centre de Recherche L'Oréal
90 rue du Général Roguet
92983 Clichy Cedex
France

Nicola Loprieno, MD
University of Pisa
Department of Environmental Sciences
Via S. Guiseppe 22
56126 Pisa
Italy

Nicholas J Lowe, MD, FRCP
Clinical Professor, UCLA, Los Angeles
Senior Lecturer, UCH, London
3 Harcourt House
Cavendish Square
London W1M 9AB
UK

Daniel H Maes, MD
Vice President
Estée Lauder Companies
Research and Development
125 Pinelawn Road
Melville, NY 11747
USA

Howard I Maibach, MD
University of California
Department of Dermatology
Medical Center Way, Surge 110
San Francisco, CA 94143–0989
USA

Danielle Marcoux, MD, FRCPC
Pediatric Dermatologist
Hôpital Sainte-Justine
3175 chemin Côte Ste-Catherine
Montréal (Quebec) H3T 1C5
Canada

Kenneth D Marenus, PhD
Executive Director
Estée Lauder Companies
Research and Development
125 Pinelawn Road
Melville, NY 11747
USA

Jean-Paul L Marty, PhD
Department of Dermopharmacology and
Cosmetology
Université de Paris Sud
5 rue Jean-Baptiste Clément
92296 Châtenay-Malabry Cedex
France

Jenette Michalak, MD
Carmel Medical Center
13450 N Meridion Street, Suite 355
Carmel, IN 46032
USA

Anne Marie Orrechioni, PhD
Professor and Chairman
Laboratoire de Pharmacie Galénique
UFR de Medecine et de Pharmacie
Université de Rouen
76803 Saint-Etienne du Rouvray Cedex
France

Jean-Paul Ortonne, MD
Professor and Chairman
Department of Dermatology
Hôpital l'Archet 2
151 Route Saint Antoine Ginestière
06202 Nice Cedex 3
France

Alessandra Pelosi, MD
Department of Dermatology
University of Pavia
IRCCS Policlinico
S. Matteo, Pavia
Italy

Georg Rajka, MD
Emeritus Professor
University of Oslo
Frederik Stangsgate 44
0264 Oslo
Norway

Albert-Adrien Ramelet, MD
2 Place Benjamin-Constant
1003 Lausanne
Switzerland

Anthony Rawlings, PhD
Department of Cell Biology and Physiology
Unilever Research
Colworth House Laboratory
Sharnbrook
Bedford, MK44 1LQ
UK

Victoria L Rayner
Clinical Cosmetrician/Dermatology Associate
Director of Camouflage
Therapy Clinic
University of California
Center for Appearance and Esteem
251 Post Street, Suite 420
San Francisco, CA 94108
USA

Henry H Roenigk Jr, MD
Department of Dermatology
Northwestern University Medical School
222 Building, Suite 240
303 East Chicago Avenue
Chicago, IL 60611-3008
USA

Randall K Roenigk, MD
Consultant, Department of Dermatology
Mayo Clinic and Mayo Foundation
Professor of Dermatology
Mayo Medical School
200 First Street SW
Rochester, MN 55905
USA

Mathias Rohr, PhD
Institute Schrader, Skin Physiology
Max-Planck-Strasse 6
D 37603 Holzminden
Germany

Timothy J Rosio, MD
Fulton Skin Institute
1617 Westcliff Drive, Suite 100
Newport Beach, CA 92660
USA

Kurt M Schilling, PhD
Skin Division
Unilever Research
Edgewater Laboratory
Edgewater, NJ 07020
USA

Liliane Schnitzler, MD
9 Bldg Inkermann
92200 Neuilly S/Seine
France

Douglas Schoon, MS
Director of Research and Development
Creative Nail Design Inc
1125 Joshua Way
Vista, CA 92083-7800
USA

Karlheinz Schrader, PhD
Institute Schrader, Skin Physiology
Max-Planck-Strasse 6
D 37603 Holzminden
Germany

Alan R Shalita, MD
State University of New York
Health Science Center at Brooklyn
450 Clarkson Avenue
Brooklyn, NY 11203
USA

F Anthony Simion, PhD
Andrew Jergens Co
2535 Spring Grove Avenue
Cincinnati, OH 45214
USA

Philippe Simonin
Cathyor Engineering
2 Blvd Jacques Dalcroze
Geneva
Switzerland

Rodney D Sinclair, MD
Skin and Cancer Foundation
95 Rathdowne Street
Carlton
Melbourne 3055
Australia

Michael S Starch, BS
Andrew Jergens Co
2535 Spring Grove Avenue
Cincinnati, OH 45214
USA

Ethel Tur, MD
Department of Dermatology
Tel Aviv University
Ichilov Medical Center
6 Weizman Street
Tel Aviv 64239
Israel

Christopher Tzermias, MD
46 Mitropoleos Strados
Thessaloniki 54623
Greece

Philip W Wertz, PhD
Associate Professor
Dows Institute for Dental Research
Iowa City, IA 52242
USA

Ronald C Wester, MD
Research Dermatologist and Adjunct Professor
Department of Dermatology
University of California at San Francisco School
of Medicine
San Francisco, CA 94143-0989
USA

Pamela S Witt, MS
Andrew Jergens Co
2535 Spring Grove Avenue
Cincinnati, OH 45214
USA

Judith K Woodford, PhD
Andrew Jergens Co
2535 Spring Grove Avenue
Cincinnati, OH 45214
USA

Gil Yosipovitch, MD
Department of Dermatology
Rabin Medical Centre
Beilinson Campus
Tel-Aviv University
Petah Tikva 49100
Israel

Comment: Drugs, cosmetics and cosmeceuticals

Robert Baran, Howard I Maibach

Current definitions of drugs and cosmetics are unworkable. An intermediate category might be introduced, and this would carry a sensible proportion of the regulations now applicable to drugs. The new category would be of low risk and proven benefit, and would be controlled by regulations commensurate with reduced risks associated with these substances.

Ten years ago, Albert Kligman termed products intermediate between pharmaceuticals and cosmetics 'cosmeceuticals'. Despite the proliferation of cosmetics with pharmaceutical activity, regulatory agencies have not accepted this category.

In the USA and the European Union, a drug is defined as

> *an article intended for the use in the diagnosis, mitigation, treatment or prevention of disease or intended to affect the structure or any function of the body*

Under the US Federal Food, Drug and Cosmetic Act, 1938, cosmetics have no therapeutic function. These rigid definitions cause difficulties.

In 1991, the Court of Justice in Hertogenbosch (The Netherlands) ruled that male-pattern baldness was not a disease and that minoxidil was not a drug (Upjohn vs Farzoo). Upjohn appealed via the Supreme High Court of the Netherlands to the European Union Court of Justice, which ruled that an article is a drug if it is intended to affect the structure or any function of the body, but it does not have to be intended to modify disease. As minoxidil alters hair growth, the Court ruled that it was a drug. In the USA, minoxidil is registered as an over-the-counter drug for treating patterned baldness, irrespective of whether this is regarded as occurring in normal or diseased skin. It is not classified as a cosmetic.

Notwithstanding prior legal judgments, regulatory agencies tend to classify a product as a drug if it modifies the structure and/or function of the skin. Therefore a manufacturer's failure to claim drug activity for a product may not prevent it being classified as a drug. A cosmetic may be reclassified in the light of increasing knowledge of its effect on normal or diseased skin – even water could affect the stratum corneum and might therefore be classified as a drug. (Informally, this view has been expressed by the FDA to one of the authors (BAG) of reference 1.) Paradoxically, the addition of penetration enhancers to topical formulae, which modifies the skin barrier, does not lead to an altered classification.

Two adverse effects of this illogical distinction are as follows:

- Manufacturers will hesitate to incorporate new technology, in order to avoid the possibility of their product being classified as a drug, with the resultant increase in costs.
- Claims for existing products may be limited and minimized because of the fear of reclassification. This would restrict information that could be made available to both consumer and expert.

Therefore definitions should be realigned with present dermatological knowledge and, as in Japan, an intermediate category of drug should be introduced, comprising products of low risk and proven benefit. The regulatory processes should be varied and commensurate with the relative risks associated with the three categories. Regulations should include terms of reference aimed at giving consumers and physicians better access to product information. Regulatory authorities should ignore financial considerations, which are the responsibility of others.

This would lead to a new regulatory approach. As all products have pharmaceutical effects, including the enhanced wound healing effects of so-called inert creams, a cosmeceutical should have a beneficial effect proven by accepted methodologies.

Products used to treat diseased skin should be classified as drugs. Nonetheless, the concept of what is disease may change with time and with other factors. Male-pattern baldness and photoaging – once regarded as normal processes resulting from age and environment – now tend to be regarded as diseases, or, at least, treatable. This provides an enormous market potential for the development of an intermediate category of cosmeceuticals, for the modification of such conditions.

The manufacturer of a proposed cosmeceutical should submit data along specified guidelines, to the official agency. Premarket testing would be a requirement. Provided that data have been presented to the authority, marketing may not necessarily require prior approval. The product could always be recalled if this became advisable. This category would fall between the rigid regulation of a drug and the lack of regulation of a cosmetic.

The regulatory agencies would protect the public from unproven claims and unsafe materials.

REFERENCE

1. Vermeer BJ, Gilchrest BA, Cosmeceuticals. A proposal for rational definition, evaluation, and regulation. *Arch Dermatol* 1996; **132**: 337–40.

1

Climatic influence on cosmetic skin parameters

Mathias Rohr, Karlheinz Schrader

INTRODUCTION

A high degree of standardization is required in order to quantify the effects of cosmetics. As the following discussion will show, it is not only normal standardization procedures, such as acclimatization of volunteers in special air-conditioned laboratories, that have to be taken into consideration when interpreting objective and subjective cosmetic parameters, but also the effect of the actual climate during the application phase and especially during the days of measurement. Based on objective investigations of, for example, moisture-retaining effects, smoothing of the skin profile, and data from regeneration tests of the stratum corneum obtained with the aid of dihydroxyacetone (DHA) colouring, we shall demonstrate that the influence of temperature and relative humidity is of great significance in quantifying and classifying results. Furthermore, effects that are felt subjectively are shown to be equally dependent on climatic conditions as objectively rated parameters. This is shown, for instance, by comparing the results of washing the bend of the elbow.

We shall be summarizing the individual results and averages of thousands of volunteers. Both positive standards (in the sense of increasing moisture and smoothness) and negative standards (in the sense of increasing dehydration, roughness or side-effects) are used to present the effect of climatic conditions on skin physiology tests.

MATERIALS AND METHODS

Climatic data

In order to correlate climatic data with skin physiology parameters, the relative humidity and outside temperature are measured continuously at a station by computer (CAN system from the Lufft company). Capturing the data by computer ensures that the climate is recorded day and night. Let us take climatic changes in Holzminden (longitude 9.27° E and latitude 51.49 N: Middle Germany) over a year as an example. As Figure 1.1 shows, temperature fluctuates between about −10°C and +25°C in a year. Relative humidity is about 50% in summer and 90% in winter.

All tests mentioned in this discussion were carried out in an electronically controlled air-conditioned laboratory, which ensures that room temperature and air humidity are kept constant. The volunteers were kept seated in this laboratory at 22°C and 60% relative humidity for 45 minutes before the test and during the complete test procedure. Transient individual side-effects that may have

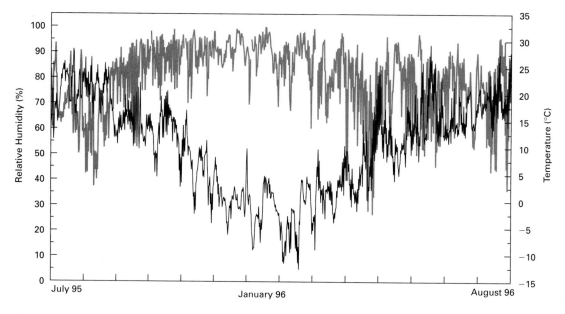

Figure 1.1 Outdoor climatic conditions at Holzminden, Germany.

an influence on the skin are standardized in this way. However, as will be shown, this procedure does not compensate for climatic conditions such as winter or summer.

Positive and negative standards

Tests have been carried out with the same products again and again over a period of several years, and these will serve to demonstrate the effect of climatic conditions on skin physiology. The positive standard is a well-accepted former brand product that is currently unavailable on the European market. However, we have now been making it at a constant quality level for years using the known formulation. This product, referred to hereinafter as *standard L* (see Table 1.1), is tolerated very well by the skin, and demonstrates a moisture-retaining and skin-smoothing

Table 1.1 Declaration of positive standard L according to INCI

Ingredients (INCI Declaration)

Aqua
Paraffinum liquidum
Caprylic/capric triglyceride
Hydrogenated coco-glycerides
Glycerine
Myristyl alcohol
Isohexadecane
Glyceryl stearate
Cetyl alcohol
Proprietary composition
4-Methylbenzylidene camphor
Tocopheryl acetate
Butyl methoxydibenzoylmethane
Aloe Barbadensis
Isopropyl myristate
Methylparaben
Polyaminopropyl biguanide
Bisabolol
Soluble collagen
Simethicone
Sodium hydroxide
EDTA

effect that can be classified well in terms of skin-physiological effectiveness. This makes it an ideal standard, because other products can be classified as better or worse than it in respect of their effectiveness. Another aspect of demonstrating the effectiveness of products on skin physiology relates to negative effects, which can be induced, for instance, by aggressive surfactants. Here, too, we have been using the same standard product for years. This is sodium dodecyl sulfate (SDS), which is referred to as the *negative standard* from now on.

Laser profilometry

The laser profilometry technique is used to investigate the antiwrinkle effect. In general, cosmetics are not allowed to be used on the test areas (volar forearm) for three days before the test begins and during the test. A silicone replica is made of each test area before the test begins in order to have a document of the volunteers. Then new replicas are made after the application phase, 12 hours after the last application. Evaluation is based on comparing the initial and final values.

Skin replicas are taken from the test areas on the volar forearms by means of a white pigmentary silicone substance (two components, Optosil Bayer). A round impression having a diameter of 18 mm is made using a label especially designed for this purpose. While the replicas are being taken, the volunteers are seated on chairs with adjustable arm-rests so that the angle between the upper arm and the forearm can be adjusted to 90°. Fixing the forearms in this way ensures that no fictitious smoothing or roughening effects, due to stretching the arms when the replicas are taken after application, are evaluated and included in the documentation.

An automated laser scanner with an optical autofocus sensor is used for contactless scanning of the skin replicas (UBM, optical mea-suring system Microfocus, UBM RC14). The laser diode ($\lambda = 780$ nm) that is used to expose the skin replica illuminates the silicone impression through a freely suspended objective lens. The diameter of the focus is about 1 µm. The light reflected by the replica falls on a differential photodiode via the sensor. If the distance between the surface and the transmitter changes during profile measurement, the light-spot image on the pair of photodiodes will move so that one or other diode will get more or less light. The necessary movement of the objective lens can be deduced from this displacement of light so that during its adjustment it is always guaranteed that the focus will coincide with the surface of the skin replica. An exact reconstruction of the profile surface can then be deduced from the movement of the objective lens.

The measuring range of the laser scanner is ± 500 µm at a resolution of less than 0.01% of the measuring range. The measuring spot (focus of the laser diode) has a diameter of about 1 µm. The Z resolution is increased to ± 25 mm by an additional shift of the Z axis if necessary.

The resolution in the X and Y directions is identical in order to be independent of any main direction of wrinkles. The skin replica taken from the volar forearm of a volunteer is scanned over an area of 8 mm $\times$ 8 mm in the X and Y directions at a resolution of 25 points/mm. This means that 40 000 individual measurements are available, permitting an exact three-dimensional reconstruction of the skin surface.[1] Changes to the skin profile are quantified according to the DIN parameters which are described below. A paired Wilcoxon test is performed[2] to establish any changes of roughness from the state of 'not treated' to the state of 'treated'.

The DIN parameters[3] described below are indicated by an R prefix, and are the two-dimensional definitions of the DIN parameters. To analyse the laser profilometry data, which are three-dimensional, the two-dimensional

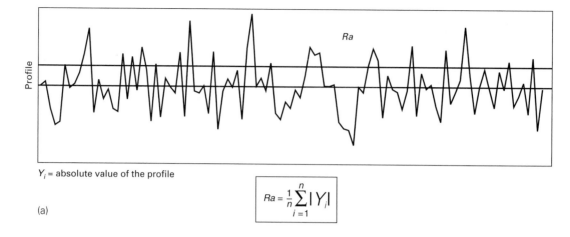

Y_i = absolute value of the profile

$$Ra = \frac{1}{n}\sum_{i=1}^{n}|Y_i|$$

(a)

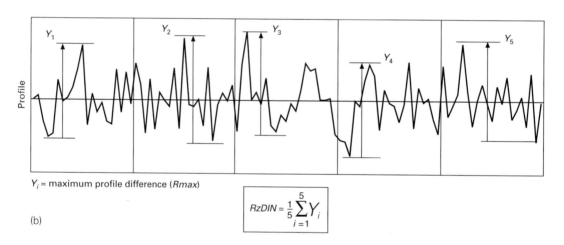

Y_i = maximum profile difference (*Rmax*)

$$RzDIN = \frac{1}{5}\sum_{i=1}^{5}Y_i$$

(b)

Figure 1.2 DIN parameters *Ra* (a) and *RzDIN* (b).

DIN parameters are transferred to the three-dimensional form (*S* parameters).[4] The two-dimensional case is explained below together with a definition of the three-dimensional case for the sake of simplification and explanation. In order to demonstrate a climatic influence, only *Ra* and *RzDIN* are summarized.

Ra/Sa (Figure 1.2a)

The DIN parameter *Ra* represents the mean roughness index according to DIN 4768. *Ra* indicates the arithmetic mean of the absolute values of the skin profile's deviations from the centre line over the total distance.

If the overall structure of the profile remains unchanged (*RzDIN* = constant) but the fine structure of the profile changes then the *Ra* parameter will indicate smoothing or roughening by a reduced or increased value respectively.

RzDIN/Sz (Figure 1.2b)

The *RzDIN* parameter represents a mean peak-to-valley height according to DIN 4768/1. Transferring this to the three-dimensional case results in the *Sz* parameter.[4]

If, in the two-dimensional case, a profile line is divided into five equal parts and the *Rmax* parameter is calculated for each part then *RzDIN* will be the arithmetic mean of these five individual values. The *RzDIN* parameter will indicate roughening of the skin profile by a significantly increased value if the profile is changed by the influence of a product.

Corneometer

Water differs markedly from most substances as far as its dielectric constant is concerned. A quantitative proof of changes to the water content of the skin can therefore be achieved by means of capacitance measurements in a non-invasive manner.[5]

A measuring capacitor reacts to the samples in the volume to be measured by way of capacitance changes (depending on water content). Those capacitance changes registered by the measuring head capacitor are processed fully automatically by the equipment to form a digital measured value. There is no conductive (galvanic) connection between the object measured and the measuring equipment. Consequently almost no electricity flows through the object measured. Properties such as ionic conductivity and polarization effects have no influence on the measurement result. The fact that the electronics adapt to the moisture circumstances almost without inertia means that the measuring process is very fast and that it is possible, to a considerable extent, to eliminate effects on the results caused by involuntary movements or moisture accumulation during the measuring process.

A corneometer (Courage + Khazaka) is used to measure the water content. The measuring sensor is square. Its active face, coated with a special glass, allows axial movement and has a range of at least 3 mm. The principle of measurement requires the face to sit evenly at a constant pressure. To ensure that this is as reproducible as possible, the face of the measuring head is very small, with an area of 7 mm $\times$ 7 mm. The inner movable part – the active face – is pressed onto the skin at 3.5 N by means of a spring. This guarantees standardized measurements, irrespective of the experimenter. The data are averaged for each volunteer (maximum 8 measurements) via computer control and archived.

Regeneration

Dihydroxyacetone (DHA) is a substance that is tolerated very well and is approved in the cosmetics industry as a suntan substance. It tans by means of the Maillard reaction, forming combinations with amino acids in the skin that do not wash off. The colour disappears within approximately 3 weeks as a result of desquamation of the coloured horny cells. The tan of the skin decreases accordingly.

For this investigation, the desquamation effect, and consequently the rate of regeneration, is measured in the laboratory colour room by measuring the decolouring with a Minolta Chromameter CR 300 (*L–a–b* colour system). The yellow value *b* differentiates best, and this is used to establish the colour-decay curves.

The region that is tested is again the volar forearm. Areas of 4 cm $\times$ 4 cm in the middle of the region of application are coloured with DHA[6] after a defined washing procedure to standardize the baseline conditions. In the colouring process, a special emulsion with 10% DHA is applied to the area to be tested. The amount applied is 6 mg/cm^2. In addition, a plaster saturated with DHA emulsion is applied for 24 hours. Over the next 18 days, the volunteers continue to use the products twice a day. The forearms are only permitted to be washed twice a day with warm water. Surfactants and abrasive cleansing agents are not allowed to be used. Measurements are taken directly before DHA colouring, and then every day over the next 18 days with the exception of weekends. For each time and area of measurement, three values are recorded at different places in the measurement area and averaged out.

Analysis and statistics

The *b*-values of all 30 volunteers per product are averaged out, and the standard deviations, percentage changes and percentage differences standardized to the colouring are calculated. The colour-decay curves can be described under normal conditions with the following exponential function:

$$b = a_1 e^{-a_2 t} + a_3$$

Further statistical treatment is described in detail in Neter et al[7] and Schrader et al.[8]

Washing test on the bend of the elbow

To assess the skin tolerance, the cleansing effect and the acceptance of surfactant products, we carry out the washing test on the bend of the elbow. In a practical test the bend of the elbow is washed under intense conditions. Twenty volunteers take part in this test. In each application, the bend of one elbow is lathered vigorously with the first sample and washed for two minutes by hand. After rinsing with lukewarm water, this bend of the elbow is again lathered and washed for two minutes. This is followed by a period of drying, also lasting two minutes. After the second rinsing with lukewarm water, the area in question is dabbed dry carefully with a towel, ensuring that there is no rubbing. The bend of the other elbow is treated in exactly the same way with the negative standard SDS.

In order to determine any side-effects induced by the test products, the volunteers are asked at the end of the test about any reactions they noticed directly after washing. The following parameters are ascertained: *reddening, stinging, skin tautness, itchiness, skin roughness, dull feeling* and *bad skin feeling*. The ratings are given on the basis of a coded volunteer questionnaire[9] (Table 1.2).

Table 1.2 Summary of experimental conditions for the various skin physiology tests	
Investigation	**Brief description**
Corneometer	• 20–30 volunteers • 2–3 weeks of application; twice a day • Baseline measurement on the forearm • Final value 12 hours after the last application • Statistical analysis of data
Laser profilometry	• 30 volunteers • 3 weeks of application; twice a day • Silicone replica of the forearm (baseline) • Silicone replica 12 hours after the last application (final value) • Robot-controlled laser profilometry • Analysis of *Ra* and *RzDIN*
Washing test on the bend of the elbow	• 20 volunteers • 5 days of application • Twice a day, 2 × 1 minute of washing • Subjective rating of side-effects in a direct comparison • Reddening/stinging/skin tautness/itchiness • Skin roughness/dull feeling/bad skin feeling • Statistical analysis of reaction points
DHA decolouring	• 20 volunteers, aged >50 years • Measurement of skin colour/chromameter (baseline) • Application of DHA/inner side of forearm • Application of test product/twice a day/18 days • Measurement of skin colour every day • Analysis of decay curves

RESULTS AND DISCUSSION

One of the major factors in cosmetic skin physiology is the moisture-retaining effect of a product. Figure 1.3 shows a summary of this for 1992 to 1995. The data have been summarized on a monthly basis in each case. Figure 1.3 shows the percentage increase in moisture that is induced by positive standard L after allowing for changes to the comparative untreated area. As the individual items of data in Table 1.3 show, the recorded averages are based on at least 100 volunteers who were tested over the years in the month indicated. Figure 1.3 – a simple representation – makes it clear that the moisture increase that can be achieved with positive standard L depends on the season. As can be seen in Table 1.3, there

is an average moisture increase of approximately 12.7% for all data that have been recorded. To make it easier to compare seasonal dependence of the achievable moisture increase, Figure 1.4 shows the difference from the overall average after the data have been standardized on the basis of the overall average. A change of 0% corresponds to the above-mentioned overall average of approximately 12.7% moisture increase. A bar in the positive direction thus shows an increase in moisture that is higher than the average, whereas a bar in the negative direction indicates a distinctly reduced level of effectiveness. Figure 1.4 shows that November to February result in a figure that is about 15% above the average moisture increase, whereas the summer months of June, July and August

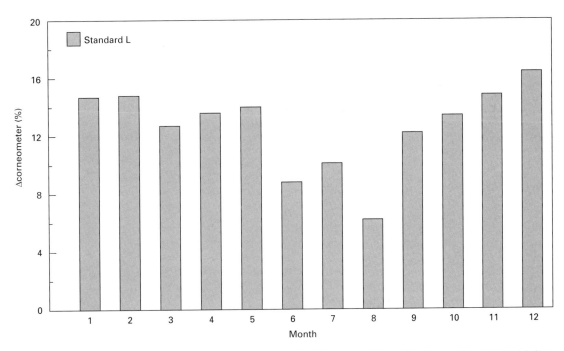

Figure 1.3 Percentage increase in moisture after allowing for the untreated area for the positive standard L in a monthly summary.

Table 1.3 Individual results of moisture retention tests. The percentage changes in the moisture of the skin 12 hours after final application of the product are recorded, allowing for the change to the untreated area that was included in the test. Each figure recorded is an average for at least 20 volunteers

| Test No. | 14 days corneometer investigation 12 h after the last application | | | | | | | | | | | |
| | Month January–December | | | | | | | | | | | |
	1	2	3	4	5	6	7	8	9	10	11	12
1	15.7	8.1	8.0	12.7	11.4	10.1	13.0	5.5	17.5	10.9	11.5	10.5
2	11.7	5.4	9.4	9.0	11.0	11.6	10.2	8.9	9.5	17.4	9.4	18.6
3	12.4	12.5	14.5	12.4	13.7	11.1	10.2	3.0	8.5	12.8	15.0	18.9
4	15.6	11.6	12.7	9.1	16.3	6.6	11.3	6.8	7.7	11.5	18.0	15.5
5	18.1	12.0	13.2	10.6	20.7	6.1	7.6	1.7	10.9	15.3	20.0	18.4
6		14.5	15.4	8.3	11.8	11.0	7.1	2.4	11.2	15.9		
7		12.1	12.8	11.3	10.7	8.8	6.9	8.0	16.3	10.2		
8		13.9	15.8	11.5	9.7	3.7	4.7	9.7	13.7			
9		17.6		11.7	6.8	4.3		8.0	14.3			
10		14.6		7.4	10.3			8.3	11.5			
11		15.9		13.7	9.4			5.8	14.6			
12		18.6		8.3	11.4				11.9			
13		22.5		25.2	12.9				11.2			
14		18.9		10.9	9.3							
15		18.3		17.1	18.9							
16		19.3		7.5	13.8							
17				16.7	20.5							
18				17.9	14.1							
19				12.7	12.7							
20				16.3	13.6							
21				15.6	18.4							
22				14.7	13.4							
23				19.8	11.6							
24				10.3	17.9							
25				20.2	18.9							
26				12.7	14.7							
27				22.5	16.4							
28					15.9							
29					16.1							
30					16.7							
Number	5	16	8	27	30	9	8	11	13	7	5	5
Mean	14.7	14.8	12.7	13.6	14.0	8.1	8.9	6.2	12.2	13.4	14.8	16.4
Standard deviation	2.6	4.4	2.8	4.7	3.6	3.0	2.7	2.8	2.9	2.8	4.4	3.5
95% CI	3.25	3.08	2.72	2.50	1.80	2.80	2.69	2.30	2.25	2.91	5.44	4.39
CI-95 (%)	22.14	20.89	21.39	18.42	12.92	34.48	30.30	37.24	18.41	21.71	36.81	26.80
No. of tests	144											
No. of volunteers	2880											
Mean overall	12.6											
SD overall	4.4											

result in a level of effectiveness that is approximately 50% below the average achievable moisture increase.

Figure 1.5 shows the relative change of the laser profilometry parameters *Ra* and *RzDIN* both for positive standard L and for the untreated area in a way that is comparable to Figure 1.3. At this juncture, we must point out that the area referred to as 'untreated' has not been treated with a cosmetic but has been subjected to a washing procedure to obtain better results as described in the 'Materials

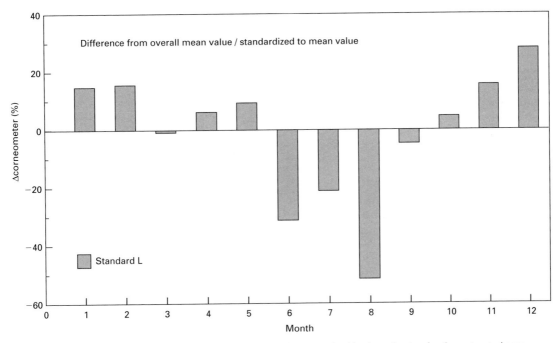

Figure 1.4 Standardized differences in moisture for the positive standard L after allowing for the untreated area.

and methods' section above. Figure 1.5 clearly shows how important this prior treatment is. Whereas the *Ra* and *RzDIN* parameters for the positive standard fluctuate between −6% and −8% from January to October 1994 to 1996 without showing a definite trend, these parameters fall noticeably for the untreated area from January to August followed by a rise in September and October. After allowing for the untreated area, the profilometry tests result in the dependence that is shown in Figure 1.6. Again, positive standard L is found to be less effective in the summer months of June, July and August than in the other months.

The data clearly show that the seasonal dependence is based both on the reduced positive effectiveness of standard L in the summer and on the reduced negative sensitivity of the untreated area (prior treatment with a surfactant of all areas tested). External climatic conditions thus have a distinct influence on the cosmetic effects that can be achieved. The basic level of the skin is increased in the summer months to such an extent that, on the one hand, skin moisture and smoothing can only be increased further by cosmetics to a limited degree, and, on the other hand, that the deliberate use of substances that are detrimental to the skin also has just a limited negative effect. All in all, this leads to an apparent reduction of cosmetic effectiveness.

In addition to these objective skin physiology parameters, subjective information gained from volunteers' answers to questions indicates a comparable dependence on external climatic conditions. Figure 1.7 shows the

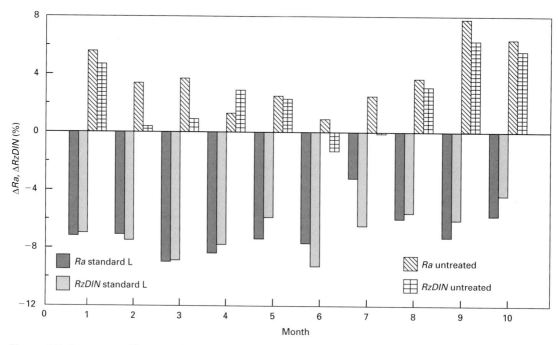

Figure 1.5 Percentage differences in the DIN parameters *Ra* and *RzDIN* for the positive standard L and the untreated area in a summary of laser profilometry data (1000 volunteers in general).

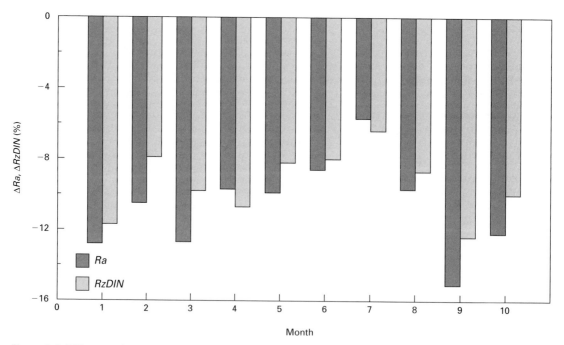

Figure 1.6 Differences in the DIN parameters *Ra* and *RzDIN* after allowing for the untreated area.

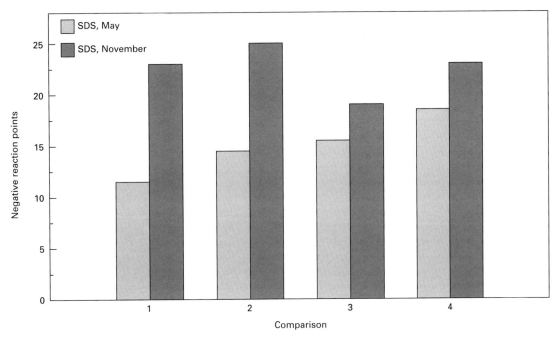

Figure 1.7 Negative reaction points in a subjective rating system for four individual comparisons of the negative standard SDS with four different products in a washing test on the bend of the elbow.

total negative reaction points that volunteers gave for reddening, stinging, skin tension, itchiness, skin roughness, dull feeling and bad skin feeling in the elbow washing test. The negative reaction points for the negative standard fluctuate between 11 and 18 in May, depending on the comparative product. Since the comparative product is of crucial importance in rating effects subjectively, the same test set-up was repeated in November with the same comparative products. Here the average total number of negative reaction points for the comparative product SDS is distinctly higher in all four panels taking part in the test. Whereas the average for May is approximately 15 negative reaction points, it rises to approximately 23 reaction points in November under otherwise identical conditions as far as the volunteers' subjective feel-

ings are concerned. These data, based on 80 volunteers, clearly show that it is possible and necessary to correlate information derived from volunteers' subjective ratings with climatic conditions, and to consider this along with the objectively demonstrable parameters for skin physiology.

Another example of how external climatic conditions make it almost impossible to evaluate the results of skin physiology investigations is given by the turnover of the stratum corneum on the basis of DHA decolouring tests. When the stratum corneum has been coloured with DHA, it can generally be expected that there will be a constant exponential reduction of skin colouring both of the untreated area and of the areas that have been treated with the test products.[1] Figure 1.8 shows average curves, which have been

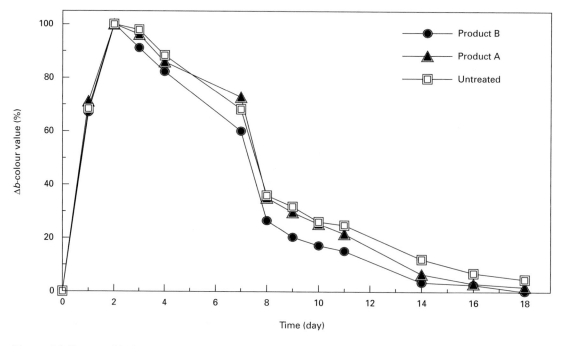

Figure 1.8 Exponential decay curves of the DHA decolouring test standardized to the maximum colouring characterized by changing of the *b*-value of the *L–a–b* colour system.

standardized to the maximum colouring, on the basis of 20 volunteers for two test products (A and B) containing α-hydroxy acid (AHA) and one untreated area. The observation period was 18 days. In contrast to theoretical expectations and preliminary experiments, this investigation revealed a fall of skin colouring from about 70% to about 30% on day 8. Both before and after this sudden change, the curve is in keeping with theoretical expectations. When all potential technical sources of error had been eliminated, the solution to this problem was found in the temperature and relative humidity data for the days of measurement as shown in Figure 1.9. As the curves show, relative humidity fell from about 90% to 60%, whereas temperature rose from

about 0°C to 6°C over the same period of just a few hours, and then fell to 1°C after a short time. Since temperature and humidity fluctuations were far less extreme in the rest of the test period, it seems reasonable to suppose that the strong fluctuations of temperature and humidity correlate with the recorded inconsistency in the DHA colour-decay curves. This inconsistency induced by extreme climatic fluctuations made it necessary to repeat the test, because it was no longer possible to carry out an exponential analysis of the decay curves.

As the measured curve was constant before and after day 8 but higher humidity fluctuations accompanied by lower temperature fluctuations were recorded on day 7, it can be

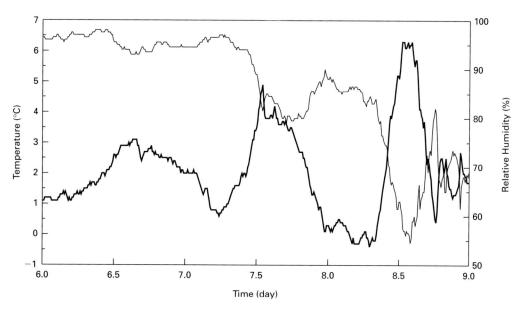

Figure 1.9 Climatic data on temperature and relative humidity from day 6 to day 8 during the DHA investigation.

assumed that humidity is of greater importance in examining the regeneration of the stratum corneum, and that the outside temperature only plays a subordinate part in the quality of this skin physiology investigation.

All of the data that have been documented so far show that skin physiology tests are influenced by external climatic conditions to a great extent. At this point, we should like to provide an example of a test for which climatic dependence is generally accepted as given but that we were unable to confirm with the results we obtained. The test in question is one to determine the sun protection factor (SPF). This is primarily based on the European COL-IPA method at our institute. In keeping with the skin physiology tests presented above, Figure 1.10 shows a monthly summary of the SPF for 1994 to 1996. The product tested was the European High Standard (P3), which is expected to lie between 14 and 17.

Whereas in 1994 there was a tendency for the SPF to fall in the course of the year followed by a rise in the winter months, this wave-like movement was not confirmed in 1995 and 1996. The recorded averages of 2814 individual results thus show that, in the framework of annual biological fluctuations, it is possible to determine a sun protection factor that lies within the specified limits of 14–17. On the basis of our data, it was not possible to demonstrate a direct correlation with climatic conditions. This conflicts with the general opinion that sun protection factors cannot be determined at all in the summer months, or can only be determined inadequately then.

SUMMARY

The data recorded, both from objective skin physiology parameters such as moisture and

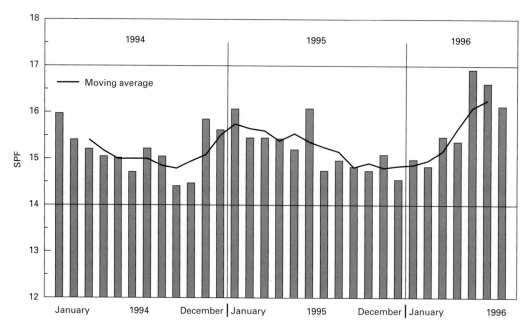

Figure 1.10 Monthly summary of SPF testing results of the European High Standard P3 with an expected SPF value of 14 to 17.

smoothness, and from subjective factors in the elbow washing test, clearly shows that such tests are influenced considerably by climatic conditions. Differences, such as between summer and winter, cannot be compensated by acclimatization in air-conditioned laboratories. Alongside standardized measurement conditions, it is therefore essential to record the quality of the test panel not only by including an untreated area but also by means of a positive or negative control. Only in this way is it possible to establish a classification system for test products that is not dependent on a particular season and allows the quality of cosmetic products to be rated objectively.

REFERENCES

1. Rohr M, Schrader A, Schrader K, The multifunctional effects of AHA. *Parfümerie und Kosmetik* 1996; **77**: 762–7.

2. Hartung J, Statistik. In: *Lehr- und Handbuch der angewandten Statistik*, 9. Auflage. Munich: Oldenbourg-Verlag, 1993.

3. DIN 4768 Ermittlung der Rauheitskenngrössen Ra, RzDIN, Rmax mit elektrischen Tastschnittgeräten, Begriffe, Messbedingungen.

4. Stout KJ, Sullivan PJ, Dong WP et al, *The Development of Methods for Characterization of Roughness in Three Dimensions*, Commission of the European Communities, Report EUR 15178EN, 1993.

5. Schrader K, Untersuchungen wasser-retinierender Kosmetika auf der Haut. *Parfümerie und Kosmetik* 1981; **62**: 265–72.

6. Piérard GE, Piérard-Franchimont C, Dihydroxyacetone test as a substitute for the dansyl chloride test. *Dermatology* 1993; **186**: 133–7.

7. Neter J, Wassermann W, Kutner MH, *Applied Linear Statistical Models, Regression, Analysis of Variance and Experimental Design*, 2nd edn. Richard D Irwin Inc, 1984.

8. Schrader A, Eckey H, Rohr M, Die Prüfung der Wirksamkeit reizlindernder Stoffe an der menschlichen Haut am Beispiel verschiedener Kamillenextrakte. *SÖFW-Journal* 1997; **123:** 3–11.

9. Schrader K, Praxisbezogene hautphysiologische Untersuchungskriterien mit Seifen und Syndets. *Parfümerie und Kosmetik* 1990; **71:** 686–95.

2

Skin and gender

Ethel Tur, Sarah Brenner

INTRODUCTION

The skin is a mirror reflecting the various characteristics of the body, including gender. Genetic and hormonal differences affect skin structure and function, resulting in variations between women and men and causing these gender variations to change with age. In addition, exogenous factors differ according to differences in lifestyle between the sexes.

During the last few decades, methodologies used in dermatological research have improved substantially, providing means of objective evaluation of skin function and characteristics. Differences between women and men, however, have not yet been systematically studied, and most of the data are by-products of studies with a different focus. This chapter outlines the various aspects of physiological differences between the skin of women and men, based on the available data.

STRUCTURAL AND ANATOMICAL CHARACTERISTICS (Table 2.1)

The skin of female frogs is thicker than that of males in all body regions[1] (whereas the oppo-

This chapter is modified from Tur E, Brenner S, *Clin Dermatol* 1997; **15**: 5–16, with permission from Elsevier Science Inc.

site is true for rat skin[2]). In humans, skin thickness is greater in men than in women,[3] whereas the subcutaneous fat thickness is greater in women.[4] The skin of men is thicker across the entire age range of 5–90 years.[5] Hormonal influence on skin thickness was demonstrated when conjugated estrogens were given to postmenopausal women.[6] Following 12 months therapy, the dermis was significantly thicker, and histologic improvement in the previously atrophic epidermis was noted.

Skin collagen and collagen density were measured in addition to dermal thickness.[7] The skin of men demonstrated a gradual thinning with advancing age (12–93 years), whereas the thickness of women's skin remained constant up until the fifth decade, after which it decreased with age. The male forearm skin contained more collagen at all ages in the range 15–93 years. In both sexes there was a linear decrease in skin collagen with age. Collagen density calculated as the ratio of skin collagen to thickness was lower in women at all ages. The rate of collagen loss was similar in both sexes. Women start with a lower collagen content; therefore they seem to age earlier than men. Collagen density, representing the packing of fibrils in the dermis, is lower in women than in men. This may be due to androgen, since skin collagen

Table 2.1 Structural and anatomical characteristics

(a) Significant differences

Ref.	Finding	Obtained by	Subjects	Conclusions
3	Skin thickness in humans greater in men than in women, except for lower back in young subjects	Echographic evaluation	24 women; 24 men; half 27–31 y, half 60–90 y	—
5	Men's skin thicker than women's across the entire age range of 5–90 y	Ultrasonic echography; forearm	69 women; 54 men; 5–90 y	—
6	Thickening of dermis following 12 months estrogen therapy	Conjugated estrogen therapy; ultrasound measurement	28 estrogen; 26 placebo; women: 51–71 y	Estrogens affect skin thickness
7	Men: gradual thinning of skin with advancing age. Women: thickness constant up to 5th decade, then decreasing with age	Skin collagen, skin thickness and collagen density, measured chemically and histologically	Collagen: 80 women; 79 men; 15–93 y Thickness: 107 women; 90 men; 12–93 y Density: 26 women; 27 men; 15–93 y	Rate of collagen loss same in men and women, although total skin collagen content is less in women than men at all ages
8	Forearm skinfold thickness decreases starting at age 35 for women and 45 for men. Starting at age 35 it is thinner in women than in men	Caliper; forearm	145 women and men; 8–89 y	—
9	Skinfold thickness lower in women	Caliper; forearm, thigh and calf	42 women; 37 men; 17–24 y	—
4	Subcutaneous fat thickness greater in women	Caliper and ultrasound	45 women; 41 men; Japanese; 18–22 y	—
10	Heel pad thickness thicker in men than in women; correlation with body weight	Ankle X-ray	113 women; 125 men; Ethiopian; 10–70 y	—
4	Skinfold compression in women is greater in the trunk and less in the limbs	Caliper and ultrasound	45 women; 41 men; Japanese; 18–22 y	—
11	Up to 12 years of age no difference between the sexes. Subcutaneous fat increases more than threefold, while internal fat mass increases less than twice. After 12 y, the relative mass of the subcutaneous fat increased in girls but not in boys	Caliper	1292 women; 1008 men; ages 6, 8, 10, 18	—
12	Lipoprotein lipase activity higher in women. Women: higher values in gluteus than abdomen. Men: higher in abdomen	Lipoprotein lipase activity and mRNA levels measured; hybridization, Northern blot	8 women; 11 men; 37 ± 4 y	Regional and sex differences in lipoprotein lipase activity might underlie the difference in fat distribution and total fat content. Variation is both at mRNA and post-translational levels.

(b) No significant differences

Ref.	Finding	Obtained by	Subjects	Conclusions
11	Up to 12 y: the mass of the subcutaneous fat increases more than threefold, while that of the internal mass increases less than twice in both sexes	Caliper	1292 women; 1008 men; ages 6, 8, 10, 18	—

density is increased in patients with virilism.

Forearm skinfold thickness, as measured by a caliper, decreases starting at age 35 for women and 45 for men. Starting at age 35, it is thinner in women than in men.[8] Another study found lower forearm, thigh and calf skinfold thickness in women compared with men in younger subjects: 17–24 years.[9]

Heel pad thickness, an indicator of soft tissue thickness in the body, was thicker in Ethiopian men than in women.[10] Skinfold compressibility in Japanese students was greater in women than in men at the pectoral site, and smaller at nuchal, submental, biceps, thigh, suprapatellar and medial calf sites.[4] The changes in the distribution of fat between the ages of 6 to 18 years were studied in 2300 subjects.[11] Up to 12 years of age, there was no difference between the two sexes: the mass of the subcutaneous fat increased more than threefold, while that of the internal mass increased less than twice. After the age of 12, the relative mass of the subcutaneous fat continued to increase in girls but not in boys.

The distribution of fat over the body is different in men and women.[12] In men, an increase in fat tends to accumulate in the abdominal region and upper parts of the body, whereas in women it is located in the lower body, particularly in the gluteal and femoral regions. In addition, the proportion of body fat is higher in non-obese women than in non-obese men. The characteristic difference in body fat distribution between the sexes exists both in non-obese subjects and obese ones. Lipoprotein lipase activity and mRNA levels were higher in women both in the gluteal and in the abdominal regions. In women, higher enzyme activity was found in the gluteus than in the abdomen, whereas in men it was higher in the abdomen. These regional and sex differences in lipoprotein lipase activity might underlie the difference in fat distribution and total fat content. Variation is both at the mRNA level and post-translational level.

BIOCHEMICAL COMPOSITION (Table 2.2)

Significant age-related differences in the stratum corneum sphingolipid composition were found in women, but not in men.[13] From prepubertal age to adulthood there was a significant increase in ceramide 1 and 2 accompanied by a decrease in ceramide 3 and 6. After maturity there was a decrease in ceramide 2 and an increase in ceramide 3. These findings indicate an influence of

Table 2.2 Biochemical composition

Significant differences

Ref.	Finding	Obtained by	Subjects	Conclusions
13	Stratum corneum sphingolipid composition differs with age in women, but not in men	Ethanolic extracts; biochemical methods of lipid identification	27 women; 26 men; 10–79 y	Female hormones influence the composition of stratum corneum sphingolipids
14	Women: higher concentrations of metals in hair. Concentrations of copper did not differ with age in men, whereas in women they increased with age	Liquid chromatography; trace metal determination	60 women; 72 men; 6–40 y	—

female hormones on the composition of stratum corneum sphingolipids. These lipids play an important role in the water permeability barrier function of the human epidermis, and thus endocrinological factors may influence this barrier.

Differences in the metal content of human hair were found between men and women: higher concentrations of metals were noted in women. Concentrations of copper did not differ with age in men, whereas an increase with increased age was noted in women.[14]

MECHANICAL PROPERTIES (Table 2.3)

Clinical assessment, as well as objective measurements of stratum corneum hydration, and grading of scaling (by adhesive tape strippings

Table 2.3 Mechanical properties

(a) Significant differences

Ref.	Finding	Obtained by	Subjects	Conclusions
21	From 15 y up to 69 y of age women exhibited longer blistering times than men. The difference was more pronounced in the age range 15–39 y than 40–69 y, and disappeared in older ages	Measuring the speed of dermal–epidermal separation utilizing the time required for blisters to form by controlled suction; antecubital and abdominal sites	178 women, 15–101 y; 209 men, 16–96 y	—

(b) No significant differences

Ref.	Finding	Obtained by	Subjects	Conclusions
15	Stratum corneum hydration, and grading of scaling showed no differences between men and women	Clinical assessment and bioengineering measurement	50 women; 22 men; 21–61 y	—
16	A positive effect of estrogens on facial skin: moisture increased, wrinkles decreased	Stratum corneum hydration and wrinkles – profilometry of skin replicas	18 women (8 applied estriol, 10 estradiol); 46–66 y	Topical treatment with estrogen seems promising
17	No difference between men and women in friction, moisture, transepidermal water loss	Bioengineering measurement	7 women, 25 y (mean); 7 men, 29 y; 7 women, 75 y; 8 men, 74 y	—
18	No difference in moisture	Bioengineering; healthy and chronic renal failure subjects	Healthy: 24 women, 21 men. Patients: 30 women, 50 men	—
22	Skin elasticity did not differ between the sexes, as measured by a suction device	In vivo suction device (bioengineering)	Young: 8 women (26 y); 8 men (28 y); Old: 9 women (75 y); 8 men (75 y)	—
5	Torsional extensibility did not differ between men and women	Twistometer	69 women; 54 men; 5–90 y	—
20	The adhesion of the stratum corneum did not differ between men and women	Biopsy; in vitro measurement of the force needed to separate cells	9–34 women and men (number varied with site studied); 20–40 y	—

Table 2.4 Functional differences

Significant differences

Ref.	Finding	Obtained by	Subjects	Conclusions
18	Men sweat more than women	Pilocarpine iontophoresis – healthy and chronic renal failure subjects	Healthy: 24 women; 21 men. Patients: 30 women; 50 men; 18–75 y	—
23	Cutaneous extensibility increased only in women after hydration	Bioengineering methods	15 women; 14 men; 23–49 y and 60–93 y	Hydration allows the effect of thinner dermis in women to be reflected in extensibility

followed by densitometry readings) showed no differences between men and women.[15] A positive effect of estrogens on stratum corneum hydration and wrinkles was demonstrated when estriol or estradiol cream was applied on the face of perimenopausal women.[16]

Frictional properties of the skin, as well as stratum corneum hydration, did not differ between men and women, in both young and old subjects.[17,18] In addition, transepidermal water loss showed no difference between the two sexes.[17] In contrast, another study[19] found lower basal transepidermal water loss values in women compared with men aged 18–39 years.

The adhesion of the stratum corneum, measured in vitro in skin biopsy samples, did not differ between men and women in several body regions.[20] But age (and probably hormonal) related differences were demonstrated in vivo by measuring the speed of dermal–epidermal separation utilizing the time required for blisters to form by controlled suction.[21] From 15 up to 69 years of age, women exhibited longer blistering times than men in both antecubital and abdominal sites. The difference was more pronounced in the age range 15–39 years than 40–69 years, and disappeared in older ages.

Skin elasticity did not differ between the sexes, as measured utilizing a suction device.[22] Similarly, torsional extensibility of the skin, as measured by a twistometer, did not differ between the sexes.[5]

Cutaneous extensibility was identical in men and women, but after hydration it increased only in women.[23] Hydration changes the properties of the stratum corneum, softening it, and thus allowing the difference in dermal thickness to express itself as a difference in extensibility. Since the dermis is thinner in women, elimination of the stratum corneum factor allows a rapid extensibility of the skin in women.

FUNCTIONAL DIFFERENCES (Table 2.4)

Sebum secretion following pilocarpine iontophoresis measured in healthy and chronic renal failure subjects revealed higher sebum secretion rates in men than in women in both subject groups.[18]

The fatty acid composition of sebum is affected by androgens in both sexes.[24]

Sex-related differences in the metabolism in the skin of topically applied compounds were found in guinea pig skin.[25]

DIFFERENCES IN RESPONSE TO EXOGENOUS TRIGGERS (Table 2.5)

The incidence of irritant dermatitis is higher in women than in men, but experimental

Table 2.5 Exogenous triggers

(a) Significant differences

Ref.	Finding	Obtained by	Subjects	Conclusions
26	Incidence of irritant dermatitis higher in women than in men			Occupational factors
19	Lower baseline transepidermal water loss in women compared with men, but after irritation similar values in both sexes	Sodium lauryl sulfate irritation; evaporimeter	15 women; 23 men; 18–39 y	Comparing the irritation index (the difference between irritated and unirritated values over unirritated): female skin more irritable
29	Higher on the day of minimal estrogen/progesterone secretion compared with the day of maximal secretion. Also higher on the day of maximal progesterone secretion compared with the day of maximal estrogen secretion	Back and forearm sites; baseline transepidermal water loss; evaporimeter	9 women; 19–46 y (mean 32)	Barrier function is less complete just prior to the onset of menses compared with the days just prior to ovulation

(b) No significant differences

Ref.	Finding	Obtained by	Subjects	Conclusions
27	No significant differences between men and women with or without hand eczema	Irritation tested for 11 irritants at several concentrations	21 women; 21 men with hand eczema; 21 women; 21 men without hand eczema; 20–60 y	No tendency to stronger reactions in either sex. Speculation: women's occupations lead to a greater exposure to irritants
28	No significant differences between men and women in developing cumulative irritant dermatitis	Repeated once-daily application of 3 concentrations of irritant (SLS), 5 days, followed by a patch test; upper back; bioengineering measurements	7 women; 7 men; 16–65 y	No sex-related susceptibility to develop cumulative irritant dermatitis. Speculation: women's occupational and domestic duties lead to a greater exposure to irritants

irritant dermatitis does not differ between men and women.[26,27] Occupational factors leading to a greater exposure to irritants by women may provide an explanation of this discrepancy. In a study of skin irritability by sodium lauryl sulfate, women showed lower baseline transepidermal water loss compared with men, but after irritation both sexes gave similar transepidermal water loss values.[19] The importance of interpretation of the results, and the lack of a standardized way of analyzing them, is illustrated in the latter study. The authors define an irritation index as the ratio of the difference between the values for irritated and unirritated skin to the value for unirritated skin. Although the value for irritated skin did not differ between men and women, this index was higher in women, since the value for unirritated skin was lower in men, and so the authors conclude that women's skin is more irritable. A review article considering the absolute values following irritation interpreted the same results as indicating no sex-related differences in sodium lauryl sulfate irritation.[26] Until a universal way of interpreting the results is established, contradictory conclusions may be reached by different analyses of the same set of data. In another study baseline transepidermal water loss did not differ between men and women.[28] This study found no significant differences between men and women in developing cumulative irritant dermatitis, when visual scoring, transepidermal water loss, skin blood flow and dielectric water content were assessed. Changes during the menstrual cycle, however, were demonstrated by measuring baseline transepidermal water loss.[29]

CUTANEOUS MICROVASCULATURE
(Table 2.6)

Hormonal factors affect the skin blood flow: differences between men and women were found during the reproductive years, and differences were found within the different phases of the menstrual cycle.[30] Moreover, vasospastic diseases, such as Raynaud's phenomenon, are more common in women, more prevalent in the reproductive years, and improve during pregnancy, suggesting an influence of female sex hormones.[30] Skin circulation varied during the menstrual cycle. There might be a direct influence of sex hormones on the blood vessel wall, or an indirect systemic hormonal action causing a cyclic pattern in women. Estrogens influence the sympathetic nervous system, inducing an upregulation of (vasoconstrictive) α_2-adrenoceptors. Thus blood flow measurements utilizing laser Doppler flowmetry revealed a reduction of basal cutaneous blood flow in women compared with men,[31–33] but these differences existed only in young women and not in women over 50 years.[34] This reduction was due to a basal increase in sympathetic tone rather than to a local structural or functional difference in the cutaneous circulation.

The vasodilatation induced by local heating occurred at a lower skin temperature in women.[35] However, the maximum skin blood flow following heating of the skin was not different between men and women, and neither was the postocclusive reactive hyperemia response in a study including a group of women aged 20–59 years.[31] In contrast, in a study that divided women according to age, the reactive hyperemia response was lower in young women compared both with women over 50 years and with young men.[34] The latter study also measured the response to cooling, which was prolonged in young women compared with the other two groups.

The skin microvascular response to acetylcholine, an endothelium-dependent vasodilator, and to nitroprusside and isoprenaline – two endothelium-independent vasodilators with different modes of action – was evaluated by a laser Doppler perfusion imager, which maps the skin blood perfusion. The substances were iontophorized into the skin. The response to nitroprusside, and to a lesser extent to acetylcholine, was higher in women before menopause than after,[36] reflecting functional and structural changes in skin vasculature with aging.

The cutaneous blood flow response to topical and intradermal administration of histamine was comparable in men and women at three anatomical sites: the back, volar side of the forearm, and ankle.[37] These observations indicate that there are no functional differences between men and women in the skin microvascular response to histamine. On the other hand, histamine administered by iontophoresis produced bigger wheals in women, as measured by laser Doppler flowmetry.[2] The bigger wheals were attributed to differnces in the stratum corneum layer, which is the main obstacle to penetration.

Transcutaneous oxygen pressure is a method that measures changes in oxygen pressure at the skin surface that are mainly determined by changes in skin blood flow. During skin surface measurement, significantly higher values of transcutaneous oxygen pressure were noted in women.[38,39] The difference might be explained by the thinner epidermis of women. Age-related sex differences were

Table 2.6 Cutaneous microcirculation

(a1) Significant differences

Ref.	Finding	Obtained by	Subjects	Conclusions
31	Reduction in basal skin blood flow in women	Bioengineering measurement	56 women; 44 men; 20–59 y	—
33	Reduction in facial basal skin blood flow in women	Laser Doppler	5 women; 5 men; 25–52 y	—
32	Reduction in basal skin blood flow in women	Bioengineering measurement; cooling and warming to change sympathetic tone	26 women; 23 men; 23–38 y	Sympathetic tone is increased – not a structural or functional difference in the cutaneous circulation
30	Skin circulation varied during menstrual cycle: basal flow lowest in the luteal phase, highest in the pre-ovulatory phase. Greatest cold-induced constriction and lowest recovery in the luteal phase	Bioengineering measurements at 4 times during the menstrual cycle	31 women; 15–45 y	Skin blood flow and its response to cold varies during the menstrual cycle
34	Reactive hyperemia response lower in young women as compared to both women over 50 y or young men. The response to cooling prolonged in young women compared with the other two groups	Bioengineering measurement; postocclusive reactive hyperemia and direct and indirect cooling	12 women, 19–39 y; 13 women, 51–67 y; 13 men, 22–47 y	Hormonal factors might explain the differences. Different dressing habits may also contribute
35	Vasodilatation induced by local heating occurs at a lower skin temperature in women	Bioengineering measurement	9 women; 6 men; age not specified	—
36	Response to nitroprusside higher in women before menopause than after	Laser Doppler perfusion imager; iontophoresis	21 women; 13 men; 18–80 y	Indicating functional and structural changes in skin vasculature of women with aging
2	Histamine produced bigger wheals in women	Histamine administered by iontophoresis	33 women; 38 men; 15–52 y	Differences in the stratum corneum layer

(a2) Significant differences: transcutaneous oxygen pressure

Ref.	Finding	Obtained by	Subjects	Conclusions
38	Significantly higher values of transcutaneous oxygen pressure in women	Bioengineering; anterior chest, forearm	18 women; 42 men; 22–88 y	—
39	Significantly higher values of transcutaneous oxygen pressure in women	Bioengineering; 23 sites on face, extremities and trunk	7 women; 12 men; 21–63 y	Might be explained by women's thinner epidermis
40	Transcutaneous oxygen pressure during postocclusive reactive hyperemia greater in adult women than in men, but did not differ between boys and girls	Bioengineering measurement; forearm; postocclusive reactive hyperemia, 35–37°C	Adults: 30 women; 37 men; 22–60 y. Children before puberty: 34	Hormonal influence is indicated

(b) No significant differences

Ref.	Finding	Obtained by	Subjects	Conclusions
37	No difference in cutaneous blood flow response to histamine	Topical and intradermal administration; bioengineering methods	10 women; 10 men; 24–34 y	—
31	No difference in postocclusive reactive hyperemia and maximum skin blood flow following heating	Bioengineering methods	56 women; 44 men; 20–59 y	—

noted in measuring transcutaneous oxygen pressure during postocclusive reactive hyperemia. Greater values were found in adult women than in men, but no differences between boys and girls.[40]

SENSORY FUNCTIONS (Table 2.7)

Thermoregulatory response

Studies of human thermoregulation were conducted by exposing subjects to various thermal environments. The importance of taking into account all the possible variables is demonstrated in studies of the physiological responses to heat stress:[41] data showed differences between women and men. But when taking into consideration the differences in the percentage of fat in the body and the ratio between the body surface and mass, the effect of gender disappeared.

In contrast to these results of heat stress, the response to cold stress of Japanese young subjects differed with gender, although body surface area-to-mass ratios were similar.[42] Subjects were exposed to cold (12°C) for 1 hour at rest in summer and in winter. Women's tolerance to cold was superior to men's in winter, whereas no significant differences between the sexes were found in the summer. Differences in the distribution of fat over the body, even though body surface area-to-mass ratios were similar in the two sexes, might have contributed to the differences in cold tolerance.

Thermal response to stimulation

The decrease in finger temperature as a response to musical stimulus was greater in women.[43] This may be due to differences between men and women in vascular autonomic sensitivity to music, or to differences in sensitivity or density of peripheral vascular adrenergic receptors.

Electrodermal responses: electrodermal asymmetry has been considered as an index of hemispheric specialization. A study recorded the magnitude and frequency of the skin conductance responses when subjects listened to tones.[44] Subjects were right-handed in order to control the effects of handedness. Men displayed more asymmetry between hands, with larger skin conductance responses on the left hand. In women, asymmetry was less marked, and larger skin conductance responses were found on the right hand. These results indicate a possible hemispheric difference in response to auditory stimuli.

Thermal and pain sensation, pressure sensitivity

Sensation in the skin can be studied in relation to pain. Pain can be induced mechanically, electrically, by chemical stimulus or by thermal stimulus. Pain sensation is best determined by the threshold at which pain begins, and the stimulus required to produce it can be quantified. Thermal and pain sensations are mediated by cutaneous receptors and travel through myelinated (Aδ) and unmyelinated (C) nerve fibers. Women were more sensitive to small temperature changes and to pain caused by either heat or cold.[45] Another study measured the threshold of the pricking sensation provoked by heat projected to the skin from a lamp.[46] The pricking pain threshold increased with age in both sexes. In addition, the threshold of women was lower at all ages in the range 18–90 years. Possible explanations to the difference between the sexes are:

(i) anatomical differences in skin thickness;
(ii) differences in blood flow and blood vessels that absorb part of the heat transmitted to the skin;
(iii) differences in nervous structure or function.

Unlike the forearm lower pricking pain sensation threshold in women, pressure threshold was lower in women than men on the palm and on the sole, but not on the forearm.[47]

Table 2.7 Sensory function

(a) Significant differences

Ref.	Finding	Obtained by	Subjects	Conclusions
45	Women more sensitive to small temperature changes and to pain caused by either heat or cold	Marstock method – quantitative	67 women; 83 men; 10–73 y	—
46	Lower threshold values in women than in men	Pricking pain sensation to heat; threshold determination, volar forearm	93 women; 165 men; 18–28 y 132 women; 135 men; 50–90 y	—
47	Women more sensitive than men: palm and sole, but not on the forearm	Pressure threshold measurement; palm, sole, forearm	68 women; 68 men; 17–30 y	—
48	Neonate girls: significantly higher conductance than boys	Skin conductance (autonomic function)	20 women; 20 men; neonates: 60–110 h	These differences may represent differences in maturation. Very young: no effect yet of training and different behavior accorded the sexes
42	Women's tolerance to cold superior to men's in winter	Exposed to cold (12°C) for 1 h at rest in summer and in winter; skin and body temperature	7 women; 8 men; Japanese; 18–26 y	Differences in fat distribution over the body, even though body surface area-to-mass ratios were similar in the two sexes, might have contributed to the differences in cold tolerance
43	Greater decrease in women in finger temperature as a response to musical stimulus	Auditory stimulation, music; skin temperature, index finger	60 women; 60 men; young students	Possible explanation: difference in vascular autonomic sensitivity to music
44	Men: more asymmetry between hands, larger skin conductance responses on the left hand. Women: less asymmetry, larger skin conductance responses on right hand	Auditory stimulus. Magnitude and frequency of skin conductance responses	15 women; 15 men; 19–27 y; right-handed	Possible hemispheric differences in response to auditory stimuli

(b) No significant differences

Ref.	Finding	Obtained by	Subjects	Conclusions
41	Physiological responses to heat stress differ with gender, but depend on fat content and body surface area	Heat stress; ergometer; oxygen uptake; body and skin temperature; sweat rate	12 women; 12 men; 20–28 y	Differences between women and men disappeared when differences in the percentage of fat in the body and the ratio between body surface and mass were taken into account

Autonomic function

Skin conductance measures one aspect of the autonomic function. Neonate girls manifested a significantly higher conductance than boys.[48] These differences may represent differences in maturation.

Table 2.8 Skin color

Significant differences

Ref.	Finding	Obtained by	Subjects	Conclusions
14	Women's skin lighter	Spectrophotometry	Review article	Not a simple hormonal effect. Differences in melanin, hemoglobin and carotene
50	Women's skin lighter	Spectrophotometry	33 women; 68 men; 8–24 y	Differential tanning; vascularity variations
51	Women's skin lighter	Spectrophotometry; upper inner arm	566 women; 578 men; 1–50 y	During puberty, males darken, females lighten. Different levels of MSH. Hereditary and environmental factors
53	Forehead: boys darker than girls. Medial upper arm: girls darker than boys during early adolescence, not different from boys during middle adolescence, and during late adolescence girls lighter than boys	Skin color, measured by reflectance of forehead and medial upper arm, in adolescents	105 women, 10–16 y; 105 men, 12–18 y	Physiologic changes during adolescence may cause these sex differences
52	Women's skin lighter. Both sexes darken with age	Spectrophotometry; inner upper arms, lateral forearms, back of hands	461 women; 346 men; 20–69 y	Different levels of MSH. Difference in sun exposure (tanning and thickening of skin)
55	In the elderly: skin of men darker and redder compared with women, but not in the young	Colorimetric measurements of forehead (sun-exposed) and forearm (protected)	8 women, 5 men, 65–88 y; 9 women, 4 men, 18–26 y	—

SKIN COLOR (Table 2.8)

An article by Tegner[49] gives several examples of artists depicting their female models as lighter skinned than males. Such differences were indeed found utilizing spectrophotometric measurements, in various ethnic populations. A lighter skin in women was demonstrated in studies from Iran,[50] India[51] and Australia.[52] In addition to hormonal influences, differences in melanin, hemoglobin and carotene might be involved, as well as differences in sun exposure. In general, both sexes darken as age increases.[52] But the changes are more intricate:[51] from the end of infancy to the onset of puberty there is a progressive skin darkening in both sexes. During adolescence they both lighten, but women lighten more. Simple hormonal effects cannot explain this difference, since both testosterone and estrogen provoke darkening rather than lightening of the skin. These changes might be partly attributed to differences in exposure to sunlight, since UV irradiation increases the number of melanocytes in both exposed and unexposed skin. Another study assessed skin color in adolescents.[53] The forehead (sun-exposed) pigmentation of boys was darker than that of girls. But the medial upper arm (less sun exposure) pigmentation varied among the different phases of adolescence: girls were darker than boys during early adolescence, during middle adolescence the pigmentation was similar in the two sexes,

Table 2.9 Hormonal influence				
Significant differences				
Ref.	Finding	Obtained by	Subjects	Conclusions
56	Hormone replacement treatment limited the age-related increase in skin extensibility. Other parameters of skin viscoelasticity were not affected	Computerized suction device measuring skin deformability and viscoelasticity; inner forearm	Women: 43 nonmenopausal (19–50 y); 25 menopausal not treated (46–76 y); 46 on hormone replacement therapy since onset of menopause (38–73 y)	Hormone replacement therapy has a preventive effect on skin slackness
57	Collagen content increased by 48% with hormone replacement therapy compared with nontreated subjects	Hydroxyproline and collagen content; biopsies of right thigh below the greater trochanter	Postmenopausal women (35–62 y); 29 untreated; 26 estradiol + testosterone	Estrogen or testosterone, or both, prevent the decrease in skin collagen content that occurs with aging
58	Increased proportion of type III collagen in the skin of postmenopausal women receiving hormone replacement therapy	Analysis of collagen types; biopsies of lateral thigh	Postmenopausal women (41–66 y); 14 untreated; 11 estradiol + testosterone	The clinical improvement in the skin following hormone replacement therapy is due not only to increase in total collagen but also to changes in the ratio of type III to type I

and during late adolescence girls were significantly lighter than boys.

The lighter skin colour of women was attributed to differences in melanin, hemoglobin (variations in vascularity) and carotene.[54] Natural selection might give an explanation of the overall visual effect of lighter skin. In addition, women are more homogenous in color than men, since regional variations in reflectance spectrophotomery were smaller in women than in men.[54] Colorimetric measurements revealed a darker and redder skin in elderly men (65–88 years) compared with elderly women, but such differences were not found in young subjects (18–26 years).[55] Another study of 461 women and 346 men aged 20–69 years found that both sexes darken with age.[52]

HORMONAL INFLUENCE (Table 2.9)

Any of the above mentioned differences between women and men might be related to hormonal effects. Some evidence for hormonal influence on the skin has already been mentioned above, like the increase of skin thickness following conjugated estrogens treatment of postmenopausal women,[6] or the positive effect of estrogens on stratum corneum hydration and wrinkles of the face of perimenopausal women,[16] or the changes during the menstrual cycle demonstrated by measuring baseline transepidermal water loss[29] and skin blood flow.[30] Hormone replacement therapy for menopause had an effect on skin extensibility:[56] in untreated women a steep increase in skin extensibility was evidenced during the menopause. Hormone replacement treatment limited this age-related increase in skin extensibility, thus having a preventive effect on skin slackness. Other parameters of skin viscoelasticity were not affected. After menopause the skin becomes thinner, associated with loss in skin collagen content. Collagen content increased with hormone replacement therapy by 48%

Table 2.10 Pilosebaceous unit

Significant differences

Ref.	Finding	Obtained by	Subjects	Conclusions
60	During January women's hair was denser and the percentage of telogen hair lower compared with men	Phototrichogram; hair count after washing	7 women, 29–49 y; 7 men, 25–47 y	—
59	Higher sebum secretion in men than in women for age ranges 20 to over 69, but not for the 15–19 age range. In the 50–70 age range the secretion in men remains unaltered, whereas in women there is a significant decrease in sebum output, probably as a result of decreased ovarian activity	Sebum production	330 women; 458 men; 15 y to over 69 y	—
59	No correlation between sebum production and plasma testosterone	Sebum production and plasma androgen levels	8 women; 28 men	—

compared with non-treated subjects.[57] Moreover, the ratio of type III to type I collagen in the skin is reduced with age. Postmenopausal women receiving hormone replacement therapy showed an increased proportion of type III collagen in the skin.[58] In the future, further hormonal manipulation might change the skin of both men and women in ways we cannot yet predict.

PILOSEBACEOUS UNIT (Table 2.10)

The sebaceous glands are hormone-dependent. The increase in their activity during puberty can be stimulated by the administration of the appropriate hormone. Androgenic steroids, of either gonadal or adrenal origin, have a direct stimulatory effect on sebaceous gland activity. Most of the hormones (TSH, ACTH, FSH, LH) act indirectly by stimulating their respective endocrine tissues. In other cases the hormones (for instance GH) act synergistically with another hormone to which the sebaceous gland is sensitive. Average values for sebum secretion were significantly higher in men than in women for age ranges 20 to over 69, but not for 15–19 years.[59] This difference in sebaceous gland activity becomes more apparent in the 50–70 age range, when the secretion in men remains unaltered whereas in women there is a significant decrease in sebum output, probably a result of decreased ovarian activity.

Beginning in young adulthood there is an age-related decline in wax ester secretion – thus hormones also affect the composition of sebum.

Obviously, the distribution of hair over the body differs between men and women. The hair follicles possess individual mechanisms controlling the evolution and triggering of successive phases, but systemic factors like hormones and external factors also play a significant part. The season of the year has an effect on hair growth and hair shedding. From data given in a study concerning this seasonal effect,[60] we calculated sex differences, which were not discussed in the study. The data refer to the month of January. Women's hair was denser and the percentage of telogen hair lower compared with men.

The diversity of male and female hair patterns is determined by a difference in the transformation of vellus to terminal hair, stimulated by androgens, but also by racial and genetic factors.

The effect of androgens on hair growth varies according to body site, and may be opposite, like transforming vellus hair on the face to terminal beard hair at puberty and the reverse on the scalp. The face, scalp, beard, axilla and pubic hair follicles are targets for androgens. Androgen affects different cells in the dermal papilla, which is also affected by melanocyte-stimulating hormone (MSH), prolactin, thyroid hormones, pregnancy and nutritional state.[61] In addition to higher serum levels of testosterone, female facial hirsutism correlated with obesity and age.[62]

Despite exposure to the same circulatory hormones, the activity of hair follicles depends on the body site, varying from no effect on the eyelashes to stimulation in many other areas. High levels of testosterone inhibit the hair papilla cells and outer root sheath keratinocytes, and have a lesser effect on fibroblasts and interfollicular keratinocytes, while low levels of testosterone have no effect. The opposite was found with estrogen and cyproterone.[63]

CONCLUSIONS

Maintaining skin health is an intricate orchestration of many variables. The need for hard data is paramount, not only for gaining knowledge about the pathophysiology of human skin, but also for the assessment and clinical management of skin diseases. The introduction of new and improved instrumentation will no doubt allow for more studies, and much more data will also be available on the subject of skin physiology as relates to gender.

We hope that this chapter will trigger further investigations of the subject.

REFERENCES

1. Greven H, Zanger K, Schwinger G, Mechanical properties of the skin of *Xenopus laevis* (Anura, Amphibia). *J Morphol* 1995; **224**: 15–22.

2. Magerl W, Westerman RA, Mohner B, Handwerker HO, Properties of transdermal histamine iontophoresis: differential effects of season, gender, and body region. *J Invest Dermatol* 1990; **94**: 347–52.

3. Seidenari S, Pagnoni A, Di Nardo A, Giannetti A, Echographic evaluation with image analysis of normal skin: variations according to age and sex. *Skin Pharmacol* 1994; **7**: 201–9.

4. Hattori K, Okamoto W, Skinfold compressibility in Japanese university students. *Okajimas Folia Anat Jpn* 1993; **70**: 69–78.

5. Escoffier C, de Rigal J, Rochefort A et al, Age-related mechanical properties of human skin: An in vivo study. *J Invest Dermatol* 1989; **93**: 353–7.

6. Maheux R, Naud F, Rioux M et al, A randomized, double-blind, placebo-controlled study on the effect of conjugated estrogens on skin thickness. *Am J Obstet Gynecol* 1994; **170**: 642–9.

7. Shuster S, Black MM, McVitie E, The influence of age and sex on skin thickness, skin collagen and density. *Br J Dermatol* 1975; **93**: 639–43.

8. Leveque JL, Corcuff P, de Rigal J, Agache P, In vivo studies of the evolution of physical properties of the human skin with age. *Int J Dermatol* 1984; **18**: 322–9.

9. Davies BN, Greenwood EJ, Jones SR, Gender differences in the relationship of performance in the handgrip and standing long jump tests to lean limb volume in young adults. *Eur J Appl Physiol* 1988; **58**: 315–20.

10. Tilahun M, Atnafu A, Heel pad thickness of adult Ethiopian patients in Tikur Anbessa hospital, Addis Abeba. *Ethiop Med J* 1994; **32**: 181–7.

11. Malyarenko TN, Antonyuk SD, Malyarenko Yu E, Changes in the human fat mass at the age of 6–18 years. *Arkh Anat Gistol Embriol* 1988; **94**: 43–7.

12. Arner P, Lithell H, Wahrenberg H, Bronnegard M, Expression of lipoprotein lipase in different human subcutaneous adipose tissue regions. *J Lipid Res* 1991; **32**: 423–9.

13. Denda M, Koyama J, Hori J et al, Age and sex-dependent change in stratum corneum sphingolipids. *Arch Dermatol Res* 1993; **285**: 415–17.

14. Sturado A, Parvoli G, Doretti L et al, The influence of color, age and sex on the content of zinc, copper, nickel, manganese, and lead in human hair. *Biol Trace Elem Res* 1994; **40**: 1–8.

15. Jemec GBE, Serup J, Scaling, dry skin and gender. *Acta Derm Venereol (Stockh)* 1992; **177**(Suppl): 26–8.

16. Schmidt JB, Binder M, Macheiner W et al, Treatment of skin ageing symptoms in perimenopausal females with estrogen compounds. A pilot study. *Maturitas* 1994; **20**: 25–30.

17. Cua AB, Wilhelm KP, Maibach HI, Frictional properties of human skin: relation to age, sex and anatomical region, stratum corneum hydration and transepidermal water loss. *Br J Dermatol* 1990; **123**: 473–9.

18. Yosipovitch G, Reis J, Tur E et al, Sweat secretion, stratum corneum hydration, small nerve function and pruritus in patients with advanced chronic renal failure. *Br J Dermatol* 1995; **133**: 561–4.

19. Goh CL, Chia SE. Skin irritability to sodium lauryl sulphate – as measured by skin water vapor loss – by sex and race. *Clin Exp Dermatol* 1988; **13**: 16–19.

20. Chernova TA, Melikyants IG, Mordovtsev VN et al, Mechanical properties of the skin in normal subjects. *Vestn Dermatol Venereol* 1984; **2**: 12–15.

21. Kiistala U, Dermal–epidermal separation. *Ann Clin Res* 1972; **4**: 10–22.

22. Cua AB, Wilhelm KP, Maibach HI, Elastic properties of human skin: relation to age, sex and anatomical region. *Arch Dermatol Res* 1990; **282**: 283–8.

23. Auriol F, Vaillant L, Machet L et al, Effects of short time hydration on skin extensibility. *Acta Derm Venereol (Stockh)* 1993; **73**: 344–7.

24. Yamamoto A, Serizawa S, Ito M, Sato Y, Fatty acid composition of sebum wax esters and urinary androgen level in normal human individuals. *J Dermatol Sci* 1990; **1**: 269–76.

25. Boehnlein J, Sakr A, Lichtin JL, Bronaugh RL, Characterization of esterase and alcohol dehydrogenase activity in skin. Metabolism of retinyl palmitate to retinol (vitamin A) during percutaneous absorption. *Pharm Res* 1994; **11**: 1155–9.

26. Wilhelm KP, Maibach HI, Factors predisposing to cutaneous irritation. *Dermatol Clin* 1990; **8**: 17–22.

27. Bjornberg A, Skin reactions to primary irritants. *Acta Derm Venereol (Stockh)* 1975; **55**: 191–4.

28. Lammintausta K, Maibach HI, Wilson D, Irritant reactivity in males and females. *Contact Dermatitis* 1987; **17**: 276–80.

29. Harvell J, Hussona-Safed I, Maibach HI, Changes in transepidermal water loss and cutaneous blood flow during the menstrual cycle. *Contact Dermatitis* 1992; **27**: 294–301.

30. Bartelink ML, Wollersheim A, Theeuwes A et al, Changes in skin blood flow during the menstrual cycle: the influence of the menstrual cycle on the peripheral circulation in healthy female volunteers. *Clin Sci* 1990; **78**: 527–32.

31. Maurel A, Hamon P, Macquin-Mavier I, Lagrue G, Flux microcirculatoire cutané étude par laser–doppler. *Presse Med* 1991; **20**: 1205–9.

32. Cooke JP, Creager MA, Osmundson PJ, Shepherd JT, Sex differences in control of cutaneous blood flow. *Circulation* 1990; **82**: 1607–15.

33. Mayrovitz HN, Regan MB, Gender differences in facial skin blood perfusion during basal and heated conditions determined by laser Doppler flowmetry. *Microvasc Res* 1993; **45**: 211–18.

34. Bollinger A, Schlumpf M, Finger blood flow in healthy subjects of different age and sex and in patients with primary Raynaud's disease. *Acta Chir Scand* 1975; **465**(Suppl): 42–7.

35. Walmsley D, Goodfield MJD, Evidence for an abnormal peripherally mediated vascular response to temperature in Raynaud's phenomenon. *Br J Rheumatol* 1990; **29**: 181–4.

36. Algotsson A, Nordberg A, Winblad B, Influence of age and gender on skin vessel reactivity to endothelium-dependent and endothelium-independent vasodilators tested with iontophoresis and a laser Doppler perfusion imager. *J Gerontol Med Sci* 1995; **50**: 121–7.

37. Tur E, Aviram G, Zeltser D et al, Histamine effect on human cutaneous blood flow: regional variations. *Acta Derm Venereol (Stockh)* 1994; **74**: 113–16.

38. Glenski JA, Cucchiara RF, Transcutaneous O_2 and CO_2 monitoring of neurosurgical patients: detection of air embolism. *Anesthesiology* 1986; **64**: 546–50.

39 Orenstein A, Mazkereth R, Tsur H, Mapping of the human body skin with transcutaneous oxygen pressure method. *Ann Plast Surg* 1988; **20**: 419–25.

40. Ewald U, Evaluation of the transcutaneous oxygen method used at 37°C for measurement of

reactive hyperaemia in the skin. *Clin Physiol* 1984; **4**: 413–23.

41. Havenith G, van Middendorp H, The relative influence of physical fitness, acclimatization state, anthropometric measures and gender on individual reactions to heat stress. *Eur J Appl Physiol* 1990; **61**: 419–27.

42. Sato H, Yamasaki K, Yasukouchi A et al, Sex differences in human thermoregulatory response to cold. *J Human Ergol* 1988; **17**: 57–65.

43. McFarland RA, Kadish R, Sex differences in finger temperature response to music. *Int J Psychophysiol* 1991; **11**: 295–8.

44. Martinez-Selva JM, Roman F, Garcia-Sanchez FA, Gomez-Amor J, Sex differences and the asymmetry of specific and non-specific electrodermal responses. *Int J Psychophysiol* 1987; **5**: 155–60.

45. Meh D, Denislic M, Quantitative assessment of thermal and pain sensitivity. *J Neurol Sci* 1994; **127**: 164–9.

46. Procacci P, Bozza G, Buzzelli G, Della Corte M, The cutaneous pricking pain threshold in old age. *Geront Clin* 1970; **12**: 213–18.

47. Weinstein S, Sersen E, Tactual sensitivity as a function of handedness and laterality. *J Comp Physiol Psychol* 1961; **54**: 665–9.

48. Weller G, Bell RQ, Basal skin conductance and neonatal state. *Child Dev* 1965; **36**: 647–57.

49. Tegner E, Sex differences in skin pigmentation illustrated in art. *Am J Dermatopathol* 1992; **14**: 283–7.

50. Mehrai H, Sunderland E, Skin colour data from Nowshahr City, Northern Iran. *Ann Hum Biol* 1990; **17**: 115–20.

51. Banerjee S, Pigmentary fluctuation and hormonal changes. *J Genet Hum* 1984; **32**: 345–9.

52. Green A, Martin NG, Measurement and perception of skin colour in a skin cancer survey. *Br J Dermatol* 1990; **123**: 77–84.

53. Kalla AK, Tiwari SC, Sex differences in skin color in man. *Acta Genet Med Gemellol* 1970; **19**: 472–6.

54. Frost P, Human skin color: a possible relationship between its sexual dimorphism and its social perception. *Perspect Biol Med* 1988; **32**: 38–58.

55. Kelly RI, Pearse R, Bull RH et al, The effects of aging on the cutaneous microvasculature. *J Am Acad Dermatol* 1995; **33**: 749–56.

56. Pierard GE, Letawe C, Dowlati A, Pierard-Franchimont C, Effect of hormone replacement therapy for menopase on the mechanical properties of skin. *J Am Geriatr Soc* 1995; **43**: 662–5.

57. Brincat M, Moniz CF, Studd JWW et al, Sex hormones and skin collagen content in postmenopausal women. *Br Med J* 1983; **287**: 1337–8.

58. Savvas M, Bishop J, Laurent G et al, Type III collagen content in the skin of postmenopausal women receiving oestradiol and testosterone implants. *Br J Obstet Gynaecol* 1993; **100**: 154–6.

59. Pochi PE, Strauss JS, Endocrinologic control of the development and activity of the human sebaceous gland. *J Invest Dermatol* 1974; **62**: 191–201.

60. Courtois M, Loussouarn G, Hourseau S, Grollier JF, Periodicity in the growth and shedding of hair. *Br J Dermatol* 1996; **134**: 47–54.

61. Randall VA, Thornton MJ, Messenger AG et al, Hormones and hair growth: variations in androgen receptor content of dermal papilla cells cultured from human and red deer (*Cervus Elaphus*) hair follicles. *J Invest Dermatol* 1993; **101**: 114S–20S.

62. Ruutiainen K, Erkkola R, Gronroos MA, Irjala K, Influence of body mass index and age on the grade of hair growth in hirsute women of reproductive ages. *Fertl Steril* 1988; **50**: 260–5.

63. Kiesewetter F, Arai A, Schell H, Sex hormones and antiandrogens influence in vitro growth of dermal papilla cells and outer root sheath keratinocytes of human hair follicles. *J Invest Dermatol* 1993; **101**: 98S–105S.

PART TWO

PHARMACOLOGY OF COSMETIC PRODUCTS

3

In vitro skin toxicity assays for predicting cosmetic-induced irritancy

Jeff D Harvell, Howard I Maibach

The safety of cosmetic products is of great concern to both manufacturer and consumer. Traditionally, the Draize rabbit assay[1] has been used by many cosmetic manufacturers in the United States and Europe as a means of predicting the ability of cosmetic ingredients and/or final formulations to produce irritancy/toxicity. These assays have been supplemented with human patch tests to further validate safety.[2]

In the past two decades, there has been a greater emphasis placed on developing non-animal, in vitro methods to predict irritation. The reasons for this relate mainly to criticisms of the Draize assay, which include

- the subjective nature of the visual scoring system employed;
- the questionable ability to extrapolate results to man;[3–5]
- the fact that the test is time consuming and costly;
- the fact that the test may result in animal distress.

There currently exist a number of in vitro alternatives designed to predict the dermal toxic/irritant capability of compounds in man (Table 3.1). These are based on a variety of methods, including cell culture, physico-chemical analysis, microorganism studies, iso-lated tissue techniques, and computer modeling. Because the process of dermal irritation is complex and its various mechanisms have yet to be fully discerned, no single parameter has emerged as a 'best predictor' of irritation. The myriad of in vitro assays therefore utilize a wide array of endpoints designed to be predictive of irritation/toxicity. Such endpoints include cell death, decreased cellular metabolic function, decreased cellular protein production, decreased mitochondrial enzyme function, decreased fluorescence capability, decreased motility of simple protoza, histologic changes, release of intracellular enzymes, release of inflammatory mediators, damage to vascular systems, and protein denaturation. The utility of these endpoints is made clearer in the following discussion of individual test methods.

Cytoxic tests using cell culture systems include the neutral red dye uptake assay, the MTT dye uptake and reduction assay, the [³H]uridine uptake system, and assays that measure the release of cellular proteins or inflammatory mediators. The neutral red dye uptake assay uses a dye that is taken up by viable cells and retained in lysosomes. Perturbations by cytotoxic agents that result in damage to either plasma membrane or lysosomal membrane uptake systems there-

Table 3.1 In vitro assays and their endpoints

Assay	Endpoint	Refs
Neutral red dye uptake system	Decreased dye uptake as a result of membrane disruption	6–8
MIT dye uptake and reduction system	Decreased mitochondrial enzyme function and/or decreased dye uptake due to membrane perturbation	8–10
[^{3}H]Uridine uptake system	Decreased uptake of nucleotide	11–13
Release of intracellular enzymes	Release of lactate dehydrogenase, β-glucoronidase, etc to extracellular space	8, 14–16
Kenacid blue method and other total protein assays	Decreased cellular protein content due to metabolic disturbances	17, 18
Release of inflammatory mediators	Release of arachadonic acid leukotrienes, and prostaglandins to extracellular space	8, 19–21
Decreased glucose utilization	Decreased glucose metabolism by cultured cells	8,22
Silicon Microphysiometer	Decreased metabolic rate as measured by decreases in lactate and [CO_2] production	23, 24
Skin equivalents	Many of the same endpoints as above	25–28
Microtox	Decreased fluorescence of bacteria	29
Tetrahymena thermophila assay	Decreased motility of protozoa	30, 31
Chorioallantoic membrane (CAM) system	Damage to vascular network	32, 33
Skintex dermal assay	Protein denaturation and disruption of other macromolecules	34

fore result in decreased dye uptake. The endpoint for this assay is known as the NR_{50} and represents the concentration of toxicant that reduces by 50% the uptake of dye as compared with control cells.[6,7] The MTT assay correlates cell viability to both intact mito-chondrial enzyme function and intact mito-chondrial enzyme function and intact plasma membrane uptake processes.[8–10] This system uses a tetrazolium salt that in viable cells is reduced to a blue formazan product by the action of mitochondrial enzyme systems.

Cytotoxic agents that interfere with mitochondrial function cause decreased formation of the blue formazan product. The measured endpoint for this system is an MTT_{50}, which, like the NR_{50}, represents the concentration of toxic agent that reduces the formation of formazan product by 50%. Similarly, the tritiated [^3H]uridine uptake assay assesses cell membrane function as well as enzyme activity. This assay measures the ability of viable cells to transport and accumulate the essential nucleotide, uridine. Sublethal alterations in cellular metabolism induced by toxicants result in a decreased ability to perform this vital function.[11-13]

Other cell-culture-based systems utilize the release of cellular proteins such as lactate dehydrogenase, β-glucuronidase, and alkaline phosphatase.[8,14-16] The release of these intracellular enzymes represents damage to plasma membrane retention systems by cytotoxic agents. Total protein assays (e.g. the kenacid blue dye method) measure the growth inhibitory effects of toxic/irritant substances.[17,18] The amount of total cellular protein in untreated wells is compared with that of treated wells, and the amount of substance that decreases total protein content by 50% is the endpoint. Measurements of inflammatory mediator release, such as histamine, serotonin, arachadonic acid, prostaglandins, and leukotrienes, represent the cells' response to perturbation by irritating (but not necessarily lethal) substances.[8,19-21] These mediators are synthesized by viable cells and released to the extracellular matrix as part of the inflammatory response to irritating substances.

Finally, other cell-culture-based systems have correlated cell viability to such endpoints as glucose utilization (i.e. depletion of glucose from the extracellular medium),[8,22] and changes in cellular metabolic activity. The latter system is marketed as the Silicon Microphysiometer (Molecular Devices, Menlo Park, CA), and represents a sensitive method capable of detecting small changes in the metabolic activity of a monolayer cell system.[23,24] The principles of this device are based on the premise that cellular metabolic activity is reflected by the concentration of extracellular, acidic byproducts such as lactic acid and carbon dioxide. Changes in the metabolic activity of the monolayer (as a result of toxic/irritant effects) are therefore represented by changes in the pH of the extracellular medium. These subtle pH changes are measured by means of a silicon-based electrode known as a light addressable potentiometric sensor (LAPS).

The aforementioned cell-culture-based methods generally use monolayer cell systems; however, there now exist commercially available multilayer cell systems, collectively known as skin equivalents.[25-27] Such systems consist of multilayers of dermal fibroblasts or keratinocytes grown on a variety of substrata. In many of these commercially available models, the cells are keratinocytes or fibroblasts derived from human tissue (for example as a result of circumcision or breast reduction surgeries). Some of the systems contain a stratified, differentiated epithelium, which forms as a result of raising the system to the air–liquid interface. In general, the same endpoints utilized for the monolayer systems can also be used in these multilayer skin equivalents.[27,28] One of the advantages of these multilayer systems is that substances can be applied directly to the dry, apical surface without regard to their physical nature. Hence solid materials and lipophilic materials can be assayed without regard to their solubility in aqueous cell culture media. In the future, the incorporation of other cell types, such as mast cells, will be the goal in making these systems even more predictive of the in vivo situation.

Other in vitro assay systems utilize the chemical processes of microorganisms as a measure of toxic effect. The Microtox system uses the luminescent bacterium *Phosphobacterium phosphoreum*. Toxic agents generally cause a decrease in the fluorescence capabilities of this bacterium, the degree of which can be quantitated and correlated to degree of toxicity.[29] The motile ciliated protozoan *Tetrahymena thermophila* has been used in toxicity studies.[30,31] The effect of a toxic substance on this unicellular organism is assessed by noting changes in its swimming pattern, such that the amount of substance that just induces a change in motility pattern defines an endpoint.

Since the primary events in inflammation (namely erythema, heat and edema) are dependent upon vascular processes, it follows that investigation of the effect of irritant/toxic compounds on a vascular network would comprise a suitable in vitro alternative. Such a model is represented by the chorioallantoic membrane system (CAM).[32,33] This uses fertilized chicken eggs, whose vascular network (or CAM) is exposed by cutting a small 'window' into the shell. Test compounds are then applied directly to the CAM and their effects graded by noting visual changes in the blood vessel network (i.e. hemorrhage, injection or coagulation).

Physico-chemical models for the prediction of dermal toxicity are rare. This is because of the paucity of knowledge regarding the effects of toxicants at the molecular level. One model, the Skintex dermal assay system, uses protein denaturation and changes in conformation of macromolecules as an endpoint.[34] The ability of toxicants/irritants to disturb the ordered array of protein components and other macromolecules in the system is measured spectrophotometrically. This model provides a quantitative response to materials that may produce irritation by protein binding, enzyme inactivation, and a variety of other pathways where macromolecular confirmation is altered in the initiation of dermal irritation.

While all of the aforementioned tests will probably show promise in predicting the ability of substances to induce acute, primary irritation (i.e. irritant contact dermatitis), few in vitro tests are available to predict immunologically mediated contact dermatitis (i.e. allergic contact dermatitis, delayed hypersen-

sitivity, or type IV allergy). Likewise, relatively less attention is given to the validation of assays for the prediction of photosensitive (i.e. phototoxic and photoallergic) reactions, even though a number of methodologies exist.

Currently, our ability to predict, in vitro, the potential of unknown substances to induce immunologically mediated contact dermatitis resides in the lymphocyte transformation test and assays that assess lymphokine production: the leukocyte migration inhibition test and the macrophage migration inhibition test. The lymphocyte transformation test discerns the ability of potential contact allergens to induce proliferation of lymphocytes in culture as measured by [^{3}H]thymidine uptake. Lymphokine assays measure the ability of potential contact allergens to induce migration inhibition of macrophages or leukocytes via the production of the lymphokine, leukocyte migration inhibition factor.[35]

Assays predictive of phototoxicity include photohemolysis of red blood cells and photosensitized killing of *Candida albicans*.[36–38] Additionally, a number of the systems already discussed have been modified to demonstrate their utility in predicting phototoxicity. Specific examples include the neutral red assay,[39] the MTT assay,[40,41] the kenacid blue test, [^{3}H]thymidine incorporation,[42] and the Skintex dermal assay system (marketed as Solatex-PI).[43] Modifications of the lymphocyte transformation test and macrophage migration inhibition test have allowed the successful reproduction of photoallergic responses in vitro with a limited number of known photoallergens.[44,45]

All of the above assays are currently in a stage of validation, the goal of which is to assess both their reproducibility (i.e. degree of interlaboratory variation) and their relevance (i.e. the degree to which these tests are predictive of in vivo irritation/toxicity).[46] The assessment of relevance is most often made by comparing the in vitro result with some in vivo result. Currently, the majority of validation projects use the Draize rabbit assay as the in vivo arm of the correlate; however, the question arises as to whether the 'standard' for in vivo irritancy should reside in a species other than man. The reasons for the use of rabbits in toxicity testing are obvious; however, their use has been criticized on the grounds of questionable ability to extrapolate results to man and other species.[3-5] With this in mind, it makes sense that at least some aspect of the validation process should attempt to correlate the results of in vitro dermal toxicity tests to in vivo human data.

One example of this approach compared the irritant capabilities of the irritants benzalkonium chloride, trichloroacetic acid, phenol, and hydrochloric acid in the human and in the Skintex dermal assay system. As can be discerned from Figure 3.1, the Skintex system was fairly sensitive in its ability to predict the irritant potential of these compounds in man (sensitivity 82%, specificity 71%, positive predictive value 82%).[47] Additionally, the in vivo dose response curves for each of the four substances was compared to the in vitro

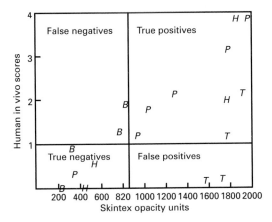

Figure 3.1 Contingency table with calculated sensitivity of 82%, specificity of 71%, and positive predictive value of 82% (B, benzalkonium chloride; P, phenol; T, trichloracetic acid; H, hydrochloric acid).

dose–response curves, and correlation coefficients calculated. The in vitro dose response for benzalkonium chloride ($R^2 = 0.987$) and phenol ($R^2 = 0.994$) were strikingly similar to those generated in vivo, possibly indicating that the mechanisms of action in vivo and in vitro are similar for these two compounds.

Part of the problem that plagues scientists involved in the validation endeavor relates to the fact that relatively little is known regarding the mechanisms by which irritation (especially primary, acute, nonimmunologic irritation) is produced. What is known is that the mechanisms of irritation production appear to be different for different chemical classes. In other words, while there may in fact be variable degrees of overlap, the mechanism by which compound A produces irritation will be different from that of compound B in terms of time course of inflammation, types of inflammatory mediators, cell types affected (damaged), and cell types recruited.[48,49]

As scientists, we have much to learn regarding the cascade of events that occurs when normal homeostatic processes are disturbed by exogenous agents. New endogenous chemical mediators of inflammation continue to be discovered, and the role of these various mediators in the inflammatory cascade is only now becoming more clear. At the cellular level, advances in the field of molecular biology now permit many key cellular functions to be 'visualized' by means of fluorescent probes, and biosensors.[50-54] By correlating the effect of toxic/irritant substances on these metabolic functions, we develop a greater understanding of the mechanistic basis of irritation/toxicity. Such advances will allow the development of in vitro tests with greater predictive power.

What then is the future for in vitro assays? First, it is apparent from already completed validation steps that a single in vitro assay will not be capable of predicting the dermal irritancy for all classes of compounds. It seems unlikely that one assay could be predictive for the array of vastly different chemical structures that induce irritation by as yet undefined mechanisms. Rather, batteries will be employed using single in vitro tests, with each test differing as to the molecular/physiological endpoint measured. Secondly, as confidence in the reproducibility and relevance of these in vitro alternatives increases, we shall see a reduction in the number of animals utilized for toxicity study. The total elimination of animal use for toxicity study is most likely far in the future. Finally, as our experience with the array of in vitro assays increases – each test having its own distinct physiological/molecular endpoint – our knowledge concerning mechanisms of dermal irritation and toxicity will expand concurrently. With this enhanced knowledge, we shall add information to the growing quantitative structure activity analysis (QSAR) database, and in the future be able to make better predictions about the effect of chemical structures on cellular and tissue function. The task appears monumental; however, each small validation step adds a piece to the puzzle.

REFERENCES

1. Draize JH, Woodard G, Calvery HO, Methods for the study of irritation and toxicity of substances applied topically to the skin and mucous membranes. *J Pharmacol Exp Ther* 1944; **82:** 377–89.

2. Jackson EM, Cosmetics: substantiating safety. In: *Dermatotoxicology*, 4th edn (Marzulli FN, Maibach HI, eds). New York: Hemisphere, 1991:835–43.

3. Kastner G, Irritancy potential of cosmetic ingredients. *J Soc Cosmet Chem* 1977; **28:** 741–54.

4. Patrick E, Maibach HI, Comparison of time course, dose response, and mediators of chemically induced skin irritation in three species. In: *Current Topics in Contact Dermatitis* (Frosch PJ, Dooms-Goossens A, Lachapelle J-M et al, eds). New York: Springer-Verlag, 1989:399–403.

5. Davies R, Harper KH, Kynoch SR, Inter-species variation in dermal reactivity. *J Soc Cosmet Chem* 1972; **23:** 371–81.

6. Borenfreund E, Puerner JA, A simple quantitative procedure using monolayer cultures for cytotoxicity assays. *J Tiss Cult Meth* 1984; **9:** 7–9.

7. Wallace KA, Harbell JW, Accomando N et al, Evaluation of the human epidermal keratinocyte neutral red release and neutral red dye uptake assay using the first 10 MEIC test materials. *Toxicol in Vitro* 1992; **6:** 367–71.

8. Osborne R, Perkins MA, In vitro skin irritation testing with human skin cell cultures. *Toxicol in Vitro* 1991; **5:** 563–7.

9. Mosman T, Rapid colorimetric assay for cellular growth and survival: application to proliferation and cytotoxic assays. *J Immunol Meth* 1983; **65:** 55–63.

10. Tada H, Shiho K, Kuoshima K et al, An improved colorimetric assay for interleukin 2. *J Immunol Meth* 1986; **93:** 157–65.

11. Shopsis C, Inhibition of uridine uptake in cultured cells: a rapid, sublethal cytotoxicity test. *J Tiss Cult Meth* 1986; **9:** 19–22.

12. Borenfreund E, Shopsis C, Borrero O et al, In vitro alternative irritancy assays: comparison of cytotoxic and membrane transport effects of alcohols. *Ann NY Acad Sci* 1983; **407:** 416–19.

13. Shopsis C, Borenfreund E, Walberg J et al, A battery of potential alternatives to the Draize test: uridine uptake inhibition, morphological cytotoxicity, macrophage chemotaxis and exfoliative cytology. *Food Chem Toxicol* 1985; **23:** 259–66.

14. Korzeniewski C, Callewaert DM, An enzyme release assay for natural cytotoxicity. *J Immunol Meth* 1983; **64:** 313–20.

15. Cornelis M, Dupont C, Wepierre J, In vitro cytotoxicity tests on cultured human skin fibroblasts to predict the irritation potential of surfactants. *Alternatives Lab Animals* 1991; **19:** 324–36.

16. Sasaki T, Kawai K, Saijo-Kurita K et al, Detergent cytotoxicity: simplified assay of cytolysis by measuring LDH activity. *Toxicol in Vitro* 1992; **6:** 451–7.

17. Shopsis C, Eng B, Rapid cytotoxicity testing using a semi-automated protein determination on cultured cells. *Toxicol Lett* 1985; **26:** 1–8.

18. Knox P, Uphill PF, Fry JR et al, The FRAME multicentre project on in vitro cytotoxicology. *Food Chem Toxicol* 1986; **24:** 457–63.

19. DeLeo V, Harber LC, Kong BM et al, Surfactant induced alteration of arachadonic acid metabo-

lism of mammalian cells in culture. *Proc Soc Exp Biol Med* 1987; **184:** 477–82.

20. DeLeo V, Hanson D, Scheide S, The effect of surfactants on metabolism of choline phospholipids in human epidermal keratinocytes in culture. *J Toxicol Cutaneous and Ocular Toxicol* 1989; **8:** 227–40.

21. Cohen C, Dossou G, Rougier A et al, Measurement of inflammatory mediators produced by human keratinocytes in vitro: a predictive assessment of cutaneous irritation. *Toxicol in Vitro* 1991; **5:** 407–10.

22. Mol MAE, Van de Ruit ABC, Kluivers AW, NAD$^+$ levels and glucose uptake of cultured human epidermal cells exposed to sulfur mustard. *Toxicol Appl Pharmacol* 1989; **98:** 159–65.

23. Parce JW, Owicki JC, Kercso KM et al, Detection of cell-affecting agents with a silicon biosensor. *Science* 1989; **246:** 243–7.

24. Hafeman DG, Parce JW, McConnell HM, Light-addressable potentiometric sensor for biochemical systems. *Science* 1988; **240:** 1182–5.

25. Naughton G, Jacob L, Naughton BA, A physiological skin model for in vitro toxicity studies. In: *Alternative Methods in Toxicology*, Vol 7: *In Vitro Toxicology: New Directions* (Goldberg AM, ed.). New York: Mary Ann Liebert, 1989:183–9.

26. Bell E, Parenteau L, Haimes HB et al, Testskin: a hybrid organism covered by a living human skin equivalent designed for toxicity and other testing. In: *Alternative Methods in Toxicoloty*, Vol 6: *Progress in In Vitro Toxicology* (Goldberg AM, ed.). New York: Mary Ann Liebert, 1988:15–25.

27. Gay R, Swiderek M, Nelson D et al, The living skin equivalent as a model in vitro for ranking the toxic potential of dermal irritants. *Toxicol in Vitro* 1992; **6:** 303–15.

28. Gay RJ, Swiderek M, Nelson D et al, The living dermal equivalent as an in vitro model for predicting ocular irritation. *J Toxicol Cutan Ocular Toxicol* 1992; **11:** 47–68.

29. Bulich AA, Bioluminescence assays. In: *Toxicity Testing Using Micro-organisms*, Vol 1 (Bitton G, Dutka BJ, eds). Boca Raton, FL: CRC Press, 1986:57–74.

30. Silverman J, Preliminary findings on the use of protozoa (*Tetrahymena thermophila*) as models for ocular irritation testing in rabbits. *Lab Animal Sci* 1983; **33:** 56–8.

31. Silverman J, Pennisi S, Evaluation of *Tetrahymena thermophilia* as an in vitro alternative to ocular irritation studies in rabbits. *J Toxicol Cutan Ocular Toxicol* 1987; **6:** 33–42.

32. Luepke NP, Kemper FH, The HET–CAM test: an alternative to the Draize eye test. *Food Chem Toxicol* 1986; **24:** 495–6.

33. Bagley DM, Rizva PY, Kong BM et al, An improved CAM assay for predicting ocular irritation potential. In: *Alternative Methods in Toxicology*, Vol 6: *Progress in In Vitro Toxicology* (Goldberg AM, ed.). New York: Mary Ann Liebert, 1988:131–8.

34. Soto RJ, Gordon VC, Evaluation of an in vitro dermal irritation assay. In: *Alternative Methods of Toxicology*, Vol 8: *In Vitro Toxicology: Mechanisms and New Technology* (Goldberg AM, ed.). New York: Mary Ann Liebert, 1991:343–9.

35. von Blomberg BME, Bruynzeel DP, Scheper RJ, Advances in mechanisms of allergic contact dermatitis: in vitro and in vivo research. In: *Dermatotoxicology*, 4th edn (Marzulli FN, Maibach HI, eds). New York: Hemisphere, 1991:255–362.

36. Daniels F, A simple microbiological method for demonstrating phototoxic compounds. *J Invest Dermatol* 1965; **44:** 259–63.

37. Hetherington AM, Johnson BE, Photohemolysis. *Photodermatology* 1984; **1:** 255–60.

38. Przybilla B, Georgii A, Berner T et al, Demonstration of quinolone phototoxicity in vitro. *Dermatologica* 1990; **181:** 98–103.

39. Lasarow RM, Rivkah Isseroff R, Gomez EC, Quantitative in vitro assessment of phototoxicity by a fibroblast-neutral red assay. *J Invest Dermatol* 1992; **98:** 725–9.

40. Duffy PA, Bennett A, Roberts M et al, Prediction of phototoxic potential using human A431 cells and mouse 3T3 cells. *Mol Toxicol* 1987; **1:** 579–87.

41. Richter AM, Waterfield E, Jain AK et al, In vitro evaluation of phototoxic properties of four structurally related benzoporphyrin derivatives. *Photochem Photobiol* 1990; **52:** 495–500.

42. Maier K, Schmitt-Landgraf R, Siegmund B, Development of an in vitro test system with human skin cells for evaluation of phototoxicity. *Toxicol in Vitro* 1991; **5:** 457–61.

43. Soto RJ, Gordon VC, Evaluation of an in vitro skin photoirritation assay. *Toxicologist* 1992; **12:** 109.

44. Herman PS, Sams WM, Carrier protein specificity in salicylanilide sensitivity. *J Invest Dermatol* 1970; **54:** 438–9.

45. Herman PS, Sams WM, Experimental results: immunologic investigations. In: *Soap Photodermatitis* (Herman PS, Sams WM, eds). Springfield, IL: Charles C Thomas, 1972:100–16.

46. Balls M, Botham P, Cordier A et al, Report and recommendations of an international workshop on promotion of the regulatory acceptance of validated non-animal toxicity test procedure. *Alternatives to Laboratory Animals* 1990; **18:** 339–44.

47. Bason MM, Harvell J, Realica B et al, Comparison of in vitro and human in vivo dermal irritancy data for four primary irritants. *Toxicol in Vitro* 1992; **6:** 383–7.

48. Patrick E, Burkhalter A, Maibach HI, Recent investigations of mechanisms of chemically induced skin irritation in laboratory mice. *J Invest Dermatol* 1987; **88:** 24s–31s.

49. Willis CM, Stephens CJM, Wilkinson JD, Epidermis damage induced by irritants in man: a light and electron microscopic study. *J Invest Dermatol* 1989; **93:** 695–9.

50. Owicki JC, Parce JW, Kercso KM et al, Continuous monitoring of receptor-mediated changes in the metabolic rates of living cells. *Proc Natl Acad Sci USA* 1990; **87:** 4007–11.

51. McConnell HM, Rice P, Wada GH et al, The microphysiometer biosensor. *Curr Opin Struct Biol* 1991; **1:** 647–52.

52. Tsien RY, Poenie M, Fluorescence ratio imaging: a new method into intracellular ionic signaling. *Trends Biochem Sci* 1986; **11:** 450–5.

53. Tsien RY, Fluorescent probes of cell signalling. *Annu Rev Neurosci* 1989; **12:** 227–53.

54. Maftah A, Petit JM, Leprat P et al, A new methodology for testing chemicals and drugs on cell activity. *Int J Cosmet Sci* 1990; **12:** 253–63.

RECOMMENDED READING

Rougier A, Goldberg AM, Maibach HI, *In Vitro Skin Toxicology: Irritation, Phototoxicity, Sensitization.* New York: MA Liebert, 1994.

4
Perfumes

Walter Larsen

Fragrances are the most common cause of allergic contact dermatitis due to cosmetics. In a five-year study of cosmetic reactions in the USA, fragrances were found to be the most common cause of contact dermatitis, followed by preservatives, *p*-phenylenediamine and glycerol monothioglycolate in that order.[1] Skin-care products, hair preparations and facial makeup were responsible for the majority of the reactions. The most common positive reactions to fragrance materials were with cinnamic alcohol, musk ambrette, hydroxycitronellal and isoeugenol. Less common reactions were due to geraniol, cinnamic aldehyde, coumarin, eugenol and oakmoss.

Perfumes are complex mixtures of fragrance ingredients of organic (plant or animal) or synthetic origin. Synthetic materials are increasingly popular because of their consistency of supply and purity. The Research Institute of Fragrance Materials (RIFM)* studies the safety of fragrance materials and reports the results in scientific journals. The International Fragrance Association (IFRA)† makes recommendations to industry on the safe use of fragrance materials based on the data published by the RIFM.

ALLERGIC CONTACT DERMATITIS

The best way to determine fragrance sensitivity is to patch test with the perfume itself or with a standard screening series of fragrance materials.[2] The following 14 chemicals are recommended for routine screening:

1.	Cinnamic alcohol	5% petrolatum
2.	Cinnamic aldehyde	1%
3.	Hydroxycitronellal	4%
4.	Isoeugenol	5%
5.	Eugenol	5%
6.	Oakmoss absolute	5%
7.	α-Amylcinnamic alcohol	5%
8.	Geraniol	5%
9.	Benzyl salicylate	2%
10.	Sandalwood oil	2%
11.	Anisyl alcohol	5%
12.	Benzyl alcohol	5%
13.	Coumarin	5%
14.	Musk ambrette	5%
	(also a photoallergen)	

The fragrance mixture is a helpful screening mixture frequently used in standard screening patch test series. The original screening mixture consisted of eight chemi-

* RIFM, 375 Sylvan Avenue, Englewood Cliffs, NJ 07632, USA.
† IFRA, 8 Rue Charles-Humbert, CH-1205 Geneva, Switzerland.

Table 4.1 Fragrance mixture	
1. Cinnamic alcohol	1% petrolatum
2. Cinnamic aldehyde	1%
3. Hydroxycitronellal	1%
4. Isoeugenol	1%
5. Eugenol	1%
6. Oakmoss absolute	1%
7. α-Amylcinnamic alchol	1%
8. Geraniol (sorbitan sesquioliate added as an emulsifier)	1%

Table 4.2 Perfume mixture results[4]			
January 1979– March 1980		Tested positive	Percent
Perfume mixture	2461	172	7
Cinnamic aldehyde		94	4
Cinnamic alcohol		61	2
Isoeugenol		48	2
Oakmoss		29	1.2
Eugenol		25	1
Geraniol		7	0.2
Hydroxycitronellal		36	1.4
α-Amylcinnamic alcohol		5	0.2

cals at 2% concentration each in petrolatum. However, this proved to be somewhat irritating, and it was later reduced to 1% in petrolatum. The addition of the emulsifying agent sorbitan sesquioliate has made this a more effective screening mixture (Table 4.1).

The fragrance mixture detects about 70–80% of fragrance sensitivity.[3] Therefore, in a patient who is perfume-sensitive but has a negative reaction to the perfume mixture, it is necessary to obtain the components of the offending perfume and test the individual components in order to determine the fragrance allergen. Calnan et al[4] tested the fragrance mixture on 2461 patients, and found the fragrance mixture to be positive in about 7%, most of which were relevant. They also tested the patients to the individual components (Table 4.2).

Balsam of Peru detects up to approximately 50% of patients allergic to fragrance materials.

PHOTOALLERGIC CONTACT DERMATITIS

The two fragrance materials most recently found to cause photoallergic contact dermatitis have been musk ambrette and 6-methylcoumarin.

Musk ambrette is a synthetic chemical that has been used widely for the last 70 years. This nitromusk compound is used as a fixative in perfume formulations in concentrations from 1% to as high as 15%. Since the late 1970s, there have been numerous reports of photoallergic contact dermatitis due to the musk ambrette in men's aftershave lotions.[5] IFRA recommends that musk ambrette not be used in fragrance compounds for cosmetics, toiletries and other products that under normal conditions of use will come in contact with the skin. These include rinse-off products. Musk ambrette sensitivity is still occasionally seen, but the epidemic has decreased.

6-Methylcoumarin is a synthetic compound related to the furocourmarins. In the late 1970s, 6-methylcoumarin was used in increased concentrations in a popular sunscreen, and an epidemic of photodermatitis occurred.[6] The reaction occurred primarily in women, and developed within several hours after they applied the suntan lotion and went into the sun. The Food and Drug Administration received many consumer complaints, and initiated a shelf recall of suntan products containing this ingredient. IFRA recommends that the methylcoumarins *not* be used as fragrance ingredients in any product.

Table 4.3 shows the fragrance materials that cause photoallergic contact dermatitis.

Table 4.3 Fragrance materials that show photoallergic contact dermatitis[7]
4,6-Dimethyl-8-butylcoumarin 7-Ethoxy-4-methylcoumarin 7-Methoxycoumarin 6-Methylcoumarin 7-Methylcoumarin Musk ambrette

Table 4.4 Fragrance materials that cause phototoxic contact dermatitis[7]
5-Acetyl-1,1,2,3,3,6-hexamethylindane Angelica root oil (*Angelica archangelic* L.) Bergamot oil expressed (*Citrus aurantium* L. subsp. *bergamia* Wright et Arn.) Cumin oil (*Cuminum cyminum* L.) Fig leaf absolute (*Ficus carica*) Lemon oil cold pressed (*Citrus limon* L. Burm. F.) Lime oil, expressed (*Citrus aurantifolia* Swingle) Methyl *N*-methylanthranilate Orange peel oil, bitter (*Citrus aurantium* L.) Rue oil (*Ruta graveolens* L.) Tagetes absolute (*Tagetes patula* L.) Tagetes minuta absolute (*Tagetes minuta* or *glandulifera*) Tagetes oil (*Tagetes erecta* L.; *T. patula* L.; *T. glandulifera* Schrank) Verbena oil (*Lippia citriodora* Kunth.)

PHOTOTOXIC CONTACT DERMATITIS

Phototoxic contact dermatitis usually occurs due to a furocoumarin derivative in fragrances. In the past, the most common cause of phototoxic contact dermatitis in cosmetics was the presence of perfumes such as Shalimar. Today, however, the furocoumarin has been removed from the oil of bergamot, so that phototoxic reactions are not commonly seen.

Recently a patient developed a severe photodermatitis on the arms and neck after applying Shalimar perfume and going into a suntan booth. The Shalimar perfume was 40 years old and apparently still contained the oil of bergamot with the furocoumarin. Berlocque dermatitis is a term used for a hyperpigmented phototoxic reaction to oil of bergamot containing the furocoumarin. It is rarely seen today. Table 4.4 gives a list of phototoxic fragrance materials.

CONTACT URTICARIA

Contact urticaria is either allergic or non-allergic. Balsam of Peru and some of its derivatives can cause non-allergic urticaria. The chief agents in balsam of Peru responsible for this are cinnamic acid, cinnamyl cinnamate, benzyl benzoate, benzoic acid and benzyl alcohol. Other fragrance materials such as terpinyl acetate and cinnamic aldehyde can also cause urticaria.

Contact urticaria is responsible for the immediate redness and itching when perfumes or cosmetics are applied to the skin.

The mechanism of action is probably a non-allergic histamine-liberating effect that may be more than a purely cutaneous phenomenon, because some individuals suffering from chronic respiratory allergies precipitate symptoms of their condition on exposure to some fragrance materials.

TREATMENT

Patients with an allergy to fragrance can avoid scents in cosmetics by using products that are labeled fragrance-free. Most hypoallergenic products have no fragrance materials. Patients can also perform a repeat open application test of the fragrance or cosmetic on their arms to see if they react. Some fragrance-sensitive patients use perfume on their clothes or put it in their hair, thus avoiding skin contact.

Patch testing is the only scientific way to ascertain if patients are sensitive to fragrance materials.

THE FUTURE

Fragrances are constantly changing in the marketplace as new synthetic materials are

Table 4.5 Fragrance materials restricted by IFRA[7]

Substance	Recommendation[a]	Reason
Acetylethyltetramethyltetralin (AETT)	Prohibited	Neurotoxicity
5-Acetyl-1,1,2,3,3,6-hexamethylindane	Restricted	Phototoxicity
Acetyl isovaleryl	Prohibited	Sensitization
Acetyl vetiver oil	Preparation	Sensitization by some samples
Alantroot oil (elecampane oil)	Prohibited	Sensitization
Allyl esters	Restricted	Irritation
Allyl heptine carbonate	Restricted	Sensitization
Amylcyclopentenone (2-pentyl-2-cyclopenten-1-one)	Restricted	Sensitization
Angelica root oil	Restricted	Phototoxicity
Anisylidene acetone (4-(*p*-methoxyphenyl)-3-buten-2-one)	Prohibited	Sensitization
Benzylidene acetone (4-phenyl-3-buten-2-one)	Prohibited	Sensitization
Bergamot oil	**Restricted**	**Phototoxicity**
Bitter orange oil expressed	Restricted	Phototoxicity
p-t-Butylphenol	Prohibited	Sensitization and depigmentation
Carvone oxide	Quenching[b]	Sensitization
Cassia oil	Restricted	Sensitization
Cinnamic alcohol	**Restricted**	**Sensitization**
Cinnamic aldehyde	**Quenching[b]**	**Sensitization**
Cinnamic aldehyde–methyl anthranilate Schiff base	**Quenching[b]**	**Sensitization**
Cinnamon bark oil, Ceylon	Restricted	Sensitization
Citral	Quenching[c]	Sensitization
Costus root oil, absolute and concrete from *Saussurea lappa* Clarke	Prohibited	Sensitization
Cumin oil	Restricted	Phototoxicity
Cyclamen alcohol (3-(4-isopropylphenyl)-2-methylpropanol)	Prohibited[b]	Sensitization
Diethyl maleate	Prohibited	Sensitization
Dihydrocoumarin	Prohibited	Sensitization
2,4-Dihydroxy-3-methylbenzaldehyde	Prohibited	Sensitization
4,6-Dimethyl-8-t-butylcoumarin	Prohibited	Photosensitization
Dimethyl citraconate	Prohibited	Sensitization
Ethyl acrylate	Prohibited	Sensitization
Ethyl heptine carbonate	Restricted	Sensitization
Farnesol	Specifications	Sensitization by impurities
Fig leaf absolute	Prohibited	Phototoxicity and sensitization
trans-2-Heptenal	Prohibited	Sensitization
Hexahydrocoumarin	Prohibited	Sensitization
trans-2-Hexenal	Restricted	Sensitization
trans-2-Hexenal diethyl acetal	Prohibited	Sensitization
trans-2-Hexenal dimethyl acetal	Prohibited	Sensitization
α-Hexylidene cyclopentanone	Restricted	Sensitization
Hydroabietyl alcohol	Prohibited	Sensitization
Hydroquinone monoethyl ether	Prohibited	Depigmentation
Hydroquinone monomethyl ether	Prohibited	Depigmentation
Hydroxycitronellal	**Restricted**	**Sensitization**
Isoeugenol	**Restricted**	**Sensitization**
6-Isopropyl-2-decalol	Prohibited	Sensitization
Lime oil expressed	Restricted	Phototoxicity
Marigold oil and absolute (Tagetes oil and absolute)	Restricted	Phototoxicity
Menthadienyl-7-methyl formate	Restricted	Sensitization
7-Methoxycoumarin	Prohibited	Sensitization
α-Methylanisylidene acetone (1-(4-methoxyphenyl)-1-penten-3-one)	Prohibited	Sensitization

Table 4.5 Fragrance materials restricted by IFRA[7] – *continued*

Substance	Recommendation[a]	Reason
6-Methylcoumarin	**Prohibited**	**Photosensitization**
7-Methylcoumarin	Prohibited	Photosensitization
Methyl crotonate	Prohibited	Sensitization
4-Methyl-7-ethoxycoumarin	Prohibited	Photosensitization
6-Methyl-3,5-heptadienone	Restricted	Sensitization
Methyl heptine carbonate	Restricted	Sensitization
p-Methylhydrocinnamic aldehyde	Restricted	Sensitization
Methyl *N*-methylanthranilate (dimethylanthranilate)	Restricted	Phototoxicity
3-Methyl-2(3)-nonene nitrile	Restricted	Sensitization
Methyl octine carbonate	Restricted	Sensitization
Musk ambrette	**Prohibited**[c]	**Neurotoxicity and photosensitization**
Nitrobenzene	Prohibited	Acute toxicity
Nootkatone	Specifications	Sensitization by impurities
Oakmoss absolute and resinoid (concrete)	**Restricted**	**Sensitization**
1-Octene-3-yl acetate (amylvinylcarbinyl acetate)	Restricted	Sensitization
Opoponax	Preparations	Sensitization by some samples
Oils from *Pinacea* family	Specifications	
Pentylidene cyclohexanone	Prohibited	Sensitization
Perilla aldehyde	Restricted	Sensitization
Peru balsam (exudation from *Myroxylon pereirae* (Royle) Klotzsh)	**Prohibited**	**Sensitization**
Phenylacetaldehyde	Quenching[b]	Sensitization
Propylidene phthalide	Restricted	Sensitization
Pseudoionone (2,6-dimethylundeca-2,6,8-trien-10-one)	Prohibited[c]	Sensitization
Pseudomethylionones	Prohibited[c]	Sensitization
Rue oil	Restricted	Phototoxicity
Safrole, isosafrole and dihydrosafrole	Prohibited[c]	Chronic toxicity
Savin oil	Specifications	Sensitization by some samples
Sclareol	Specifications	Sensitization by some samples
Styrax American and Asian	Preparation	Sensitization by some samples
Verbena absolute (*Lippia citriodora*)	Restricted	Sensitization
Verbena oil (*Lippia citriodora*)	Prohibited	Phototoxicity and sensitization

Bold entries are commonly used materials.
[a] For more information, such as the reasons for the recommendations and the limits of restrictions, see the IFRA Code of Practice (obtainable from IFRA, 8 Rue Charter-Humbert, CH-1205 Geneva, Switzerland).
[b] Quenching means the substance should only be used in a quenching agent.
[c] Special exemptions exist.

developed. Therefore ongoing epidemiological studies are important to determine which fragrance materials are causing allergic reactions. Table 4.5 lists fragrance materials that IFRA recommends not be used, or used only in restricted amounts.

Table 4.6 lists some of the fragrance materials that have caused allergic contact dermatitis and should be investigated in the future.

In 1992, a three-year worldwide multicenter (USA, Europe, Japan) investigation was launched to expand the information on fragrance sensitization.[8] The purpose was to determine the prevalence of responses to

Table 4.6 Fragrance materials that need epidemiological investigation
Anethole
Benzyl salicylate
Citral
Citronellal
Galoxilide
Hedione
Heliotropine
Ionone, gamma
Jasmine absolute/synthetic
Lilial
Limonene
Linalool
Lyral
Phenylethyl alcohol
Santolol, alpha
Terpineol
Ylang-Ylang oil

Table 4.7 Responses to fragrance ingredients (n = 167)	
Fragrance mix 8%	47.3%
Balsam of Peru 25%	27.2%
Ylang-Ylang oil 10%	17.4%
Cinnamic aldehyde 1%	14.4%
Hydroxycitronellal 4%	13.8%
Isoeugenol 4%	13.8%
Hydroxycitronellal 7%	13.8%
Oakmoss absolute 5%	13.2%
Eugenol 5%	7.8%
Narcissus absolute 2%	6.6%
Cinnamic alcohol 5%, lanolin	6.6%
Sandela (Givaudan) 5%	6.6%
Sandalwood oil 10%	6.6%
Majantol (Drom) 5%	5.4%
Benzyl salicylate 5%	4.8%
Galbanum resin 2%	4.8%
Geraniol 5%	3.0%
Sandalore (Givaudan) 5%	3.0%
α-Amylcinnamic aldehyde 5%	3.0%
Benzyl salicylate 2%	3.0%
Patchiouli oil (CV Kaimun Medan) 10%	3.0%
Helional (IFF) 5%	2.4%
Cedramber 5%	1.8%
Anisyl alcohol 5%	1.8%
Benzyl alcohol 5%	1.2%
Violet leaves absolute 2%	1.2%
Lilial 5%	1.2%
Coumarin 5%	1.2%
Lanolin (purified) as is	1.2%
Floropal 5%	1.2%
Musk ambrette 5%	1.2%
Ligustral (Schiff's base) 5%	0.6%
Helional (Schiff's base) 5%	0.6%
Cashmeran 5%	0.6%
Petrolatum as is	0.6%
Sorbitan sesquioleate 20%	0.6%

selected fragrance materials in patients with known fragrance allergy, and to further evaluate the risk factors and associations with such responses. In 1992, 167 subjects were evaluated in seven centers worldwide with the 8% FM, the eight ingredients in the fragrance mixture, six other well-known fragrance allergens, balsam of Peru, and 15 less well-studied fragrance materials (Table 4.7). By design, one-half of these patients were fragrance-sensitive by history only, and the other half were fragrance-sensitive by past positive patch tests to fragrance materials. Of the patients, 85% were female. The face and hands were the most common sites of clinical involvement.

Of the patients tested, 47.3% reacted to the fragrance mixture. There were fewer positive responses elicited to the 8% FM, isoeugenol and oakmoss absolute in Asians when compared with Caucasians. In contrast, Asians were more likely to exhibit a response to benzyl salicylate. The response to the 8% FM in the USA and Europe was similar. Oakmoss absolute produced more responses in Europe than in the USA or Japan.

Frequent reactions were seen to the 8% FM, balsam of Peru, Ylang-Ylang oil, narcissus absolute and sandalwood oil. Reactions to the

8% FM were concordant with 290 of a total of 328 positive responses to the individual test materials (i.e. 88.4% of all positives). Sensitivity to Ylang-Ylang oil, narcissus and sandalwood oil as a possible second group of screening test substances to be formulated as a mixture was evaluated. Testing with these three natural materials would pick up 19 positives that would have been missed with the 8% FM alone, yielding an attributable improvement in positive response frequency of 6.6%. Thus using both mixtures gave a detection rate of 309 positives, or 94.2%, of the responses obtained by testing with all individual fragrance ingredients. Balsam of Peru was tested on only 148 of the study patients (not tested in Japan). Balsam of Peru elicited six positive responses that were missed by the two mixtures. Thus balsam of Peru improved the proportion of positive responses to individual ingredients that were predicted to 315, or 96%. The data thus suggest that using a second fragrance mixture consisting of the natural materials Ylang-Ylang oil, narcissus and sandalwood oil might be useful in extending the usefulness of the 8% FM.

The second study in 1993 showed a significant number of reactions to jasmine absolute 10% in petrolatum, and spearmint oil 5% in petrolatum. The final study in 1994 showed a significant number of reactions to clove bud oil 10% in petrolatum.

In 1996, an international study comparing the 8% FM with a newly designed natural fragrance mixture was started. This new natural fragrance mixture consists of five natural fragrance materials in petrolatum:

1. Ylang-Ylang oil 2%
2. Narcissus absolute 2%
3. Sandalwood oil 2%
4. Jasmine absolute 2%
5. Spearmint oil 2%

The composition of the natural fragrance mixture is based on the results obtained in the three-year international study. The natural fragrance mixture is being used to determine if it will extend the screening ability of the original 8% FM. The disadvantage of natural materials is that such substances are not chemically defined and may vary from batch to batch, depending on where and when they were processed. Balsam of Peru is also being tested, as is a newly designed synthetic jasmine.

There has been a renaissance of interest in perfumes during the last several years. Several comprehensive reviews of fragrances have recently been published.[9–11]

REFERENCES

1. Adams RM, Maibach HI, A five year study of cosmetic reactions. *J Am Acad Dermatol* 1985; **13:** 1062–9.

2. Larsen W, Perfume dermatitis. In: *Contact Dermatitis*, 3rd edn (Fisher AA, ed). Philadelphia: Lea & Febiger, 1986:394–404.

3. Larsen WG, Perfume dermatitis. *J Am Acad Dermatol* 1985; **12:** 1–9.

4. Calnan CD, Cronin E, Rycroft R, Allergy to perfume ingredients. *Contact Dermatitis* 1980; **6:** 500–1.

5. Raugi GJ, Storrs FJ, Larsen WG, Photoallergic contact dermatitis to men's perfumes. *Contact Dermatitis* 1979; **5:** 251–60.

6. Jackson RT, Nesbitt LT Jr, DeLeo VA, 6-Methylcoumarin photocontact dermatitis. *J Am Acad Dermatol* 1980; **2:** 24–7.

7. Ford R, The toxicology and safety of fragrances. In: *Perfumes: Art, Science and Technology* (Muller, PM, Lamparsky D, eds). New York: Elsevier, 1991: 441–63.

8. Larsen W, Nakayama H, Fischer T et al, Fragrance contact dermatitis – a worldwide multicenter investigation. *Am J Contact Dermatitis* 1996; **7:** 77–83.

9. Scheinman PL, Allergic contact dermatitis to fragrance: a review. *Am J Contact Dermatitis* 1996; **7:** 65–76.

10. DeGroot AC, Frosch PJ, Adverse reactions to fragrances. A clinical review. *Contact Dermatitis* 1997; **36:** 57–86.

11. Nethercott JR, Larsen WG, Contact allergens. What's new – fragrance. In: *Clinics in Dermatology* 1997; **15:** 499–504.

5

Regulation

Nicola Loprieno

INTRODUCTION

In the European Union (EU) production and marketing of cosmetic products are regulated by Council Directive 76/768/EEC (1976); a recent amendment to this Directive was approved in June 1993 (the Sixth Amendment) introducing several innovations that will be applied during 1997. Such innovations refer to

1. the establishment of the European Inventory of ingredients employed in cosmetic products on the basis of information supplied by the European Cosmetic Industry;
2. the availability of a technical dossier for each product, reporting information on the composition, manufacturing and, primarly, the assessment of safety of the final product;
3. a full labelling information system, including a statement of the function of the product, a list of ingredients and the efficacy of the product;
4. the safety testing of cosmetics and a ban of the use of animals, starting from January 1998.*

*See page 21, Commission Directive 97/18/EC, Article 1.

This chapter presents information on the development of the European procedures for implementing the Sixth Amendment, discussing the contribution provided to the European Commission (EC) from the Scientific Committee on Cosmetology (SCC) created by the EC in 1978 with the task of assisting the legislator with the technical issues concerning the safety of cosmetic products and cosmetic ingredients.

INVENTORY

On 8 May 1996, the European Commission established an inventory and a common nomenclature of ingredients employed in cosmetic products (96/335/EC).[1] The inventory contains information concerning the identity of the ingredients, notably the INCI (International Nomenclature Cosmetic Ingredient name), the Ph.Eur (European Pharmacopoeia name), the INN (International Non-Proprietary name), the IUPAC (International Union of Pure and Applied Chemistry name), the ELINCS (European List of Notified Chemical Substances name), the CAS (Chemical Abstract Service name) and the Colour Index number.

This nomenclature established by the EC represents the support for the implementation of the full labelling information system, as requested by the Sixth Amendment, and will make it possible to identify substances by using an unique name in all the EU Member States. As a result, consumers will be easily able to recognize substances that they have been advised to avoid (for example because of allergies), no matter where they buy cosmetic products within the European Union.

The European Inventory includes the two sections provided for in Directive 93/35/EEC, namely

1. a list of cosmetic ingredients other than perfume and aromatic raw materials (Section 1);
2. a list of perfume and aromatic raw materials (Section 2).

The first list covers all items foreseen under Article 5a of the Cosmetic Products Directive concerning identity, usual function and restrictions on cosmetic ingredients. These are listed in the alphabetical order of their INCI names, which together constitute the common nomenclature for labelling throughout the EU. The restrictions refer to the ingredients covered under the Annexes of the Cosmetic Products Directive. The list covers all references to the Annexes up to and including the 17th Commission Directive 94/32/EEC adapting Annexes of the Cosmetic Products Directive to technical progress. The function refers to the usual function of the ingredient as used in cosmetic products; an ingredient may, however, have several functions.

The listed functions are defined as follows:

Abrasives Substances that are added to cosmetic products either to remove materials from various body surfaces or to aid mechanical tooth cleaning or to improve gloss.

Absorbents Substances that are added to cosmetic products to take up water- and/or oil-soluble dissolved or finely dispersed substances.

Additives Substances that are added to cosmetic products, often in relatively small amounts, to impart or improve desirable properties or suppress (or minimize) undesirable properties.

Anticorrosives Substances that are added to cosmetic products to avoid corrosion of the packaging.

Antidandruff agents Substances that are added to hair care products to control dandruff.

Antifoaming agents Substances that are added to cosmetic products either to suppress foam during manufacturing or to reduce the tendency of finished products to generate foam.

Antimicrobials Substances that are added to cosmetic products to help reduce the activities of microorganisms on the skin or body.

Antioxidants Substances that are added to cosmetic products to inhibit reactions promoted by oxygen, thus avoiding oxidation and rancidity.

Antiperspirant agents Substances that are added to cosmetic formulations to reduce perspiration.

Antistatic agents Substances that are added to cosmetic products to reduce static electricity by neutralizing electrical charge on a surface.

Binders Substances that are added to solid cosmetic mixtures to provide cohesion.

Biological additives Substances derived from biological origin that are added to cosmetic products to achieve specific formulation features.

Bleaching agents Substances that are added to cosmetic products with the intention of lightening the shade of hair or skin.

Botanicals Substances derived from plants, mostly by physical means, that are added to cosmetic products to achieve specific formulation features.

Buffering agents Substances that are added to cosmetic products to adjust or stabilize their pH.

Chelating agents Substances that are added to cosmetic products to react and to form complexes with metal ions that could affect the stability and/or appearance of cosmetics.

Cosmetic colorants Substances that are added to cosmetic products to colour them and/or to impart colour to the skin and/or its appendages. All colours listed are substances of the positive list of colorants (Annex IV of the Cosmetic Products Directive).

Denaturants Substances that are added mostly to cosmetic products containing ethanol, in order to render them unpalatable.

Deodorant agents Substances that are added to cosmetic products to reduce or mask unpleasant body odours.

Depilatory agents Substances that are added to cosmetic products to remove unwanted body hair.

Emollients Substances that are added to cosmetic products to soften and smooth the skin.

Emulsifying agents Substances that are added to cosmetic products and that are surface-active and promote the formation of intimate mixtures of immiscible liquids.

Emulsion stabilizers Substances that are added to cosmetic products to help the process of emulsification and to improve formulation stability and shelf life.

Film formers Substances that are added to cosmetic products to produce, upon application, a continuous film on skin, hair or nails.

Hair dyes Substances that are added to cosmetic products to colour hair.

Humectants Substances that are added to cosmetic products to hold and retain moisture.

Opacifiers Substances that are added to transparent or translucent cosmetic products to render them more impervious to visible light and near-visible radiation.

Oral care agents Substances that are added to cosmetic products for the care of the oral cavity.

Oxidizing agents Substances that are added to cosmetic products to change the chemical nature of another substance by adding oxygen.

Preservatives Substances that are added to cosmetic products for the primary purpose of inhibiting the development of microorganisms therein (Annex VI of Cosmetic Products Directive).

Propellants Gaseous substances that are added to cosmetic products under pressure in pressure-resistant containers for expelling the contents of the containers when the pressure is released.

Reducing agents Substances that are added to cosmetic products to change the chemical nature of another substance by adding hydrogen or removing oxygen.

Solvents Substances that are added to cosmetic products to dissolve other components.

Surfactants Substances that are added to cosmetic products to lower the surface tension as well as to aid the even distribution of the cosmetic product when it is used.

UV absorbers Substances that are added to cosmetic products specifically intended to filter certain ultraviolet rays in order to protect the skin or the products from certain harmful effects of these rays. In order to protect the skin from these effects, only the use of substances listed in Annex VII of the Cosmetic Products Directive is allowed.

Viscosity controlling agents Substances that are added to cosmetic products to increase or decrease the viscosity of the finished product.

The second list is representative of the basic materials used in perfumes and aromatic compositions. The lists were compiled mainly on the basis of information provided by EFFA (European Flavour and Fragrance Association). They constitute the Inventory of Fragrance Ingredients.

Fragrance ingredients do not need a common nomenclature, because the fragrance or its ingredients (perfume and aromatic compositions and their raw materials) must be indicated on the labels using the words 'perfume' or 'flavour' (Article 6 (1) (g) of the Cosmetic Products Directive). Hence the information on the identity of these substances consists of a chemical name identifying the substances in the clearest possible way. Such a system already exists in the *'acquis communautaire'* – namely the EINECS Inventory (European Inventory of Existing Commercial Chemical Substances),[2] and the ELINCS (European List of Notified Chemical Substances).[3] These publications mainly contain the information necessary to describe a chemical substance in an unequivocal manner, i.e. a chemical name, a CAS number and an EINECS number.

These lists also include substances of unknown structure, of variable composition or of biological origin (so-called UVCB substances). This is why the Inventory of Fragrance Ingredients was compiled on the basis of the EINECS system. The other identifiers mentioned in Directive 93/35/EEC cannot be applied (CTFA name, European Pharmacopoeia name, names recognized by the World Health Organization, Colour Index number). The IUPAC identifier is covered by the EINECS identifier.

When substances have not been included in the EINECS system, only the CAS number and CAS name have been indicated.

The function of all ingredients included in this inventory is as perfumes. Certain ingredients, however, may have several functions.

Substances used in fragrances for their properties in mixtures (solvents, excipients, etc.) are also included in the list. According to Article 6 (1) (g) of the Cosmetic Products Directive, these substances may be considered as part of the fragrance and do not have to be declared as a cosmetic ingredient, provided they are not used in excess of the recommended levels.

Restrictions on the use of a given ingredient are identified wherever relevant. These restrictions are set out in the Directive itself or in the IFRA (International Fragrance Association) Code of Practice. These restrictions may take the form of a quantitative limitation (expressed as a percentage of the final product or as a concentration for application to the skin), or the ingredient may have to meet certain specifications or may only be used in conjunction with certain specified ingredients.

These substances are marked in the list with one asterisk (*) (IFRA restrictions) or two asterisks (**) (restrictions in the Cosmetic Directive).

It should be noted that in this inventory the various qualities of a given ingredient, such as geramol, have not been recorded separately; the same applies to different qualities of natural products with the same botanical origin. For example, orange oils from Brazil, Florida, California, etc., concentrated or otherwise, are all indicated under a single entry, namely 'sweet orange extractives', CAS 802848-6, EINECS 232-433-8. This rubric is defined as follows: 'Extractives and their physically modified derivates such as tinctures, concretes, absolutes, essential oils, oleoresins, terpenes, terpene-free fractions, distillates, residues, etc. obtained from *Citrus sinensis*, Rutaceae'.

Neither does the inventory include ingredients whose chemical identity is secret and constitutes the intellectual property of a fragrance manufacturer. These substances are not sold as such but are used exclusively in fragrance compositions, generally at low concentrations, to give them a certain characteristic and/or exclusiveness.

The SCC, during its Plenary Meeting of 19 April 1995, recognized that for the time being an available version of the inventory could be accepted. However, certain aspects needed to be reconsidered in the near future; moreover, certain disputed questions needed to be discussed in order to produce improved versions at regular intervals. In particular, the following aspects should be considered:

- more precise nomenclature for the identification of some cosmetic ingredients;
- alternative classification for some polymers and copolymers;
- the need for a better specification of functions;
- identification problems associated with extracts from plants and animal sources.

DOSSIER (PRODUCT INFORMATION)

The manufacturer or his agent or the person to whose order a cosmetic product is manufactured or the person responsible for placing an imported cosmetic product on the Community market shall for control purposes keep the following information readily accessible to the competent authorities of the Member State concerned at the address specified on the label in accordance with Article 6(1)(a), Council Directive 93/35/EEC (Sixth Amendment).

(a) The qualitative and quantitative composition of the product; in the case of perfume compositions and perfumes, the name and code number of the composition and the identity of the supplier.

(b) The physico-chemical and microbiological specifications of the raw materials and the finished product and the purity and microbiological control criteria of the cosmetic product.

(c) The method of manufacture complying with the good manufacturing practice laid down by Community law or, failing that, laid down by the law of the Member State concerned; the person responsible for manufacture or first importation into the Community must possess an appropriate level of professional qualification or experience in accordance with the legislation and practice of the Member State that is the place of manufacture or first importation.

(d) Assessment of the safety for human health of the finished product. To that end the manufacturer shall take into consideration the general toxicological profile of the ingredients, their chemical structures and their levels of exposure. Should the same product be manufactured at several places within Community territory, the manufacturer may choose a single place of manufacture where that information will be kept available. In this connection, and when so requested for monitoring purposes, the manufacturer shall be obliged to indicate the place so chosen to the monitoring authority/authorities concerned.

(e) The name and address of the qualified person or persons responsible for the assessment referred to in (d). That person must hold a diploma as defined in Article I of Council Directive 89/48/EEC in the field of pharmacy, toxicology, dermatology, medicine or a similar discipline.

(f) Existing data on undesirable effects on human health resulting from use of the cosmetic product.

(g) Proof of the effect claimed for the cosmetic product, where justified by the nature of the effect or product.

(B2) The assessment of the safety for human health referred to in Paragraph 1(d) shall be carried out in accordance with the principles af good laboratory practice laid down in Council Directive 87/18/EEC of 18 December 1986 on the harmonization of laws, regulations and administrative provisions relating to the application of the principles of good laboratory practice and the verification of their application for tests on chemical substances.

(B3) The information referred to in Paragraph I must be available in the national language or languages of the Member State concerned, or in a language readily understood by the competent authorities.

Authorities' requirements for a Product Information (PI), as from the text cited, is clearly related to the requirement to have all information that could be needed 'for control purposes' available promptly on the technical characteristics and safety of every cosmetic product placed on the market. The (PI) is in fact set out so that information is easily accessible for an overall assessment of the safety of the cosmetic product on the basis of all relevant knowledge.

The assessment of the safety of any cosmetic product clearly relates to the manner of use. This factor is important, since it determines the amount of substance that may be ingested, inhaled or absorbed through the skin or mucous membranes. Consideration of the quantity of ingredients applied in the different products is also important, as the following examples illustrate. For example, soaps are applied in dilute form, and although the area of application may be extensive, the product is rapidly washed off. Products used on the lips and mouth will be ingested to some extent. Cosmetics used around the eyes and genital regions may come into contact with the conjunctiva or mucosa respectively, resulting in reaction due to the thin epithelial lining of these areas. Sun-tanning products, body lotions or body creams may be applied over a large surface of the body, and the ingredients, often at appreciable concentrations, may remain in contact with the skin for several hours. Sun-tanning products, owing to their extensive skin contact, combined with direct exposure to UV radiation for prolonged periods, require a distinct type of safety evaluation.

Thus, before any safety evaluation and risk assessment of a finished product is made, the degree and route of consumer exposure must be known. This needs to be carried out on a case-by-case basis, but the following may provide guidance. In calculating the exposure at least the following factors must be considered:

1. class of cosmetic product(s) where the ingredient may be used;
2. method of application, (rubbed-in; sprayed, applied and washed off; etc.);
3. concentration of ingredients in product;
4. quantity of product used at each application;
5. frequency of application;
6. total area of skin contact;
7. site of contact (e.g. mucous membrane, sunburnt skin);
8. duration of contact (e.g. rinse-off products);
9. foreseeable misuse that may increase exposure;
10. nature of consumers (e.g. children, people with sensitive skin);
11. quantity likely to enter the body;
12. projected number of consumers;
13. application on skin areas exposed to sunlight.

The relevant exposure depends upon the toxicological effects under consideration. For example, for skin irritation or phototoxicity the exposure per unit area of skin is important, while for systemic toxicity the exposure per unit of body weight is of more significance.

The route or routes of exposure (skin, mucous membranes, ingestion, inhalation, skin exposed to sunlight) must be considered in designing any test programme and in risk analysis. The possibility of secondary exposure by routes other than those resulting from the direct application should be considered (e.g. inhalation of hairsprays, ingestion of lip products).

The levels of use of of cosmetic products are subjected to several factors, some of which will vary with time, such as age group, seasonal variation, local habits, fashion trends, disposable income, and product innovation.

According to the Sixth Amendment of the European Cosmetic Directive, the safety assessor must provide the person responsible for the marketing of a given product (manufacturer or importer within the European Union) with a safety assessment for each cosmetic product put on the market (PI).

The assessment is not represented by and limited to a simple certificate: it must be based on serious scientific reasons resulting from well-documented sources. In order to do so, a clear identification of the toxicological profile of the ingredients, complex ingredients when justified, and specific fragrance ingredients present in the fragrance compound, as well as information concerning the formulation of the finished product, its degree and route of application and any available toxicological data, are important factors to be taken into consideration. As part of the information may not be available or needed, it is therefore the responsibility of the safety assessor to report and justify the scientific reasoning adopted for accepting the formulation.

The SCC adopted during its Plenary Meeting of 20 December 1996 the second revision of a document entitled 'Notes of Guidance for Testing of Cosmetic Ingredients for Their Safety Evaluation' (doc XXIV/1878/96), in which it presents a set of suggestions for the safety assessor on how to proceed while defining the 'assessment'. The SCC's Guidance should not be used as a checklist, but adopted on a case-by-case basis when assessing the safety of a finished product.

1 Transparency of the ingredient's identity

Terminology
Cosmetic ingredient means

(1) any chemically defined substance with a molecular formula and a structural formula;
(2) any complex substance, requiring a definition, corresponding to substances of unknown or variable composition and to biological substances;

(3) mixtures of (1) and (2);

used in the composition of cosmetic products.

1.1 Qualitative and quantitative formula (dir 93/35/EEC, art 7a, l(a))
Precise identification and description of the ingredients is crucial for a toxicological assessment.

The finished product's formula will be supplemented for each ingredient and for each complex ingredient by a 'definition' statement comprising all the particulars not included in the inventory. The definition will be sufficiently precise to identify a given ingredient with regard to its composition and its effects.

Ingredients should be defined in particular in terms of manufacturing and purification process: chemical synthesis, isolation and purification by chemical processes, or physical, enzymatic, biotechnological or microbiological processing using material of biological origin.

Most biotechnologically derived ingredients are well-defined chemicals covered by the general requirements (e.g. acids, alcohols and amino acids), and a series of excipients, additives and foodstuffs.

The molecular formula and the structural formula of the chemically defined substance will be given.

Ingredients should also be characterized by their analytical specifications.

1.2 Physical, chemical and microbiological specifications of ingredients (dir 93/35/EEC, art 7a, 1, (b))
Appropriate physical, chemical and microbiological specifications should be defined for each ingredient. The factors with an important bearing on safety for cosmetic purposes must be taken into account.

1.2.1 As regards general problems of identification, ingredients requiring a 'definition' including any impurities that they contain that are of toxicological significance (e.g. toxic subcomponents, residual solvents, and heavy metals) and the ingredients authorized in the annexes to the Cosmetics Directive should be specified using discriminant analytical techniques such as HPLC, GC/MS and NMR.

1.2.2 Microbiological specifications are essential. For ingredients of biological origin (e.g. derived from plants, animals or other sources), specifications must be adapted with appropriate regard to the source material.

1.3 Examples of complex ingredients

A. Ingredients of mineral origin
B. Ingredients of animal origin
C. Ingredients of plant origin
D. Special ingredients derived from biotechnology
E. Commercial addition mixtures, including perfumes
• Reaction mixtures
• Ingredients of variable composition

A. Ingredients of mineral origin

According to the type of ingredient under consideration and the extent to which it is modified, full identification particulars should be considered in the safety assessment. The following are given as examples:

• Starting material
• Description of
  The preparation process
  – physical processing (e.g. destructive distillation)
  – chemical modifications
  – possible purification
  Characteristic elements of the composition
  – characteristic components
  – toxic components (with percentage)
• Physical and chemical specifications
• Microbiological quality

B. Ingredients of animal origin

According to the type of ingredient under

consideration and the extent to which it is modified, full identification particulars should be considered in the safety assessment. The following are given as examples:

• Species (bovine, ovine, crustacean, etc.)
• Organs, tissues or liquids (placenta, serum, cartilage, etc.)
• Country of origin
• Description of
  The preparation process
  – conditions of extraction (solvent, pH, temperature etc.)
  – type of hydrolysis (acid, enzyme, etc.)
  – other chemical modifications
  – possible purification
  Commercial form
  – powder product
  – product in solution (solvent and concentration)
  – lyophilisate, etc.
  Characteristic elements of the composition
  – characteristic amino acids
  – total nitrogen
  – polysaccharides
  – molecular mass
• Physical and chemical specifications
• Microbiological quality including viral contamination
• Xenobiotic contamination

C. Ingredients of plant origin

According to the type of ingredient under consideration and the extent to which it is modified, full identification particulars should be considered in the safety assessment. The following are given as examples:

• Botanical name and family (Linnaean system)
• Part of the plant processed
• Description of:
  The preparation process
  – extraction
  – distillation
  – destructive distillation (e.g. wood tars)

– possible purification
Commercial form
– powder product
– product in solution (solvent and concentration)
Characteristic elements of the composition
– characteristic components
– toxic components (with percentage)
• Physical and chemical specifications
• Microbiological quality including fungi
• Xenobiotic contamination

D. Special ingredients derived from biotechnology

For special biotechnologically derived ingredients, where a modified microorganism or a potential toxin has not been fully removed, specific data must be available, which can comprise:

• Description of organisms
  – donor organism
  – recipient organism
  – modified microorganism
• Pathogenicity of the host
• Pathogenicity of the modified organism
• Toxicity and, when possible, identity of metabolites (toxins) produced by the organism
• Fate of viable organism in the environment, survival, potential for transfer of characteristics to, e.g., natural bacteria
• Physical and chemical specifications
• Microbiological quality
• Xenobiotic contamination

E. Commercial addition mixtures

Any ingredient, according to INCI name when available, occurring in the composition of commercial mixtures supplied as 'raw materials' must be given in the qualitative and quantitative formula of the finished product. The following are given as examples:

• Main component(s)
• Preservatives
• Antioxidants
• Buffering agents
• Solvents
• Other additives

2 Transparency of the assessment of the safety for human health of the finished cosmetic product

Each cosmetic finished product is an individual and unique combination of ingredients. The number of finished products is extremely large compared with the number of cosmetic ingredients.

In general, the safety evaluation of the finished product can be obtained from knowledge of the toxicity of the cosmetic ingredients (Council Directive 93/35/EEC). Toxicity information on the ingredients should include the evaluation of the most relevant toxicological end points.

In some cases, however – for instance when the formulations used in the finished product are different from the solvents employed in the toxicity studies of the ingredients and they are likely to considerably increase the *penetration* or the *irritancy* of some of the ingredients – additional information on finished products to allow a better safety evaluation will be needed.

If there could be potentiation of the toxic effects of the ingredients, or if toxic effects resulting from chemical interaction between individual ingredients are likely to occur, specific toxicological information on the finished products should be considered. Conversely, as indicated previously, any claim of decreased absorption or potential hazard of some ingredient, due to the formulation, should be supported by adequate information.

When the combination of ingredients present in the finished product makes the formation of new substance of toxicological concern highly probable, additional toxicological information on the finished product will be needed.

2.1 Toxicological profile of the ingredients (dir 93/35/EEC, art 7a, 1, (d))

The safety assessor must take account of all the toxicological data available for each ingredient in the final product, including those from (natural) biological origin. Sources of the respective data should be given.

Toxicological data available may be obtained from:

- tests on animals or recognized/validated alternative methods of testing; whenever data on clinical human observations are available, they are to be included;
- specific toxicological studies or studies conducted for other regulatory purposes;
- the raw material suppliers, and completed with data available to the person responsible for the safety assessment through databases or published literature.

Toxicological data must enable a determination of the possible toxic effect(s), including the allergenic potential of all ingredients, including those from biological origin.

2.2 Assessment of the safety of the finished product

Details of the scientific reasoning adopted by the safety assessor must be set out in the assessment. This should consider all intended and likely routes of human exposure during use.

All toxicological data available on the formulation and its ingredients, either favourable or unfavourable, should be taken into account, including an assessment of the potential for chemical or biological interaction of/in the formulated product. The safety assessor must take into account the acceptability of the inclusion in the formulation of particular ingredients that may have a low threshold of safety.

2.3 Qualifications of the safety assessor (dir 93/35/EEC, art 7a, 1, (e))

The curriculum vitae of the safety assessor described in the directive must be added to the dossier.

The safety assessors may be external consultants. If the safety assessors are employed by the manufacturer, they must have no connection with the production or the marketing sides. As well as having the requisite training, they must also provide evidence of relevant experience in the fields of toxicology.

3 Fragrances

According to the Code of Practice for the fragrance industry:

> Fragrance manufacturers should provide customers with all available information to ensure that fragrance materials are used in accordance with standards of good practice.

In its guidelines for communicating the IFRA status of a fragrance compound (i.e. a blend of fragrance ingredients representing a specific formula), IFRA recommends consideration, in particular, of

- a statement that the fragrance complies with the IFRA guidelines for the mentioned application and used concentration,
- a reference to the bases of the IFRA guidelines, RIFM data and other available sources.

Without questioning the principle of intellectual property underlying the derogation concerning the qualitative and quantitative formula of fragrance compounds (dir 93/35/EEC, art 7a, 1, (a)), several measures should be considered with a view to providing something more than a safety guarantee of a purely legal nature and to informing the person responsible for safety with regard to human health.

3.1 Certificate of comformity

The existing certificate of conformity with IFRA standards attached to a fragrance compound should be systematically supplemented by

- a semiquantitative declaration naming the

fragrance ingredients that have been subject to restrictions in the IFRA Code of Practice and, in a more general way, those that have an established potential to cause contact sensitization and (or) phototoxic reactions (e.g. F.I. listed in the European Standard Fragrance Mix), for example

- essential oil from the bark of cinnamonum zeylanicum < 1%
- *Evernia prunasti* concrete (oakmoss extract) < 3%
- methyloct-2-ynoate < 0.01%
- geraniol ...%
- eugenol ...%
- α-amylcinnamaldehyde ...%

• an indication of the cosmetic product types in which it may be used

While safeguarding the formula's confidentiality, the safety assessment should be confirmed on the fragrance compound considered as a whole, and the data and the scientific reasoning should be included in the conformity certificate.

3.2 Safety assessment of perfumed cosmetics

The exact concentration of the perfume composition (= fragrance compound in the cosmetic product) should be indicated (dir 93/35/EEC, art 7a,1,(a)).

In the safety assessment of the cosmetic product for human health (dir 93/35/EEC, art 7a, I, (d)),

• reference should be made to the semiquantitative formula of the fragrance compound naming the fragrance ingredients declared in the certificate of conformity (see 3.1 above), and account should be taken of their toxic potential;

• reference should be made to the safety assessment of the fragrance compound considered as a whole.

LABELLING INFORMATION SYSTEM

Article 6/1 of Cosmetic Directive 76/768/EEC, amended by Directive 93/35/EEC states that:

Member States shall take all measures necessary to ensure that cosmetic products may be marketed only if the container and packaging bear the following information in indelible, easily legible and visible lettering; particular precautions to be observed in use, especially those listed in column 'Conditions of use and warnings which may be printed on the label' in Annexes III, IV, VI and VII, which must appear on the container and packaging. The label of cosmetic products must contain:

- the function of the product, unless it is clear from the presentation of the product;
- a list of ingredients in descending order of weight at the time they are added. That list shall be preceded by the word 'ingredient'. Where that is impossible for practical reasons, an enclosed leaflet, label, tape or card must contain the ingredients to which the consumer is referred either by abbreviated information or the symbol.

Perfume and aromatic compositions and their raw materials shall be referred to by the word 'perfume' or 'flavour'. Ingredients in concentrations of less than 1% may be listed in any order after those in concentrations of more than 1%. Colouring agents may be listed in any order after the other ingredients, in accordance with the colour index number or denomination adopted in Annex IV.

For decorative cosmetic products in several colour shades, all colouring agents used in the range may be listed, provided that the terms 'may contain' are added.

An ingredient must be identified by the common name referred to in the European Inventory (93/35/EEC, art 5a).

SAFETY TESTING OF COSMETICS

A cosmetic product that is put on the market within the European Union must not cause damage to human health when applied under normal or reasonably foreseeable conditions of use, taking into account, in particular, the product's presentation, its labelling, any instructions for its use and disposal as well as any other indication or information provided by the manufacturer or his authorized agent or by any other person responsible for placing the product on the Community market (Art 2: Directive 76/768/EEC amended by Directive 93/35/EEC).

Council Directive 76/768/EEC, as modified by Council Directive 93/35/EEC intends to protect consumers' health from possible deleterious effects due to the presence of specific substances that could cause damage to humans, because of their intrinsic unsafe properties.

Several mechanisms have been triggered by this Directive in order to fulfil its main requirements regarding consumers' health protection:

- identifying chemicals that must not be contained in finished products (Annex II);
- identifying substances that cosmetic products must not contain except those subject to restrictions and conditions laid down in Annex III;
- authorizing substances of particular function such as antioxidants, colouring agents (Annex IV) hair dyes, preservatives (Annex VI) and UV filters (Annex VII).

As for other sectors of toxicity testing (pesticides, drugs, food additives, industrial chemicals, etc.), the relevant test procedures are those reported in the Commission Directive 84/449/EEC and in the Annex to Commission Directive 92/69/EEC; OECD Guidelines for testing of chemicals are also suitable information for the safety evaluation of cosmetics.[4]

The majority of these official and international test procedures are based on the use of animal models; thousands of studies have been performed during the last 30 years and their results have been discussed, interpreted and applied for the identification and management of human risk as a consequence of human exposure to those chemicals (Commission Regulation 1488/94). The Sixth Amendment to Cosmetic Directive 76/768/EEC has inserted the new sentence:

> Assessment of the safety of use of the ingredients employed in cosmetics and of the finished product should take into account the requirement of Directive 86/609/EEC which concerns protection of animals used for experimental and other scientific purposes.

Within the scope of the European Community, Directive 86/609/EEC affirms a few general principles that must regulate the use of animals in toxicity experiments on chemicals. These principles, although at variance with those of previous regulations, have stimulated the development of strategies of research and of methodologies for determining the toxic effects of chemical substances, in agreement with alternative, scientifically valid principles.

Directive 86/609/EEC affirms that all experiments on animals are forbidden unless they are carried out with the object of:

- research aimed at preserving the species at issue; or
- essential biomedical purposes, provided that the species employed in experiments represent the only specific ones for attaining that purpose.

This means, in principle, a restriction on animal experimentation in toxicity studies and, above all, in those cases where the predictive significance of studies of similar effects on humans is rather low.

The above mentioned rule firmly maintains (art 7.2) that 'an experiment shall not be performed if another scientifically satisfactory method of obtaining the result sought, not entailing the use of an animal, is reasonably and practically available'.

As a consequence of this position, Council Directive 76/768/EEC was amended by Council Directive 93/35/EEC, by imposing a ban on the testing on animals of ingredients or combinations of ingredients as from 1 January 1998 (Council Directive 76/768/EEC amended, Art 4(1) (i)).

The Sixth Amendment states, however, that if there has been insufficient progress in developing satisfactory methods to replace animal testing, and in particular in those cases where alternative methods of testing, despite all reasonable endeavours, have not been scientifically validated as offering an equivalent level of protection for the consumer, taking into account OECD toxicity test guidelines, then the Commission shall by 1 January 1997 submit draft measures to postpone the date of implementation of this provision, for a sufficient period and in any case for no less than two years. Before submitting such measures, the Commission shall consult the Scientific Committee on Cosmetology.

Clearly, the legislator has intended to ban the testing on animals of cosmetic ingredients or finished products, in relation to the problem of the toxicity or safety evaluation of these specific chemicals, or their combinations, only provided that there are alternative methodologies available.

'Alternative methodology' means any modification to the present toxicity assay testing protocols that are internationally and scientifically approved and based on animal models, in such a way as to introduce a different mode of conducting toxicological studies necessary to assess the safety of ingredients employed in the manufacture of finished cosmetic products.

Alternative methodologies must offer a level of protection to consumers equaling that presently offered by toxicological studies performed on animals: this implies that the alternative methods must be scientifically validated.

The in vitro methodologies for evaluating the toxic potential of cosmetic ingredients that have been reported in the scientific literature or those that have been submitted to validation studies during the past three years have not yet been demonstrated to be useful in the prediction of toxic risk to humans. Their precision is so low that the practical utility of such prediction is questionable.[5]

The in vivo studies allow the possibility of investigating the toxicological profile of a cosmetic ingredient when applied to an animal by a route of exposure similar to that of human exposure. They provide for the determination of the non-observed adverse effect level (NOAEL) and also the adverse effects at higher exposures.

Studies in humans are the ideal in the case of cosmetics. Contemporary ethical standards may prevent the use of toxic or radiolabelled compounds in such studies. However, at the present time sufficiently sensitive methods for the detection of unlabelled compounds in the plasma are under active investigation. For instance, the absorption of a chemical following dermal application may also be investigated by studying its excretion or its metabolites.

In 1993, the European Commission established the European Centre for Validation of Alternative Methods (ECVAM), whose task is 'to promote the scientific and regulatory acceptance of alternative methods'. ECVAM considered, among priority sectors, the safety testing of cosmetics as a consequence of the issue of the Sixth Amendment.

It is ECVAM's opinion that the introduction of bans on animal testing may not be the best way to secure the acceptance and use of validated alternative methods. It might be preferable, for ECVAM, in line with Directive 86/609/EEC, to insist that an alternative method must be used, except in circumstances where a convincing scientific case for using an animal procedure is presented to the relevant authorities in advance of the conduct of the testing of a particular material. Since the end of 1996, the interim position of ECVAM on different types of cosmetics' safety testing has been the following:

Finished products The testing in animals of finished cosmetic products that are manufactured and/or marketed in the EU should cease to be acceptable with effect from 1 January 1998. Nevertheless, it should be recognized that a convincing scientific case for research involving animal procedures could be made in certain circumstances, for example if a product showed unexpected human toxicity after marketing or in the case of an unexpected chemical interaction between the components of a product that could not have been predicted. Such events are very rare, but there might be occasions when it would be useful to investigate what had happened, in the hope of avoiding similar events in the future.

Phototoxicity Phase II of the EU/COLIPA international validation study on in vitro tests for phototoxicity (photoirritancy) has been very successful. Those concerned are confident that an acceptable OECD guideline can be drafted within the next two years, i.e. after the final report on the study has been published and minor refinements to protocols have been made. Of the 38 materials tested in Phases I and II of the study, 18 were relevant to the cosmetics industry. ECVAM would consider funding a small study on some types of chemicals of particular interest to the SCC, because information about their potential toxicity and safety is specifically required under the terms of Directive 76/768/EEC.

Percutaneous absorption ECVAM and the OECD recently organized a discussion aimed at solving differences between European and North American agencies in relation to the acceptance of in vitro methods for evaluating percutaneous absorption. The meeting was also attended by individuals connected with COLIPA, DGXXIV/4, ECETOC, the US FDA, the UK Department of Health and the SCC. It was

agreed that a draft guideline currently before the OECD should be redrafted, in order to promote clarification and to resolve the intercontinental differences. It is hoped that this new draft guideline will be acceptable to all concerned. If not, the EU may want to consider whether or not to proceed with its own in vitro test guideline.

Skin corrosivity An ECVAM validation study on in vitro tests for corrosivity is about to take place, and there is confidence that the acceptability of one or more relevant and reliable in vitro tests will be confirmed. With new ingredients, an evaluation of potential for corrosivity must precede a consideration of potential irritancy.

Skin irritancy An ECVAM-style workshop is needed on the circumstances in which in vitro tests for skin irritancy are likely to be needed, and also on what basic information is required, before it is ethically acceptable to conduct studies with human volunteers.

Eye irritation Attempts to validate in vitro tests for ocular irritancy have so far been very disappointing. However, this is more likely to be due to the inability of the Draize eye irritancy test to provide reproducible, quantitative data than to the inadequacy of some or all of the main in vitro methods under consideration. Urgent action is needed to determine the best way forward on this issue.

Summary of ECVAM position

The proposed ban spelled out in the Sixth Amendment to Directive 76/768/EEC could be applied as follows:

1 January 1998
- Finished product testing

1 January 2000
- Phototoxicity testing
- Percutaneous absorption testing
- Skin irritancy testing

In addition, efforts should be put into making bans on the following possible:

- Eye irritancy testing, by 1 January 2000
- Sensitization testing, by 1 January 2003

Cosmetic Industries in the European Union (COLIPA) in collaboration with cosmetic industries in the USA (CTFA) and Japan (JCIA), the UK Home Office, the European Commission and ECVAM, have been heavily involved in validation studies: the focus of efforts has been to find alternatives to those tests normally associated with the use of cosmetics: skin and eye irritation, skin sensitization, phototoxicity and percutaneous absorption.

Strategies

Percutaneous absorption Industry is applying in vitro protocols for more than 10 years. COLIPA has developed a guideline: industry is prepared to rely on in vitro testing for testing of cosmetic ingredients.

Skin irritation COLIPA has prepared a guideline on using human volunteers rather than animals for finished product testing. COLIPA will develop a similar guideline on ingredients, expected to be available at the beginning of 1998.

Photoirritation A joint EU/COLIPA validation programme has been in place since 1991. Phase I has been completed; the results of Phase II were available by mid-1996. Preliminary results indicate that in vitro assays provide data at least as reliable as those generated from animal experiments. COLIPA strongly supports the development of an OECD test guideline on in vitro testing rather than on in vivo testing.

Eye irritation This has been the focus of the greatest effort by the cosmetic industry from the beginning, with contributions from cosmetic companies to all the major validation studies. The results of the two most recent

and major validation studies demonstrate the complexity and challenges of replacing the in vivo assay for ingredient testing. Industry is continuing its efforts with a new validation study which was started at the end of 1997; results are expected to be available by the end of 1999.

Sensitization Research focusing on mechanistic studies and protocol development is ongoing. COLIPA proposes to the Commission to enter into discussions on a research programme in collaboration with EC-DGXII.

The cosmetics industry is contributing to finding alternatives for other types of safety testing, with, for example, systemic toxicity and developmental toxicity and carcinogenicity, but it believes efforts in these areas have to be made jointly with others involved (i.e. ECVAM, ZEBET, FRAME, the chemical industry and the pharmaceuticul industry and the food industry). Some cosmetic companies are also involved in other activities such as food, chemicals and pharmaceuticals, and thus contribute in this way.

Finished product testing Many companies are already applying in vitro assays in their product safety evaluation procedures.

Potential animal test ban: position of the cosmetic industry

Table 5.1 lists the tests that could be carried out on cosmetic ingredients or combinations of ingredients to perform a proper safety evaluation.

The tests have been classified according to current scientific knowledge on the possibilities of replacing them partially or totally by methods not making use of animals.

On the basis of the present scientific knowledge on the development and validation of adequate alternative methodologies to the use of animals in the safety testing of cosmetics, the Scientific Committee on Cosmetology of

Table 5.1 Testing of cosmetic ingredients for safety evaluation

Good prospect for alternatives
- Skin irritation
- Percutaneous absorption
- Photoirritation
- Eye irritation

Some prospect for alternatives
- Skin sensitization

Little prospect for alternatives
- Acute toxicity
- Systemic toxicity
- Developmental toxicity
- Mutagenicity in vivo
- Immunotoxicity
- Carcinogenicity
- Neurotoxicity
- Reproductive toxicity

the European Commission, as a fulfillment of the Sixth Amendment's requirements, adopted the following opinion on 20 December 1996:

1. On the basis of the EC/HO International Validation Study on Alternatives to the Draize Eye Irritation Test[5] and the COLIPA International Validation Study on Alternatives to the Rabbit Eye Irritation Test,[6] 'at the present time there are no adequate and reliable alternative methodologies to substitute the eye irritation testing protocol'.

2. After having considered the results of the EU–COLIPA International Validation Study on in vitro tests for phototoxicity, the SCC recommends that the cosmetic industries test new UV filters for their potential by using the neutral red uptake phototoxic assay, in order to develop a database that could support the use of this in vitro methodology. It seems reasonable and scientifically justified to predict that more in vitro methodologies will be available in the near future.

3. Knowledge on in vitro testing procedures for percutaneous absorption has improved considerably during the last few years: many cosmetic ingredients have been tested, and some of them were accepted by the SCC. A recent meeting organized by ECVAM and OECD has discussed the possibility of an in vitro guideline for percutaneous absorption.

   In order to document the adequacy and relevance of in vitro methods for percutaneous absorption, data available in the scientific literature are being collected and evaluated.

   It is the opinion of the SSC that, especially for cosmetic ingredients, relevant studies for assessing percutaneous absorption are chiefly important, and that alternative methods for the study of percutaneous absorption will be available in the near future.

4. The SCC confirms its opinion adopted in 1990[7] that the safety evaluation of finished cosmetic products in general could be obtained by knowledge of the toxicity of the cosmetic ingredients. In some cases additional information on finished products is needed.

The European Commission, in fulfillment of the Sixth Amendment, has approved a Directive[8] postponing the deadline of 1 January 1998 for the ban on animal testing. This Directive is reproduced as an appendix to this chapter; the explanatory memorandum is also included.

SAFETY REGULATIONS IN THE USA AND JAPAN

Table 5.2 reports the indications given in Japan and the USA for toxicity studies, requested or frequently expected for cosmetics and compared with similar requests from the European Union.

US cosmetic regulations

A cosmetic may be distributed in, or imported into, the USA only if it is in compliance with

Table 5.2 Toxicity studies for the evaluation of cosmetics in different countries

Studies	EU[a]	USA[b]	Japan[10]
Acute toxicity	Yes	Yes	Yes
Dermal absorption	Yes		
Dermal irritation	Yes	Yes	Yes
Mucous membrane irritation eye irritation	Yes	Yes	
Skin sensitization	Yes	Yes	Yes
Subchronic toxicity	Yes		
Mutagenicity	Yes	Yes	Yes
Phototoxicity	Conditional (in the case of UV filters)		Conditional (in the case of UV filters)
Photomutagenicity	Conditional (in the case of UV filters)		
Photosensitization	Conditional	Conditional	
Toxicokinetics	Conditional		
Teratogenicity, reproduction toxicity, carcinogenesis, additional genotoxicity	Conditional		
Human data	Conditional		Yes

[a] Recommended by EC-SCC.[7]
[b] Frequently expected.[9]

the cosmetic provisions of Chapter VI of the Federal Food, Drug and Cosmetic Act and with the Fair Packaging and Labeling Act and regulations published under these laws.

Cosmetics are regarded as articles other than soap that are applied to the human body for cleansing, beautifying, promoting attractiveness or altering the appearance. This definition includes products such as skin creams, lotions, perfumes, lipsticks, fingernail polishes, shampoos, eye and face make-up, permanent waves and hair colouring preparations, toothpastes, and deodorants.

Articles that are cosmetics but that are also intended to treat or prevent disease or affect the structure or functions of the human body are drugs as well as cosmetics, and must comply with both the drug and cosmetic provisions of the law and regulations. Examples of this class, namely over-the-counter (OTC) products, are anticaries drug products, oral health care products, hormone creams, sunscreens, topical acne preparations, antiperspirants, antidandruff shampoos, skin bleaching drug products, skin protectants and vaginal drug products.

The Food, Drug and Cosmetic Act prohibits the distribution of cosmetics that are adulterated or misbranded. A cosmetic is misbranded if its labelling is false or misleading, if it does not bear the required labelling information or if it is deceptively packaged.

The Food, Drug and Cosmetic Act does not require cosmetic firms to register manufacturing establishments or formulations with the FDA or make available safety data or other information before a product is marketed in the USA.

With the exception of colour additives (regulated and revised by the FDA), a cosmetic manufacturer may, on its own responsibility, use essentially any ingredient or market any cosmetic until the FDA can demonstrate that it may be harmful to consumers under customary conditions of use.

In fact, the list of banned substances is limited to 14 ingredients/categories.

Labelling

The label of a cosmetic must give

- a statement of identity;
- the name and address (street address, city, state and zip code) of the manufacturer, packer or distributor;
- an accurate statement of the net amount of the cosmetic in the package in terms of weight, measure, numerical count or their combination;
- the ingredients, listed in descending order of their predominance;
- warning statements, when necessary;
- the English name of the country of origin if the article is imported.

All information must be in English, and must be shown in a manner that makes it easily noticed and readily understood.

Japanese cosmetic regulations

In Japan cosmetics are regulated by the Ministry of Health and Welfare (MHW) under the Pharmaceutical Affairs Law, which requires manufacturers or importers to submit complete formulations before a licence (*kyoka*) to manufacture or import a product can be granted. A cosmetic (*keshohin*) is defined by law as:

Any article intended to be used by means of rubbing, sprinkling or by similar application to the human body for cleansing, beautifying, promoting attractiveness and altering the appearance of the human body, and for keeping the skin and hair healthy, provided that the action of the article on the human body is mild.

Products intended to affect the structure or any function of the body are not considered as cosmetics (rather they are quasidrugs or medical devices or drugs).

The basic regulation published in 1967 requires all ingredients used to conform to certain standards approved by the MHW and published in the Japanese Standards of Cosmetic Ingredients (JSCI). This official list has been expanded through the years, and now contains close to 600 entries. If a cosmetic formulation contains only ingredients on the list and if they meet the standards, then no further safety data are required for approval.

In 1986 the MHW also issued a note on banned cosmetic ingredients, and a number of different MHW Ordinances list approved colours.

Because of the limited number of chemicals in the JSCI list, the MHW has approved other ingredients on a case-by-case basis. This list was secret until its release in recent years by the MHW and its publication by the Japanese Cosmetic Industry Association (CIA) as its dictionary (CID), containing about 1300 ingredients.

In order to have a faster licensing system the Comprehensive Licensing System (CLS or *sAubetsu kyoka*) was introduced in 1985. This is a pre-marketing notification applied to cosmetics containing only approved ingredients within specified limits. In fact, however, the CLS, with its 35 cosmetic categories and strict concentration ranges, has proved to be too complex to have more than limited usefulness.

Post-marketing monitoring of a licensed cosmetic containing a new ingredient is actually regulated by the MHW on a case-by-case basis, but a 1987 policy draft specifies that the safety examination period is two years for completely new developed ingredients and one year for ingredients already in use in other countries.

Quasidrugs comprise a category of cosmetics including medicated cosmetics (including products for the prevention of acne and itchy skin rash, and disinfectants), special bath preparations, body deodorants, talcum powders, mouthwashes, antiperspirants, hair growth products, hair dyes, UV filters (depending on the claims made), and permanent waving and hair products, for which licensing still requires at least six months.

Labelling

The following information must be printed on containers or packaging:

- the name and address of the manufacturer or importer;
- the name of the product;
- the production number or code;
- the name of the ingredient designated by the MHW, if any (there is a list of ingredients that may cause skin disorders, e.g. hormones, coal-tar colours, benzoic acid, lanolin, parabens and *p*-aminobenzoic acid (PABA) esters);
- the shelf life – only for those cosmetics that may change in appearance, condition and quality under proper storage conditions within three years following manufacture or import.

It should be noted that Article 66 of the Pharmaceutical Affairs Law bans any advertisement containing false, misleading or exaggerated information.

REFERENCES

1. *Official Journal of the European Communities* 1 June 1996; L132, **39:** 684.
2. *Official Journal of the European Communities* 15 June 1990; No. C, 146A.
3. *Official Journal of the European Communities* 17 December 1994; No. C, 361.
4. *OECD Guidelines for the Testing of Chemicals*, Vols 1 and 2, Paris 1993.
5. Balls M, De Klerck W, Baker F et al, Development and validation of non-animal tests and testing strategies: The identification of a co-ordinated response to the challenge and the opportunity presented by the Sixth Amendment to the Cosmetics Directive (76/768/EEC). ATLA 1995; **23:** 398–409.
6. COLIPA, Draft, 1996.
7. Loprieno N, Guidelines for safety evaluation of cosmetic ingredients in the EC countries. *Food Chem Toxicol* 1992; **30:** 809–15.
8. Commission Directive 97/18/EC of 17th April 1997. *Official Journal of the European Communities* 1 May 1997; L114, 43–4
9. McEwen GM, Cosmetic regulation and safety substantiation in the USA. In: *Proc V World Congress of the International Society of Cosmetic Dermatology, Montecatini, Italy, 26–29 October 1995.*
10. Loprieno N, Bruner LH, Carr GJ et al, Alternatives in cosmetic testing. *Toxicology in Vitro* 1995; **9:** 827–38.

APPENDIX

COMMISSION DIRECTIVE 97/18/EC OF 17TH APRIL 1997

postponing the date after which animal tests are prohibited for ingredients or concentrations of ingredients of cosmetic products

THE COMMISSION OF THE EUROPEAN COMMUNITIES,

Having regard to the Treaty establishing the European Community,

Having regard to Council Directive 76/768/EEC of 27 July 1996 on the approximation of the laws of the Member States relating to cosmetic products,* as last amended by Directive 96/41/EC,† and in particular Article 4(1)(i) thereof,

After consulting the Scientific Committee on Cosmetology,

* OJ No L262, 27.9.1976, p.169
† OJ No L 198, 8.8.1996, p.36

Whereas the main objective of Directive 76/768/EEC is to protect public health; whereas to this end, it is indispensable to carry out certain toxicological tests to evaluate the safety for human health of ingredients and combinations of ingredients used in cosmetic product formulations;

Whereas pursuant to Article 4(1)(i) of Directive 76/768/EEC Member States must ban the placing on the market of cosmetic products containing ingredients or combinations of ingredients tested on animals after 1 January 1998 in order to meet the requirements of the Directive;

Whereas the second sentence of this provision provides that the Commission shall submit draft measures to postpone the date of implementation if there has been insufficient progress in developing satisfactory methods to replace animal testing, and in particular in those cases where alternative methods of testing, despite all reasonable endeavours, have not been scientifically validated as offering an equivalent level of protection for the consumer, taking into account OECD toxicity test guidelines;

Whereas progress has been made in research into alternative methods of testing, in particular in the fields of percutaneous absorption and local risks to the eyes and skin; whereas it has not yet been possible to validate scientifically any alternative testing method; whereas the OECD has not yet adopted pertinent guidelines for toxicity tests in the field of alternative testing methods;

Whereas it is unlikely that the state of the art will change before 1 January 1998; whereas, therefore, the date provided for in Article 4 (1)(i) of Directive 76/768/EEC should be postponed, in compliance with the second sentence of this provision;

Whereas Directive 76/768/EEC provides that the date be postponed for a sufficient period, and in any case for no less than two years; whereas, therefore, it is necessary to stipulate a date later than 1 January 2000; whereas at this stage it is extremely difficult to foresee the date by which certain alternative methods for testing certain ingredients or combinations of ingredients for the presence of certain risks for human health will have been scientifically validated;

Whereas, however, it can be foreseen that alternative methods will progressively become available in regard to percutaneous absorption, photoirritation, eye irritation and skin irritation;

Whereas, likewise, taking into account the provision's objective, scientific reassessment should not be excessively delayed; whereas therefore it is necessary to lay down at this stage a date before which it can be foreseen that no alternative method of testing will have been adequately scientifically validated;

Whereas it is therefore appropriate to postpone the date to [1 June 2000];

Whereas, in these circumstances, it is not possible to lay down a time limit offering the certainty that it will be possible to implement the ban on animal experiments on a specified date; whereas, therefore, the Commission is not in a position to exercise the powers endowed on it by virtue of Article 4(1)(i) of the Directive except in part;

Whereas it is therefore necessary to provide that the Commission shall submit new draft measures under the conditions provided for in this Article;

Whereas everything must be done to ensure that alternative methods to animal experiments are developed, validated and accepted; whereas, pursuant to the provisions of Article 130f(3) of the Treaty and the Fourth Framework Programme for Research, the Commission must take the necessary measures to promote research for the validation of alternative methods to animal experiments in the field of ingredients and combinations of ingredients used in cosmetic product formulations;

Whereas the measures provided for in this Directive are in accordance with the opinion of the Committee on the Adaptation to Technical Progress of the Directive on the Removal of Technical Barriers to Trade in the Cosmetic Products Sector;

HAS ADOPTED THIS DIRECTIVE;

Article 1

The date of 1 January 1998 shall be replaced by 30 June 2000, in the first sentence of Article 4(1)(i) of Directive 76/768/EEC.

Article 2

If there has been insufficient progress in developing satisfactory methods to replace animal testing, and in particular in those cases where alternative methods of testing, despite all reasonable endeavours, have not been scientifically validated as offering an equivalent level of protection for the consumer, taking into account OECD toxicity test guidelines, the Commission shall, by 1 January 2000, submit draft measures to postpone the date referred to in Article 1 for those testing methods, in respect of which there has been insufficient progress in developing alternative methods, in accordance with the procedure laid down in Article 10 of Directive 76/768/EEC. Before submitting such measures, the Commission will consult the Scientific Committee on Cosmetology.

Article 3

1. Member States shall bring into force the laws, regulations and administrative provisions necessary to comply with this Directive no later than 31 December 1997. They shall forthwith inform the Commission thereof.

   When Member States adopt these provisions, these shall contain a reference to this Directive or shall be accompanied by such reference at the time of their official publication. The procedure for such reference shall be adopted by Member States.

2. Member States shall communicate to the Commission the provisions of national law which they adopt in the field covered by this Directive.

Article 4

This Directive shall enter into force on the third day following its publication in the Official Journal of the European Communities.

Article 5

This Directive is addressed to the Member States.

Done at Brussels, 17th April 1997
For the Commission
Ms Emma BONINO
Member of The Commission

EXPLANATORY MEMORANDUM

1. GENERAL CONTEXT

Article 4(1)(i) of Directive 76/768/EEC on cosmetic products as amended by Council Directive 93/35 of 14 June 1993 provides that Member States shall ban the marketing of cosmetic products containing 'ingredients or combinations of ingredients tested on animals after 1 January 1998 in order to meet the requirements of this Directive'.

However, this article specifies that '[i]f there has been insufficient progress in developing satisfactory methods to replace animal testing, and in particular in those cases where alternative methods of testing, despite all reasonable endeavours, have not been scientifically validated as offering an equivalent level of protection for the consumer, taking into account OECD toxicity test guidelines, the Commission shall, by 1 January 1997, submit draft measures to postpone the date of implementation of this provision, for a sufficient period, and in any case for no less than two years, in accordance with the procedure laid down in Article 10. Before submitting such measures, the Commission will consult the Scientific Committee on Cosmetology.'

This is the context of this proposal for a Directive.

The progress made in the development, validation and legal acceptance of alternative methods has been described in the Commission's annual reports presented to the European Parliament and Council, also on the basis of Article 4(1)(i). These are the 1994, 1995 and 1996 reports on the development, validation and legal acceptance of alternative methods to animal experiments in the field of cosmetic products.

2. CONSTRAINTS AND OBJECTIVES

In this connection the Commission has to consider two main objectives:

(a) consumer safety and
(b) the reduction and, wherever possible, elimination of animal suffering.

3. CONSUMER SAFETY

Consumer safety must be the prime consideration. Here it should be noted that the notion of 'cosmetic products' encompasses not only so-called 'decorative' products. such as lipstick or nail varnish, but also articles such as soap, shampoos, toothpaste which are used throughout a lifetime from early childhood on. It is essential that these products should not cause harmful, immediate and visible effects, such as irritation, or long-term, latent effects such as carcinogenicity or teratogenicity.

To evaluate the safety of cosmetic products in this respect, it is necessary to evaluate not only the safety of the finished product but above all that of the ingredients used in its manufacture. It is for the manufacturer to ensure that the ingredients are harmless, in compliance with Article 2 of the Cosmetic Products Directive, according to which cosmetic products '... must not be liable to cause damage to human health when they are applied under normal conditions of use'; manufacturers may also be held liable in the event of damages on the basis of Council Directive 85/374/EEC on liability for defective products.

Pursuant to Council Directive 93/35/EEC of 14 June 1993 amending for the sixth time the basic Cosmetic Products Directive, the manufacturer must, as of 1 January 1995, keep certain information readily accessible to the competent authorities, including 'assessment of the safety for human health of the finished product. To that end the manufacturer shall take into consideration the general toxicological profile of the ingredient, its chemical structure and its level of exposure.'

The Cosmetic Products Directive also includes a series of annexes featuring positive and negative lists of substances. The general principle is that substances may be used freely, unless they are prohibited (Annex II), or subject to certain limitations and conditions (Annex III). There are three exceptions to this general principle; the only colouring agents, preservatives and UV filters authorised are those featuring in positive lists (Annexes IV, VI and VII). A substance can only be included in these lists, which are adapted to technical progress each year by a Commission Directive, if it has been the subject of an opinion delivered by the Scientific Committee on Cosmetology concerning the toxicity for human health. This SCC opinion is delivered on the basis of all the existing scientific data and notably the test results furnished by industry, which may concern sensitisation, mutagenicity, eye irritation, skin irritation, photoirritation, carcinogenicity, teratogenicity, and acute, subchronic and chronic toxicity.

While some 7000 substances are already used in cosmetic products and while for many cosmetic substances new tests are not generally required, it should however be stressed that such tests may sometimes be crucial in reevaluating, on the basis of technical progress and new scientific knowledge, certain substances that have been in use for a very long time.

Hence each year the SCC examines a series of existing substances and on the basis of its opinions the Commission supplements the list of prohibited substances (approximately 400) and substances subject to particular limitations and conditions (approximately 50).

It must also be possible to examine the risks associated with the use of these products in combination. Thus for safety reasons it is not possible to dispense entirely with animal trials, even for substances already in use. Moreover, in the cosmetic products sector as in all other industrial sectors, it would be neither wise nor reasonable to bring innovation to a standstill. Apart from the fact that consumers are quite entitled to seek ever better products, a blanket ban on innovation by outlawing the use of new substances would certainly put numerous European cosmetic product manufacturers out of business, mainly the employment-generating SMEs (Small and Medium Enterprises).

4. REDUCTION AND ELIMINATION OF ANIMAL SUFFERING

Reduction – both by alleviating animal suffering during tests and by reducing the number of tests – and, where possible, elimination of animal suffering is an objective that merits the closest attention and one in respect of which resources should be mobilised at all levels. This objective reflects ethical imperatives concerning respect for life, a deep-seated desire on the part of public opinion, and the aspirations of the European Parliament. It is enshrined in several European instruments including Directive 86/609/EEC on the protection of animals used for experimental and other scientific purposes and Directive 93/35/EEC (the Sixth Amendment to the initial Cosmetic Products Directive).

While consumer safety must be assured, we must also do our utmost to ensure that animal tests are replaced by alternative tests as soon as possible, provided these provide an equivalent level of protection. It is true that animal tests in the cosmetics field account for a mere 0.03% of all animal tests and that all chemical substances already have to be tested in order to provide the toxicity data required under Directive 93/35/EEC. Moreover cosmetic products have been prioritised and there has been a big drive in recent years, notably since the adoption of Directive 93/35/EEC, to promote the development of alternative methods.

These endeavours, as well as progress to date and the outlook for the future, are described in the 1994 and 1995 annual reports on the development, validation and legal acceptance of alternative methods to animal experiments in the field of cosmetic products, already presented by the Commission to the EP and the Council. The 1996 annual report is currently being drafted.

Notably, these reports describe the work done by ECVAM (European Centre for the Validation of Alternative Methods), a unit of the Ispra Joint Research Centre, with an eye to coordinating the validation of alternative methods at Community level, creating a forum for pooling information, and developing, updating and managing a database and promoting dialogue between all interested parties.

ECVAM has organised numerous workshops whose reports have been published and has regular contacts with the OECD, which is developing its work on the drafting and adoption of guidelines on alternative methods.

DG XI has partly funded an EU/HO study to validate methods to substitute the Draize eye irritancy test and an international EU/COLIPA validation study on in vitro phototoxicity. DG XII has also subsidised in vitro alternative methods to pharmaco-toxicological animal tests in the context of the Community research programmes since 1985 (first framework programme), including research into cell cultures for the development of new tests (which are a priority of the fourth framework programme which runs until 1998) for amounts that already exceed 10 million ECUs. Validation of the tests developed under the research programmes is the task of ECVAM at the Joint Research Centre. But it should be noted that no alternative test has yet been validated by the JCR. DG XXIV has recruited a high-level consultant, has funded research work, and participates in meetings between all the partners. The Scientific Committee on Cosmetology, responsible for delivering scientific opinions to DG XXIV on ingredients featuring in the annexes to the Cosmetic Products Directive and on the applicability of alternative methods validated in the process of evaluating the safety of cosmetic products, has held numerous plenary meetings and meetings of its Alternative Methods Subcommittee, sometimes together with European industry. The SCC has prepared a document which is a direct contribution to future validation studies.

The European cosmetics industry has devoted considerable resources to researching and developing in vitro methods. COLIPA (the European Cosmetics, Toiletry and Perfume Association) has also created a Steering Committee on Alternatives to Animal Testing (SCAAT). Work has also been done at international level.

It is important to note that the preparation, validation and acceptance of alternative methods cannot be achieved overnight, despite all the efforts being made. Again, the validation phases – i.e. the complex process by which the pertinence, reliability and reproducibility of a test developed for routine application and legal acceptance are evaluated and monitored – have turned out to be more numerous and complex than initially foreseen, and new phases have had to be fitted in.

Moreover, as in the case of all scientific research, it is well-nigh impossible to guarantee a precise result by a given date, and certain studies, which were thought to be on the verge of completion – such as the EU/HO study on alternatives to the Draize test – turned out to be disappointing as regards the predictability of the risk.

As regards alternative tests on human volunteers, for example in the field of skin irritation, the greatest possible prudence is required; such tests should only be countenanced in the proven absence of real risks.

For all that, progress to date has already made it possible to substantially reduce the number of animals used as well as their suffering, by alleviating pain during animal tests.

5. INTERNATIONAL ASPECTS

Directive 93/35 refers to the OECD.

OECD Guidelines for the Testing of Chemicals and the Principles of Good Laboratory Practice (GLP) are developed in the broader context of the concept of mutual acceptance of data. Both of these instruments for ensuring harmonized data generation and data quality are an integral part of the 1981 OECD Council Decision on the Mutual Acceptance of Data (MAD). In accordance with this decision, OECD's 28 Member Countries agree that data generated in the testing of chemicals in any OECD Member Country, when in accordance with OECD Test Guidelines and Principles of GLP, shall be accepted in any other Member Country for the purpose of assessment and other uses relating to the protection of man and the environment.

The practical consequence of this decision is that data developed in a Member Country under these conditions and submitted for fulfilling regulatory requirements in another Member Country, cannot and will not be refused. Consequently, OECD Test Guidelines are globally accepted as the standard methods for safety testing and as such enhance the validity and international acceptance of test data. Recognizing the significance of OECD Test Guidelines, the European Commission strongly supports work on the development of new test guidelines and the updating of existing ones. In order to avoid the development of EC testing methods as referred to in Annex V to Directive 92/69/EEC leading to any overlap of work with the OECD, the European Commission refrains from the development of EC testing methods and instead adopts OECD Test Guidelines as EC testing methods. In addition, the European Commission financially supports the OECD Test Guidelines Programme with one staff post.

Relations with the OECD are important because the European Union must operate in the broader framework of international trade.

6. RATIONALE FOR A DIRECTIVE

This Directive takes into account the objectives described above.

While progress has been made in research into alternative test methods, notably in the fields of percutaneous absorption and local risks to the eyes and skin, the fact remains that no alternative method has yet been scientifically validated and that the OECD has not yet adopted pertinent guidelines on toxicity tests in the field of alternative testing methods.

The state of the art is unlikely to change before 1 January 1998.

Hence the Directive proposes the postponement of the date mentioned in Article 4(1)(i) of Directive 76/768/EEC, in compliance with the second sentence of that provision, for not less than two years.

Currently it is difficult to predict precisely when certain alternative methods for testing certain ingredients or combinations of ingredients will be scientifically validated. However as it is likely that alternative methods will progressively become available in the field of percutaneous absorption, photoirritation, eye irritation and skin irritation, and whereas, besides, the Commission is mindful of the

objective of Article 4(1)(i), the proposal postpones the deadline to a date before which no alternative method of testing is likely to have been adequately scientifically validated, viz. 1 June 2000. It also stipulates that before 1 January 2000 the Commission shall present draft measures taking into account progress made by that date.

Finally, in the context described above, and also in compliance with the provisions of Article 130f(3) of the Treaty and Fourth Research Framework Programme,* the Commission will take the necessary measures to promote research into and the validation of alternative methods to animal testing in the field of ingredients and combinations of ingredients in cosmetic product formulations.

7. FINISHED COSMETIC PRODUCTS

As regards finished cosmetic products, progress to date suggests that it will generally be possible to evaluate their safety on the basis of available knowledge on the toxicity of their ingredients and their physicochemical properties, using methods which do not involve the use of animals, even if these methods are not liable to be the subject of an OECD guideline dealing only with ingredients and combinations of ingredients.

Hence it will only be necessary to resort to animal testing in rare, exceptional cases, where there are grounds to fear that the toxic effects of the ingredients may be potentiated, notably when skin penetration of the ingredients is facilitated by the vehicle used or when such effects result from the interaction of the ingredients. The SCC has emphasised this fact in its Guidelines on the use of alternative methods to animal studies in the safety evaluation of cosmetic ingredients or combinations of ingredients of 20 December 1996.

Certain cosmetics firms already very often use methods which do not involve the use of animals to test their finished products.

COLIPA (the European Cosmetic, Toiletry and Perfumery Association) has announced that it could progressively establish a voluntary ban on animal testing for finished cosmetic products –

---

* Decision No 111°/94 of the European Parliament and Council of 26 April 1994 concerning the Fourth Framework Programme of the European Community activities in the field of research and technological development and demonstration (1994–1998) OJ No L 126, 18.5.94.

except in the exceptional cases referred to above – for the entire European cosmetics industry, and that it would be willing to organise technology transfer in this respect. COLIPA would ensure the widest possible dissemination of findings in this area and promote training in European companies and laboratories; this training could be coordinated by the Commission's services, and in particular by ECVAM. The Commission, in particular will promote the dissemination of methods not involving these animals among the SMEs. It could also endeavour to promote such measures at international level.

In the context described above, the Commission will in the coming months present a proposal for a European Parliament and Council Directive amending Article 4(1)(i) in order to address, in a legally appropriate text, the ban on animal testing in regard to finished cosmetic products – banning

exceptional cases – as of 1.1.1998, in compliance with the requirements of Directive 76/768/EEC. These exceptional cases must be foreseen to take into account particular health requirements and the international obligations deriving from the GATT/TBT rules.

Since the Directive will be based on Article 100a, this Commission proposal requires the approval of the European Parliament and the Council.

8. CONSULTATIONS

The SCC was consulted as regards the postponement of the date of the ban because of the non-availability of alternative methods to animal tests in evaluating the safety of ingredients and combinations of ingredients at its plenary meeting of 2 October 1996.

PART THREE

CUTANEOUS ABSORPTION AND COSMETOLOGY

6

Cosmetic percutaneous absorption

Ronald C Wester, Howard I Maibach

INTRODUCTION

Percutaneous absorption is a complex biological process. The skin is a multilayered biomembrane that has certain absorption characteristics. If the skin were a simple membrane, absorption parameters could easily be measured, and these would be fairly constant provided there was no change in the chemistry of the membrane. However, skin is a dynamic, living tissue, and as such its absorption parameters are susceptible to constant change. Many factors and skin conditions can rapidly change the absorption parameters. Additionally, skin is a living tissue and it will change through its own growth patterns, and this change will also be influenced by many factors. When dealing with percutaneous absorption, the skin should not be regarded as an inert membrane. Instead, it should be viewed as a dynamic, living biomembrane with unique properties. In this chapter we review some of the more relevant factors that influence the percutaneous absorption of cosmetics.

METHODS FOR MEASURING PERCUTANEOUS ABSORPTION

Ideally, information on the dermal absorption of a particular compound in humans is best obtained through studies performed in humans. However, since many compounds are potentially toxic, or it is not convenient to test them in humans, studies can be performed using other techniques. Percutaneous absorption has been measured by two major methods:

- in vitro diffusion cell techniques;
- in vivo determinations, which generally use radiolabeled compounds.

To insure their applicability to the clinical situation, the relevance of studies using these techniques must constantly be challenged.

In vitro techniques involve placing a piece of human skin in a diffusion chamber containing a physiological receptor fluid. The compound under investigation is applied to one side of the skin. The compound is then assayed at regular intervals on the other side of the skin. The skin may be intact, dermatomed or separated into epidermis and dermis; however, separating skin with heat will destroy skin viability. The advantages of the in vitro techniques are that they are easy to use and results are obtained quickly. Their major disadvantage is the limited relevance of the conditions present in the in vitro system to those found in humans.

Percutaneous absorption in vivo is usually

determined by the indirect method of measuring radioactivity in excreta following the topical application of a labeled compound. In human studies, the plasma level of a topically applied compound is usually extremely low – often below assay detection. For this reason, a tracer methodology is used. After the topical application of the radiolabeled compound, the total amount of radioactivity excreted in urine or in urine plus feces is determined. The amount of radioactivity retained in the body or excreted by a route not assayed (CO_2) is corrected for by determining the amount of radioactivity excreted following parenteral administration. Absorption represents the amount of radioactivity excreted, expressed as a percentage of the applied dose. Percutaneous absorption can also be assessed by the ratio of the areas under the concentration-versus-time curves following the topical and intravenous administration of a radiolabeled component. The metabolism of a compound by the skin as it is absorbed will not be detected by this method. A biological response, such as vasoconstriction after the topical application of steroids, has also been used to assess dermal absorption in vivo.

Percutaneous absorption has been defined as a series of steps.[1] Table 6.1 lists our current knowledge of these steps. Step 1 is the vehicle containing the chemical(s) of interest. There is a partitioning of the chemical from the vehicle to the skin. This initiates a series of absorption and excretion kinetics that are influenced by a variety of factors such as regional and individual variation. These factors moderate the absorption and excretion kinetics.

Once a chemical has been absorbed through the skin, it enters the systemic circulation of the body. Here the pharmacokinetics of the chemical define body interactions. This is illustrated for [14C]hydroquinone in vivo in man, where plasma radioactivity was measured ipsilaterally (next to the dose site) and contralaterally (in the opposite arm)

Table 6.1 Steps to percutaneous absorption

1. Vehicle
2. Absorption kinetics
   (a) Skin site of application
   (b) Individual variation
   (c) Skin condition
   (d) Occlusion
   (e) Drug concentration and surface area
   (f) Multiple dose application
   (g) Time
3. Excretion kinetics
4. Effective cellular and tissue distribution
5. Substantivity (nonpenetrating surface adsorption)
6. Wash and rub resistance/decontamination
7. Volatility
8. Binding
9. Anatomical pathways
10. Cutaneous metabolism
11. QSAR
12. Decontamination
13. Dose accountability
14. Models

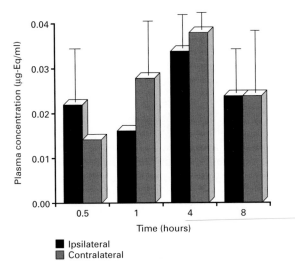

Figure 6.1 Plasma radioactivity is detected in human volunteers 30 minutes after [14C]hydroquinone is applied to skin. 'Ipsilateral' is blood taken near the site of dosing, and 'contralateral' is from the other arm. Hydroquinone is rapidly absorbed into and through human skin.

after a topical dose. In 30 minutes following the dose, the hydroquinone has been absorbed through skin and reached a near-peak plasma concentration (Figure 6.1).

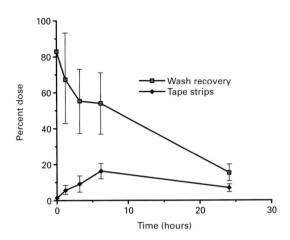

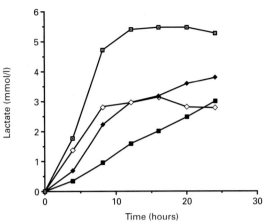

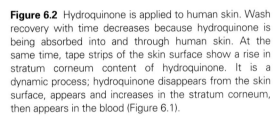

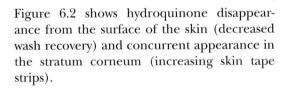

Figure 6.2 Hydroquinone is applied to human skin. Wash recovery with time decreases because hydroquinone is being absorbed into and through human skin. At the same time, tape strips of the skin surface show a rise in stratum corneum content of hydroquinone. It is a dynamic process; hydroquinone disappears from the skin surface, appears and increases in the stratum corneum, then appears in the blood (Figure 6.1).

Figure 6.3 Human skin in vitro will show viability by producing lactate from glucose circulating in the receptor fluid. Thus human skin viability in vitro can be monitored. The above is illustrated by skin from four different individuals.

Figure 6.2 shows hydroquinone disappearance from the surface of the skin (decreased wash recovery) and concurrent appearance in the stratum corneum (increasing skin tape strips).

SKIN VIABILITY

The skin of a living person is viable. When this skin is removed from the body for scientific research (tummy tuck, cadaver skin) the question of skin viability arises. An example would be skin used for in vitro percutaneous absorption. Viable skin in vitro is able to utilize glucose and produce lactate (anaerobic energy metabolism). Figure 6.3 illustrates this for four human skin sources shortly after removal from the body, and this viability can be maintained in the in vitro diffusion cell system for 24 hours. However, this requires near-

immediate access to human skin at the time of death, maintenance of skin viability with refrigeration (*not* freezing) and properly balanced physiological fluids. Storage time will decrease skin viability, heat treatment for epidermis and dermis separation will greatly decrease skin viability, and freezing for storage will completely destroy skin viability.

DISEASED SKIN

The assumption has been that percutaneous absorption through diseased or damaged skin is enhanced, and that the skin's ability to protect against intrusion by chemicals is impaired. The picture of skin flood gates opening and chemicals pouring in is certainly not warranted (except perhaps in severe burn cases). The data suggest that diseased skin can retain barrier properties, and that differences will exist for different drugs and for different disease conditions. In psoriasis, there are definite formulation effects, and treatment (e.g. salicylic acid scrub) will probably affect drug delivery into the skin. However, even for a compound such as hydrocortisone where skin absorption is low for diseased and damaged skin, enhanced absorption will occur in severe conditions. For more potent corticosteroids, the risk of systemic side-effects such as adrenal suppression remains real. Finally, it should be pointed out that the total data package for percutaneous absorption in diseased human skin is limited. Certainly, more research in this area is warranted.[2]

COSMECEUTICS OF VITAMIN E

The biological activities of vitamin E in cosmetics are supported by several studies of its percutaneous absorption. In data obtained in vitro on rat skin six hours after the application of a 5% vitamin E alcoholic solution, 38.6% of the applied dose was recovered in the viable epidermis and dermis; the amount detected in the horny layer was 7.12%, and the residual fraction persisting on the surface of the integument represented 54.3% of the applied dose. Both the alcohol and acetate forms of vitamin E are readily absorbed through the human scalp, and within 6–24 hours after treatment they concentrate in the dermis. These results substantiate the claim that vitamin E can be used as an active ingredient in cosmetology with the possibility of efficacy in the deeper structures of the skin (see Chapter 7).

Several patients have developed allergic contact dermatitis from the use of so-called vitamin E soaps and hand lotions. There is a mistaken notion that vitamin E can 'toughen' and 'soften' and have an 'emollient' effect on the skin of the hands. However, there is no evidence that topical applications of vitamin E achieve any of these miracles. It is of interest that, although the systemic administration of vitamin E practically never produces any allergic reaction, various topical preparations containing vitamin E have produced allergic sensitivity.[3] And now in the newsprint comes word that vitamin E slows the development of

atherosclerosis by preventing the oxidation of LDL cholesterol – the oxidized form more likely to form plaque. This brings the delivery of vitamin E back to skin. Drugs and hormone supplements are delivered to the internal human system from transdermal patches and topical cream or gel formulations. Then, why not vitamin E? A study was done where radioactive vitamin E acetate, in cream formulations differing only in slight variations in pH, was applied to human skin in vitro, and the absorption into and through skin was determined.

Table 6.2 summarizes the in vitro percutaneous absorption of vitamin E acetate into and through human skin. Each formulation was tested in four different human skin sources. The percent dose absorbed for a 24-hour dosing period is given for receptor fluid accumulation (absorbed), skin content, and surface wash (soap-and-water wash recovery after the 24-hour dosing period).

Totals of $0.63 \pm 0.45\%$ and $0.78 \pm 0.87\%$ were absorbed for formulations A and B respectively. Skin contents were $1.56 \pm 1.69\%$ for the two formulations. Thus both formulations were able to deliver vitamin E acetate into and through human skin, but statistically (paired *t*-test) there was no difference in

Table 6.2 In vitro percutaneous absorption of vitamin E acetate into and through human skin			
	Percent dose absorbed		
	Receptor fluid	Skin content	Surface wash
Formula A:			
Skin source 1	0.34	0.55	74.9
Skin source 2	0.39	0.66	75.6
Skin source 3	0.47	4.08	89.1
Skin source 4	1.30	0.96	110.0
Mean ± SD	0.63 ± 0.45[a]	1.56 ± 1.69[b]	87.4 ± 16.4
Formula B:			
Skin source 1	0.24	0.38	—
Skin source 2	0.40	0.64	107.1
Skin source 3	0.41	4.80	98.1
Skin source 4	2.09	1.16	106.2
Mean ± SD	0.78 ± 0.87[a]	1.74 ± 2.06[b]	103.8 ± 5.0

[a] $p = 0.53$ (non-significant; paired *t*-test).
[b] $p = 0.42$ (non-significant; paired *t*-test).

vitamin E acetate absorption between the two formulations. The majority of the vitamin E acetate was recovered in the soap-and-water skin surface wash.

There was individual variation in the skin absorption of vitamin E acetate between human skin sources. Note in Table 6.2 the consistency of low or high absorption and low or high skin content over the two formulations. This accounted for most of the variation that exists for each calculated mean. However, a careful examination of the individual values in Table 6.2 shows consistency within individuals. Analysis of variance (ANOVA) for individual variation showed statistical significance for receptor fluid ($p = 0.02$) and skin content ($p = 0.000$) (Figure 6.1); therefore, when comparing treatments for in vitro percutaneous absorption, it is recommended that each treatment be a part of each skin source.

This study shows that vitamin E acetate can be delivered into human skin and into the systemic circulation with a simple topical formulation. Clinically, both the skin and systemic systems should benefit. Individual variation occurs with most clinical treatments, and skin delivery of vitamin E acetate is no exception. Skin has metabolic properties, and it is not known if skin delivery of vitamin E acetate would be any different from the vitamin in food or in a pill. This needs to be determined. However, it is an intriguing thought that a simple topical formulation might benefit several human organ systems.

In a related study, Podda et al[4] showed that the antioxidant α-lipoic acid is absorbed into the skin, and metabolically converted to the even more potent antioxidant dihydrolipoic acid. This could potentiate skin antioxidant protection.

PERCUTANEOUS ABSORPTION AND PRODUCT DEVELOPMENT

Drugs are applied to skin to test local skin conditions (and for transdermal delivery and systemic effect). Drug efficacy is balanced against toxicity. This is illustrated for a controlled release of benzoyl peroxide, which retains efficacy but lessens irritancy (toxicity) in acne treatment.[5] Skin absorption of benzoyl peroxide from a topical lotion containing freely dispersed drug was compared with that from the same lotion in which the drug was entrapped in a controlled-release styrene–divinylbenzene polymer system. In an in vitro diffusion system, statistically significant ($p = 0.01$) differences were found in the content of benzoyl peroxide in excised human skin and in percutaneous absorption (Table 6.3). In vivo, significantly ($p = 0.002$) less benzoyl peroxide was absorbed through Rhesus monkey skin from the polymeric system. This controlled release of benzoyl peroxide to skin can alter the dose relation that exists between efficacy and skin irritation. Corresponding studies showed reduced skin irritation in cumulative irritancy studies in rabbits and human beings, whereas in vivo human antimicrobial efficacy studies showed that application of the formulations containing entrapped benzoyl peroxide significantly reduced counts of *Propionibacterium acnes* ($p < 0.001$) and aerobic bacteria ($p < 0.001$) and the free fatty acid/triglyceride ratio in skin lipids. These findings support the hypothesis that, at least for this drug, controlled topical delivery can enhance safety without sacrificing efficacy.

COSMETIC CHEMICALS, PERCUTANEOUS ABSORPTION AND TOXICITY

The potential toxicity of cosmetics has in the past been dismissed as an event unlikely to occur. The argument was put forth that cosmetics did not contain ingredients that could prove harmful to the body. The argument went further to say that, because cosmetics were applied to skin with its 'barrier' properties, the likelihood that a chemical would

Table 6.3 In vitro percutaneous absorption of benzoyl peroxide in human skin

| Parameter[a] | Percent applied dose[b] | | Statistical comparison[c] |
	Formulation A (freely dispersed)	Formulation B (entrapped)	
Skin	6.1 ± 4.4	1.4 ± 0.8	$p = 0.01$
Epidermis	5.2 ± 4.1	1.1 ± 0.7	$p = 0.02$
Dermis	0.4 ± 0.4	0.1 ± 0.1	$p > 0.05$ (NS)
Skin edge[d]	0.6 ± 0.7	0.2 ± 0.3	$p > 0.05$ (NS)
Receptor fluid	17.1 ± 15.7	3.5 ± 3.4	$p < 0.05$
Surface wash	85.6 ± 29.0	83.2 ± 19.9	$p > 0.05$ (NS)
Total	108.9 ± 22.3	88.1 ± 18.4	$p > 0.05$

[a] $N = 10$ for each parameter.
[b] Data presented as mean ± SD.
[c] Student's *t*-test. NS, Not statistically significant.
[d] Edge where system is clamped together.

become systemically available was remote. The argument was proven false when carcinogens were shown to be present in cosmetics, and subsequent studies showed that these carcinogenic chemicals could be percutaneously absorbed.[6]

N-Nitrosodiethanolamine (NDELA) is an impurity that was found in several cosmetic products. It appears to be formed by a reaction between an amine such as diethanolamine or triethanolamine and a nitrosating agent. In rat feeding tests, NDELA was shown to cause liver cancer. Syrian hamsters injected with NDELA developed liver and skin cancer. Percutaneous absorption studies showed that NDELA readily penetrated swine and monkey skin. When applied in an acetone vehicle or commercial lotion, it readily penetrated excised human skin. In a human study with contaminated facial makeup, NDELA was detected in the subjects' urine. The information thus showed the presence of a carcinogen in cosmetics that would become systemically available when the cosmetic was applied to skin. Analytic procedures

are available to detect nitrosamines, and every effort should be made in the quality assurance of cosmetics to see that these compounds are not present in the final product.

1,4-Dioxane is an impurity that was detected in some cosmetic raw materials. It can be formed in the synthesis of ethylene glycol polymers, and, unless removed by vacuum distillation, will subsequently be detected in commercial products. 1,4-Dioxane is also a carcinogen. Determining its percutaneous absorption has been difficult because the chemical is volatile. With in vitro penetration using diffusion cells and human skin, the absorption was increased 10 times when the application side of the skin was occluded. Dioxane dissolved in a popular lotion and applied to waxed paper disks had evaporated by 90% in 15 minutes, and there was no trace of dioxane present within 24 hours.

Coal tar derivatives used in hair dyes have been implicated as potential carcinogens. Chemicals such as 4-methoxy-1,3-phenylenediamine, 2,4-toluenediamine, 2-nitro-1,4-phenylenediamine, and 4-amino-2-nitrophenol have been shown to cause cancer in animals, and some data on skin absorption have been generated for each of these chemicals. To assess the potential risk of these chemicals, it is necessary to have the best estimate of the percutaneous absorption, preferably in humans and under normal-use conditions. This was done using radiolabeled 2,4-diaminoansole (DAA) in Miss Clairol Creme Formula #52, black azure; using radiolabeled *p*-phenylenediamine (PPD) in Nice n Easy, blue black; and using radiolabeled HC blue #1 in Loving Care Lotion #795, darkest brown. The study was done in human subjects, and, most importantly, procedural instructions specific for each hair color product were followed. The percutaneous absorption, expressed as percentage of applied dose, was 0.015 for DAA, 0.14 for PPD and 0.09 for HC blue #1. These are reliable numbers from which the potential risk to humans can be assessed. In addition, the same dyes and procedures were used to dye the hair on Rhesus monkey scalps. The percutaneous absorption in the Rhesus was 0.02 for DAA, 0.14 for PPD and 0.12 for HC blue #1. The Rhesus monkey is therefore a reliable animal model for percutaneous absorption relevant to humans.

Table 6.4 shows the relationship between percutaneous absorption and erythema for several oils used in cosmetics. The authors attempted to correlate absorbability with erythema. The most absorbed oil, isopropyl myristate, produced the most erythema. The lowest absorbing oil, 2-hexyldecanoxyoctane, produced the least erythema. Absorbability and erythema for the other oils did not correlate.[7] The lesson to remember with percutaneous toxicity is that a toxic response required both an inherent toxicity in the chemical and percutaneous absorption of the chemical. The degree of toxicity will depend on the contributions of both criteria.

In the Rhesus monkey, the percutaneous absorption of safrole, a hepatocarcinogen, was 6.3% of applied dose. When the site of application was occluded, the percutaneous absorption doubled to 13.3% Occlusion is a covering of the application site, either intentionally as with bandaging or unintentionally as by putting on clothing after applying a cosmetic. The percutaneous absorption of cinnamic anthranilate was 26.1% of the applied dose, and this increased to 39.0% when the site of application was occluded. The percutaneous absorption of cinnamic alcohol with occlusion was 62.7%, and that of cinnamic acid with occlusion was 83.9% of the applied dose. Cinnamic acid and cinnamic aldehyde are agents that elicit contact urticaria,[8] and cinnamic aldehyde is positive for both Draize and maximization methods.[9,10]

We have thus learned that common cosmetic ingredients can readily penetrate skin and become systemically available. If the cosmetic chemical has inherent toxicity then that chemical will get into the body of a user and exert a toxic effect.

PERCUTANEOUS ABSORPTION AND TOXICITY TESTING

The development of topical drug products requires testing for skin toxicology reactions. A variety of patch test systems are available with which chemicals are applied to skin. The purpose of this study was to determine the skin absorption of *p*-phenylenediamine (PPDA) from a variety of such systems.

Table 6.4 Relationship of percutaneous absorption and erythema for several oils used in cosmetics

Absorbability (greatest to least)	Erythema
Isopropyl myristate	++
Glycerol tri(oleate)	−
n-Octadecane	±
Decanoxydecane	+
2-Hexyldecanoxyoctane	−

Table 6.5 Percutaneous absorption of PPDA from patch test systems

	Total load in chamber (mg)	Concentration in chamber (mg/mm²)	Absorption	
			Percent[a]	Total (mg)
Hill top chamber	40	2	53.4 ± 20.6	21.4
Teflon (control)	16	2	48.6 ± 9.3	7.8
Small Finn chamber	16	2	29.8 ± 9.0	4.8
Large Finn chamber	24	2	23.1 ± 7.3	5.5
AL-test chamber	20	2	8.0 ± 0.8	1.6
Small Finn chamber with paper disc insert	16	2	34.1 ± 19.8	5.5

[a] Each value is the mean ± standard deviation for three guinea pigs.

[^{14}C]PPDA (1% pet. UDP) was placed in a variety of patch test systems at a concentration normalized to equal surface area (2 mg/mm²). Skin absorption was determined in the guinea pig by urinary excretion of ^{14}C. There was a sixfold difference in the range of skin absorption $(p < 0.02)$. In decreasing order, the percentage skin absorption from the systems were Hill Top chamber (53.4 ± 20.6) > Teflon control patch (48.6 ± 9.3) > small Finn chamber with paper disc insert (34.1 ± 19.8) > small Finn chamber (29.8 ± 9.0) > large Finn chamber (23.1 ± 7.3) > AL-test chamber (8.0 ± 0.8). Thus the choice of patch system could produce a false negative error if the system inhibits skin absorption, with a subsequent skin toxicology reaction (Table 6.5).[1]

CONCLUSIONS

In the interaction of a cosmetic chemical with the skin, percutaneous absorption (bioavailability) is the initiator of subsequent biological events. The interrelationships of dose and response in dermal absorption are defined in terms of accountability, concentration, surface area, frequency of application, and time of exposure. *Accountability* is an accounting of the mass balance for each dose applied to skin. *Concentration* is the amount of applied chemical per unit skin surface area. *Surface area* is usually defined in square centimeters of skin application of exposure. *Frequency* is either intermittent or chronic exposure. 'Intermittent' can be one, two, and so on exposures per day. Chronic application is usually repetitive and on a continuing daily basis. *Time of exposure* is the duration of the period during which the skin is in contact with the chemical before washing. Such factors define skin exposure to a chemical and subsequent percutaneous absorption.

REFERENCES

1. Wester RC, Maibach HI, Percutaneous absorption of drugs. *Clin Phamacokin* 1992; **23**: 253–66.
2. Wester RC, Maibach HI, Percutaneous absorption in diseased skin. In: *Topical Corticosteroids* (Surber C, Maibach HI, eds). Basel: Karger, 1991:128–41.
3. Fisher AA, Contact dermatitis in medical and surgical personnel. In: *Occupational and Industrial Dermatology* (Maibach H, Gellin G, eds). Chicago: Year Book Medical Publishers, 1982:219–28.
4. Podda M, Rallis M, Traber MG et al, Kinetic study of cutaneous and subcutaneous distribution following topical application of [7,8-^{14}C]-*rac-*

α-lipoic acid onto hairless mice. *Biochem Pharmacol* 1996; **52:** 6227–33.

5. Wester RC, Patel RT, Nacht S et al, Controlled release of benzyl peroxide from a porous microsphere polymeric system can reduce topical irritancy. *J Am Acad Dermatol* 1991; **24:** 720–6.

6. Wester RC, Maibach H, Comparative percutaneous absorption. In: *Neonatal Skin: Structure and Function* (Maibach HI, Boisits EK, eds). New York: Marcel Dekker, 1982:137–47.

7. Suzuki M, Asaba K, Komatsu H, Mockizuki M, Autoradiographic study on percutaneous absorption of several oils useful for cosmetics. *J Soc Cosmet Chem* 1978; **29:** 265–71.

8. von Krogh G, Maibach HI, The contact urticaria syndrome. In: *Dermatotoxicology* (Marzulli FN, Maibach HI, eds). Washington, DC: Hemisphere, 1983:301–22.

9. Marzulli FN, Maibach HI, Contact allergy: predictive testing in humans. In: *Dermatotoxicology* (Marzulli FN, Maibach HI, eds). Washington, DC: Hemisphere, 1983:279–99.

10. Marzulli FN, Maibach HI, Allergic contact dermatitis. In: *Dermatotoxicology* Marzulli FN, Maibach HI, eds). Washington, DC: Taylor & Francis, 1996:143–6.

11. Kim OH, Wester RC, McMaster JA et al, Skin absorption from patch test systems. *Contact Dermatitis* 1987; **17:** 178–80.

7

Percutaneous penetration and diffusion of cosmetic ingredients: Implications for safety and efficacy

Jean-Paul L Marty

INTRODUCTION

The skin is a remarkable membrane, maintaining the body fluids and preventing the passage of foreign compounds into the circulation. For decades it was considered as an impenetrable barrier for topically applied chemicals. In fact, compared with most tissues, the skin surface is only slightly permeable. Nearly all substances can penetrate the intact stratum corneum to some degree, and are then able to diffuse into the viable epidermis and the dermis, and finally to enter the blood or lymphatic vessels, i.e. to be absorbed. The degree of absorption will depend on the physico-chemical properties of the substance and on the composition of the vehicle. Generally, the faster and greater penetrating compounds are relatively non-polar small molecules.

In Europe the most recent definition of a cosmetic product was published in the Sixth Amendment (93/35/CEE of 14 June 1993) of the European Directive 76/768/CEE (published 27 July 1976):

> A cosmetic product means any substance or preparation intended to be placed in contact with the various external parts of the human body (epidermis, hair system, nails, lips and external genital organs) or

> with the teeth and the mucous membranes of the oral cavity with a view exclusively or principally to cleaning them, perfuming them, changing their appearance and/or correcting body odours and/or protecting them and/or to keep them in good condition.

This definition specifies the objective of a cosmetic product, and does not restrict the functions of cosmetics to cleansing and make-up products. Annex 1 to the Directive gives a list of product categories satisfying the above definition, for example, 'skin-whitening products' and 'anti-wrinkle products'. If one accepts that cosmetics act on the tegument and are able to exhibit some pharmacological or physiological activities then such effects are a direct consequence of the percutaneous penetration of the active ingredients to a specific pharmacological target. One can reasonably assume that the active components are able to penetrate the skin more or less deeply to obtain a biological response.

So, when any cosmetic product is applied on the surface of the skin, all the components are theoretically able to penetrate the skin layers – at least in small amounts. The availability of any ingredient for the skin and its degree of penetration can induce a biological effect that can be beneficial or not (i.e. toxic – locally, and systematically if it is absorbed).

In this chapter cosmetics are considered in the wide meaning of the term, including cosmetics for medical use, which are, depending on locality, considered to be real cosmetics, quasi-drugs or over-the-counter (OTC) products. Differences between drugs and cosmetics are basically due to the fact that different countries give different legal definitions. Finally, the same product (e.g. an antiperspirant) may be classified as a cosmetic in the European Union (EU), a drug in the USA and a quasi-drug in Japan. The distinction between cosmetics and drugs is increasingly important. On the one hand, classification as a drug may exempt a product from local luxury taxes and permit trade claims. On the other hand, however, drug distribution may be limited and premarket clearance difficult because of registration procedures and the corresponding delays. So, understanding how different countries distinguish between cosmetics and drugs is significant. We shall discuss here, how percutaneous penetration can justify the activity and safety of active ingredients. The objective of these studies is to give a scientific demonstration of the activity desired by consumers and to estimate risk factors.

A TOOLBOX FOR THE DEMONSTRATION OF COSMETIC EFFICACY

Advertising efficacy is extremely important for marketing cosmetics. One of the principles of the Federal Trade Commission in the USA is that a claim that cannot be substantiated by appropriate data or information is deceptive. The same concept is developed in the EU through Article 7bis.1g of the Sixth Amendment of the European Directive, where 'proof of the effect claimed for the cosmetic product, where justified by the nature of the effect or product' *should be substantiated.*

So, in order to satisfy any check by the competent national authorities, each manufacturer, importer or organization responsible for the marketing of a cosmetic product should be able to keep and show substantiation of any effects claimed. Of course, too much claim substantiation can be harmful, because it could push a cosmetic product over into the drug category. Such a product would be subject to health authority regulation. This alternative – to declare it as a drug product and get approval – is a priori difficult when a product is not intended to treat a disease but just to improve physiology.

Claims on skin moisturization were the first to appear, some 20 years ago. Many products have focused on dry skin and its relation with aging, and it has been accepted that elasticity, smoothness and suppleness of the horny layer are closely related to its water content. A dry skin is inflexible and inelastic, so small damages like wrinkles or fissures appear. Reliable non-invasive techniques like electrical capacitance and impedance, infrared spectroscopy, water diffusion measurement, extensometry, laser or mechanical profilometry, nuclear magnetic resonance, confocal microscopy, and scanning electron microscopy have been suggested for measuring the efficacy of moisturizing products. Such objective methods are needed to characterize the skin properties – most of them are currently essential instruments present in the toolbox of the dermopharmacologist and cosmetologist.

The best way to objectively substantiate a cosmetic claim is to associate clinical observations, self-evaluation by the consumer and/or instrumental measurements for quantifying the phenomenon under investigation. Thus, according to the nature of the cosmetic product, the evaluation can be made after short-term use (e.g. facial make-up, fragrances) or long-term use (e.g. skin care products). The combination of the results from subjective evaluation (in a controlled study, the same person can be evaluated for how he or she feels before and after using a product) and objective measurements should provide a more effective substantiation of claims than each alone. The physiological or morphological modifications related to cosmetic activity are, by nature, of a relatively low degree – in particular, of a lower degree than those found in pathological conditions. So, interpretation of the results in terms of cosmetic properties is difficult, and the combination of several techniques of evaluation is really useful.

Industry has concentrated its efforts during the last decade on utilizing modern technology and instrumentation for increasing knowledge of skin physiology and for substantiating at least some of the claims and understanding better how cosmetic products affect the skin. Obtaining scientific data to prove claims has given rise to the enormous development of skin bioengineering.

As an example, products that exhibit real activity on the viable epidermal cells or on the dermal fibroblasts are, by definition, able to penetrate and diffuse through the whole skin to reach their target(s). Many active ingredients readily penetrate the skin, and so, when investigating products containing such ingredients, it is necessary to measure percutaneous penetration and absorption in order to obtain pharmacokinetic proof of their pharmacological efficiency and parallel safety. Under these circumstances, methodologies used to study the percutaneous absorption of chemicals are part of the toolbox of dermopharmacologists.

SAFETY AND EFFICACY OF COSMETICS

Although a substance is not a priori defined as a drug or a cosmetic, the choice of active ingredients is relatively limited because they must satisfy rather limited criteria:

- to exhibit a very large safety margin under normal and even exaggerated conditions of use, with neither cutaneous side-effects nor systemic effects;
- to act only on the site of application, i.e. on the skin surface or in viable malpighian epi-

dermis and/or on the dermis and hypodermis, and on the hair, sebaceous glands and sweat glands;
- to constitute neither a limitation nor a risk for subsequent therapy.

The question is to demonstrate the activity or efficiency of the product and to evaluate the associated safety. Furthermore, it is important to consider whether there is a risk of the ingredient being ingested (e.g. lipstick), inhaled (powders or aerosols) or absorbed through the skin. Depending on the route of administration, the amount absorbed and the rate of absorption will be very different, and will have to be evaluated for safety assessment. We shall limit our discussion of absorption here to the problems that occur with the percutaneous route.

COSMETIC TOXICITY AND PERCUTANEOUS ABSORPTION

When a cosmetic product is applied to the skin, some penetrates into and diffuses within the skin layers and is absorbed, while some is lost by evaporation or removed by washing and by contact with clothes and the environment. The adverse reactions that one can expect are local, and arise at the application site (irritation, sensitization, phototoxicity and photosensitization) or systemic, appearing at other sites in the body than the skin. Such effects are undesirable or harmful, and in cosmetology are considered toxicological effects.

If a chemical is absorbed through the skin and reaches the general circulation, the damage that may occur is governed by the same principles that are valid in toxicology for all routes of administration. Loomis[1] has emphasized the two basic toxicological principles regulating the access to the receptor systems that are most applicable to the occurrence of systemic toxicity:

1. The rate of percutaneous absorption must be greater than the rate of inactivation

and/or excretion, thereby leading to an accumulation of the agent and/or its metabolites at the receptor site or target organ.

2. The toxicological potency must be sufficient that the total amount of agent at the receptor site reaches the toxicological threshold.

Thus knowledge of the pharmacokinetic parameters – absorption, distribution (target organs), metabolism and excretion of a compound – is relevant for evaluating its toxicological potential when applied on the skin. If the rate of elimination is less than the rate of absorption, the chemical will accumulate in the body. In contrast, if elimination is faster than absorption, the amount of material in the body will decrease rapidly as the rate of output is high. The intermediate situation when the rates of absorption and elimination are equal will lead to a constant level of chemical in the organism.

The skin is only a special site of exposure, and the systemic toxicity that would occur should be the same after exposure to any route of administration unless the epidermal and dermal tissues confer especially toxic properties to a compound,[1] because of either a specific metabolism (first-pass effect) or a lack of inactivation during diffusion. The metabolic activity of the skin is considered less important (2–6%) than that of the liver, but nevertheless the skin possesses a variety of enzymes involved in oxidation, reduction, hydrolytic or conjugation reactions.[2] So the skin is able to metabolize compounds, and may exert a first-pass metabolic effect towards topically applied cosmetic ingredients during their penetration, especially since the diffusion process is slow. Such an effect will be important for systemic and local toxicity if the metabolite thus formed is present in considerable amounts and if it is not produced in any other organs in the body.

The lack of skin metabolism has been reported as being responsible for the difference in toxicity that exists for hexachlorophene between topical and oral administration.[3] Hexachlorophene when ingested is metabolized and detoxified intensively by the liver. In contrast, it does not appear to be biotransformed in the skin, and is delivered unchanged to the general circulation. Under these conditions, the systemic toxicity of a compound can be more important via the transdermal route than via the oral one when its hepatic first-pass metabolism is very high.

Although, in general, the influence of skin metabolism on systemic toxicity is weak, biotransformations of chemicals within the skin are of interest for local toxicology studies. Metabolites can react with cellular components and bind to macromolecules, inducing irritation and/or sensitization reactions – even carcinogenesis. The latter is clearly demonstrated with polycyclic aromatic hydrocarbons, for which metabolic activation is the first step towards induction of skin cancers.[2] It may be possible to develop antimetabolic agents that could be co-administered with a potential irritant or allergen to inhibit these biotransformations and to decrease statistically the risk of local side-effects.

For a new ingredient intended for use in cosmetic formulations, classical safety evaluation during development is focused on assessing its local toxicology (on skin, eyes and mucous membranes). Ideally, toxicological determinations should be performed with the material applied on intact or abraded skin. Then, according to the results obtained, systemic toxicological studies are undertaken. Therefore skin pharmacokinetics is of interest in both local and systemic toxicological studies. The distribution and rate of penetration of the applied material in the skin allows one to define its substantivity and/or accumulation in particular areas of the tegument. Absorption, reflected by blood levels or amounts excreted, allows one to compare the dermal route with other routes of administration (oral and parenteral). If these pharmacokinetic data are documented by the ingredient manufacturer, the user can easily define with a single bioavailability study the potential effect of a formulation on the release and relative bioavailability of the active ingredient(s) and evaluate the toxicity of the final product.

It has been clearly demonstrated that the formulation of a dermatological preparation can appreciably affect the penetration of the active component by changing its release rate and bioavailability and/or by modifying some aspects of skin structure.[4] There are a large number of possible cosmetic products (in the form of creams, lotions, sticks, foams, shampoos, and so on), formulated from a great number of raw materials (more than 4000 ingredients are listed in the Cosmetic, Toiletry and Fragrance Association Dictionary and in the Inventory of Ingredients of the European Union), so a complete cosmetic formulation can contain up to 40 different 'inactive chemicals' and one or more 'pharmacologically active components'. Each of these compounds is able by itself to penetrate into the skin and to interact with the others during this process. Finally, the total impact of the full formulation on the diffusion of any ingredient is extremely difficult to predict, and needs to be evaluated experimentally. Experimental protocols in vivo or in vitro should relate closely to in-use circumstances, and the following parameters have to be investigated:

- concentration of the ingredient in the formulation;
- mode and frequency of administration (open and occluded);
- surface of application and anatomical site;
- length of exposure (rinse-off or non-rinse-off).

COSMETIC EFFICACY AND PERCUTANEOUS ABSORPTION

The ability of cosmetic ingredients to penetrate the skin has repercussions not only for systemic and local toxicity but also for local pharmacological activity. If the biological effect of an active component can be determined by very different methodologies involving biochemical, physiological or physicochemical reactions, then the measurement of any biological response in vitro on whole skin specimens or on cell cultures would have no predictive value of the clinical activity if the concentration of the active component in the experimental medium was different from that obtained in the skin when the product is applied topically. This concentration can be estimated by measuring more particularly the amount of material that penetrates into the different skin layers – stratum corneum, viable epidermis, dermis and subcutaneous tissue – and is distributed and eventually accumulated within them. A complete analysis of the local pharmacokinetics of the considered ingredients gives information that can help the cosmetologist to select the optimal formulation.

Caffeine

Caffeine is a good example of this relation between in vitro pharmacology, skin pharmacokinetics and pharmacological activity in vivo.[5] Like other methylxanthines, it increases lipolysis (breakdown of triglycerides into free fatty acids and glycerol) both in vitro and in vivo. By inhibition of phosphodiesterase, caffeine is able to raise levels of cyclic AMP, which activates triglyceryl lipase, and is used topically as a local slimming ingredient. When caffeine is applied topically, its concentration detected after 100 minutes in the dermis is close to 10^{-4} M. The lipolytic effect found in vitro on isolated adipocytes, with a caffeine concentration of 10^{-4} M, can be obtained in vivo, where the repeated application of a 5% caffeine emulsion on rat skin for 3 weeks leads to a fall of more than 15% in the concentration of subcutaneous lipids in the treated area. These data confirm that percutaneous pharmacokinetic methodology allows one to link a biological activity demonstrated in vitro with the effect obtained in vivo.

Sunscreens

Sunscreen agents are also good examples of widely used cosmetic ingredients. They are included in a number of skin care products to prevent damage induced by excessive exposure to the sun, i.e. the possible dangers of premature aging of the skin and skin cancer. Sunscreens correspond very well to the definition of cosmetic products in the EU. Claims on the skin protection against sunburn or aging are allowed if they are backed by proofs. Furthermore, information is given to the public on the positive protective role of sunscreen products against skin cancer. To date, nine chemical entities and their salts or esters, if any exist, have been approved and recognized as safe and effective filters. Eleven more ingredients are registered on a special list awaiting final classification when enough data on their safety (including pharmacokinetic information) are available.

Sunscreens are incorporated not only in 'suntan' products but also in everyday products such as lipsticks, face lotions, body moisturizers and hair products in order to provide constant protection against UVA and UVB radiation. Following the choice of UV filter and the specification of the desired sun protection factor, the most important element is the vehicle. The choice of vehicle depends on the UV filter used and the final formulation desired: lotion, emulsion, gel, stick or aerosol. Two objectives govern the formulation of a suncare product. The first is to obtain a final product, with good cosmetic properties, in which the filter is solubilized for good homogeneity of application and good photochemical stability. The second objective is to maintain the filter on the skin surface, and to avoid any loss either by diffusion through the skin or by elimination from the skin after a bath (water resistance) or sun exposure (evaporation or photodegradation).

The photostability of the UV filters in the formulation after application on the skin as a thin film (corresponding to a maximum dose of 2 mg/cm^2) is a criterion of choice. Low stability, related to the dissipation of the energy absorbed by the filter, can lead to a decrease in the protection against radiation and to poor tolerance of the product (because of irritation and/or sensitization, as well as phototoxicity and/or photoallergic reactions that could be induced by the various products of filter photodegradation).

Most available data on the behaviour of sunscreens under UV radiation have been obtained in vitro using a solar simulator. An interesting in vivo experimental approach in human volunteers, using the stripping technique from the skin surface after exposure to artificial light or 'natural' sun, has been described by Marginean-Lazar et al.[6] The filter persisting in the horny layer is removed with several pieces of adhesive tape (10 or more strips can be performed under controlled contitions of adhesivity and pressure) and assayed by HPLC. Such an analysis is particularly interesting because it gives information from the surface of the skin (first strip) and from the depth of the tissue (other strips), so one can define, according to time, both the penetration profile of the filter and its photostability under the same experimental conditions.

Vitamins

Vitamins are well known for their functions in normal growth and maintenance of body functions. Many skin disorders are related to vitamin deficiencies. Dry skin has been observed for patients with deficiencies in vitamins A or B_8, pigmentation disorders have been described for deficiencies in vitamins C, PP, B_2 or B_5, skin ulceration has been linked to vitamins A, B_1, B_2 and PP deficiencies, hair loss has been related to deficiencies in vitamins B_5 and B_8, and nail disorders have been observed when vitamins B_5 and B_{12} are absent.

In cosmetic products the main claim for the use of vitamin E during the last decade has been as a natural moisturizer to treat dry skin and to aid indirectly in concealing wrinkles. Its principal biochemical activity is to protect cell membranes against the damaging effects of free radicals by its antioxidant activity; in the skin the formation of these free radicals is induced by UV radiation. Vitamin E after topical application was reported to be useful in reducing UV light damage, and was also found to be active in reducing cell membrane phospholipid peroxidation. Peroxides are implicated in the aging process, and one of their known breakdown products, malondialdehyde, has been shown to cross-link collagen. This effect could explain the decreased elasticity of aged skin.[7] The biological activites of vitamin E in cosmetics are supported by several studies of its percutaneous absorption, showing that within 6–24 hours after a topical treatment, it clearly concentrates in the dermis, substantiating the claim that vitamin E can be used as an active ingredient in cosmetology with a real efficacy in the deeper structures of the skin. Furthermore, the combination of the beneficial effects of vitamins E and A on several parameters of skin aging is of interest. A product containing these two vitamins would be able to improve skin hydration, free-radical protection, regulation of epidermal cell growth, and regulation of keratinization.

The oral pharmacokinetics of vitamins is well documented, and it has been reported that, because of poor absorption, metabolic dysfunction and/or aging, orally ingested vitamins are not always transported to the skin in sufficient amounts.[8] Under these circumstances, the local delivery of vitamins after a topical application is a necessity. Using the skin as a route of administration offers the following advantages: the compound is delivered to the site where its activity is required, the local concentrations are high because no preliminary dilution in the body takes place, the metabolic activity of the keratinocytes may be important in the activation of provitamins like provitamin B_5 (panthenol), esters of vitamin E (palmitate, linoleate and nicotinate) and esters of retinol and retinal (for vitamin A). These 'old' ingredients, so important in skin biology, have been the subjects of a tremendous amount of research work in order to demonstrate their efficacy in cosmetic products from pharmacological models in vitro and in vivo, and during clinical trials. Panthenol and vitamins C, E and A are, together with the α-hydroxy acids, cosmetic ingredients of great interest at the present time.

α-Hydroxy acids

Van Scott et al[9] reported the effects of α-hydroxy acids (AHAs), more specifically glycolic, lactic, malic, tartaric and citric acids, in the treatment of abnormal keratinization – specifically ichthyosis. The specificity of the biological action of AHAs appears to be related to their chemical structure, not their acidity. AHAs are currently used for various cosmetic and dermatologic conditions, including dry skin, dandruff, acne, keratoses, warts, wrinkles and photoaging.[10]

AHAs are organic carboxylic acids having one hydroxyl group (OH) in the α-position to the acidic function. This structure allows these compounds to be dissociated when they are dissolved in water according to the value of their dissociation constant (pK_a), conferring a specific pH to the medium in relation to their concentration. The value of pK_a makes the difference, in terms of strength, between the acids: the lower the pK_a, the stronger the acid. Like other acids, AHAs can be neutralized with bases (of mineral or organic origin), leading to the formation of salts.

Because of the lipophilicity of the stratum corneum, when an ionizable chemical is applied on the skin barrier, the non-ionized moiety, which is more lipophilic by definition, is better absorbed than the ionized one (which is more hydrophilic). So, in the special case of AHAs, the vehicle is of primary importance for the delivery of the compound to the skin. The lower is the pH, the higher is the amount of the non-ionized form capable of diffusing. The higher is the pH, the lower is the diffusion. The skin irritation induced by AHAs and the pharmacological response are two independent phenomena related only to the capacity of the chemical to diffuse through the skin barrier and reach the viable epidermis. Thus the formulator can adjust and optimize the pH of a formulation and the concentration of AHAs in order to find a compromise between the two different biological effects of the same molecule and modulate the penetration of the compound through the skin.

DYNAMICS OF COSMETICS APPLIED ON THE SKIN

Because of their poor cosmetic qualities and lack of elegance, old oily formulations have largely been replaced by hydrophilic gels and emulsions (simple or multiple) in which many components are added to the fundamental water, oil and emulsifying agents. When formulations such as creams and lotions are applied to the surface of the skin, water and volatile components evaporate rapidly (within 5–10 minutes). The rate of evaporation of the volatile components (i.e. primarily water but eventually others like alcohols and glycols) for a given formulation depends on the environmental conditions (relative humidity and outside temperature), the temperature of the skin, and the amount of preparation applied – or, more precisely, the thickness of the film formed on the skin surface.

As a consequence, the structure and composition of the formulation originally applied to the skin change, and only a residue containing principally non-volatile material persists on the tegument. This phenomenon may have profound effects on the release of the active ingredient incorporated into the original formula, and the subsequent percutaneous penetration and absorption, by changing the following.

- *The viscosity of the product and the associated diffusivity of the penetrant.* Evaporation induces changes in the physical structure of the residual materials present on the skin surface.
- *The partition coefficient of the active material between the horny layer and the residual vehicle.* In an emulsion, tensioactive agents are able to modify partitioning of both lipophilic and hydrophilic compounds by changing their solubility parameters in the persistent phases.
- *The thermodynamic activity of the penetrant* – by increasing its concentration up to saturation. The solubility of any ingredient in the residual material can be completely different (more or less important) than that in the complete formulation. If the solubility is considerably decreased, crystals can be formed on the tegument, and absorption is generally decreased.
- *The hydration level of the horny layer.* The residual material on the skin can be occlusive, so the penetration will be enhanced by the increase in horny-layer water content, with repercussions on both the solubility and diffusivity parameters of the ingredients in the stratum corneum.
- *The stucture and properties of the barrier itself.* Slowly evaporating solvents like glycols (often used as co-solvents and humectants in formulations) can increase the penetration of compounds into the horny layer, and at high concentration (as when the other components have evaporated) can be considered as percutaneous absorption enhancers. Surfactants, like glycols, which are among the major groups of adjuvants used in cosmetic formulations, are not volatile, and since their concentration increases during the evaporation of volatile compounds, they can induce damage to the

skin. This effect has been demonstrated with concentrations as low as 1% with anionic and cationic tensioactives. Acute histological modification of the skin may follow single and/or chronic applications of these compounds. Non-ionic tensioactives are less irritant than others, but are nevertheless able to penetrate the skin. The increased penetration induced by surfactants is largely related to strong interactions with the stratum corneum components – particularly with binding to keratin filaments, which induces a denaturation of the proteinaceous matrix, and with disorganization of the lamellae intercellular lipids. Surfactants also interact with the penetrant, which can be solubilized by the micelles, inducing changes in both its thermodynamic activity and solubility/partitioning parameters.

The effects of the vehicle on the absorption of active components are complex, and it is easy to see why published experimental data regarding the advantages of one vehicle over another are often conflicting. Each formulation – by the physiochemical nature of the different elements involved and their relative proportion – is a unique delivery system with highly specific characteristics.

CONCLUSIONS

Cosmetics contribute to beauty – but also to health in the widest sense, with all its psychological and social implications. Advertising claims emphasize particularly the performance of products, so consumers seek effective skin care products that can exert a beneficial action with the greatest safety, i.e. that offer no risk. Numerous chemicals commonly found in cosmetic formulations have been shown to diffuse through the stratum corneum. This penetration may result in irritant and/or allergic reactions, but it may also induce a positive pharmacological response.

If a cosmetic ingredient really does act on the skin, it must penetrate the tegument. Depending upon the formulation, the nature of the components, the conditions of use, and whether or not the product remains on the skin in a sufficient amount and for a long enough time, the subsequent penetration and absorption will be more or less intense. In order to predict the safety and efficacy of these ingredients, it is important to measure their rate of penetration into and absorption through the skin – either directly by the determination of the amount of the active material that reaches a certain anatomical level of the skin and/or the blood flow, or indirectly by an objective evaluation of the induced biological effect. In this case skin-penetration measurements are useful tools to substantiate advertising and labelling claims, and a good way to evaluate the safety of a product.

REFERENCES

1. Loomis TA, Skin as a portal of entry for systemic effects. In: *Current Concepts in Cutaneous Toxicology* (Drill VA, Lazar P, eds). New York: Academic Press, 1980:153–69.

2. Noonan PK, Wester RC, Cutaneous metabolism of xenobiotics. In: *Percutaneous Penetration: Mechanisms, Methodology, Drug Delivery* (Bronaugh RI, Maibach HI, eds). New York: Marcel Dekker, 1985:65–85.

3. Marzulli FN, Maibach HI, Relevance of animal models: the hexachlorophene story. In: *Animal Models in Dermatology* (Maibach HI, ed). New York: Churchill Livingstone, 1975:156–67.

4. Barry BW, *Dermatological Formulations: Percutaneous Absorption.* New York: Marcel Dekker, 1983.

5. Wepierre J, Courtheoux S, Thevenin M, Evaluation of the lipolytic effect of drugs applied percutaneously. In: *Cosmetic Technology and Science. Proceedings of the 12th IFSCC Congress, Paris, 1982,* Vol 2, 139–43.

6. Marginean-Lazar G, Fructus AE, Baillet A et al, Sunscreens photochemical behavior: in vivo evaluation by the stripping method. *Int J Cosmet Sci* 1997; **19:** 87–101.

7. Idson B, Vitamins in cosmetics, an update. II. Vitamin E. *Drug Cosmet Ind* 1990; **147:** 20–5, 60–1.

8. Idson B, Vitamins in cosmetics, an update. I. Overview and vitamin A. *Drug Cosmet Ind* 1990; **146:** 26–8; 91–2.

9. Van Scott EJ, Yu RJ, Control of keratinization with α-hydroxy acids and related compounds. I. Topical treatment of ichthyotic disorders. *Arch Dermatol* 1974; **110:** 586–90.

10. Ditre CM, Griffin TD, Murphy GF et al, Effects of α-hydroxy acids on photoaged skin: a pilot clinical; histologic and ultrastructural study. *J Am Acad Dermatol* 1996; **34:** 187–95.

8

Transungual drug delivery systems: What's new and relevant?

Jean-Paul L Marty, Robert Baran

INTRODUCTION

Historically, nail topical therapy has met with little success – partly because of the poor penetration of drugs into nail tissue. This is a pity, since there are nail conditions such as psoriasis and onychomycosis that look unsightly and where potent systemic therapy may sometimes be limited by severe adverse reactions. Moreover, the new systemic drugs that penetrate the nail keratin in a few days via the nail bed give a poor response when there is fungal involvement of the lateral nail edge or of the subungual tissue leading to onycholysis.[1] In addition, some patients are unable or unwilling to take oral drugs. They often prefer topical therapy because they perceive the infection to be trivial and not to merit systemic treatment. Therefore an attractive alternative would be topical application directly onto the nail plate.

WHY IS CONVENTIONAL TOPICAL THERAPY INEFFECTIVE?[2]

The formulations are not specifically adapted to the nails.

1. Conventional formulations of antifungal agents do not promote diffusion across the nail barrier.

2. Conventional formulations are not adapted for the usual treatment duration required for the growth of a healthy nail.

3. Conventional formulations do not remain in contact with the site of application for long periods and do not induce sustained release of drugs.

WHAT ARE THE REQUIREMENTS FOR SUCCESSFUL LOCAL THERAPY?

- Potent active (antifungal) agent
- High concentration of the drug in the formulation
- Diffusion at levels exceeding MIC
- Adequate method of delivery
- Ease and convenience of application.

Transungual diffusion of the appropriate chemical is the necessary and limiting condition for all local applications, and nail diffusion will depend on three factors:

(i) the physico-chemical properties of the nail;
(ii) the properties of the chemical;
(iii) the physico-chemical characteristics of the vehicle containing the active agent.

PHYSICO-CHEMICAL PROPERTIES OF THE NAIL

The entire nail fabric is hard keratin, and the most external dorsal layer is especially dense.[3] The hardness of the nail plate not only depends on the junctions between the cells and their architectural arrangement, but may also depend on the transverse orientation of the keratin filaments with respect to the axis of nail growth. Moreover, the multiplicity of the lateral bonds between keratin fibres (disulfide bridges, hydrogen bonds, acid–base bonds, electrostatic bonds) also account for the high resistance of nail keratin to the diffusion of active principles.

The nail plate is hardly remarkable chemically, given that it is a cornified epithelial structure, but the nail plate is, compositionally, more like hair than stratum corneum.[3] Its major component is nitrogen. The nail plate contains cholesterol as its principal lipid; it is also a plasticizer. Solvent extraction of cholesterol leaves the nail dry and brittle. In fact, the main nail plasticizer is water. The ideal concentration of water in nail tissue is 18%, and is directly related to ambient relative humidity, given the relative thickness of the stratum corneum and nail. The permeability of nail to water is some 1000-fold greater than that of the stratum corneum.[4,5]

The hydrophilic pathway as opposed to the lipophilic pathway explains the rapid diffusion of water and highly water-soluble compounds such as urea and methanol.[3]

THE PROPERTIES OF THE CHEMICAL

The chemical chosen should be an appropriate keratinophilic drug. Molecular weight and size as well as lipophilic/hydrophilic profile should be considered. The nail is breachable by many polar and non-polar substances with widely differing molecular weights (30–665).[3]

The use of a transungual diffusion promoter such as dimethyl sulfoxide (DMSO) is equivocal. Stüttgen and Bauer[6] claim that DMSO enhances the permeation inside the deeper keratin layers. On the other hand, Walters et al[7] found no indication that DMSO can accelerate permeability across the nail plate. At least theoretically, on the basis of diffusion across the lipids of the horny layer, solvents that tend to promote diffusion through the stratum corneum have little promise as enhancers of nail plate permeability. Moreover, DMSO was even found to retard the permeation of methanol and hexanol, while isopropanol reduces only the permeation rate of hexanol across the nail plate.

There are indications, however, that sodium lauryl sulfate, sodium sulfide and sodium thioglycolate are penetration enhancers.[3] The water solubility of these compounds is consistent with their penetrating properties across an hydrophilic structure.

THE VEHICLE CONTAINING THE ACTIVE AGENT

We know that the method of delivery in use on skin is inappropriate for releasing active agents onto the nail despite the penetration enhancers. This explains the following approaches.

1. To improve conventional topical treatments, the vehicle pH can be modified, as in the case of miconazole, where a high concentration of the active agent is achieved by decreasing the pH of the formulation, thereby increasing drug solubility in the vehicle for maximal diffusion.[7]
2. New simple formulations such as Faergeman's solution (lactic acid, urea, propylene glycol), 28% tioconazole or 40% urea can be used. However, the first two of these have produced only moderate results, and urea paste acts principally on the pathologic nail plate–nail bed attachment.
3. A real step forward has been achieved with the development of a new vehicle in the form of a cosmetic nail lacquer that will

reduce transungual water loss by an occlusive effect. Because of the formulation, the nail lacquer maintains the active agent in a polymer film on the nail surface, from which the chemical diffuses evenly through the nail keratin to reach the nail bed. Interestingly, after evaporation of the solvent, the concentration of the diffusion molecule in the film increases, which in turn enhances penetration by the laws of diffusion.[8,9] 8% ciclopirox nail lacuquer[9] increases concentration to 34.8%, and 5% amorolfine increases it to 19.8%.[10,11] Release and rate of diffusion can be optimized by selecting the components of the lacquer formulation to help modulate the release of the antifungal drug into the nail plate and to maintain it at a high level. This new method of delivery solves the problem of retaining the active agent in contact with the substrate for a sufficiently long time to produce the desired antifungal action.

CONCLUSION

In conclusion, it does not seem unreasonable to predict that it may soon be possible for pharmaceutical manufacturers to chemically tailor drugs that will prove more effective in the topical management of some nail conditions.[12]

REFERENCES

1. Baran R, de Doncker P, Lateral edge nail involvement indicates poor prognosis for treating onychomycosis with the new systemic antifungals. *Acta Derm Venereol* 1996; **76:** 82–3.

2. Marty JP, Amorolfine nail lacquer: a novel formulation. *JEADV* 1995; **4**(Suppl 1): S17–21.

3. Walters KA, Flynn GL, Permeability characteristics of the human nail plate. *Int J Cosmet Sci* 1983; **5:** 231–46.

4. Spruit D, Measurement of water vapor loss through human nail in vivo. *J Invest Dermatol* 1971; **56:** 359–61.

5. Walters KA, Flunn GL, Marvel JR, Physichochemical characterization of the human nail: 1. Pressure sealed apparatus for measuring nail plate permeability. *J Invest Dermatol* 1981; **76:** 76–9.

6. Stüttgen G, Bauer E, Bioavailability, skin- and nail-penetration of topically applied antimycotics. *Mykosen* 1982; **25:** 74–80.

7. Walters KA, Flynn GL, Marvel JR, Penetration of the human nail plate: the effects of vehicle pH on the permeation of miconazole. *J Pharm Pharmacol* 1985; **37:** 418–19.

8. Marty JP, Dervault AM, Voie percutanée. In: *Therapeutique dermatologique* (Dubertret L, ed). Paris: Médecine Sciences, Flammarion, 1991: 649–63.

9. Cesquin-Roques CG, Hanel H, Pruja-Bougaret SM et al, Ciclopirox nail lacquer 8%. In vivo penetration into and through nails and in vivo effect on pig skin. *Skin Pharmacol* 1991; **4:** 89–94.

10. Baran R, Amorolfine nail lacquer. A new transungual delivery system for nail mycoses. *JAMA Southeast Asia* 1993; **9**(Suppl 4): 5–6.

11. Polak A, Kinetics of amorolfin in human nails. *Mycoses* 1993; **36:** 101–3.

12. Walters KA, Penetration of chemicals into, and through, the nail plate. *Pharm Int* 1985; **6**(April): 85–9.

PART FOUR

COSMETOLOGY FOR NORMAL SKIN

9

Ceramides and the skin

Anthony V Rawlings, Clive R Harding, Kurt M Schilling

INTRODUCTION

Prevention of desiccation is the major function of the skin. This function is performed for the most part by the skin's epidermis, with a particularly crucial contribution by the outermost layer, the stratum corneum (SC) (Figure 9.1). At the skin's surface there is a delicate balance between the water content of the SC and the air itself, and although the SC contains relatively little water, a critical level of moisturization is essential for the normal barrier function and health of the skin. To maintain the proper level of moisturization, the skin's epidermis has evolved a finely tuned differentiation programme, which generates and maintains a SC composed of cellular and macromolecular components that provide the required structure, humectancy and barrier to water loss (for a review see reference 1). This structure has been compared to a brick wall,[2] with the 'bricks' representing the corneocytes (i.e. terminally differentiated keratinocytes of the SC) and the 'cement' representing the highly specialized and uniquely organized intercellular lipids (Figure 9.1).

These lipids are primarily ceramides, cholesterol and fatty acids, together with smaller amounts of phospholipids, glucosylceramides, free sphingoid bases and cholesterol sulfate.[3,4]

These lipid species, together with specialized lipids that are covalently bound to the corneocyte envelope,[5,6] form the major permeability barrier to the loss of water from the underlying epidermis.[7] They also form part of the intercellular cement that helps to maintain the integrity of the tissue.[8,9] This chapter will review recent developments in our understanding of the biological functions of ceramides, the major polar species from which the extracellular lipids of the SC are organized.

STRATUM CORNEUM CERAMIDES

It is now well established that within the SC there are six major classes of 'free' ceramides (non-corneocyte-bound) and two major classes of ceramides covalently bound to the corneocyte surface.[10,11] The ceramide backbone is a long-chain sphingoid base (C16–C22), which is most commonly sphingosine, and less frequently dihydrosphingosine, phytosphingosine or 6-hydroxysphingosine. These sphingoid bases are amide-linked with long-chain non-hydroxy and α-hydroxy fatty acids (Figure 9.2 and Table 9.1). In some cases, these amidated fatty acids are ω-hydroxylated and may be further esterified with other fatty acids, as is found in ceramides 1 and 6. Ceramide 1 is the predominant ceramide containing unsaturated

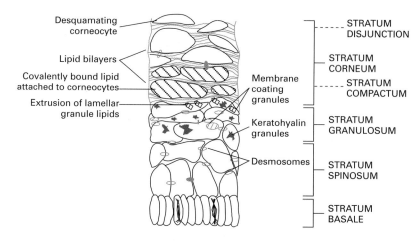

Figure 9.1 Schematic representation of the epidermis. Modified from reference 1.

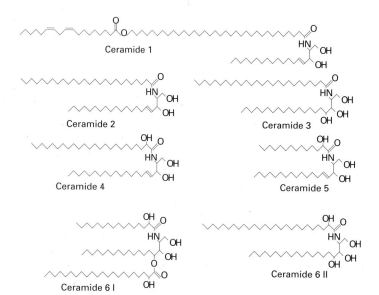

Figure 9.2 Chemical structures of stratum corneum ceramides. Modified from reference 1.

fatty acids in the SC; it is remarkably enriched in linoleic acid, which comprises a minimum of 20–30% of the ω-esterified fatty acid. The epidermis has a requirement for linoleic acid in order to maintain a correctly functioning barrier. This is most likely due to a pivotal role for ceramide 1 linoleate, with its unusual, long-chain fatty acid species providing unique physi-cal properties (see below). The physiological roles of the other individual ceramide species are largely unknown.

The two covalently bound species of ceramide (A and B) make up some 80% of the total bound lipid. Ceramide A, the major component (53%), consists of C30–C34 ω-hydroxy acids amide-linked to sphingosine.

Table 9.1 Stratum corneum ceramide types and levels[6,40]

Stratum corneum intercellular lipids		Covalently bound lipids	
Ceramide	Proportion of each species expressed as % of total mass of ceramides	Lipid	Proportion of each species expressed as % of total mass of lipid
1	10.6 ± 1.8	Ceramide A	53.5 ± 2.1
2	20.2 ± 4.2	Ceramide B	24.8 ± 2.1
3	18.0 ± 2.9	ω-Hydroxy fatty acid	9.4 ± 2.1
3a[a]	10.6 ± 4.6	Fatty acids	12.7 ± 1.2
4/5	21.8 ± 5.1		
6I	7.0 ± 3.5		
6II	12.4 ± 3.7		

[a] Ceramide 3a is believed to be de-esterified ceramide 1.
Modified from references 6 and 40.

The more polar ceramide B contains the same hydroxy acids linked to the novel sphingoid base 6-hydroxy-4-sphingenine.[11] The precise role of these lipids remains unclear, but they may be important for maintaining the correct orientation of the intercellular lipid bilayers.

Recently, ceramide-hydrolysing enzymes have been identified in the SC that may contribute to the formation of the ceramide degradation products.[12] A lipid species called acyl acid, which appears to be the ω-esterified *N*-acyl fatty acid portion of ceramide 1, and free sphingoid bases were shown to be present in human epidermis.[13,14] It is possible that both of these lipid species could be derived from hydrolysis of ceramide 1 or acylglucosylceramides. Although the role of these degradation products is uncertain, sphingosine and other sphingoid bases may be involved in a SC–epidermis signalling function, since they have been reported to inhibit keratinocyte proliferation.[15] Recent studies have reported that sphingosine is also a potent antimicrobial, and its presence in the SC may well form part of the skin's defences against invading microorganisms.[16]

VARIATIONS IN STRATUM CORNEUM CERAMIDE LEVELS

The total amount of ceramides in SC, as well as individual ceramide species, are influenced by disease status, diet, age, race, external environment, and, as has been shown more recently, by circannual variation. These variations in the levels and types of lipids present in the SC can influence barrier function, water content and ultimately skin condition.

Psoriasis and lamellar ichthyosis

Of the genetic diseases impacting on skin condition, only lamellar ichthyosis and psoriasis have been fully investigated for the levels of SC ceramides. In both of these conditions dramatic changes in SC lipid structure are observed,[17,18] including increases in ceramides 2, 3a and 4 and decreases in ceramides 3b and 5. These changes in ceramides, together with the altered cholesterol and fatty acid levels, are believed to contribute towards some of the aberrations in SC function that are characteristic of these conditions, including corneocyte cohesion and faulty desquamation.

It has also been reported that the composition of the covalently bound lipids in psoriatic SC differs from that of healthy SC. In psoriatics, ceramide B decreases, whilst other components such as ω-hydroxy acids and fatty acids, particularly the covalently bound oleate and linoleate, are seen to increase.[19]

Although the SC lipid profiles in other ichthyotic diseases have not been fully determined, reduced levels of sphingosine have been found in a variety of subjects with various ichthyoses.[20] This decrease in sphingosine could partly explain the cellular hyperproliferation observed in these conditions, since sphingosine has been proposed to feed back to the epidermis and downregulate keratinocyte turnover.[15]

Atopic dermatitis

Atopic dermatitis is also associated with decreases in SC ceramide levels, particularly with low levels of ceramide 1 linoleate.[21] Lowered levels of ceramides in atopics have been linked to an altered expression of the enzyme sphingomyelin acylase.[22] Xerosis and reduced barrier function measured by transepidermal water loss (TEWL) and corneosurfametry are apparent in these subjects. The inflammation in this disorder appears to be due in part to altered metabolism of sphingomyelin. In atopics, sphingomyelin is hydrolysed to release free fatty acid and sphingosyl phosphatidyl choline.[23] This latter compound is known as a potent modulator of epidermal function.

Abnormalities in lamellar granule structure have been shown in atopic individuals,[24] which could be directly due to a reduction in epidermal linoleoyl-acylglucosyl ceramide. Alternatively, modified epidermal differentiation may be the underlying problem in atopics, since this molecule has been shown to influence corneocyte envelope formation in vitro.[25]

Acne

Alterations in lipid species are also evident in acne. Downing et al[26] found reduced proportions of linoleate bound to ceramide 1 in acne patients, and postulated that this reflected a localized decrease in the bioavailability of the essential fatty acid due to a dilutional effect of increased sebum production. More recently, Yamamoto et al[27] have shown that the general decrease in both ceramides and free sphingosine in acne patients correlates with diminished water barrier function. Therefore altered barrier functionality leading to epidermal hyperkeratinization and poor desquamation within the follicular epithelium may be responsible for comedone formation in susceptible individuals.

Senile xerosis

It is widely experienced that as we age we suffer from more skin problems. Although these problems arise from a combination of many factors, an age-related reduction in the levels of SC ceramides may contribute to senile xerosis and other skin conditions. The most likely cause of an age-related decline in lipid levels is a reduced epidermal lipid biosynthesis capability, as recently reported by Ghadially et al.[28] The increased activity of ceramidase reported by Akimoto et al[29] may also contribute to declining ceramide levels. Age-related declines in SC ceramide have been reported in both Japanese[30] and Caucasian[31,32] subjects. In the latter study, although the relative levels of the main ceramide subtypes did not change, overall SC lipid levels diminished with increasing age on face, leg and hand skin. In addition, the same group reported an age-related decline in ceramide 1 linoleate levels, which may have a dramatic effect on SC barrier function. In another study with French Caucasians, a selective depletion of sterol esters and triglycerides, but not ceramides, was reported in ageing leg stratum corneum.[33] Ceramide subtypes have also been reported to change with age in Japanese women.[30] Surprisingly, increases in ceramides 1 and 2 but decreases in ceramides 3 and 6 were found on going from prepuberty to adulthood. These studies and others suggest that the impact of age on ceramide levels is likely to be influenced by ethnic background. For instance, in comparing SC lipid levels in several racial groups, Sugino et al[34] recently reported that SC ceramide levels were lowest in African Americans compared with other racial types. Although considerable progress has been made, our understanding of the influences of race, gender and age on SC lipids remains incomplete.

Effects of environmental factors on the expression of winter xerosis

It has become apparent that many factors influence the levels and types of SC lipids, and it is possible that their reduction leads directly to poor skin condition. Levels of lipids differ on different body sites, which may make those sites more or less prone to environmental damage.[35] For instance, lower levels of SC lipids will be more susceptible to extraction (e.g. during hand washing) or perturbation of their structural organization, which could lead to abnormalities in SC function and overall skin condition, resulting in a visibly dry and flaky skin surface. Indeed, a picture is emerging that lipids influence the expression of this common problem. Lipids are easily extracted from the SC by solvents[36] and surfactants,[37] leading to their depletion from the intercellular spaces of the SC, and resulting in skin scaling. In studies employing aggressive acute treatment regimes, solvent and surfactant extraction leads to changes in the relative amounts of the different lipid species in the outer layers of the skin, due to selective removal of lipids. However, during chronic treatments, particularly with surfactants, differences in SC lipid composition, but not total lipid levels, have been reported.[38] Following chronic exposure to surfactants, increases in ceramides 1 and 2 and cholesterol were observed, whereas ceramides 3–6, cholesterol esters and long-chain fatty acids all decreased in concentration. Similar changes in SC ceramide profiles have been reported in other experimental models for scaly skin (e.g. tape-stripping), indicating that the changes in SC lipid composition are related to changes in epidermal lipid biosynthesis rather than lipid extraction from the SC.[39] In skin suffering from soap-induced winter xerosis, the total levels of SC ceramides are decreased[40,41] and the levels of fatty acids are increased.[40,42]

Although the effects of climate on skin condition are well known, there have been very few studies examining circannual variation in SC lipids. One study has shown a general decrease in epidermal cerebrosides in winter compared with summer.[43] More recently, SC lipids from the face, hand and leg skin of female Caucasians in the winter, summer and spring months of the year were analysed, and decreases in all major lipid classes were seen on all body sites during the winter months.[31] Although the levels of ceramide subtypes were unchanged, the amount of linoleate esterified to ceramide 1 was reduced. These changes are likely to result in reduced barrier function. For instance, an increased susceptibility to treatment with sodium lauryl sulphate (SLS) has been reported for the winter months of the year,[44] and an inverse correlation has been shown between ceramide levels and TEWL following an SLS patch.[45]

Thus SC ceramides show marked biological variation. As lipids influence the permeability barrier to water and natural moisturizing factor loss together with the mechanical and desquamatory properties of the SC, changes in their levels or composition can lead to disturbances in SC functioning. In this respect, ceramide 1 – specifically ceramide 1 linoleate – appears to play a vital role, and disturbances in its levels are common to acne, atopic dermatitis, and age-related and winter-induced xerotic skin. Ceramide 1 linoleate has been proposed as playing a membrane-organizing role in the SC by spanning adjacent lipid bilayers and acting as a 'molecular rivet'.[46] More recent studies have indicated that this molecule influences SC extensibility behaviour by increasing flexibility at low environmental relative humidity.[47] Further studies on the behaviour of model lipid mixtures containing ceramide 1 linoleate led Oldroyd et al[48] to conclude that ceramide 1 linoleate, unlike the oleate derivative, helped to maintain a fluid lipid phase, and prevented the crystallization of other SC lipids at physiological temperatures. Thus ceramide 1 linoleate may be a naturally occurring 'lipid crystallization inhibitor', and this property may be vital, not only for the mechanical properties of the tissue, but also in facilitating the desquamatory process.

THE IMPORTANCE OF CERAMIDES FOR STRATUM CORNEUM STRUCTURE AND FUNCTION

Effect of ceramides on SC barrier function

Imokawa and co-workers[36,37] were the first to investigate the effects of topical application of human SC ceramides to solvent- and surfactant-induced scaly skin. When the extracted lipids – in particular the ceramide fraction – were reapplied to the damaged skin, reductions in scaling and improvements in skin moisturization, as measured by skin conductance, were observed. This amelioration of skin condition was superior to placebo and corresponding formulations containing sebaceous lipids. In these studies the ceramides were either solubilized in squalene or emulsified in a water-in-oil cream containing monomethylheptadecylglyceryl ether. Interestingly, these effects were not observed in the absence of the glyceryl ether. Although the

latter may aid penetration of the ceramides into the SC, it is also likely that it influences SC lipid-phase behaviour. Agents such as glycerol and glyceric acid are known to influence the physical properties of the ceramide-containing SC lipids. Thus it has been proposed that SC ceramide lipid mixtures have to maintain a liquid-crystalline state in order to reduce water loss.

Beradesca et al[49] and Linter et al[50] have demonstrated that exogenously supplied ceramide 1 and ceramide 2 respectively reduced the detrimental effects of SLS on disturbing skin barrier function.[51] In addition, Nardo et al[45] demonstrated an inverse correlation between various SC ceramide species and the erythema and TEWL that follow barrier insult by SLS. These studies indicate that low levels of particular ceramides may determine proclivity to SLS irritant contact dermatitis.

Elias and co-workers[51] have also focused on the use of exogenously supplied lipids to repair water barrier function. Although equimolar mixtures of ceramides, cholesterol and fatty acids allow the barrier to repair at normal rates, an optimized mixture (cholesterol, ceramide, palmitate and lineolate: 4.3 : 2.3 : 1 : 1.08) was seen to accelerate barrier repair following disruption of the murine water barrier by acetone. Although this mixture was seen to accelerate barrier repair following a range of barrier insults (tape-stripping, treatment with *N*-laurosarcosine or dodecylbenzenesulfonic acid), the mixture was not effective after barrier damage with SLS or ammonium laurylsulfosuccinate.[52] These studies suggest that customized mixtures of the critical lipid species may be required to repair barrier damage resulting from differing insults. Further studies are required to relate the significance of these observations to human skin.

Effect of ceramides on desquamation

Although the prime function of lipids in the stratum corneum is to provide the water bar-

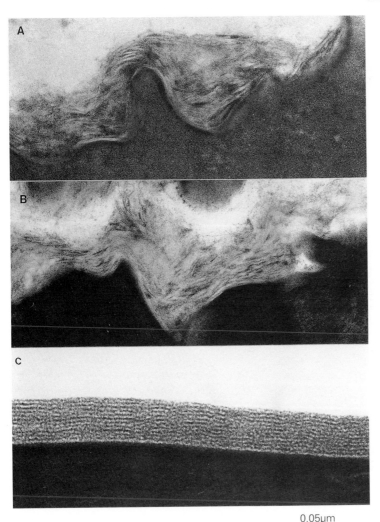

Figure 9.3 Structure of stratum corneum lipids in tape strippings of subjects with winter xerosis. Electron micrograph of tape strippings of subjects with severe xerosis. Aberration in lipid organization toward the surface of the stratum corneum. (A) First strip: disorganized lipid lamellae. (B) Second strip: disorganized lipid lamellae. (C) Third strip: normal lipid lamellae. × 200 000. Modified from reference 40.

0.05μm

rier, lipid abnormalities associated with altered cornification have been reported in many common dermatological disorders (e.g. psoriasis and atopic dermatitis). Structural abnormalities in SC lipid lamellae also occurs in the outer layers of the SC in dry skin (Figure 9.3). However, at present there is not a detailed understanding of how changes in the lipid composition, or specifically the ceramide composition, influence corneocyte cohesion and ultimately desquamation. There is indirect evidence for SC lipids being involved in cell cohesion from corneocyte reaggregation studies in vitro. Numerous workers have reaggregated previously dispersed corneocytes in the presence of SC lipids and found the physical properties of the reconstituted SC lipid-cell films to be similar to those of the intact tissue.[53,54] In marked contrast, Chapman et al[55] suggested that lipids may actually play an anticohesive role, preventing close opposition of adjacent corneocytes. In those particular studies, when SC lipids were completely extracted, the intercorneocyte forces were dramatically increased and SC cells became tightly opposed. Taken

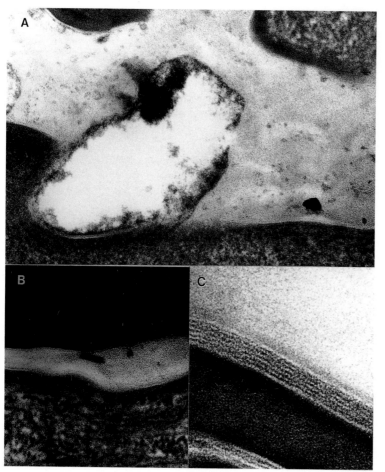

Figure 9.4 Structure of stratum corneum lipids in tape strippings of subjects with clinically normal skin. Electron micrographs of tape strippings of normal skin. Morphological changes in lipid organization towards the surface of the stratum corneum. (A) First strip: absence of bilayers and presence of amorphous lipid material. (B) Second strip: disruption of lipid lamellae. (C) Third strip: normal lipid lamellae. × 200 000. Modified from reference 40.

0.05μm

together, these observations indicate that both the intercellular and covalently bound lipids may play a role in SC integrity.

Changes in the physical properties of the SC ceramide lipids may also be important in promoting cell dyshesion towards the skin surface. It is known that there is a decreasing gradient of ceramide levels towards the outermost layers of the SC and that the fine ultrastructure of the ceramide bilayers is dis-turbed in the superficial layers in normal skin (Figure 9.4). This loss of structure, critical for normal desquamation, may reflect hydrolysis by ceramidases.[12] Degradation of ceramide 1 may be particularly relevant in this respect, since the intact molecule has been proposed to act as a molecular rivet holding lipid bilayers together.[38] Alternatively, surfactant-like sebaceous fatty acids may lead to bilayer disruption.

Ultimately it is the corneodesmosome (the modified desmosome of the SC) that is primarily responsible for intercorneocyte cohesion,[56–58] and it is this structure that must be effectively hydrolysed to ensure desquamation. Ceramides, together with other lipid species, may play an important role in this process. Although the precise mechanism is far from understood, the phase behaviour and organization of the intercellular lipids controls the water content in the SC, and may influence the activity of the hydrolytic enzymes[59] present within the intercellular space that are responsible for desmosomal degradation.

BIOSYNTHESIS OF STRATUM CORNEUM CERAMIDES AND BARRIER REPAIR

Endogenous regulation of ceramide synthesis and barrier function

Several models of barrier repair have been developed by Elias and co-workers to decipher the biochemical control mechanisms of barrier homeostasis (reviewed in reference 60). That all major species of SC lipids are synthesized during barrier repair and are required for full barrier homeostasis is suggested by studies using inhibitors to the key rate-limiting enzymes (Figure 9.5). In contrast to the synthesis of cholesterol and fatty acids, which increase almost immediately after barrier disruption, synthesis of glucosylceramides, the precursors of the SC ceramides, is delayed until approximately 7 hours later.[61] It is possible that the synthesis of the other lipids occurs more quickly, since the rate-limiting enzymes (hydroxymethylglutaryl CoA reductase and fatty acid synthetase) involved in their synthesis are subjected to acute metabolic control mechanisms such as phosphorylation, whereas serine palmitoyl transferase (SPT) is not subjected to such control and requires the transcription and translation of further enzymes. Furthermore, recent studies on transcriptional control of lipid synthesis in mammalian cells have shown that the expression of genes involved in cholesterol and fatty acid synthesis and uptake is regulated by the sterol regulatory binding proteins (SREBP 1 and 2); ceramide synthetic machinery, in contrast, does not appear to be regulated by this system.[62]

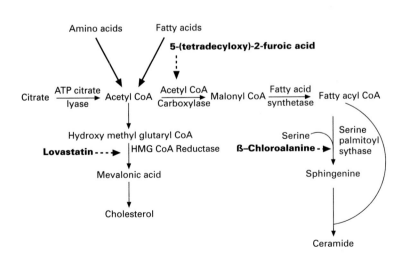

Figure 9.5 Generalized summary of stratum corneum lipid biosynthesis pathways. Inhibitors of rate-limiting enzymes are shown in bold.

Although altered water flux is a key factor in initiating barrier repair following stratum corneum perturbation,[63] the precise signal is not understood. As ionic gradients (i.e. calcium) downregulate lipid biosynthesis, it is possible that a disturbance in such a gradient allows an increase in lipid biosynthetic activity.[64] On the other hand, a variety of cytokines are released/secreted by the epidermis during such conditions, and they equally may contribute as key lipid biosynthetic switches.[65,66]

Enhanced ceramide synthesis through delivery of ceramide precursors

Several groups have investigated the potential to increase lipid biosynthesis using lipid precursors. The earliest work relates to the correction of ceramide levels and barrier function in essential fatty acid deficiency by the application of linoleic and linolenic acids.[67] Similarly, it has also been demonstrated that the low ratio of ceramide 1 linoleate to ceramide 1 oleate, which is characteristically seen in skin in the winter months, and which may predispose such skin to winter xerosis, can be improved by up to 85% through the topical application of formulations containing linoleic acid in the form of natural oils.[68] Brod et al[69] have also demonstrated similar effects on dry skin. Thus increasing the proportion of SC ceramide 1 linoleate may improve SC function in such conditions.

Lactic acid, especially L-lactic acid, can also function as a general precursor to ceramides, and this may explain the improvements in SC resilience observed following treatment with this α-hydroxy acid. The L-chiral isomer improved SC barrier function, as measured both by reduction in TEWL values following a challenge with SLS and by improved resistance to the appearance of dry skin in moisturization efficacy studies.[70] These improvements were related to the overall increase in SC ceramide levels – especially ceramide 1 linoleate levels – following use of

the prototype formulation. Furthermore, in vitro studies with keratinocytes established that lactic acid was utilized for lipid biosynthesis, and it is possible that this also occurs in vivo, leading to increased ceramide levels and a more effective barrier.

Other precursors, such as serine, the primary substrate for SPT (the rate-limiting enzyme in the ceramide biosynthesis pathway), are utilized by keratinocytes in the presence of thiols (lipoic acid and N-acetylcysteine) to stimulate ceramide biosynthesis.[71] These thiols presumably activate SPT by thiol–disulfide exchange mechanisms, and might be expected to provide benefit to the skin of subjects with a perturbed barrier.

Another option for enhancing ceramide biosyntheses is to use substrates that can feed into the ceramide biosynthesis pathway beyond the rate-limiting enzyme (SPT). Carlomusto et al[72] have shown that the modified sphingoid base tetraacetylphytosphingosine (TAPS) is a substrate for ceramide biosynthesis in vitro.[72] Furthermore, in studies where TAPS have been applied to the skin topically, a majority of subjects showed an increase in ceramide biosynthesis in vivo as measured by lipid analysis of tape-stripped stratum corneum.[73] Moreover, in those subjects whose skin showed increased ceramide levels with TAPS, a corresponding increase in resistance to surfactant damage was observed. In further studies, a synergistic improvement in SC ceramide levels and a corresponding increase in barrier function was achieved when TAPS was combined with ω-hydroxy acids and linoleic acid. This triple-lipid combination preferentially increased ceramide 1 levels above those of other ceramides, supporting its proposed mode of action as a ceramide 1 precursor.[73]

Influence of ceramides on keratinocyte differentiation

Ceramides may also improve SC resilience by improving differentiation. Ceramides and other sphingolipids are known to be important intracellular signalling agents that are involved in cellular decisions on proliferation, differentiation and apoptosis.[74-76] Extracellular or exogenously added ceramides may play an important pro-differentiation role. For instance, exogenously supplied short-chain ceramides are known to induce keratinocyte differentiation in vitro.[77] Short-chain ceramides and pseudoceramides also potentiate the effects of vitamin D, which is essential for keratinocyte differentiation.[77] Furthermore, vitamin D is known to activate keratinocyte sphingomyelinase, leading to increased intracellular levels of ceramide.[78] The structure/function requirements for ceramide-induced keratinocyte differentiation remain to be elucidated. However, hydroxy-acid-containing ceramides have been shown to be superior to non-hydroxy-acid-containing ceramides in inducing keratinocyte differentiation. In addition, of four ω-esterified fatty acid variants of ceramide 1 evaluated in vitro, ceramide 1 linoleate has been found to be the most potent differentiation enhancer.[79] Similar effects have been reported for glycated forms of these molecules.

CONCLUSIONS

Research into the structure and function of skin ceramides has increased substantially over the past two decades. These complex lipids have been shown not only to influence the barrier function of the SC, but also to impact upon its mechanical and desquamatory properties. All three elements influence the integrity, performance and ultimately the appearance of the outermost layers of the skin. In this respect, our understanding of the relationship between stratum corneum lipids and xerotic skin conditions has been essential for our ability to begin to improve these abnormal skin conditions, through the use either of defined barrier lipid species or of their biosynthetic precursors. However, as we move towards a new millennium, it is becoming increasingly evident that our understanding of these molecules is in its infancy, and that there remains much to learn about the role of ceramides in epidermal signalling and differentiation.

REFERENCES

1. Rawlings AV, Scott IR, Harding CR, Bowser PA, Stratum corneum moisturization at the molecular level. *J Invest Dermatol* 1994; **103**: 731-40.

2. Elias PM, Epidermal lipids, barrier function and desquamation. *J Invest Dermatol* 1983; **80**(Suppl): 44-9.

3. Yardley HJ, Epidermal lipids. *Int J Cosmet Sci* 1987; **9**: 13-19.

4. Elias PM, Menon GK, Grayson S, Brown BE, Membrane structural alterations in murine stratum corneum. Relationship to the localisation of polar lipids and phospholipases. *J Invest Dermatol* 1988; **91**: 3-10.

5. Swartzendruber DC, Wertz PW, Madison KM et al, Evidence that the corneocyte has a chemically bound lipid envelope. *J Invest Dermatol* 1987; **88**: 709-13.

6. Wertz PW, Madison KM, Downing DT, Covalently bound lipids of human stratum corneum. *J Invest Dermatol* 1989; **92**: 109-11.

7. Elias PM, Menon GK, Structural and lipid biochemical correlates of the epidermal permeability barrier. In: *Advances in Lipid Research*, Vol 24 (Elias PM, ed.). New York: Academic Press, 1991:1-26.

8. Epstein EH, Williams ML, Elias PM, Steroid sulphatase, X-linked ichthyosis and stratum corneum cohesion. *Arch Dermatol* 1981; **117**: 761-3.

9. Ranasinghe AW, Wertz PW, Downing DT, Mackenzie IC, Lipid composition of cohesive and desquamated corneocytes from mouse ear skin. *J Invest Dermatol* 1986; **86**: 187-90.

10. Wertz PW, Miethke MC, Long SA et al, Composition of ceramides from human stratum corneum and comedones. *J Invest Dermatol* 1985; **84**: 410-12.

11. Robson KJ, Stewart ME, Michelsen S et al, 6-Hydroxy-4-sphingenine in human epidermal ceramides. *J Lipid Res* 1994; **35**: 2060-8.

12. Wertz PW, Downing DT, Ceramidase activity in porcine epidermis. *Biochim Biophys Acta* 1989; **1002:** 213–17.

13. Bowser PA, Nugteren D, White RJ et al, Identification, isolation and characterisation of epidermal lipids containing linoleic acid. *Biochim Biophys Acta* 1985; **834:** 429–36.

14. Wertz PW, Downing DT, Free sphingosine in human epidermis. *J Invest Dermatol* 1990; **94:** 159–61.

15. Gupta AK, Fischer GJ, Elder JT et al, Sphingosine inhibits phorbol ester-induced inflammation, ornithine decarboxylase activity and the action of protein kinase C in mouse skin. *J Invest Dermatol* 1988; **91:** 486–91.

16. Bibel DJ, Aly R, Shinefield HR, Antimicrobial activity of sphingosines. *J Invest Dermatol* 1992; **98:** 269–73.

17. Lavrijsen APM, Bouwstra JA, Gooris GS et al, Reduced skin barrier function parallels abnormal stratum corneum lipid organisation in patients with lamellar ichthyosis. *J Invest Dermatol* 1995; **105:** 619–24.

18. Menon G, Ghadially R, Morphology of lipid alterations in the epidermis: a review. *Microsc Res Tech* 1997; **37:** 180–92.

19. Wertz PW, Madison KC, Downing DT, Covalently bound lipids of human stratum corneum. *J Invest Dermatol* 1989; **92:** 109–11.

20. Paige DG, Morse-Fisher N, Harper JI, Quantification of stratum corneum ceramides and lipid envelope ceramides in the hereditary ichthyoses. *Br J Dermatol* 1994; **131:** 23–7.

21. Yamamoto A, Swerizawa S, Ito M et al, Stratum corneum lipid abnormalities in atopic dermatitis. *Arch Dermatol Res* 1991; **283:** 219–23.

22. Imokawa G, Abe A, Jin K et al, Decreased levels of ceramides in stratum corneum of atopic dermatitis: an etiological factor in atopic dermatitis. *J Invest Dermatol* 1991; **96:** 523–6.

23. Murata Y, Ogata J, Higaki Y et al, Abnormal expression of sphingomyelin acylase in atopic dermatitis: an etiological factor for ceramide deficiency? *J Invest Dermatol* 1996; **106:** 1242–9.

24. Fartasch M, Bassukas ID, Diepgen TL, Disturbed extruding mechanism of lamellar bodies in dry non-eczematous ski of atopics. *Br J Dermatol* 1992; **127:** 221–7.

25. Uchida Y, Iwamori M, Nagai Y, Activation of kera-tinization of keratinocytes from fetal skin with *N*-(linoleoyl)ω-hydroxy fatty acyl sphingosyl glucose as a marker of epidermis. *Biochim Biophys Acta* 1990; **179:** 162–8.

26. Downing DT, Stewart ME, Wertz PW, Strauss JS, *J Am Acad Dermatol* 1986; **14:** 211–15.

27. Yamamoto A, Takenouchi K, Ito M, Impaired water barrier function in acne vulgaris. *Arch Dermatol Res* 1995; **287:** 214–18.

28. Ghadially R, Brown B, Sequiera-Martin SM et al, The aged epidermal permeability barrier: structural, functional, and lipid biochemical abnormalities in humans and a senescent murine model. *J Clin Invest* 1995; **95:** 2281–90.

29. Akimoto K, Yoshikawa N, Higaki Y et al, Quantitative analysis of stratum corneum lipids in xerosis and asteatitic eczema. *J Dermatol* 1993; **20:** 1–6.

30. Denda M, Koyama J, Hori J et al, Age- and sex-dependant changes in stratum corneum sphingolipids. *Arch Dermatol Res* 1993; **285:** 415–17.

31. Saint-Leger D, Francois AM, Leveque JL, Stratum corneum lipids in skin xerosis. *Dermatologica* 1989; **178:** 151–5.

32. Rogers JS, Harding CR, Mayo A, Rawlings AV, Stratum corneum lipids: the effect of ageing and the seasons. *Arch Dermatol Res* 1996; **288:** 765–70.

33. Saint-Leger D, Francois AM, Leveque JL et al, Age associated changes in stratum corneum lipids and their relation to dryness. *Dermatologica* 1988; **177:** 159–64.

34. Sugino K, Imokawa G, Maibach HI, Ethnic differences of varied stratum corneum function in relation to stratum corneum lipids. *J Invest Dermatol* 1993; **102:** 482.

35. Lampe MA, Burlingame AL, Whitney J et al, Human stratum corneum lipids: characterisation and regional variations. *J Lipid Res* 1983; **24:** 120–30.

36. Imokawa G, Akasaki S, Minematsu Y et al, Importance of intercellular lipids in water retention properties of the stratum corneum: induction and recovery study of surfactant dry skin. *Arch Dermatol Res* 1989; **281:** 45–51.

37. Imokawa G, Akasaki S, Minematsu Y et al, Selective recovery of deranged water-holding properties by stratum corneum lipids. *J Invest Dermatol* 1986; **87:** 758–61.

38. Fulmer AW, Kramer GJ, Stratum corneum abnor-

malities in surfactant induced dry scaly skin. *J Invest Dermatol* 1986; **80**: 598–602.

39. Denda M, Koyama R, Horii I et al, Sphingolipids and free amino acids in experimentally induced scaly skin. *Arch Dermatol Res* 1992; **284**: 363–7.

40. Rawlings A, Hope J, Rogers et al, Abnormalities in stratum corneum structure, lipid composition and desmosomal degradation in soap-induced winter xerosis. *J Soc Cosmet Chem* 1994; **45**: 203–20.

41. Saint-Leger D, Francois AM, Leveque JL et al, Stratum corneum lipids in winter xerosis. *Dermatologica* 1989; **178**: 151–5.

42. Nappe C, Delesalle G, Jansen A et al, Decrease in ceramide II in skin xerosis. *J Invest Dermatol* 1993; **100**: 530.

43. Nieminen E, Leikola E, Kolijonen M et al, Quantitative analysis of epidermal lipids by thin layer chromatography with special reference to seasonal variation. *Acta Derm Venereol* 1967; **47**: 327–38.

44. Agner T, Serup J, Seasonal variation of skin resistance to irritants. *Br J Dermatol* 1989; **121**: 323–8.

45. Nardo A, Sugino K, Wertz P et al, Sodium lauryl sulphate induced irritant contact dermatitis: a correlation study between ceramides and in vivo parameters of irritation. *Contact Dermatitis* 1996; **35**: 86–91.

46. Swartzendruber DC, Wertz PW, Kitco DJ et al, Molecular models of intercellular lamellae in mammalian stratum corneum. *J Invest Dermatol* 1991; **92**: 251–7.

47. Rawlings A, Critchley P, Ackerman C et al, The functional roles of ceramide one. In: *Proceedings of the 17th International Federation Society of Cosmetic Chemists Congress*, Vol 1, 1992:14.

48. Oldroyd J, Critchley P, Tiddy G, Rawlings AV, Specialised role for ceramide one in the stratum corneum water barrier. *J Invest Dermatol* 1994; **102**: 525.

49. Berardesca E, Vignoli GP, Oresago C et al, Prevention of barrier function damage by topically applied ceramides. In: *Proceedings of the 17th International Federation Society of Cosmetic Chemists Congress*, Vol 1, 1992:881–9.

50. Linter K, Mondon P, Girard F et al, The effect of a synthetic ceramide 2 on transepidermal water loss after stripping or SLS treatment: an in vivo study. *Int J Cosmet Chem* 1997; **19**: 15–25.

51. Mao-Qiang M, Feingold KR, Elias PM, Exogenous lipids influence permeability barrier recovery in acetone-treated murine skin. *Arch Dermatol* 1993; **129**: 728–38.

52. Yang L, Mao-Qiang M, Talbeni M et al, Topical stratum corneum lipids accelerate barrier repair after tape-stripping, solvent treatment and some but not all types of detergent treatment. *Br J Dermatol* 1995; **133**: 679–85.

53. Abraham W, Downing DT, Interaction between corneocytes and stratum corneum lipid liposomes in vitro. *Biochim Biophys Acta* 1990; **1021**: 119–25.

54. Smith WP, Christensen MS, Nacht S, Gans EH, Effects of lipids on the reaggregation and permeability of human stratum corneum. *J Invest Dermatol* 1982; **78**: 7–11.

55. Chapman SJ, Walsh A, Jackson S et al, Lipids, proteins and corneocyte adhesion. *Arch Dermatol Res* 1991; **283**: 1679–732.

56. Menon GK, Ghadially R, Williams ML, Elias PM, Lamellar bodies as delivery systems of hydrolytic enzymes: implications for normal and abnormal desquamation. *Br J Dermatol* 1992; **126**: 337–45.

57. Rawlings A, Hope J, Rogers J et al, Skin dryness – what is it? *J Invest Dermatol* 1993; **100**: 510.

58. Skerrow CJ, Cleland DG, Skerrow D, Changes to desmosome antigens and lectin binding sites during differentiation in normal epidermis: a quantitative ultrastructural study. *J Cell Sci* 1989; **92**: 667–77.

59. Egelrud T, Purification and preliminary characterisation of stratum corneum chymotryptic enzyme: a protease that may be involved in desquamation. *J Invest Dermatol* 1993; **101**: 200–4.

60. Feingold KR, The regulation and role of epidermal lipid synthesis. In: *Advances in Lipid Research*, Vol 24 (Elias PM, ed.). New York: Academic Press, 1991:57–82.

61. Holleran WM, Man MQ, Wen NG et al, Sphingolipids are required for mammalian epidermal barrier function-inhibition of sphingolipid synthesis delays barrier recovery after acute perturbation. *J Clin Invest* 1991; **88**: 1338–45.

62. Harris IR, Farrell AM, Grunfeld C et al, Identification of sterol regulatory element binding protein in epidermis: modulation in parallel to changes in key enzymes of cholesterol and fatty acid synthesis. *J Invest Dermatol* 1997; **108**: 553.

63. Grubauer G, Elias PM, Feingold KR, Transepidermal water loss: the signal for recovery of barrier structure and function. *J Lipid Res* 1989; **30:** 323–33.

64. Lee SH, Elias PM, Proksch E et al, Calcium and potassium are important regulators of barrier homeostasis in murine epidermis. *J Clin Invest* 1992; **89:** 530–8.

65. Wood LC, Jackson SM, Elias PM et al, Cutaneous barrier perturbation stimulates cytokine production in the epidermis of mice. *J Clin Invest* 1992; **90:** 482–7.

66. Nickoloff BJ, Naidu Y, Perturbation of epidermal barrier function correlates with initiation of cytokine cascade in human skin. *J Am Acad Dermatol* 1994; **30:** 535–46.

67. Prottey C, Hartop PJ, Press M, Correction of the cutaneous manifestations of essential fatty acid deficiency in man by application of sunflower seed oil to the skin. *J Invest Dermatol* 1975; **64:** 228–34.

68. Conti A, Rojers J, Verdejo P, Rawlings AV, Seasonal influences on stratum corneum ceramide 1 fatty acids and the influence of topical essential fatty acids. *Int J Cosmet Sci* 1996; **18:** 1–12.

69. Brod J, Traitler H, Studer A, de LaCharrière O, Evolution of lipid composition in skin treated with blackcurrant seed oil. *Int J Cosmet Sci* 1988; **10:** 149–59.

70. Rawlings AV, Conti A, Verdejo P et al, The effect of lactic acid isomers on epidermal lipid biosynthesis and stratum corneum barrier function. *Arch Dermatol Res* 1996; **288:** 383–90.

71. Zhang K, Kosturko R, Rawlings AV, The effect of thiols on epidermal lipid biosynthesis. *J Invest Dermatol* 1995; **104:** 687.

72. Carlomusto M, Pillai K, Rawlings AV, Human keratinocytes in vitro can utilise exogenously supplied sphingolipid analogues for keratinocyte ceramide biosynthesis. *J Invest Dermatol* 1996; **106:** 919.

73. Davies A, Verdejo P, Feinberg C, Rawlings AV, Increased stratum corneum ceramide levels and improved barrier function following treatment with tetraacetylphytosphingosine. *J Invest Dermatol* 1996; **106:** 918.

74. Spiegel S, Merrill AH, Sphingolipid metabolism and cell growth regulation. *FASEB J* 1996; **10:** 1388–97.

75. Hunnan YA, functions of ceramides in coordinating cellular responses to stress. *Science* 1996; **274:** 1855–9.

76. Merrill AH, Schmelz E-M, Dillehay DL et al, Sphingolipids – the enigmatic lipid class: biochemistry, physiology and pathophysiology. *Toxicol Appl Pharmacol* 1997; **142:** 208–25.

77. Pillai K, Frew L, Cho S, Rawlings AV, Synergy between the vitamin D precursor, 25 hydroxyvitamin D and short chain ceramides on human keratinocyte growth and differentiation. *J Invest Dermatol* 1996; Suppl 1 (Symp Proc):39–45.

78. Carlomusto M, Mahajan M, Pillai S, Vitamin D-mediated keratinocyte differentiation does not involve sphingomyelin hydrolysis. *J Invest Dermatol* 1997; **108:** 660.

79. Bosko C, Samares S, Santanastasio H, Rawlings AV, Influence of fatty acid composition of acylceramides on keratinocyte differentiation. *J Invest Dermatol* 1996; **106:** 871.

10

Main finished products: Moisturizing and cleansing creams

Daniel H Maes, Kenneth D Marenus

INTRODUCTION

When one looks at the history of cosmetics – especially back to the time of Cleopatra, who was already using perfumed ointments, eye makeup and lip colors – one may have the dubious feeling that there has not been much progress made in the formulation of cosmetic products, since, even today, the net result of the application continues to be to hide some of the skin's defects in order to temporarily improve its appearance.

As a matter of fact, the definition of a cosmetic product as conceived by the US Food and Drug Administration[1] corresponds to the initial idea that was at the origin of this type of product, since the Federal Food Drug and Cosmetic Act clearly stipulates that the term 'cosmetic' means articles intended to be rubbed, poured, sprinkled or sprayed on, introduced into, or otherwise applied to the human body or any part thereof for cleansing, beautifying, promoting attractiveness, or altering the appearance of the skin. However, today's cosmetic products provide not only immediate gratification to the consumer by improving the appearance of the skin, but in addition improve the structure and morphology of the skin through the activity of very specific ingredients that have been intro-duced through modern scientific achievements. These effects, however, are not permanent, and cannot be compared with the effects of drugs, which may permanently influence the activity of the skin's cells.

Even though modern cosmetic products induce some physiological changes in the skin, these changes are not permanent. Any interruption of a treatment with a cosmetic product will ultimately result in the reappearance of the skin problems the consumer was originally trying to alleviate. In other words, the modern cosmetic product is half way between the old concept of temporarily hiding skin defects, and the effect of a drug that permanently resolves an abnormal condition.

The art of designing a modern cosmetic product therefore requires not only the addition of the proper fragrance and color to a blend of excipient, but additionally the ability to incorporate the right combination of active ingredients into a vehicle that will deliver not only the desired cosmetic effects but also the longer-lasting benefits expected by the modern consumer.

The successful combination of the large variety of oils, waxes, humectants, moisturizers, solubilizers, emulsifiers, preservatives, antioxidants and any other components that will have a more significant benefit differentiates the high-quality cosmetic product from the lesser ones.

All the modern technology that comes along in the form of an ever-increasing amount of new instrumentation and new ingredients will never replace the fine art of cosmetic formulating, which consists in mixing all these ingredients in a form that not only will remain stable for a long period of time but will also provide the consumer with an ever-recurring satisfaction each time the cosmetic preparation is applied to the skin.

In this chapter, we shall review the function and composition of various cosmetic products such as cleansers and moisturizers. We shall examine the functions of these products, what they are made of, and how the manufacturer ensures that they are safe, stable, well preserved and efficacious.

CLEANSERS

In order to keep the skin healthy and of good appearance, it is necessary to eliminate grime, sebum, dead cells, applied make-up and other particulates that cover the skin surface after a full day's exposure to the environment. This task is performed by the large variety of cleansers and toners that are nowadays on the market.

Several types of cleansers have been developed to cleanse different skin types. For example, cream or lotion cleansers are perfectly suited to remove makeup and other solid residues from dry skin, since they are basically emulsions that use the solvent action of oils to dissolve makeup and other products left on the skin's surface, while at the same time leaving behind an emollient film preventing excessive delipidation. Alternatively, oily, acne-prone skin will be better treated with a surfactant-based cleanser and/or eventually with a toning lotion in order to eliminate all the oily residue and cellular debris from its surface.

One very important point to consider when formulating cleansers is that ideally these products are supposed to remove oils and other lipidic secretions originated from the sebaceous glands in the skin, but at the same time they should not remove any of the constitutive lipids like the cerebrosides or the ceramides, which play a key role in preventing excessive water loss from the skin. As we are going to see later when we examine the mechanism of action of soaps and detergents in cleansing the skin, this distinction between sebaceous lipids and the more polar epidermal lipids (ceramides and cerebrosides) is quite marginal as far as cleansing is concerned. Evidently, the choice of the right surfactant is critical in achieving such a balance.

There are four types of surfactants or surface-active agents that are used in cleansers, selected for their functionality as detergents, wetting agents, foaming agents, emulsifiers and solubilizers. The detergent and foaming properties of these surfactants are the most important factors to consider when formulating a cleanser.

- *Anionic surfactants* are those in which the surface-active ion is negatively charged in solution. Soaps are the most important category in this class, and are the most frequently used cleansers for oily skins because of their outstanding oil-removal properties.
- *Cationic surfactants* have a positive charge on the surface-active ion, which confers upon them some interesting properties such as binding to the surface of the skin, since the skin's overall negative surface charge has a tendency to attract the positive moiety of the cationic emulsifier.
- *Nonionic surfactants* are composed of a multiplicity of small uncharged polar groups such as hydroxyl groups or ethylene oxide chains, which confer the necessary hydrophilicity to the molecule but do not create a positive or negative overall charge.
- *Ampholitic surfactants* are characterized by the presence of positive and negative charges at each end of the molecule, which

confer interesting tensio-active properties while at the same time making them some of the mildest surfactants used in cleanser preparations.

Based on this description, it is obvious that these surfactants have quite a wide pH range, hence potentially affecting the pH balance of the skin. As is well known, the skin is at a slightly acidic pH (around 5.3),[2] and most surfactants, especially soaps, have a strongly alkaline pH. The utilization of large concentrations of soap or other anionic surfactants does have a strong influence on the skin's pH.[3] Measurements in the Estée Lauder laboratories show that washing the skin with soap increases the skin's pH by more than two pH units – a condition that lasts more than four hours. In addition, we have correlated this increase in skin pH with a significant stiffening of the skin surface, mostly the stratum corneum, as measured with the gas-bearing electrodynamometer, which evaluates in vivo the pliability of the outermost layer of the epidermis.

Evidently such effects should be avoided, since cleansing the skin should not induce skin tightness or stiffness. Consequently, we recommend the use of detergents that have a pH as close as possible to that of the skin (mostly nonionic detergents), and that can be easily rinsed away from the skin's surface.

Cleansers for dry skin

Let us now review the different types of cleansing regimens that are best suited for dry or oily skin conditions.

The cleansing of dry skin is best achieved with cleansing creams that are spread on the skin surface with the fingers and then wiped from the skin with a tissue, although some are water-rinsable – a characteristic that seems to be preferred by most women today. These products use the solvent effect of ingredients such as mineral oils to dissolve makeup and dirt present on the skin. A very well known category of cleansers belonging to this group are cold creams, which are made of natural waxes and mineral oils and use borax as an emulsifier.[4]

More modern products use some nonionic emulsifiers such as sorbitan fatty acid esters, resulting in a lighter-textured product. The advantage of these types of cleansers is that they are less likely to strip the skin of its essential lipids such as the ceramides and cerebrosides. For this reason, they are perfectly adapted to dry or very dry skin types, which often suffer their condition owing to the lack of these specific lipids between the cells of the stratum corneum. Higher-quality cleansers incorporate these lipids directly as protectants for dry skin. The combination of refatting agents such as fatty acids and wax esters, with the ceramides or cerebrosides, in a light emulsion base, provides the gentlest method for cleansing dry, sensitive skin.

As can be seen thus far, the most important decision in the development of a cleanser for dry sensitive skin consists in the proper choice of a surfactant that will have sufficient surface activity to remove dirt, sebum and make-up residues without affecting the lipids in the stratum corneum that provide the skin with its barrier properties.

The integrity of the skin barrier property goes far beyond the retention of water, since this important skin property prevents the penetration into the skin of molecules that may induce irritation or even a sensitization reaction. In fact, the utilization of poorly formulated cleansers may not only induce skin dryness, but can increase the risk of subsequent skin reactions from products used after cleansing.[5] For example, the extent of skin reactions to moisturizers containing vitamin A palmitate is directly related to the type of cleanser used prior to its application. Cleansers with strong anionic surfactants and no refatting agents will undoubtedly not only cause skin dryness but also increase the penetration into the skin of all the ingredients that are applied subsequently onto the skin surface, and as a result increase significantly any irritation potential they may possess.

In clinical studies of moisturizers, we have observed that in many cases the skin reactions observed were due not to the moisturizer itself but rather to subclinical damage created by the cleanser used by the panelist prior to the application of the moisturizer.

Cleansers for mixed skin

For subjects with skin conditions closer to normal, wash-off emulsions have been created, i.e. emulsions that contain a lower level of oils and waxes, and a higher amount of surfactant. These products, based on triethanolamine stearate or sorbitan fatty acid ester emulsifiers, are easily rinsable from the skin's surface and provide the sensation of thorough cleanliness. However, it is sometimes necessary to add some mild detergents such as sodium cetyl sulfate to these products, in order to improve the rinsability of calcium salts, which can be deposited onto the skin's surface if the cleanser is rinsed with hard water.

It is important to remember that an oily skin condition can be juxtaposed to a dry skin condition as often seen in individuals with mixed skin (i.e. subjects with oily forehead and nose, and dry cheeks and chins). In such cases, it will be important to choose a light oil-in-water emulsion cleanser in order to efficiently remove the excess of oils from the T-zone area, while at the same time adding lipids to some of the dryer parts of the face such as the cheeks and the chin.

In some cases, high levels of sebum and skin dryness may occur on the same sites. This observation has been made many times in the Estée Lauder laboratories, where we have measured high transepidermal water loss values (indicative of dry skin) on subjects who had an excessive sebum excretion and were rating themselves as having oily skin. In fact, this observation contradicts the accepted fact that sebum does retain water inside the skin,

and as a consequence increase the skin's moisturization. The fact that dry skin covered with a high level of sebum does not *look* dry is only due to the fact that the sebum keeps the dry skin cells glued onto the skin surface, hence reducing the grayish, scaly appearance characteristic of dry skin.

Cleansing of skin that has a mixed condition must be done with care, since the detergency needed to remove the large amount of sebum covering the skin's surface may induce more skin dryness by removing lipids that provide the skin with its barrier properties.

Cleansers for oily skin

The most logical method of cleansing oily skin is to use a simple solution of surfactant containing no oils, waxes or any other superfatting agents that could aggravate the oily condition of the skin.

Oily skin is often prevalent in younger individuals, and may be accompanied by an acne condition.

Again the same problem arises, where it is necessary to remove large quantities of oils and waxes from the skin surface and from the follicular opening, while at the same time not affecting the integrity of the skin's barrier by removing the ceramides and cerebrosides.

Cleansers formulated for oily skin are based on mixtures of various surfactants, mostly cationic and nonionic detergents that are known for their mildness and good detergency (sodium cocoyl methyl taurate, sodium cocoyl sarcosinate, decyl polyglucose).

In addition to sebum and dirt removal, cleansers for oily skin are expected to control to some extent the skin's regreasing rate, in order to limit the degree of shininess and oiliness that usually occur three hours after the skin has been cleansed. One well-accepted way to reduce the extent of skin shininess is to incorporate oil-absorbing materials like bentone or nylon powder, which remain on the skin surface after the excess of cleanser has been wiped off. This technology has some limitations, since it does not function in rinse-off cleansers, because the absorbing material will be completely washed away when the skin is rinsed with water.

Some more modern technology is now being introduced in the latest cleansers for oily skin. For example, some ingredients like polyquaternium compounds (e.g. Ceraphyl 60) have the ability to affect the superficial tension of the skin surface, making the skin more lipophobic. As a result, sebum spreading across the skin surface is reduced, the effect being that most of the sebum is confined to the skin's furrows and the appearance of shine is greatly diminished.

Measurements of the casual sebum level (i.e. the amount of sebum found on the surface of the skin three hours after cleansing) indicated a 18% reduction with a cleanser containing 0.5% Ceraphyl 60, as compared with a placebo cleanser.

These results demonstrate that it is possible to significantly reduce the oily appearance of the skin by affecting only the distribution of sebum on the skin surface without changing the amount of sebum excreted by the sebaceous glands.

The combination of sebum absorption technology with control of sebum spreading provides the most efficacious method of reducing the shiny appearance of skin, which is the most unpleasant feature associated with this condition.

Another unpleasant consequence of the presence of large quantities of sebum on the skin surface is the development of acne lesions, which are caused in part by the occurrence of anaerobic bacteria called *Propionium acnes* in the large oil pool existing in the follicles. These bacteria release specific enzymes called lipases, which hydrolyze the sebum's triglycerides into free fatty acids. These irritating free fatty acids initiate an inflammatory reaction in the follicular infundibulum, resulting in the development of an acne lesion. Obviously other events must take place at the same time to generate such a serious inflammatory reaction, but it has been well established that the presence of large numbers of *P. acne* colonies in the sebum is one of the most important steps in the development of acne lesions.

For this reason, it is customary to incorporate into cleansers for oily skin antibacterial compounds such as hexamidine diisothionate or Irgasan DP200, which will significantly reduce the bacterial counts on the skin surface, hence reducing the risk of developing an acne lesion. In addition, the thorough removal of the sebum from the skin surface and follicular openings will undoubtedly result in a significant reduction in the development of bacterial colonies, further reducing the potential for additional acne lesions.

It should be kept in mind, however, that even the most sophisticated cleanser for oily/acne-prone skin will not completely eliminate all the lesions on the skin surface, but will rather reduce the predisposition to the development of new comedones. Only products specifically formulated for this purpose, such as lotions or creams containing keratolytic agents like salicylic acid or antibacterial agents such as benzoyl peroxide, will provide the necessary therapy to rapidly reduce the number of existing lesions on the skin.

Despite all the science and technology that has been recently used in the development of modern cleansers, these products suffer a major drawback. Since they are rinsed away, they do not allow for a sufficient contact time between the active ingredients and the skin to deliver an efficient therapy, thereby limiting their effectiveness.

A good cleanser will only prepare the skin for a subsequent treatment, but will not replace leave-on over-the-counter (OTC) products containing active ingredients that exert their effects through prolonged contact time.

Testing of cleansers

As discussed previously, the most important quality of a cleanser, in addition to the cleansing of the skin surface, is to not damage the skin's barrier properties by removing the polar lipids, such as the cerebrosides and ceramides, which play such an essential role in maintaining an appropriate level of moisture in the skin, and preventing the uncontrolled penetration into the skin of substances that induce irritation or sensitization.

There are different ways to evaluate the degree of gentleness of a cleanser. One method is to measure if the cleanser adversely affects the skin barrier properties, which can result in a higher than normal transepidermal water loss.[6] Such a parameter can now be measured efficiently with an instrument such as the Servomed, which gives a fairly accurate indication of the rate of water loss from the skin after cleansing, thus providing useful information on the condition of the skin barrier.[7,8]

Other instrumental methods have been developed to measure the extent of skin irritation generated by a cleanser. For example, instruments that measure the blood flow in the skin, such as the laser Doppler blood flow monitor, can detect even the slightest increase of blood flow in the skin, which would occur from irritation induced by harsh detergents. These instruments allow the clinician to detect a level of irritation that could not be seen by the most well trained observer.[9–11]

Another useful methodology in the evaluation of the gentleness of a cleanser consists in the measurement of skin color using instruments called chromameters. These give a precise quantification of slight changes in the color of the skin, especially in the red region of the visible spectrum, allowing an exact determination of any erythema induced by a cleanser.[12,13]

Finally, the development of polarized light photography or video recording allows for a sensitive visualization of sites where some irritation still invisible to the most well trained observer might exist. In fact, this technique is the most sensitive and the most practical

Figure 10.1 Unpolarized (top) and polarized (bottom) photographs of skin, showing the presence of irritation.

method to detect early signs of subclinical irritation, although it does not provide a quantification of the severity of the skin reaction, which at this time is still invisible to the naked eye. (See Figure 10.1.)

These highly sensitive techniques allow the detection of subclinical irritation while testing under conditions of normal use. This subclinical irritation will undoubtedly turn into visible erythema accompanied by skin dryness and flakiness if the product was used on a regular basis.

These tests are an indispensable complement to the standard safety testing regularly used to assess the irritation potential of a cleanser. Tests like the soap chamber test, the cumulative irritancy test or the repeated-insult patch test challenge the skin under some exaggerated conditions, and, as such, do not provide a trustworthy picture of the irritation potential of a cleanser as used in a normal-life situation.

Although in the Estée Lauder laboratories, we evaluate our products using these well-established safety tests, we now also perform the instrumental evaluations described here in order to obtain a more accurate picture of the irritation potential of cleansers.

Finally, the last word must lie with the user, since, in addition to all the safety and instrumental testing described above, we believe it is critical to run safety-in-use studies on panelists with a dry skin condition for a period ranging between two and four weeks, during which time any subject who perceives a skin reaction such as itching or burning or who develops red patches is seen by a dermatologist to evaluate the causal relationship. Such tests should be run on groups of 200 subjects in order to obtain results with some statistical significance.

Only the proper balance of emulsifiers, refatting agents, sebum-absorbing compounds and antibacterial agents, all incorporated in a formula with a pH as close as possible to that of the skin, will result in the creation of a product that will satisfy a large number of customers with various skin types.

However, as we have already mentioned, there are no magic recipes in the art of formulating a good cleanser, and only the most thorough testing under stringent in-use situations will provide the quasi-certitude that the product is ready to be distributed to consumers.

MOISTURIZERS

Dry skin, although not a medical condition, is an uncomfortable affliction that affects many people. Characteristics of dry skin include flaking, scaling, cracking, tightness, redness and occasionally bleeding.

The causes of dry skin, although not completely defined, are centered around three overlapping areas: lack of water in the stratum corneum, overactive epidermal turnover, and barrier damage. If the stratum corneum is desiccated, the result is a dry, tight cracked surface where the squames are lifted at the edges. The resultant skin is ashen and flaky in appearance and uncomfortable for its owner.

Chronic low-level irritation from either chemicals or UV exposure can increase turnover as part of the inflammatory process. When this occurs, there is often inadequate time for the keratinocytes to differentiate properly or for the appropriate lipids to be produced. This results in a defective barrier that cannot hold water, further intensifying the dry skin condition.

The third major cause of dry skin is barrier damage. When there is depletion of the intercellular lipids, such as with detergent exposure during dishwashing, the barrier is damaged, and the rate at which water traverses the skin from within is markedly increased. If the water cannot be stopped at the upper layers of the stratum corneum then desiccation of that outer surface will occur.

Treatment of skin dryness

The simplest way to moisturize is to add water back to the skin. This is achieved through two basic approaches: occlusion and water delivery. Emulsions are the most common form of moisturizers. These are of the oil-in-water or water-in-oil varieties.

The water-in-oil emulsion works primarily by creating an occlusive film on the skin surface. This serves to slow the rate at which water is traversing the skin thus trapping it in the upper layers of the stratum corneum and allowing for softening. The water-in-oil emulsion is less widely preferred than other product forms owing to its tendency to create a heavy afterfeel, since a major constituent of these products is often petrolatum. It is this product form, however, that is widely appreciated by the individual with very dry skin or by the person who is frequently exposed to the winter elements, since it offers quick relief through occlusion.

The most common type of emulsion found today is of the oil-in-water variety, because consumers prefer the aesthetic qualities of this form. Existing as either a lotion or a cream, it is ideally suited for the population with neither excessively dry nor oily skin.

These emulsions do not work through occlusion but rather by delivering and building water in the stratum corneum. In terms of water delivery, the oil-in-water emulsion is capable of carrying up to 85% water, and, as such, can give quick and effective plasticization of the skin.

A typical curve illustrating the ability of such a product to soften the skin surface is illustrated in Figure 10.2. Using the gas-bearing electrodynanometer, an instrument that measures skin surface extensibility with a fixed force,[14] it is possible to objectively detect, quantify and evaluate the ability of such products to provide skin softening over time. As can be seen from the curve, there is an initial softening effect seen within the first few minutes. This is from the water itself. As

the water from the emulsion dries, there is a gradual return of the skin surface to its original state. The true effect of a moisturizer in softening the skin is then evaluated through the longer-term effects, which are related to the ability of the moisturizer to keep water bound to the skin surface.

Binding of water at the skin surface is accomplished by humectants that are capable of retaining large amounts of water relative to their weight. Traditional humectants such as glycerol and the glycols are now being replaced with more biocompatible agents such as hyaluronic acid and mucopolysaccharides. These have also replaced the soluble agents used in the past, including urea and certain amino acids collectively known as natural moisturizing factors (NMFs). Water-binding agents of any type are important to the formula in that they slow the evaporative rate of the water being delivered from the product.

The presence of water against the skin surface can serve to plasticize and smooth the uppermost layers of the stratum corneum. Further, it can act to temporarily soothe discomfort associated with dry tight skin. Delivering and binding water at the surface does not solve the problem of dry skin. Rather, the dry skin condition is more dramatically improved by increasing internal water-binding capacity.

Modern moisturizers can increase water retention in both the epidermis and the dermis by stimulating the synthesis of glycosaminoglycans. This is accomplished by incoporating derivatives of vitamin A such as retinyl palmitate in the formula. Glycosaminoglycans, long-chain amino-sugars, bind water at concentrations many times their weight, resulting in increased internal water retention within the skin. This 'internal moisturization' complements the delivery of water externally as described above.

An example of such an effect is shown in Figure 10.3 where we can readily observe the presence of large clumps of dry skin cells in

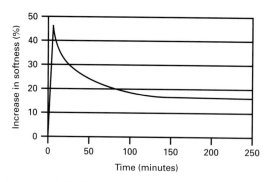

Figure 10.2 Effect of oil-in-water emulsion on skin surface extensibility.

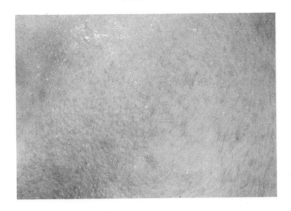

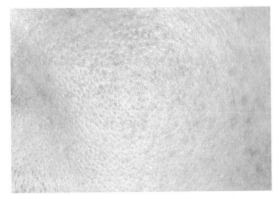

Figure 10.3 Photographs of skin before (top) and after (bottom) treatment with a moisturizer, showing the reduction of skin dryness.

the periorbital region in the picture taken before application of the moisturizer (top), whereas the picture taken one hour after treatment shows a complete remission of the dryness.

Excessive cell renewal

As noted above, chronic irritation – whether it be derived from UV, chemicals or even the dry skin condition itself – can lead to an increased turnover rate of the epidermal cells. The keratinocytes shed before there has been sufficient time for adequate differentiation to occur. This in turn prevents formation of a

proper barrier, with the result that the skin surface becomes dry, tight, flaky and cracked.

This aspect of the dry skin condition can be effectively handled by incorporating agents that help to regulate the differentiation process so that equilibrium can be re-established. The combination of vitamin A palmitate together with 7-dehydrocholesterol seems to optimize this condition.

Vitamin A as a retinoid is known as a de-differentiating agent,[15,16] and topical application can cause an increased number of cell layers together with an increase in the size of the average keratinocyte.[17] 7-Dehydrocholesterol, known as a precursor of vitamin D_3 and 1,25-dihydroxyvitamin D_3, act to accelerate the terminal differentiation process.[18,19] This in turn also results in an increase in the thickness of the epidermis.

Examples of some of the benefits observed from the rebalance between the cellular differentiation and the cellular division process are shown in Figure 10.4, where a noticeable reduction in the depth and length of the lines and wrinkles can be seen in the picture (bottom) taken after two months of daily application of a product containing both vitamin A palmitate and 7-dehydrocholesterol, compared with the picture taken before treatment (top).

When applied together, these two agents appear to work to re-establish within the epidermis a new equilibrium in terms of cell turnover that improves both the barrier condition as well as the degree of internal moisturization.

Barrier condition

If barrier condition is not optimal, water moves rapidly through the epidermis and exits the stratum corneum, leading to a desiccated surface as well as perturbation of the entire epidermis. Recent work by Elias has shown that increasing the rate at which water traverses the stratum corneum after barrier disruption is a key event in altering the

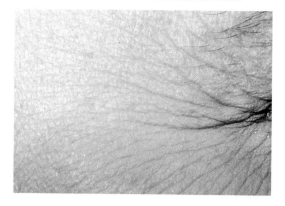

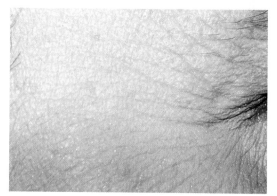

Figure 10.4 Photographs of the periorbital area of the face before (top) and after (bottom) treatment with a moisturizer.

metabolism of the underlying keratinocytes.[20–22]

One method for approaching the problem of barrier repair is the inclusion in the formula of lipids that are specifically compatible with those found within the interstices of the stratum corneum. The specific lipids often include cholesterol, cerebrosides and other glycolipids. These materials are more efficient in barrier repair than undefined fractions of hydrocarbons such as in mineral oil.

Although it is of great help, it does not suffice to add lipids to the barrier directly from the cream or lotion. It is equally important to stimulate the epidermal cells to create the lipids, which can then percolate into the stratum corneum and fill the gaps in the normal manner. Agents such as retinyl palmitate that can act to stimulate the rate of glycolipid synthesis should be included in the formula.

A key reason for hastening to repair the barrier with specific lipids and other agents is that, with the dry skin condition, unwanted materials penetrate more rapidly. This increases the potential for irritant and allergic responses. Since a defective barrier often accompanies the conditions that drive the consumer to seek the help of a moisturizing product, the defective barrier must be kept in mind when designing such products. Ingredients that have the potential for creating either an irritant or allergic response must be scrupulously avoided.

A chronic condition of low-level irritancy can also contribute to the continuation of the dry skin condition through increased epidermal cell turnover. In order to treat dry skin effectively, it is important to reduce the general degree of irritancy in the skin.

Improving the condition of the barrier can reduce the penetration of irritants and reduce low-level inflammation in the skin. This repair process takes time, however, and before barrier repair takes place there is often a lag period; thus it is of value to include in the moisturizer anti-irritants and antioxidants. These agents (vitamin E, vitamin C or botanically derived elements such as extract of chamomile) can act to reduce the irritancy process. In this way, immediate relief can be provided to the consumer during the time that it takes to repair the barrier.

After the barrier has been repaired, antioxidants and anti-irritants make an excellent second line of defense to provide additional protection from other environmental materials that might eventually penetrate.

UV protection

Any product that deals with skin care must also consider UV damage. It is now widely accepted that the majority of skin aging is due primarily to actinic damage. In addition, the increasing incidence of basal and squamous cell carcinoma also emphasizes the need for even better UV protection. Therefore most modern moisturizers contain some degree of UV-B and UV-A protection.

The level of UV protection should be commensurate with the intended use of the product. For most causal exposure an SPF of 6 or 8 should be adequate, since the individual receives little exposure other than walking to or from the car, factory or office. On the other hand, moisturizers used during longer exposure times, such as outdoor sports activities, should contain a minimum of SPF 15 protection in order to insure that very little of the damaging UV-B or UV-A irradiation penetrates into the skin.

Summary

Today, calling a product a 'moisturizer' can mean many things. In some cases, products called moisturizers do the bare minimum of occluding the skin and trapping water. Still others are sophisticated skin care products offering not only moisturization but also a variety of other consumer benefits. The modern moisturizer does more than simply deliver water to the skin. This class of product has become the all-purpose skin conditioning agent that is concerned with barrier repair and protection. It is obviously a key component of any good skin care practice.

REFERENCES

1. Federal Food, Drug, and Cosmetic Act. Title 21, Part 1, Section 201, US Department of Health, Education, and Welfare, Food and Drug Administration. FDC Act and Part 1 Regulations, 1964.
2. Zlotogorski A, Dickstein S, Measurement of skin surface pH. In: *Handbook of Non-Invasive Methods and the Skin* (Serup J, Jemec, GBE, eds). Boca Raton, FL: CRC Press, 1995:223–5.
3. Bechor R, Zlotogorski A, Dikstein S, Effect of soaps and detergents on the pH and casual lipid levels. *J Appl Cosmetol* 1988; **6:** 123.
4. Martin EW, Cook EF (eds), *Remington's Practice of Pharmacy.* Easton, PA: Maek Publishing, 1956:8 and 624.
5. Wilkinson JD, The skin as a chemical barrier. In: *The Physical Nature of the Skin* (Marks RM, Barton SP, Edwards C, eds). MTP Press, 1988:73–8.
6. Pinnagoda J, Tupker RA, Measurement of transepidermal water loss. In: *Handbook of Non-Invasive Methods and the Skin* (Serup J, Jemec GBE, eds). Boca Raton, FL: CRC Press, 1995: 173–8.
7. Kajs TM, Gartstein V, Review of the instrumental assessment of skin: effects of cleansing products. *J Soc Cosmet Chem* 1991; **42:** 249–71.
8. Lévêque JL, Measurement of transepidermal water loss. In: *Cutaneous Investigation in Health and Disease* (Lévêque JL, ed). New York: Marcel Dekker, 1989:135–52.
9. Stuttgen G, Ott A, Flesh U, Measurement of skin microcirculation. In: *Cutaneous Investigation in Health and Disease* (Leveque JL, ed). New York: Marcel Dekker, 1989:359–84.
10. Bircher AJ, Laser Doppler measurement of skin blood flux: variation and validation. In: *Handbook of Non-Invasive Methods and the Skin* (Serup J, Jemec GBE, eds). Boca Raton, FL: CRC Press, 1995.
11. Belcaro G, Nicolaides AN, Laser–Doppler flowmetry: principles of technology and clinical applications. In: *Handbook of Non-Invasive Methods and the Skin* (Serup J, Jemec GBE, eds). Boca Raton, FL: CRC Press, 1995.
12. Muizzuddin N, Marenus K, Maes D, Smith WP, Use of a chromameter in assessing the efficacy of anti-irritants and tanning accelerators. *J Soc Cosmet Chem* 1990; **41:** 369–78.
13. Takiwaki H, Serup J, Measurement of erythema and melanin indices. In: *Handbook of Non-invasive Methods and the Skin* (Serup J, Jemec GBE, eds). Boca Raton, FL: CRC Press, 1995.
14. Maes D, Short J, Turek BA, Reinstein JA, In-vivo measurement of skin softness using the gas bearing electrodynamometer. *Int J Cosmet Sci* 1983; **5:** 189–200.

15. Giudice GJ, Fuchs EV, Vitamin A mediated regulation of keratinocyte differentiation. *Meth Enzymol* 1990; **190:** 18–29.

16. Tannous-Khuri L, Talmage D, Decreased cellular retinol-binding protein expression coincides with the loss of retinol responsiveness in rat epithelial cells. *Exp Cell Res* 1997; **230:** 33–44.

17. Counts DF, Skreko F, McBee J, Wich AG, The effect of retinyl palmitate on skin composition and morphometry. *J Soc Cosmet Chem* 1988; **39:** 235–40.

18. Holick MF, Photobiology, physiology and clinical applications of vitamin D. In: *Physiology, Biochemistry and Molecular Biology of Skin* (Goldsmith LA, ed). New York: Oxford University Press, 1991:942–3.

19. Tomic M, Jiang CK, Connoly D et al, Vitamin D3, its receptor, and regulation of epidermal keratin gene expression. *Epithelial Cell Biol* 1992; **1:** 70–5.

20. Grubauer G, Feingold KR, Elias PM, Transepidermal water loss: the signal for recovery of barrier structure and function. *J Lipid Res* 1990; **30:** 323–33.

21. Ghadially R, Brown BE, Hankley K et al, Decreased epidermal lipid synthesis accounts for altered barrier function in aged mice. *J Invest Dermatol* 1996; **106:** 1064–9.

22. Proksch E, Holleran WM, Menon GK et al, Barrier function regulates epidermal lipid and DNA synthesis. *Br J Dermatol* 1993; **128:** 473–82.

11

Skin care products for normal, dry and greasy skin

David Black, Stéphane Diridollou, Jean-Michel Lagarde, Yvon Gall

INTRODUCTION

The application of products to the skin goes back a long way. Originally, this consisted essentially in the use of makeup and perfumed oils after bathing, with the intention of disguising body odour in the days before soap. Meanwhile, because of the influence of Hippocrates in Greece, there was, in parallel to medicine, the development of new types of products specifically intended for skin care. Owing to lack of knowledge in skin biology, the development of these products was purely empirical, and the situation remained unchanged until quite recently.

Advances in the biochemistry and physiology of the skin have enabled the development of specific products for different skin types. Simultaneous advances in electronics and computing have allowed the development of instruments for measuring certain parameters of the skin. Quantification of these parameters has enabled the evaluation, comparison and hence improvement of the efficacy of skin care products.

THE DIFFERENT TYPES OF SKIN

Normal skin

Normal skin is defined as having no visible lesions or sensations of discomfort. It results from an equilibrium of various continuous biological processes (including keratinization, desquamation, water loss, sebum secretion and sweating), which create a harmoniously balanced state of suppleness, elasticity and colour. 'Normal' skin is defined by functional criteria. However, it is important to realize the heterogeneity that exists in so-called normal skin. For example, in a given individual with 'normal' skin the structure and physiology of the latter will differ from one part of the body to another, and will change with time.

Variation with age[1–10]

During aging, the skin undergoes certain changes arising from external causes (in particular UV radiation) as well as the general aging process that affects the entire organism. These phenomena affect the dermis in particular. These age-related skin changes have recently been demonstrated using in vivo exploratory techniques, in particular high-frequency ultrasound.

Our findings using this technique agree

with those in the literature. Firstly, an onset in the reduction of dermal thickness is observed for both sexes at the age of 50. Secondly, there is an echolucent band in the papillary dermis, which increases in homogeneity with age. Some authors have suggested that this structure may correspond to an amorphous water–glycosaminoglycans mixture that progressively replaces deteriorated fine collagen bundles. Data acquired from UV-exposed and protected anatomical sites show this echolucent band to be present on both, but to be more pronounced on the photoexposed sites. Thus it would seem to be indicative of both solar elastosis and chronological aging.[2]

According to certain authors, these changes with age are manifested as changes in chemical structure, the quality and quantity of structural proteins, proteoglycans and hyaluronic acid.[7] For example, type III collagen, which represents a significant proportion of embryonic collagen content, is partly replaced by type I collagen during early development. Also, during adult life, dermal collagen content (all types) progressively decreases, correlating with a reduction in skin thickness.[8] A simultaneous decrease in the amount of proteoglycans and hyaluronic acid is also seen.[7]

These phenomena, which are markedly aggravated by solar (UV) exposure, are for the most part the root cause of the change in the skin's mechanical properties seen with aging, one aspect of which is the appearance of wrinkles. In fact, the flaccid, wrinkled appearance of aged skin coincides with a deterioration in its mechanical properties. In a study carried out on the inner forearms of 210 subjects aged 0.5–95 years, we have shown the following specific changes in the skin's mechanical properties:[1]

- a linear decrease in suppleness with age;
- increasing skin tension up to adolescence, followed by a more rapid decrease in tension with age;
- increasingly less elasticity from puberty.

This indicates that the skin, when mechanically stressed, takes longer to return to its initial state in older subjects than younger subjects.[1]

Elsewhere, hormonal changes occurring during adolescence and then aging account for the respective increases in sebum secretion seen in puberty, then its progressive decrease during adult life, declining considerably in postmenopausal women.[9] With aging, a decrease in the rate of corneocyte desquamation is also seen.[10]

Variation with anatomical site

In the same individual, certain characteristics of the skin show variation with anatomical site. This is particularly true for sebaceous glands, whose number per unit area of skin is particularly high in the upper part of the body (forehead $> 300/cm^2$; chest $60/cm^2$; upper back $80/cm^2$).[7] Skin permeability is another parameter whose heterogeneity has been studied frequently with respect to body site. The data vary according to the substances used, but one can quote the following examples:[11]

- for hydrocortisone, palm < forearm < scalp = axilla < forehead < scrotum;
- for the insecticide parathion, forearm < palm < scalp < forehead < axilla < scrotum.

Corneocyte exfoliation rates also vary with body site, being higher on the forearm and back than on the upper arm and abdomen.[10] These few examples illustrate the fact that the concept of normal skin tends to gloss over the reality of a tissue that is extremely heterogeneous, and ill-defined anatomically, biochemically and physiologically. Furthermore, it undergoes subtle but definite changes from one body site to another, with age, and from greasy to dry skin states, this latter point being covered in the next section.

Greasy skin

Greasy skin appears at puberty. It involves only the upper part of the body, where greater numbers of sebaceous glands are found. Clinically, greasy skin can be sub-divided into two main types, to which one can also add the case of scalp seborrhoea.[12]

Simple greasy skin

This type of skin is particularly common in adolescents and young adults. It is character-ized by skin thickening and an increase in sebaceous secretion, giving the face a shiny appearance, especially on the nose and fore-head. In extreme cases, the follicular ducts are often dilated (kerosis). However, they can also be plugged by minuscule cornified spicules, which protrude and give a sensation of roughness to the touch. Mixed skin consti-tutes a frequent variant of this type of skin. It is characterized on the face by the association of seborrhoeic plaques (thickened skin with a shiny aspect and slightly marked kerosis), with plaques of dry skin (epidermal atrophy and slight desquamation).

Clinically greasy skin

The associated complications of greasy skin consist of two types.

Acne

This is a frequent complication, but is not necessarily due to seborrhoea. It can be due to the following:[12,13]

- disruption of androgen metabolism, modi-fying its bioavailability and leading to ele-vated levels of circulating free testosterone; increase in the level of 5-α reductase in the sebaceous glands (responsible for conver-sion of free testosterone to an active metabolite, dihydrotestosterone, which binds to a cytosolic receptor, penetrating the nucleus and activating mRNA);
- proliferation of *Propionibacterium acnes* (*P. acnes*), responsible for an inflammatory reaction due to the diffusion of chemotac-tic factors in the dermis, as well as free fatty

acids arising from enzymatic hydrolysis of sebum triglycerides;
- problems in keratinization (hyperkerato-sis), responsible for sebum retention, and also implicated in the irritant action of free fatty acids produced by *P. acnes*.

Acne is characterized by the presence of open comedones (blackheads) and closed comedones (microcysts).

The inflammation seen with acne may arise from several causes:

- infection by *P. acnes* which produces free fatty acids by enzymatic hydrolysis of trigly-cerides;
- irritation of the dermis by keratin and free fatty acids released by comedones;
- immune reactions with sensitization of acne subjects to *Propionibacterium* antigens.

Seborrhoeic dermatitis

This is also a frequent problem of seborrhoeic skin, the causes of which are still unknown but may include *Pityrosporum* yeasts (mainly *P. ovale*), chemical agents (detergents) and, most of all, nervous factors (stress, etc.). It is characterized by the presence of erythe-matosquamous plaques, made up of greasy squames, localized mainly on the hairline and eyebrows, nasal folds, chin and presternal region. The scalp is often affected, with the formation of crusty plaques covering the bases of the hair shafts. These lesions are often slightly pruritic.

Seborrhoea of the scalp[9,14]

This shows the same features as skin sebor-rhea – but, with the added effect of sebum overproduction, the hair appears drab and greasy. It is often associated with facial sebor-rhea, but this is not always the case. When it is only mild, it is considered as simple greasy skin. On the other hand, severe cases are con-sidered as seborrhoeic dermatitis, being typi-fied by abundant greasy scales corresponding to excessive desquamation, with large aggre-gates often accompanied by pruritis.

Associated with this there is often a significant amount of *P. ovale*, whose precise role remains controversial since its presence could be the cause of the increase in desquamation or may only be consequential to it.

Dry skin

Dry skin is characterized by a sensation of tightness, with the skin feeling rough and scaly and appearing cracked. It is usually synonymous with a decrease in stratum corneum barrier function, shown by an increase in the passive rate of transepidermal water loss (TEWL).

Two principal factors may be involved in this phenomenon:

- dehydration of the stratum corneum – once its water content falls below 10%, its plasticity is greatly reduced;
- keratinization problems, leading to changes in structure or corneocyte cohesion, which in turn could account for abnormal cutaneous metabolism.

Two types of dry skin can be distinguished.[15]

Acquired dry skin

This may arise from normal, or sometimes even greasy, skin, which is rendered temporarily and locally dry by external factors, including

- solar (UV) radiation;
- exposure to extremes of climate: cold, heat, wind, dryness;
- exposure to chemicals (detergents, solvents);
- various therapeutic measures (e.g. retinoids).

Constitutional dry skin

This type includes many varieties of dry skin, of which the most severe form is pathological.

Non-pathological skin

Constitutional dry skin of this type is also affected by the external factors already mentioned.

Fragile skin – This is intermediate between dry and normal skin, and is most often found on women or those people with delicate, fine-grained skin. Often there is erythema or rosacea, and a sensitivity to external agents.

Senile skin – Dryness accounts for one of the properties of senile skin, within which changes are manifested at all levels.

Minor dry skin (xerosis vulgaris) – Probably of genetic origin, this is found frequently in women, usually those with a pale phototype. Xerosis affects in particular, the face, backs of hands, and limbs.

Pathological skin[16]

The ichthyoses – The ichthyoses result from a genetic defect in keratinization, which manifests itself as abnormal desquamation, altering the barrier function. Lesser forms of this disease resemble ichthyosis vulgaris.

Dry skin of atopic dermatitis – Atopic dermatitis is associated with a genetic defect in the metabolism of essential fatty acids (lack of δ-6 desaturase). It presents as a continuous diffuse xerosis, with the appearance of inflamed, plaque-like, pruritic lesions.

METHODS FOR EVALUATING SKIN CHARACTERISTICS (BIOENGINEERING)

The main parameters characteristic of different skin types that can be used to evaluate product efficacy are those related to skin surface morphology, stratum corneum hydration and sebum secretion. Because of parameter variation between different anatomical zones on the same subject and, a fortiori, between different subjects, these techniques are used mainly to measure the change in a parameter with time, on the same zone. For example, a comparison can be made between the initial state (pre-treatment) and the final state (post-treatment).

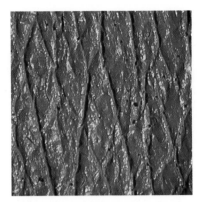

Figure 11.1 Close-up view of silicone rubber replica used for subsequent analysis of relief.

Study of skin surface morphology

Skin surface relief [17]

The principle of this method is the three-dimensional reconstruction of the skin surface using sufficient magnification to allow the observation of the microrelief. This reconstruction enables certain roughness parameters to be measured, as defined originally by the metallurgical industry, giving a quantitative analysis of relief (Figure 11.1). In practice, the first step involves replicating the skin surface by means of silicone rubber polymers. Various techniques can be used for the subsequent analysis of its relief. The first technique used is directly adapted from the metallurgical sciences, and consists in traversing a positive replica along its length (x axis) with a contact stylus. The vertical displacement of the stylus, corresponding to skin relief or height (z axis), is amplified and recorded. The profile obtained is thus the exact representation, albeit magnified, of the skin surface relief along a given axis. This allows the calculation of different roughness parameters (including area under the curve, curve length, and peak and valley height). If this process is repeated for numerous parallel scans (x axis) equidistant from each other (y axis), the scanned skin surface can be reconstructed and its average characteristics determined.

The advantage of this technique is that it gives absolute data. The disadvantages are mainly those of complexity due to the multi-step procedure. Recent improvements have replaced the mechanical scanning with optical scanning by laser beams, thus reducing operating time. However, being an extremely sophisticated technique, its availability is limited. Another approach involves digitization of an image of the replica, when obliquely illuminated with incident light at an angle of 45°. A video camera coupled with a computer shows a digital image of the skin replica. Reconstruction of the relief from each scan line is made indirectly using the grey-level intensity of each point, which, by applying appropriate algorithms, is used to calculate the slope of the feature, thus the z-axis information. From these profile reconstructions, parameters analogous to those of mechanical profilometry can be calculated. Thus this technique allows rapid measurement of skin surface relief without the need for cumbersome equipment. However, it only provides a reconstruction and not an exact image of the surface relief (for example, smaller features may be overshadowed by larger ones, and thus omitted from the analysis). An example of three-dimensional reconstruction obtained using this method is given in Figure 11.2.

Skin surface relief studies can demonstrate changes in the amount of wrinkling and in the state of hydration of the stratum corneum. An increase in hydration amounts to an increase in turgour, seen as attenuation of the relief.

Skin surface biopsies [18]

As its name implies, a skin surface biopsy is a sample of the superficial stratum corneum. It is a simple, non-invasive and painless

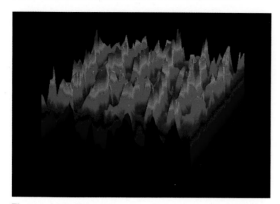

Figure 11.2 Three-dimensional reconstruction of skin surface relief from a silicon rubber replica, using an optical scanning technique.

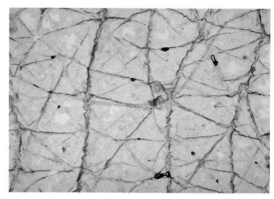

Figure 11.3 Stained skin surface biopsy from a normal individual, showing skin furrows, hairs and pilosebaceous orifices (original magnification ×200).

technique, which can be done in two ways. The first uses cyanoacrylate glue spread onto a flexible plastic slide, which is applied firmly to the skin for about 30 seconds. Removal of this slide after this time detaches about 3–5 layers of corneocytes (Figure 11.3). The second method uses small, transparent adhesive discs (D-Squames), which remove the superficial corneocytes. Whatever the technique used, the samples can be subsequently stained and viewed with a microscope.

The images obtained can illustrate various states of xerosis characterized by the roughness and abnormal desquamation of the skin surface. Using the cyanoacrylate technique, a xerosis classification has been established, consisting of five grades (Figure 11.4). Samples obtained with the adhesive film (D-Squame), allows quantitative assessment of xerosis:

- Corneocytes thus obtained are stained, and the intensity of stain measured (Chromameter, Minolta).
- More precise information regarding desquamation (number, thickness, size of squames, texture of the samples, mean opti-

cal density) can also be obtained directly and automatically by image analysis of D-Squames.[19] These parameters highlight the differences between a desquamation

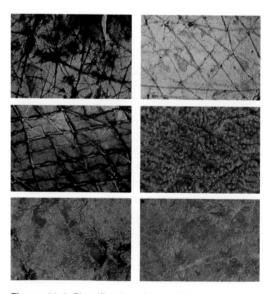

Figure 11.4 Classification of xerosis from skin surface biopsies. (After Pierard et al.[18])

consisting of thin homogenous corneocyte layers, and a thick, clustered, non-homogenous desquamation, with similar optical densities but dramatically different textures and squame numbers.

Finally, the superposition of a Sebutape over a skin biopsy taken from the same site allows the determination of the ratio of active to quiescent follicles.

Skin hydration measurements[20]

Objective assessment of skin (stratum corneum, SC) hydration remains the preoccupation of most cosmetic scientists and dermatologists. The methods and techniques used vary in complexity and have been fully described elsewhere.[20] No technique as yet can directly measure in vivo the mass of water in terms of dry weight of SC, but some are closer to others in estimating this, and are broadly split into categories of direct and indirect methods. Direct methods are those based on spectroscopy such as Fourier-transform infrared (FTIR) spectroscopy and nuclear magnetic resonance (NMR) spectroscopy, while indirect techniques involve mainly mechanical and electrical approaches. Another technique that is often associated with those previously mentioned is that entailing the direct measurement of water loss from the skin's surface, termed transepidermal water loss (TEWL). With this technique, measurement of SC hydration per se is not possible, but useful information on its hygroscopic potential and barrier properties may be obtained.

Electrical measurements[21,22]

The dielectric constants of keratin and epidermal lipids are very small compared with that of water. Therefore the dielectric constant of the stratum corneum is principally determined by its level of hydration: the greater the water content, the larger the dielectric constant. The corneometer[21] is an apparatus with a probe that is placed in contact with the skin. The probe acts as a capacitor, in which the dielectric material is the skin on which it is applied. The capacitance thus measured is proportional to the dielectric constant of the skin, and varies according to its state of hydration. The device measures capacitance in arbitrary units, which in theory are proportional to stratum corneum water content. On the forearm the following data are obtained:[22]

- <75:   dehydrated skin
- 75–90: skin with a tendency to dehydration
- >90:   normal skin

In practice, owing to the absence of a physical significance of this unit of measurement, this technique is confined to the measurement of variation in SC hydration between initial and final states (before and after). The advantage of this device is its simplicity of operation and reproducibility. Its main disadvantage is the artefactual increase in the dielectric constant of the skin due to the presence of electrolytes.

Technical improvements in the corneometer have resulted in the availability of the new CM 825 version[21] (Courage & Khazaka, Germany).

Another device used for measuring the electrical properties of the skin with regard to its hydration, is the skin surface hygrometer[23,24] (Skicon 200; IBS Ltd Japan). This uses a fixed frequency (3.5 MHz) for measuring skin conductance, unlike the corneometer, which uses a multiple frequency range of 40–75 kHz. Other multiple-frequency devices have been developed more recently: the Dermal Phase Meter[25] (DPM, Nova Technology Corporation, USA) and the SCIM[26] (ServoMed, Sweden). These use higher frequency ranges that are believed to largely negate the effects of variables such as sweat gland activity and skin temperature, which confound the true hydration state of the actual SC.

For more information on skin electrical

measurements the reader is referred to a comprehensive review by Salter.[27]

Fourier-transform infrared spectroscopy[28,29]

Groups of molecules with a dipolar structure will vibrate (i.e. undergo extension or deformation) under suitable excitation. These vibrations are specific for certain frequencies, and for certain types of molecule, and correspond to a particular excitation energy level. Since these levels are found in a range of excitation energies provided by infrared (IR) photons, the exposure of dipolar groups to IR radiation will cause a certain frequency of vibration corresponding to the photon energy absorbed. Thus the IR transmission spectrum gives bands of absorption centred on the wavelengths of absorbed photons (since photon energy is defined by its wavelength). Since the area of these bands (peaks) is proportional to the concentration of dipolar groups, IR spectroscopy can identify and quantify them at the same time.

Determination of IR absorption spectra on the skin surface in vivo has been made possible by the development of reflectance IR spectroscopy. A beam of polychromatic IR light is shone through a crystal (zinc or germanium selenide) applied to the skin surface. The crystal produces a series of reflections (between 5 and 20, depending on type) between its upper surface and that of the skin, after which the light beam is relayed back to the spectrophotometer. At each reflection on the skin, the beam penetrates a short distance into the stratum corneum, where it is absorbed. On leaving the crystal, the reflected beam has thus undergone as many reflections as absorptions. Fourier transformation of this reflected beam gives the IR spectrum with bands of absorption in the stratum corneum. Among these bands, there are two that are used to evaluate hydration. These relate to amide and protein properties (Figure 11.5):

• The 1645 cm^{-1} band, corresponding to the

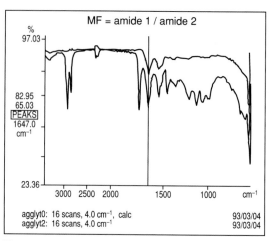

Figure 11.5 Infrared transmission/adsorption curve obtained from skin in vivo, showing peaks corresponding to amides I and II.

carbonyl ($C=O$) absorption band of the amides, I. This band is peculiar in being partially overlapped by a band of protein associated water, situated at 1640 cm^{-1}. Thus it will change according to protein water content in the stratum corneum.

• The 1545 cm^{-1} band corresponding to the absorption by $C-N$ groups of amides, II. In contrast with the 1645 cm^{-1} band, this band is not influenced by the presence of water. Thus it serves as a reference band whose vibrational properties are similar to those previously described.

The ratio of the areas of these two bands (peaks) provides a relative measure of stratum corneum water content. The main interest in this technique comes from the specific measurement of water by direct means. It is limited in the fact that these absorption bands may be obscured by neighbouring bands arising from the application of certain products. Furthermore, owing to weak IR beam penetration (5–20 μm), the data obtained pertain only to the superficial stratum corneum.

Measurement of transepidermal water loss [22,30]

Measurement of transepidermal water loss (TEWL) determines the continual flux of water vapour diffusing across the stratum corneum. Therefore, strictly speaking, it does not measure skin hydration, but does allow the evaluation of the efficacy of hydrating products whose mode of action relies on occlusivity: after evaporation of the water contained in the product, the TEWL will fall. TEWL is measured using an evaporimeter (Figure 11.6). This device consists of a probe that measures the partial water vapour pressure at two points respectively 3 and 9 mm above the skin surface, with the aid of two pairs of humidity transducers and thermistors. The difference in partial water vapour pressure between these two points enables the rate of evaporation to be calculated and displayed by the device as g/m^2 per hour. Normal TEWL values are between 2 and 5 g/m^2 per hour. They can reach values of 90–100 g/m^2 per hour after skin stripping or in the case of atopic lesions.

Owing to the non-occlusive nature of TEWL measurement, the technique lends itself to dynamic SC hydration measurement using the sorption/desorption test (SDT). This was first described by Tagami using an electrical conductance measuring device.[31] In contrast to the electrical conductance and capacitance methods, the TEWL approach has the advantage that continuous monitoring of the desorption curve is possible, as opposed to data acquisition using longer time intervals. However, the main disadvantage of the TEWL method is its more complex utilization and sensitivity to fluctuations in ambient conditions. Whatever the technique employed, the sorption/desorption curve can be quantified, giving simple parameters of SC hygroscopicity and water-holding capacity, and as such appears more informative than single-point measurements.[32,33]

An adaptation of this method for use with the simpler electrical capacitance devices has been reported, which exploits their occlusive mode of skin hydration measurement. This is called the moisture accumulation test (MAT). In a similar way to the SDT, the curve of water absorption (as opposed to desorption), while occluded by the probe head, can be quantified in terms of dynamic SC hydration.[33–35]

Mechanical measurements [3,36]

Based on the assumption that a hydrated SC is more supple than a dehydrated one, various attempts have been made to characterize this property using mechanical techniques. Perhaps the most reliable technique (and also the only one commercially available) is that based on torsional analysis[36] (Dermal Torque meter, Diastron Ltd, UK). Based on the previously described Twistometer,[3] the principle of the technique involves the stepwise application and removal of a constant torque to the skin of approximately 10 mN m. This is done by attaching a rotating central disc and fixed concentric guard ring to the skin using double-sided adhesive tape. Using different guard-ring sizes, the disc–guard-ring gap can be varied from 1 to 5 mm, thus altering the surface area of skin under test. The assumption is that by reducing this area, angular deformation will be more limited, implying shallower 'depth' of tissue involvement, i.e.

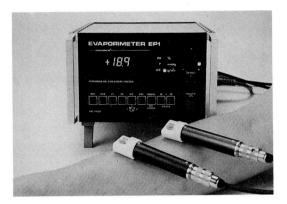

Figure 11.6 The evaporimeter.

proportionally more SC and epidermis than dermis.

Subsequent analysis of the angular deformation-against-time curves allows the quantification of the viscoelastic properties of the skin. This varies in complexity from simple extrapolation of indices[3] to curve-fitting using sophisticated models that give parameters relating more directly to skin structure and physiology.[36]

Nuclear magnetic resonance[37–40]

Since its initial intended use for chemical analysis, the technique of nuclear magnetic resonance (NMR) has revolutionized medical imaging in the 1980s. In the last five years, it has been adapted and applied to the in vivo exploration of skin.

The principle of this technique is based on the gyromagnetic properties of atomic nuclei (spin or magnetic moment). When a sample is placed in an intense magnetic field, the resulting nuclear spin will be aligned with the field axis. The nuclei are then excited by a radiofrequency wave, causing vibration or resonance perpendicular to the field axis. When the excitation ceases, the induced spin progressively returns to a state of equilibrium. This return or relaxation is the NMR signal, which is used as the parameter for characterizing the atomic and molecular properties of the sample in question.

The NMR signal may be processed to give the spectrum of resonance (magnetic resonance spectroscopy, MRS), or an image (magnetic resonance imaging, MRI).

With MRI, each point on the image corresponds to a certain signal intensity arising from a given small volume of tissue (Figure 11.7). This intensity depends on the com-

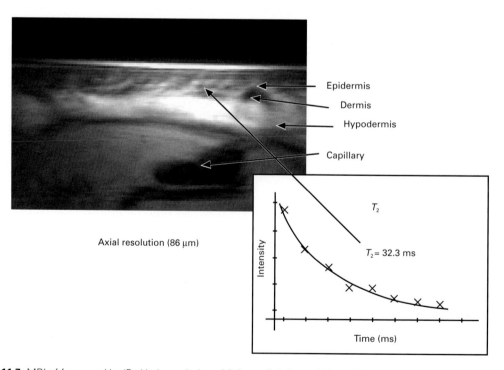

Axial resolution (86 µm)

Epidermis
Dermis
Hypodermis
Capillary

T_2
$T_2 = 32.3$ ms
Intensity
Time (ms)

Figure 11.7 MRI of forearm skin. (By kind permission of P Beau, SpinControl, Tours, France.)

bined effect of three physical parameters that are characteristic of the tissue being studied. These are the density of free protons and their longitudinal (T_1) and transverse (T_2) relaxation times. These two parameters depend on the physicochemical properties of the tissue.

The advantage of MRI over other medical imaging techniques like radiography and ultrasound is thus one of combined tissue imaging and physicochemical characterization (e.g. water content). These latter two techniques only give information on tissue density and mechanical interface differences respectively.

Current NMR technology, used for its intended purpose of large-scale medical imaging, is highly sophisticated. Needless to say, among the typical devices available, none are suitably adapted for skin imaging, which requires a minimum resolution of 100 µm since the skin thickness varies from approximately 0.5 to 3 mm.

Bittoun et al[37] have developed a micro-imaging probe that can be used with a whole-body NMR scanner, giving images with an axial resolution of 70 µm. The high-resolution images obtained clearly differentiate the epidermis, dermis and hypodermis from various anatomical regions. From such images, a tentative approach to measuring skin hydration in young and old subjects has been made using proton-density data, which correlate with free (unbound) water content.[38] Significant differences in this water content in the superficial dermis were observed between these two populations. The same authors also showed that, by measuring mobile proton density, changes in the hydration of the stratum corneum of the heel could be observed.[39]

Another way of measuring skin hydration by MRI has been reported by Franconi et al.[40] They used a BIOSPEC imager (Bruker), which, when coupled with the use of a specific probe and image acquisition sequence, resulted in images of forearm skin with an axial resolution of 86 µm (Figure 11.7). In the same study, the relaxation time T_2 was measured at the epidermal level, and showed an increase following the application of a hydrating cream. Since this parameter is directly dependent on free water content, its increase signifies an improvement in epidermal hydration. Subsequent monitoring of this parameter with time gives important information on the pharmacokinetic properties of the test product.

Despite its cost and complexity, NMR shows great future potential for skin biology research. Such applications may include measurements of hydration (free and bound water), aging and the effects of solar irradiation.

Current developments in spectroscopic imaging (e.g. water proton imaging), or localized spectroscopy, should enable the elucidation of even greater detail when studying the skin, particularly hydration.

Sebum measurement[41,42]

Measurement of sebum refers principally to the following:

- quantitation of the amount of sebum on the skin surface, which is roughly constant with time and body site for a given individual; this value is known as the 'casual level';
- determination of the refatting or sebum excretion rate (SER) on the skin surface, after removal of surface sebum under controlled conditions;
- counts of active sebaceous follicles in relation to passive ones.

Earlier techniques of sebum quantitation relied on rather impractical methods of sampling by bentonite clay or cigarette papers, with subsequent solvent extraction, before being analysed chemically or gravimetrically. Fortunately, these have been largely superseded by more recent techniques that are rapid and simple. These rely on optical measurements of an opalescent film, which is rendered transparent by sebum lipids.

The Sebumeter

The Sebumeter (Courage and Khazaka, Cologne) incorporates a probe that presses a plastic opalescent film on the skin (renewed each time) for a certain time. The sebum lipids are adsorbed on this film, and render it transparent. Next the probe is inserted into the Sebumeter, which shines a light beam onto the film. A reflective metal plate behind the film reflects the light back, passing a second time through the film, before entering a photomultiplier. The greater the film transparency, the greater the amount of light reflected. Thus the ratio of reflected to incident light, which is measured, increases proportionally to the quantity of sebum sampled. Since each application of the probe is preceded by a basal measurement with unused tape, the device automatically determines the increase in film transparency as a function of skin surface sebum. The result is shown as a lipid index.

The Lipometer

The Lipometer (L-Oréal, Paris) functions in a similar way to the Sebumeter. Its principal differences are:

- the plastic film is replaced by a ground-glass disc mounted on a dynamometer to standardize the application pressure;
- a series of standard calibrated values are used to convert readings into absolute data (e.g. µg lipid/cm^2).

Sebutape

Sebutape (Cuderm Corp., Dallas) is a film of hydrophobic microporous polymer, with an adhesive backing for skin attachment. After the skin is cleansed, the tape is applied for a fixed time, normally 20–30 minutes. When sebum is secreted from the follicles, the lipids cross the adhesive layer and fill the micropores of the film, creating a small transparent spot in contrast to the white, opaque background of the polymer. The size (area) of the spot is proportional to follicular excretion activity. Sebutape can thus evaluate the amount of sebum excreted by individual follicles. Morphometric study of Sebutapes by image analysis allows automatic counting of spots (number of active follicles), and also measurement of surface area (amount of sebum secreted).[43] Therefore, with these three techniques, the objectives stated at the beginning of this section can be satisfied. Application of the Sebumeter or Lipometer on unwashed skin allows measurement of the casual level of sebum. Four successive samples on the same site are taken to guarantee complete sebum removal.

Data for the forehead using the Lipometer are on average

- between 100 and 200 µg/cm^2 for normal skin
- >500 µg/cm^2 for greasy skin
- <50 µg/cm^2 in hyposeborrhoeic cases

Data given for the Sebumeter on the forehead are between 60 and 80 for normal skin. Without units, the data are difficult to interpret; thus the Sebumeter is mainly used for comparative studies.

The Sebumeter, Lipometer and Sebutape can be used to determine the SER after a certain time following degreasing of the skin.

With Sebutape, the quantity of sebum secreted is expressed by the total area of spots. As for the Sebumeter, this is only possible on a comparative basis. However, the Sebutape gives an idea of the heterogeneity of individual follicular secretion. For normal skin, SER varies between 0.6 and 2 µg/cm^2 per minute. It is greatly affected by external conditions, in as much that an increase in temperature of 1°C will lead to a 10% increase in SER. It has been shown that repeated measurements of sebum on the same site, using Sebutape, can be made without removing the tape, by means of colorimetric measurements in situ with a Minolta Chromameter.[44] This avoids artefacts that may arise from multisampling.

The combined use of Sebutape and the skin surface biopsy (SSB) on the same site can distinguish (and thus quantify) active sebaceous follicles visible only on Sebutape, and quiescent follicles visible only on the SSB.[18]

SKIN CARE PRODUCTS

Care of normal skin[45]

Normal skin does not require any modification, since it is already well balanced with respect to its physiological and mechanical integrity. Nevertheless, this balance can be relatively unstable, and therefore two essential approaches to care of normal skin must be considered:

- maintenance of this balance (*primum non nocere*);
- protection from external injury.

The first aim is a passive one: it is more particularly concerned with products that are not active treatments as such, but may be harmful to the skin (e.g. hygiene products). The second plays more of an active role, involving protective products such as sun creams and to a lesser extent hydrating agents.

Hygiene products

Hygiene products may have compositions potentially hazardous to skin. Whether soaps or shampoos, they all have surfactants allowing dispersion of hydrophobic material (mainly greases) in water.

Surfactants

Surfactants are amphiphilic molecules, characterized by having a polar group (hydrophilic) and a non-polar group (lipophilic). Owing to the presence of the latter, they are only slightly soluble in water. Above a certain concentration, called the critical micellar concentration, they clump together to form a micelle, a kind of aggregate in which all the molecules are orientated in the same way, with

- polar groups facing outwards in contact with water, and
- non-polar groups facing into the micelle.

The lipophilic interior of the micelle allows lipid dissolution. The micelle is thus transformed into a miniscule drop of lipid surrounded by a membrane made up of surfactants, which are anchored in their lipid phase by their lipophilic groups. Because of their double affinity, surfactants are capable of dispersing hydrophobic substances in water, from which arises their cleansing properties. Surfactants are classified according to the structure of their polar groups, since the non-polar groups are made up of aliphatic chains of variable length. Four classes of surfactant can thus be defined:

- *Cationic surfactants* (polar head, positively charged; e.g. quaternary ammonium compounds). Owing to poor tolerance, these compounds are practically no longer used.
- *Anionic surfactants* (polar head, negatively charged; e.g. sodium lauryl sulphate). These are most often used because of good lathering and detergent properties. Some are not well tolerated (sodium lauryl sulphate), but this has been remedied by the formulation of new derivatives (hemisulphosuccinates and isothionates among others).
- *Amphoteric surfactants* (polar head with pH-dependent polarity; e.g. betaines and alkyl amino acids). These are well tolerated and lather well.
- *Non-ionic surfactants* (non-charged polar head; e.g. Tweens, sucrose esters/ethers). These are tolerated best, but have mediocre lathering ability.

Cleansing products: soaps, syndets and shampoos

Soaps are made by hydrolysis of natural triglycerides (oils, tallows and greases), and neutralization of fatty acids released by sodium; thus they are sodium fatty acid salts (anionic surfactants). They are good emulsifiers, having emollient action and increased lathering power. However, two problems are associated with them:

- On the one hand, because of their powerful detergent action, overuse may completely eliminate the protective surface lipid film, which helps maintain the skin's physiological balance, and thus may engender irritation.
- On the other hand, since the saponification process is reversible, some soaps will revert back, by hydrolysis in water, to fatty acid and sodium, resulting in a soap with high pH ($\approx$10). Since skin pH is about 5, use of soaps leads to pH increases in the skin lasting for up to two hours, to which has been attributed a proliferation of microbial flora.[46]

Oily soaps (enriched in glycerol, fatty acids or oils), can leave the skin softer than ordinary soap by avoiding total delipidization of the skin surface, but they suffer from the same pH problem. Syndets, however, only contain synthetic surfactants: mainly mixtures of anionic surfactants (to improve tolerance) and, to a lesser extent, amphoteric surfactants. Their potential lies in the fact that their pH may be adjusted to that of skin. Like the soaps, they can be enriched with oily compounds. To best maintain the skin surface's physiological balance, it is advisable to use syndets rather than soaps for all toilet procedures. This advice is most appropriate in young children, whose skin is more delicate than adult skin. A similar problem is seen with the scalp. The solution to this lies in the use of a frequent-use mild shampoo, consisting mainly of non-ionic surfactants.

Protective products
Photoprotective products
Of all the environmentally noxious stimuli, that of ultraviolet radiation is the most serious, since, as well as aesthetic damage linked to premature skin aging, there is also the risk of cancer. This problem is particularly exacerbated by the current fashion for sunbathing in summer. In winter, skiing can also lead to

high UV exposure. Even though this is limited to the face, it must be borne in mind that there is an increase in UVB intensity with altitude (4% every 300 m), and significant reflection of UV by the snow (87% of incident rays).[47] In this context, photoprotection has an important role for all skin types, including normal skin. The ideal photoprotector must[48]

- effectively absorb noxious radiation (mainly UVB, but also UVA);
- be substantive to the stratum corneum, and be water- and sweat-resistant;
- be stable in daylight and in air, and to heat and water;
- be totally innocuous.

The absorptive properties of a product are defined by its protection factor PF:

$$PF = \frac{\text{MED with photoprotector}}{\text{MED without photoprotector}}$$

where MED is the mean erythemal dose (i.e. the smallest exposure dose that produces a perceptible erythema, expressed in J/cm^2, but corresponding in practice to the duration of exposure to a certain fixed level of radiation). If one knows the time to onset, TO, of erythema in an unprotected individual, and the protection factor PF for the substance in question, then T, the theoretical time during which the said individual can remain exposed before onset of the same intensity of erythema, can be calculated as

$$T = \text{TO} \times \text{PF}$$

Substantivity for the stratum corneum is determined mainly by the excipient, which must be resistant to water while pleasant to use. The photoprotective ability of sun products is determined by two types of substance: chemical filters and physical screens.

Chemical filters[48] – These are synthetic chemical substances with the following properties:

- powerful absorption of UV radiation owing

to the measure of double bonds (and benzene rings in particular;
- relative stability when excited, so the absorbed energy is released slowly.

These filters are formulated with other compounds in order to obtain highly effective products with protection factors varying from 2 to 30. However, as with all products applied to the skin, there is modest diffusion of these filters across the stratum corneum and some percutaneous absorption. This phenomenon may eventually cause some irritation due to the reactive nature of these molecules. Thus they are prone to give rise to unknown degradation by-products, which may be similarly absorbed. Since transcutaneous diffusion of these filters is determined mainly by the excipient, the formulation of this requires much thought to avoid significant changes in the absorption spectra of the filters incorporated.

Physical screens – Physical screens are mineral particles that, instead of absorbing UV rays, reflect them like a mirror. The main type used is ultrafine titanium dioxide (TiO_2), made up of particles of size 20–30 nm.[49] The attraction in using this type of sunscreen is tolerance, since they are inert particles, well tolerated, and not susceptible to percutaneous absorption because of their insolubility. The reduced size of ultrafine particles confers better reflection in the UVB and short UVA wavelengths, and better transparency in the visible wavelengths.

Hydration products

These products are primarily intended to protect the skin against climatic stress: cold, wind and so on. They consist of light oil-in-water emulsions, whose hydrating properties rely on the characteristics described below in the section on care of dry skin.

Care of greasy skin[50]

For greasy skin care, one has to consider whether one is treating simple or complex greasy skin. Hair care will be dealt with separately.

Care of simple greasy skin

Being generally less prone to external stress, simple greasy skin tends to age less quickly than other skin types. Thus it requires less protection, and treatment, if any, is often restricted to that concerning personal hygiene. The essential requirement is of course to reduce excess skin surface sebum without total delipidization. Severe degreasing treatments can lead to an exacerbation of sebaceous secretion, which defeats the desired aim. Facial washing may be carried out with either an oily soap (ordinary soap being too detergent) or a syndet. This must be followed by copious rinsing. In cold weather, the protection afforded by a continuous-aqueous-phase, light emulsion (oil-in-water) suffices. However, the oils used in such preparations must be non-comedogenic.

Care of complex greasy skin

To current personal hygiene practices, one can add treatments that are more dermatological than cosmetic. With acne, secondary effects associated mostly with treatment (such as dryness and irritation) require appropriate cosmetic remedies. Once remission has occurred and the treatment has been stopped, the skin must be considered as simple, greasy skin, with meticulous avoidance of all comedogenic products.

Hygiene[51,52]

In contrast with the case of simple, greasy skin, which is mainly typified by a certain robustness vis-à-vis external agents, in the present case inflammatory reactions render the skin more liable to irritation, and thus more sensitive. Furthermore, most treatments are themselves often irritant. The use of mild cleansing products (oily soaps and syndets) is of much benefit. For women, the use of cleansing milk is advised, with rinsing afterwards. Whatever the product used, energetic rubbing of the skin must be avoided in order to reduce irritation, and the skin must be thoroughly dried.

Acne treatments

Topical treatment[13,53]

- *Benzoyl peroxide* is a powerful oxidizing agent with anti-inflammatory properties deriving from its bactericidal action on *P. acnes*. It also has a certain keratolytic activity, but little effect on sebum production. It is effective in cases of moderate inflammatory acne. Application of this agent in the evening reduces the risks of irritation and photosensitization.
- *Tretinoin* (all-*trans*-retinoic acid or vitamin A acid) is a powerful keratolytic, which increases keratinocyte turnover and reduces intercorneocyte cohesion, facilitating the expulsion of comedones and microcysts. However, it has no anti-seborrhoeic or bactericidal activity. It is effective in microcystic and/or comedonal acne. It is, by and large, an irritant, frequently inducing transitory erythema and desquamation, often associated with burning or itching sensations at the start of treatment. Tretinoin is also a photosensitizer. Since it is teratogenic, in spite of its low percutaneous absorption, pregnancy has been one of its contraindications in some countries.
- Of the *topical antibiotics*, the most frequently used is erythromycin. Its bactericidal action on *P. acnes* results in an anti-inflammatory activity; thus it is effective for inflammatory acne, and poses no problems of tolerance. However, the risk of resistant cutaneous flora developing with prolonged use of topical antibiotics may favour the alternating use of benzoyl peroxide, which has the same activity level as the preferred treatment.
- *Azelaic acid* is a straight-chain dicarboxylic acid, whose mode of action is not yet completely known. It seems to have a keratolytic

activity, as well as a bacteriostatic activity on *P. acnes*. After 4–6 months of treatment, its activity would be the same as that of tretinoin or benzoyl peroxide, but with better tolerance.

- *Topical isotretinoin* is the 13-*cis* isomer of tretinoin, recently put on the French market and available in Europe and the USA. It acts on inflammatory and non-inflammatory lesions by altering follicular keratinization. It has the advantage of being well tolerated.

Systemic treatment[12,54]

- *Isotretinoin* (Roaccutane) is the 13-*cis* isomer of tretinoin, which
  (a) inhibits sebum production via sebaceous gland atrophy;
  (b) regulates keratinization of the pilosebaceous follicle by preventing the formation of keratin plugs;
  (c) has anti-inflammatory properties (inhibition of polymorphonuclear cell chemotaxis) and immunoiodulatory action (stimulation of Langerhans cells and regulatory effects on lymphocytes and macrophages).
- Even though it is very effective, its use must be limited to severe and extensive forms of acne because of its side-effects. The most important of these is its high teratogenicity, which requires women undergoing treatment to use suitable contraception at least one month before the start and one month before the end of the treatment period. Among other side-effects is the frequent occurrence of cheilitis and general skin dryness, requiring the concomitant use of cosmetic hydrating agents (which will be described in the paragraph relating to dry skin care).
- *Anti-androgen hormone therapy* (Diane 35) is obviously reserved for women. This treatment works at the level of sebum production, which is in part under hormonal control. We know already that sebaceous secretion is stimulated by dihydrotestos-

terone (DHT), which results from conversion of testosterone by 5-α reductase. This stimulation allows binding of DHT to cytosolic receptors for penetration into the nucleus and activation of mRNA. The antiandrogenic effect of the product (cyproterone acetate), which is due to competitive inhibition of binding of DHT to target cell cytosolic receptors, slows down the production and excretion of sebum. The moderate activity of this kind of therapy requires a treatment period of at least six months. It is important to check on any previous or current oestrogen therapy received by the patient.

Additional products – The irritant and dehydrational actions of benzoyl peroxide and of tretinoin require the concurrent use of non-greasy and non-comedogenic hydrating cosmetics. These will be described in a later section on dry skin care.

In case of exposure to the sun while using these photosensitizing products, it is advisable to use a total sun-block.

Treatment of seborrheic dermatitis[12,55]

Essentially, this consists of daily treatment, with topical antifungals (topical imidazoles), which act on *Pityrosporum.*

Treatments using products with 5-α reductase inhibitors (acetamide and unsaponifiable plant oils) may also be used to combat seborrhea.

In parallel, treatments for greasy skin will also be used.

Hair care[14,56,57]

Most treatments for hair are cosmetic, in the form of shampoos. However, some commercial medical treatments are available as lotions.

Shampoo treatments

First and foremost, shampoos are used to clean the hair. In the case of scalp seborrhea, frequent shampooing is needed, which is often a cause of irritation. Therefore a mild-based shampoo is required, formulated with anionic surfactants chosen for their high tolerability, such as amphoteric and non-ionic surfactants. Recent trends have seen the exclusive use of polyglycerol non-ionic surfactants, which allow very frequent use.

With regard to their applications, these shampoos are generally divided into two types:

- shampoos for greasy hair;
- anti-dandruff shampoos.

Among the principal ingredients in shampoos for greasy hair are

- plant extracts such as
  - Panama wood (natural pine extracts for reactive seborrhoea)
  - dead nettle (antiseptic and keratolytic properties);
- sulphur-rich amino acids (cysteine, methionine);
- coal tar extracts (for reduction of microbial proliferation);
- vitamins B_6 or PP;
- glycolic derivatives (sebum solvents).

Among the active anti-dandruff ingredients are found the following:

- *Quaternary ammonium compounds* (e.g. benzalkonium chloride), which are cationic surfactants (and thus incompatible with anionic surfactants) having antimicrobial properties. They reduce the production of free fatty acids responsible for the irritating effect of sebum.
- *Zinc pyridine thione*, which was used initially for its anti-*Pityrosporum* activity, but also has an anti-mitotic effect on epidermal cells, which would slow down squame production and corneocyte turnover. It is a well-tolerated and efficacious product, being used in many anti-dandruff shampoos.
- *Tars*, which have antiseptic, antipruritic and keratolytic properties (reduction of corneo-

cyte aggregates). Forms of coal tars used previously have tended to be replaced with tars of plant origin.

Lotions

These are lotions containing antifungals or corticosteroids, such as

- *imidazole derivatives* – antifungals and sometimes antibacterials;
- *corticosteroids*, which inhibit keratinocyte mitosis and possess antipruritic action; they are frequently combined with salicylic acid, which causes scalp stratum corneum to be shed, thus facilitating penetration.

Dry skin care

Treatment of dry skin depends on whether it is of pathological or non-pathological origin. Care of the latter is down to cosmetic science. The former often requires medical intervention (corticosteroids or retinoids), and needs to be accompanied by cosmetic treatment similar to that of non-pathological skin. Because barrier function is altered and/or inflammatory reactions are often associated, this type of skin is always delicate and often sensitive. Thus it requires specific treatment:

- avoidance of harsh washing;
- protection from external agents.

Hygiene products[15,16]

Use of mild surfactants is most important for dry skin, since it is very sensitive. Ordinary soap must therefore be avoided. Only syndets with oily ingredients (fatty acids, glycerol and oils) and very mild surfactants can be recommended. Following this, the skin must be carefully rinsed of all remaining surface detergents (however mild).

Cosmetic care/treatment[15,16]

The aim of this type of treatment is to minimize the extent of the disturbance found in the stratum corneum of dry skin. This includes

- dehydration
- delipidization
- eventual hyperkeratosis (ichthyosis).

Hydration can be done in two ways: either

- by the input of external water, which is retained in the stratum corneum by the addition of humectants; or
- by the slowing down of stratum corneum water loss due to evaporation (reducing TEWL), by means of an occlusive lipid film.

The lipids in the latter can combat the delipidization associated with dry skin, and protect against external agents. Formulation of a hydrating product involves both of these principles, but with different emphasis placed on them depending on the type of skin and conditions of use envisaged. Hydrating agents for dry skin in winter will include humectants, but stress is always placed on a protective occlusive film. The opposite approach will be adopted for the same type of product aimed at summer use, or for a winter product for greasy skin. In the latter case, particular care is taken to avoid the use of comedogenic lipids.

Humectants

These are many and varied.

Natural moisturizing factor (NMF) components – These include hygroscopic and hydrosoluble substances in the stratum corneum, which are most likely enveloped by cell membrane lipids. These substances play an important role in water retention, since it has been shown that their extraction results in a 25% loss in stratum corneum water content and 66% loss in elasticity.[58]

NMF agents include the following:

- *Pyrrolidone carboxylic acid (PCA)* is one of the principal components of NMF (approximately 12%), in the form of sodium or potassium salts. It is synthesized from glutamic acid in the epidermis. It has a hydrating effect at concentrations of 3–5%.

- *Urea* represents 7% of the NMF. It hydrates at concentrations of less than 10%. At concentrations over this, it is keratolytic. However, it is a substance that may not be well tolerated, even in low concentrations, on the delicate skin of young children, or on the face because of stinging.
- *Lactic acid* is present as sodium lactate in the NMF, accounting for 12% of its content. As a humectant, it is used at concentrations between 5% and 10%. It is part of the α-hydroxy acid family.

Polyols – These consist of small molecules in which numerous hydroxyl groups (hydrophilic) confer strong hygroscopicity. The following are principally used:

- *glycerol*, which has excellent hydrating ability;
- *sorbitol*, with moderate hydrating ability;
- *propylene gylcol*, which has good hydrating ability at low concentrations (<10%) and keratolytic activity at high concentrations (>40%).

Macromolecules – Certain macromolecules of biological origin are incorporated in hydrating products, owing to their high content of hydrophilic groups. Because of their large size, these molecules cannot penetrate the stratum corneum, but form a hygroscopic, semipermeable surface film. This category includes the following:

- *Glycosaminoglycans* are found in the ground substance of all connective tissue (dermis, cartilage), in which they form hydrated gels. This class includes hyaluronic acid and chondroitin sulphate, which are polysaccharides. The large number of hydroxyl groups that they possess allows considerable water sorption and retention.
- *Collagen and elastin* are the two main structural proteins of the connective tissue (including the dermis). The hygroscopic property of collagen enables it to form gels with water. Further hydrolysis turns it into gelatin. These proteins are generally used in denatured or hydrolysed form.
- *DNA* has hygroscopic properties derived from its large numbers of phosphate groups. It is used in a denatured and partially hydrolysed form in cosmetology.

Liposomes – These are small vesicles (50–500 nm in diameter), surrounded by one or several phospholipid bilayer membranes, similar to biological membranes. The interior of these vesicles, like the external medium in which it is suspended, is aqueous. In a particular category of liposomes, called the 'niosomes', the phospholipids are replaced by synthetic, non-ionic amphiphilic lipids. Originally developed by the pharmaceutical industry as medicinal vectors, they have been found to have great potential in cosmetology because of their high affinity for the stratum corneum and their increased hydrating power. Liposomes containing ^{14}C-labelled phospholipids have been applied to human skin in vitro.[59] Thirty minutes after application, the amounts found were as follows:

- stratum corneum   1013.6 μM
- epidermis   3.5 μM
- dermis   0.91 μM

Thus it can be seen that the phospholipids are found mainly in the stratum corneum, in which a significant concentration gradient has been observed, decreasing towards the deeper layers.

Another study using human volunteers has shown that twice-daily application of liposomes rich in phosphatidylcholine causes an increase in the hydration of the stratum corneum (measured with a corneometer), reaching a plateau after five days of treatment.[60] These properties could be linked to the similarity between liposome membranes and the bilayer structure of lipids of the stratum corneum intercorneocyte cement. Further evidence of this link can be seen in the case of delipidization of the skin, which removes the lipid bilayer structures.

Application of non-ionic liposomes to this delipidized skin has resulted in the observation of bilayer structures that closely resemble those of intact skin.[61]

Filmogenic products[15]

These are substances making up the oily phase of emulsions. After evaporation of the water in the aqueous phase, they form a more or less occlusive film on the skin surface, thus reducing TEWL. Water-in-oil emulsions, which are the oiliest type, are generally the most occlusive. The occlusive properties of oil-in-water emulsions depend on the type and amount of oils used. New possibilities in filmogenic products may result from the formulation of new types such as triple emulsions.[62] These are emulsions made in two stages, and include three distinct phases:

- emulsions of the O/W/O type are made up of oil-in-water emulsions, themselves emulsified in oil;
- emulsions of the W/O/W type are made up of water-in-oil emulsions, themselves emulsified in water.

These emulsions may have superior hydrating properties to ordinary emulsions. The following filmogenic products are among those used for the oily phase of cosmetic emulsions:

- *hydrocarbons:* vaseline, paraffin, perhydrosqualene;
- *silicones*;
- *natural oils:* plant or animal (oils rich in polyunsaturated fatty acids will be dealt with in detail below);
- *fatty alcohols:* cetyl, stearic, palmitic;
- *waxes:* these are fatty acid esters and long-chain alcohols;
- *lanolin:* secreted by sebaceous glands of the sheep, this is a complex mixture of esters, polyesters, 33 high-molecular-weight alcohols and 36 fatty acids – it has the combined properties of occlusivity and humectance, and can be mixed with up to twice its weight of water without separation.

Oils rich in polyunsaturated fatty acids[16]

Oils rich in polunsaturated fatty acids (PUFAs) occupy a particular place in cosmetology. As with other oils, they are occlusive, but their potential lies in their high PUFA content. PUFAs are long-chain fatty acids, unsaturated at ω-3 or ω-6, of which some are classed among the essential fatty acids (EFAs). The precursor of ω-6 fatty acids is linoleic acid (C 18 : 2 ω-6), which is an EFA. This itself is the precursor to two other EFAS: γ-linoleic acid (C20 : 3 ω-6) and arachidonic acid (C20 : 4 ω-6), which themselves are the respective precursors of prostaglandins PG_1 and PG_2. The precursor of ω-3 fatty acids is α-linolenic acid (C 18 : 3 ω-3). This gives rise to eicosapentaenoic acid (C20 : 5 ω-3), itself the precursor to prostaglandin-3 synthesis.

These PUFAs are found in large quantities in certain animal oils (fish oil) and plants (evening primrose, borage, grape seed). They are involved in several important physiological functions.

- They play a role in the metabolism of prostaglandins and leukotrienes, which are mediators of inflammation and regulators of keratinization.
- Linoleic acid is present systemically in six types of ceramides in man. The ceramides account for 40% of intercellular lipids. They are the origin of lamellar structures found in the intercorneocyte spaces, which play a significant role in barrier function and thus the maintenance of stratum corneum hydration. It has been shown that EFA deficiency is linked to xerosis: in the hairless rat, dietary lack of linoleic acid induces increased TEWL, which can be reduced by topical linoleic acid application.[63] In humans, EFA deficiency may result from enzymatic malfunction of δ-6 desaturase, which converts linoleic acid to γ-linolenic acid.

Keratolytic substances

These are used for treatment of hyperkeratosis, which is frequently associated with xerosis (ichthyosis). The principal keratolytic substances currently used are as follows.

α-Hydroxy acids[16] – These are organic acids, and include lactic, glycolic, malic, tartric, citric, gluconic and mandelic acids, as well as salicylic acid. The latter is an effective keratolytic in concentrations as low as 1%. The other acids of this group show hydrating action at weak concentrations (<10%), and a tendency to reduce corneocyte cohesion at the base of the stratum corneum. This makes them interesting compounds for the treatment of dry and ichthyotic skin, as well as in cases of cracked and fissured skin (atopic skin). At high concentrations (30–70%), their keratolytic action predominates: they act on the deeper epidermal layers, and even the papillary and reticular dermis. Therefore at these concentrations they are suggested for the treatment of hyperkeratosis and pre-epitheliomatous keratoses.

Propylene glycol[16] – At concentrations over 40%, this shows keratolytic properties, which enables it to be used in certain ichthyotic treatments. It can also be used with salicylic acid.

Urea[15] – This is keratolytic from 10%, but is not always well tolerated.

Topical corticosteroids[64]

These treatments are exclusively for pathological dry skin, and are thus beyond the scope of this chapter. For the record, mention will only be made of them in the case of atopic dermatitis.

Systemic treatments

These concern mainly the treatment of certain congenital ichthyoses by etretinate,[65] and thus will not be dealt with in this chapter. However, mention may be made that systemic administration of oils rich in PUFAs may be advocated for constitutionally dry skin. In fact, as previously mentioned, skin xerosis could be related to essential fatty acid deficiency (in particular, of γ-linolenic acid), resulting in an alteration of δ-6-desaturase activity, which is responsible for the conversion of linoleic acid to γ-linolenic acid. This treatment may also be recommended for cases of atopic dermatitis, in which this phenomenon seems to occur.[64]

TOLERANCE OF PRODUCTS

Whether a product is destined for personal hygiene or skin care, it must, first and foremost, be totally innocuous. Until fairly recently, product tolerance was tested using animals (primary irritation index, occular irritation). For ethical reasons, alternatives to these tests have been sought and evaluated for some time. An unexpected consequence of this research has been questioning of the validity of animal testing: i.e. rodent skin is not the same as human skin, since the permeability and metabolism of certain substances is different.

Current opinion favours two new types of testing:

- in vitro tests
- in vivo human tests.

In vitro tests

These tests are subdivided into several types, relating to models of increasing complexity, from solutions of biological macromolecules to the living skin cell. Obviously, these models are more reliable and realistic the closer they resemble actual skin. A list of the most up-to-date tests (not exhaustive), arranged in order of increasing complexity is as follows.

Tests using inert biological models (Eytex, Skintex)

Eytex contains a protein complex that undergoes a degradation process, seen as precipitation, when in contact with an irritant. The irritancy potential of the product is thus determined by the opacity of the reaction. Skintex relies on the same principle, except that the protein complex is covered by a collagen–elastin membrane, on which the product in question is applied. Thus the product reacts with the protein complex after having first diffused through this membrane.

Tests using prokaryotic cells (bacteria)

This is a test where the cytotoxicity of the product is evaluated by a living, but primitive, single-celled organism – a bacterium. The test uses bacteria that are fluorescent when alive (*Phosphobacterium phosphoreum*), thus allowing the product's toxicity to be determined simply by the amount of loss of fluorescence.

Tests using hen's eggs (Het-Cam)

Here the product under test is applied to the membrane of a hen's egg. After 20 seconds contact with the product, the membrane is rinsed and observed for signs of injection, haemorrhage and coagulation, which are recorded as scores.

Tests using bovine cornea

The product is applied to bovine cornea, which are prepared from freshly collected eyes and maintained in cell culture medium. Corneal opacity is measured by means of an opacitometer after 10 seconds contact, then re-evaluated 2 hours later. Following this, the permeability can be estimated by spectrophotometric determination of the amount of fluorescein having diffused across the cornea in 90 minutes. Using these two parameters, a global score of toxicity is calculated.

Tests using cell cultures

There are numerous types of these, which are based on dermal (fibroblast) viability after contact with the product. Application of the product may be done via diffusion in the surrounding liquid culture media or by diffusion through an agarose gel in contact with the culture ('agar overlay'). In the latter case, the product is spread on the surface of the gel,

which is covering the cell culture. This allows emulsions to be tested. After a certain contact cell viability, can be determined in one of two ways: either

- using a vital stain (neutral red), which is only taken up by living cells and which is released back into the culture medium on cell lysis; or
- by the introduction of a yellow tetrazolium salt, which is metabolized into the form of blue formazan crystals by the mitochondrial enzymes of living cells.

In vivo human testing[66]

In France, as in most other countries, these tests are carried out under medical supervision with the approval of the regional medical ethics committee, for the protection of persons involved in biomedical research. This type of testing represents a considerable step forward in medical research, and has two big advantages over animal and in vitro tests:

- data are directly applicable to humans, with no need for extrapolation;
- certain tests can reveal subclinical reactions, perceptible only by sensor-based techniques.

Several tests have been described, some of which simulate normal application conditions while others are concerned with greatly increased dosing regimes.

Patch testing

In this type of test, of which there are many variants, the product is applied under an occlusive patch. According to the methods used, there may only be a single application of the product during 24 hours, or two successive applications of 24 hours each. Application conditions are thus greatly exaggerated with this type of application, which serves to enhance transcutaneous diffusion. Products are normally tested against a negative control (water) and a positive control, usually consisting of sodium lauryl sulphate. Tolerance may be measured either by clinical scoring or with bioengineering techniques sensitive to the measurement of inflammatory changes such as skin blood flow, transepidermal water loss or skin colour (erythema).

Open repeated tests

The product is applied to the forearm under cosmetic conditions (i.e. left open to the air or unoccluded). This may be done several times a day, for several weeks. Thus the administered dose is exaggerated, but the application conditions are normal. Evaluation of tolerance may be made in a similar fashion as for that of patch tests, but clinical evaluation is generally preferred.

The stinging test

The stinging test is very sensitive, and is used to evaluate subjective sensations of burning or stinging, resulting from the application of a product that may not normally be associated with signs of clinical intolerance. This test is only carried out on preselected subjects. Subjects first undergo a facial sauna for 5–10 minutes, then have an aqueous lactic acid solution applied (5% or 10%, according to different methods) to the naso-labial fold on the side of the face, with the other side receiving a water control. Only subjects who perceive a definite stinging on the side that received the lactic acid are selected for further testing. The test product is then applied on these same individuals under the same conditions, and the intensity of the stinging sensation is quantified on an interval scale.

Use tests

In this type of test, a panel of volunteers apply the test product to the skin in the normal way, as recommended by the manufacturer. A medically qualified investigator regularly examines the panel, and records their comments and any adverse effects that arise. The idea of this test is to evaluate the product under conditions identical to those of actual use. Its main drawback is that it requires large numbers of volunteers to attain any reasonable sensitivity of testing. In contrast, tests that use exaggerated application conditions are much more sensitive. Even with small numbers of volunteers, intolerance may be seen. However, the 'artificial' mode of application may lead to bias in the results.

CONCLUSIONS

In recent years, considerable progress has been made in cosmetics, which was originally mainly concerned with perfume and make-up. Nowadays, the emphasis is much more on the development of veritable medical cosmetics of increasingly high performance, specifically adapted for all kinds of skin types, and backed up by rigorous scientific testing procedures for efficacy and tolerance. Whether one considers the various protective roles of all these products, or looks more specifically at, say, the corrective properties of treatments for dry or greasy skin, all have the common aim of maintaining or restoring the skin to its 'normal' state. At the same time, these products can also be used as complementary treatments for more classical therapy, particularly where side-effects occur. In the near future, thanks to studies of cutaneous pharmacokinetics, a better understanding of the distribution of the active ingredients in skin will be possible. This will enable more precise targeting of products, which will increase their activity, while improving their tolerance.

REFERENCES

1. Diridollou S, Etude du comportement mécanique cutané par technique ultrasonore haute résolution. Thèse, Tours, 1994.
2. De Rigal J, Escoffier C, Querleux B et al, Assessment of aging of the human skin on vivo ultrasonic imaging. *J Invest Dermatol* 1989; **5:** 621–5.
3. Escoffier C, Age related mechanical properties of human skin: an in vivo study. *J Invest Dermatol* 1989; **93:** 353–7.

4. Callens A, Vaillant L, Lecomte P et al, Does hormonal skin aging exist? A study of the influence of different hormone therapy regiments on the skin of postmenopausal women using non-invasive measurement techniques. *Dermatology* 1996; **193:** 289–94.

5. Edwards C, The acoustic properties of the epidermis and stratum corneum. In: *The Physical Nature of the Skin* (Marks RM, Barton SP, Edwards C, eds). Lancaster: MTP Press, 1988:201–7.

6. Hoffmann K, Dirsckka T, El Gammal S, Altmeyer P, Assessment of actinic elastosis by means of high-frequency sonography. In: *The Environmental Threat to the Skin* (Marks R, Plewig G, eds). London: Martin Dunitz, 1991:83–90.

7. Pierard GE, Lapiere ChM, Structures et fonction du derme et de l'hipoderme. In: *Précis de cosmétologie dermatologique* (Prunieras M, ed). Paris: Masson, 1989:37–50.

8. Shuster S, Black MM, McVitie E, The influence of age and sex on skin thickness, skin collagen and density. *Br J Dermatol* 1975; **93:** 639–43.

9. Agache P, Seborrhea. In: *The Science of Hair Care* (Zviat C, ed). New York: Marcel Dekker, 1986:469–99.

10. Roberts D, Marks R, The determination of regional and age variations in the rate of desquamation: a comparison of four techniques. *J Invest Dermatol* 1980; **74:** 13–16.

11. Wester RC, Maibach HI, Regional variation in percutaneous absorption. In: *Percutaneous Absorption* (Bronaugh RL, Maibach HI, eds). 1989:111–15.

12. Daniel F, La peau séborrhéique. *Dermatologie* 1985; **35:** 3215–24.

13. Zavaro-Colonna A, Traitements locaux de l'acné. *Bull Esthét Dermatol Cosmétol* 1992; **79:** 45–50.

14. Drouot-Lhoumeau D, Chivot M, Topiques antipelliculaires. *Bull Esthét Dermatol Cosmétol* 1985; **8:** 24–8.

15. Curtil L, Améliorer les peaux sèches. *Rev Eur Dermatol MST* 1991; **3:** 457–64.

16. Gougerot A, Enjolras O, Améliorer les peaux sèches pathologiques. *Rev Eur Dermatol MST* 1992; **4:** 75–82.

17. Grove GL, Grove MJ, Objective methods for assessing skin surface topography noninvasively. In: *Cutaneous Investigation in Health and Disease* (Lévêque JL, ed). New York: Marcel Dekker, 1989:1–32.

18. Pierard GE, Pierard-Franchimont C, Dowlati A, La biopsie de surface en dermatologie clinique et expérimentale. *Rev Eur Dermatol MST* 1992; **4:** 455–66.

19. Schatz H, Kligman AM, Manning S et al, Quantification of dry (xerotic) skin by image analysis of scales removed by adhesive discs (Dsquames). *J Soc Cosmet Chem* 1993; **44:** 53–63.

20. Elsner P, Berardesca E, Maibach HI (eds), *Bioengineering of the Skin: Water and the Stratum Corneum.* Boca Raton, FL: CRC Press, 1994.

21. Courage W, Hardware and measuring principle: corneometer. In: *Bioengineering of the Skin: Water and the Stratum Corneum* (Elsner P, Berardesca E, Maibach HI, eds). Boca Raton, FL: CRC Press, 1994:171–5.

22. Marty JP, Vincent CM, Fiquet E, Etude des propriétés hydratantes de la crème hydratante visage Neutrogena. *Réalités thérapeutiques en Dermato-Vénérologie* 1992; **15:** 37–40.

23. Tagami H, Impedance measurement for evaluation of the hydratation state of the skin surface. In: *Cutaneous Investigation in Health and Disease* (Lévêque JL, ed). New York: Marcel Dekker, 1989:79–111.

24. Tagami H, Hardware and measuring principle: skin conductance. In: *Bioengineering of the Skin: Water and the Stratum Corneum* (Elsner P, Berardesca E, Maibach HI, eds). Boca Raton, FL: CRC Press, 1994:197–203.

25. Gabard B, Treffel P, Hardware and measuring principle: the NOVA™ DPM 9003. In: *Bioengineering of the Skin: Water and the Stratum Corneum* (Elsner P, Berardesca E, Maibach HI, eds). Boca Raton, FL: CRC Press, 1994:177–95.

26. Nicander I, Ollmar S, Eek A et al, Correlation of impedance response patterns to histological findings in irritant skin reactions induced by various surfactants. *Br J Dermatol* 1996; **134:** 221–8.

27. Salter DC, Further hardware and measurement approaches for studying water in the stratum corneum. In: *Bioengineering of the Skin: Water and the Stratum Corneum* (Elsner P, Berardesca E, Maibach HI, eds). Boca Raton, FL: CRC Press, 1994:205–15.

28. Triebskorn A, Gloor M, Infrared spectroscopy. A method for measurement of moisture in the stratum corneum using the ATR method. In: *16èmes Journées Internationales de Dermocosmétologie de Lyon, 18–20 mai 1988*:47–55.

29. Davin E, Mille G, Roux-Alezais D et al, Etude 'in vivo' des propriétés hydratantes d'un complexe à base d'urée par spectroscopie infrarouge à transformée de Fourier. *Nouv Dermatol* 1988; **7**(Suppl 3): 279–83.

30. Wilson DR, Maibach HI, Transepidermal water loss: a review. In: *Cutaneous Investigation in Health and Disease* (Lévêque JL, ed). New York: Marcel Dekker, 1989:113–33.

31. Tagami H, Hashimoto-Kumasaka K, Hara M et al, In vivo and in vitro measurements of water holding capacity of the stratum corneum. In: *The Biology of the Epidermis* (Ohkawara A, McGuire J, eds). Amsterdam: Elsevier, 1992:37–47.

32. Borroni G, Zaccone C, Vignati G et al, Dynamic measurements: sorption–desorption test. In: *Bioengineering of the Skin: Water and the Stratum Corneum* (Elsner P, Berardesca E, Maibach HI, eds). Boca Raton, FL: CRC Press, 1994:217–22.

33. Treffel P, Gabard B, Stratum corneum dynamic function measurements after moisturizer or irritant application. *Arch Dermatol Res* 1995; **287**: 474–9.

34. van Neste D, In vivo evaluation of unbound water accumulation in stratum corneum. *Dermatology* 1990; **181**: 197.

35. Berardesca E, Elsner P, Dynamic measurements: the plastic occlusion stress test (POST) and the moisture accumulation test (MAT). In: *Bioengineering of the Skin: Water and the Stratum Corneum* (Elsner P, Berardesca E, Maibach HI, eds). Boca Raton, FL: CRC Press, 1994:97–102.

36. Salter DC, McArthur HC, Crosse JE, Dickens AD, Skin mechanics measured in vivo using torsion: a new and accurate model more sensitive to age, sex and moisturizing treatment. *Int J Cosmet Sci* 1993; **15**: 200–18.

37. Bittoun J, Saint Jalmes H, Querleux B et al, In vivo high resolution MR imaging of the skin in a whole-body system at 1.5 T. *Radiology* 1990; **176**: 457–60.

38. Richard S, Querleux B, Bittoun J et al, Characterization of the skin in vivo by high resolution resonance magnetic imaging: water behaviour and age related effects. *J Invest Dermatol* 1993; **100**: 705–9.

39. Querleux B, Richard S, Bittoun J et al, In vivo hydration profile in skin layers by high resolution magnetic resonance imaging. *Skin Pharmacol* 1994; **7**: 210–16.

40. Franconi F, Akoka S, Guesnet J et al, Measurement of epidermal moisture content by magnetic resonance imaging: assessment of hydration cream. *Br J Dermatol* 1995; **132**: 913–17.

41. Saint-Leger D, Quantification of skin surface lipids and skin flora. In: *Cutaneous Investigation in Health and Disease* (Lévêque JL, ed). New York: Marcel Dekker, 1989:153–82.

42. Agache P, Evaluation de la production sébacée. In: *Biologie de la peau* (Thivolet J, Schmitt D, eds). *Séminaire INSERM* 1987; **148**: 93–100.

43. Pierard GE, Pierard-Franchimont C, Le T et al, Patterns of follicular sebum excretion rate during lifetime. *Arch Dermatol Res* 1987; **279**: S104–7.

44. Pierard GE, Pierard-Franchimont C, Kligman AM, Kinetics of sebum excretion evaluated by the Sebutape–Chromameter technique. *Skin Pharmacol* 1993; **6**: 38–44.

45. Curtil L, Richard A, Maintenir en bon état les peaux normales. *Rev Eur Dermatol MST* 1991; **3**: 403–10.

46. Korting HC, Kober M, Mueller M et al, Influence of repeated washings with soap and synthetic detergents on pH and resident flora of forehead and forearm. *Acta Derma Venereol (Stockh)* 1987; **67**: 41–7.

47. Marguery MC, Les risques solaires aux sports d'hiver. *Bull Esthét Dermatol Cosmét* 1992; **83**: 31–40.

48. Jeanmougin M, Filtres et écrans solaires. *Bull Esthét Dermatol Cosmét* 1983; **7**: 11–21.

49. Msika PH, Boyer F, Efficacité et sécurité de l'oxyde-de titane ultrafin en photoprotection. *BEDC* 1993; **1**: 231–40.

50. Roger F, Les cosmétiques de la peau grasse. *Bull Esthét Dermatol Cosmét* 1985; **5**: 13–18.

51. Olivieres-Ghouti C, L'hygiène des peaux acnéiques. *Bull Esthét Dermatol Cosmét* 1985; **9**: 35–8.

52. Roger F, La cosmétologie des acnéiques. *BEDC* 1993; **1**: 131–6.

53. Schmidt-Pillet S, Maniement pratique des topiques anti-acnéiques. *Bull Esthét Dermatol Cosmét* 1991; **70**: 7–12.

54. Chivot M, L'Isotrétinoïne. *Bull Esthét Dermatol Cosmét* 1990; **55**: 31–6.

55. Poirier JP, La dermite séborrhéique. Formes frontières et traitement. *Bull Esthét Dermatol Cosmét* 1991; **74**: 47–50.

56. Carron P, Nettoyer les cheveux et la cuir chevelu. *Rev Eur Dermatol MST* 1991; **3:** 351–8.

57. Aschieri M, Garigue J, Quoi de neuf en matière d'hyperséborrhée? *BEDC* 1993; **1:** 287–90.

58. Ramette G, Produits cosmétiques de protection et de correction. In: *Précis de cosmétologie dermatologique* (Prunieras M, ed). Paris: Masson, 1981:103–22.

59. Wohlrab W, Lachmann U, Lasch J, Penetration of lecithin from hydrocortisone-containing liposomes into human skin. *Dermatol Monatschr* 1989; **175:** 344–7.

60. Chyczy M, Roding J, Hoff E, Control of skin humidity by liposomes. *Cosmetics and Toiletries Manufacture* 1991/1992: 148–52.

61. Handjani-Vila RM, Guesnet J, Les 'liposomes'. Un avenir prometteur en cosmétologie. *Ann Dermatol Venereol* 1989; **116:** 423–30.

62. Seiller M, Un concept nouveau: les émulsions triphasiques. *Réalités thérapeutiques en dermatovénérologie* 1991; **6:** 24–8.

63. Elias PM, Brown BE, Ziboh VA, The permeability barrier in essential fatty acid deficiency: evidence for a direct role for linoleic acid in barrier function. *J Invest Dermatol* 1980; **74:** 230–3.

64. De Prost Y, Dermatite atopique. In: *Thérapeutique dermatologique* (Dubertret L, ed). Paris: Flammarion, 1991:129–32.

65. Blanchet-Bardon C, Ichtyoses héréditaires. In: *Thérapeutique dermatologique* (Dubertret L, ed). Paris: Flammarion, 1991:273–8.

66. Jenkins HL, Adams MG, Progressive evaluation of skin irritancy of cosmetics using human volunteers. *Int J Cosmet Sci* 1989; **11:** 141–9.

12

Self-tanning products

Daniel H Maes, Kenneth D Marenus

INTRODUCTION

The growing awareness of the deleterious effects of sun on the skin, and the compelling need by much of the population to look tanned, has recently brought the category of self-tanning products to the top of the list of most successful cosmetic products on the market.

With the development of new technologies, the cosmetic industry is now able to create products that induce a skin coloration similar to the color resulting from the exposure of the skin to UV light.

Today, all self-tanning products found on the market contain the active ingredient dihydroxyacetone (DHA) which produces the brown skin coloration. Dihydroxyacetone is a keto-sugar of the following structure:

$$HOCH_2 \diagdown \atop C=O \atop HOCH_2 \diagup$$

Other sugars of the same family as dihydroxyacetone, such as glyceraldehyde, 6-aldo-D-fructose, erythrulose and glucose, have been shown to induce skin coloration to a lesser extent.

MECHANISM OF ACTION

Through a series of complexation and condensation reactions, DHA reacts with the amine groups of the skin's amino acids, to create a by-product having a natural tan-induced brown color. This reaction is not immediate, and usually takes 2–3 hours to fully develop on the skin. Once the coloration has developed, it will remain and resist wash-off, since it is part of the skin cells' amino acid structure. The color gradually fades as the cells themselves are eliminated through the natural desquamation process. Based on the number of stratum corneum cell layers that are colored through the reaction with DHA, it will take 5–6 days for the color to completely disappear.

Although DHA has been shown to be non-toxic, there have recently been questions as to the likelihood of penetration of this molecule into the living layers of the skin, and its systemic absorption into the body. Testing done in the Estée Lauder laboratories on human volunteers, using the cellophane tape stripping technique, has shown that the DHA does not penetrate to the glistening layer of the epidermis.[1] It remains within the dead layer structure of the stratum corneum.

Most self-tanning products on the market

use a concentration of DHA ranging from 2.5% to 10%, with the most usual concentration being 5%.

The development of a line of products with different concentrations of DHA provides the consumer with degrees of color intensity for the face or the body. Additionally, it allows for the gradual darkening of skin color, avoiding the rapid change that is frequently commented upon.

Usually, the color resulting from the reaction between DHA and the skin's amino acids is very similar to a natural tan color, i.e. a deep brown, with very little yellow component present. However, we have observed that the pH of the skin before application of the product has a significant effect on the tonality of color. For example, if DHA is applied on skin that has been previously washed with a very alkaline soap, the resulting color will tend toward the yellowish-orange rather than the brown. Similarly, if DHA is incorporated into an emulsion with an alkaline pH, the color development will not be satisfactory. In order to obtain the proper color, the skin surface should be cleansed of any oily residue (which will interfere with the reaction between the amino acids and DHA), and free of any alkaline residues such as soaps or detergents.

We have found that, after washing the skin with a soap or a cleanser, it is a good practice to wipe the skin surface with a hydroalcoholic, acidic pH toner, which solubilizes the residues left on the skin surface (mostly calcium salts of soaps).

In order to prolong the duration of skin coloration, we have tested the effect of mild exfoliation prior to the application of the self-tanning product. Indeed, the removal of a layer of dead skin cells from the surface of the skin results in an increase in the duration of the 'tan' by almost one day. Obviously this scrubbing should not be carried out after the self-tanning preparation has been applied on the skin, since it will result in the removal of the cells that have already reacted with the DHA, and will significantly reduce the intensity of the skin coloration.

FORMULATION WITH DHA

Until recently, DHA was always incorporated into oil-in-water emulsions rather than in the water-in-oil type, since the large amount of oils and waxes used in the latter reduce the darkness of the color. Now, with the advent of silicone technology, it is possible to formulate a product with a large amount of silicones, which improve the spreadability of the product, thereby reducing the risk of streaking.

Whatever the type of emulsion chosen, it is imperative that the particle size of the micelles be as small as possible, in order to improve the uniform spreading of the DHA on the skin's surface. We have observed that two similar emulsions could provide drastically different results if one emulsion has been passed through a homogenizer.

In addition to emulsions, it is now possible to incorporate DHA into hydroalcoholic vehicles and obtain an even application on the skin, again reducing the spotty or streaky look. Such technology has been used recently in the development of a self-tanning spray, which is a very convenient way to apply this type of product.

During the production of self-tanning creams and lotions, it is necessary to take a few specific precautions in order to reduce the risk of degradation of DHA. In solution, DHA is in equilibrium with its isomer, glyceraldehyde, which degrades into formaldehyde and formic acid – two unwanted ingredients in a skin care product. We have found that in order to eliminate the generation of formaldehyde and formic acid, it is necessary to maintain the pH of the emulsion at around 4, since the isomerization of DHA into glyceraldehyde is minimal in acidic solutions.

Because of the labile character of DHA, it is necessary to store it in a cool dry place, and to test frequently for the presence of formaldehyde and formic acid.

During the manufacture of the product, the DHA must not be heated to more than 40°C. Once the DHA solution has been emulsified with oils, we have observed a significant stabilization over long time periods, providing that the pH of the emulsion has been buffered to around 4.

We thus see that the acidity of a self-tanning product is important for two reasons: first because it develops a more natural color (less yellow) and second because it stabilizes the DHA by reducing its degradation into formaldehyde and formic acid.

Because of the risk of formaldehyde and formic acid generation, it is imperative to test the final product in a repeat insult patch test and a cumulative irritancy test. In the Estée Lauder laboratories, we follow the stability of the product not only by measuring the eventual amount of formaldehyde and formic acid formed in the emulsion, but also by running cumulative irritancy tests on aging samples.[2] The results we have obtained so far clearly show a good correlation between the amount of formic acid found in the emulsion and the score obtained with the cumulative irritancy test, reinforcing the importance of keeping these unwanted ingredients to a minimum level in self-tanning formulations.

Finally, it is important to realize that the color that develops on the skin does not provide any significant protection from UVB light, and cannot be considered as a sunscreen that will reduce the intensity of sunburn. It is necessary to let the consumer know that the application of a self-tanning product will not prevent sunburn, and should not be considered as a sunscreen.

However, a recent study[3] has shown that the coloration resulting from the reaction between DHA and the skin does absorb a significant portion of the UVA spectrum, resulting in a significant amount of photoprotection in the UVA region, although very little protection could be seen in the UVB region of the spectrum.

One approach to this problem would be to include UVB sunscreens into self-tanning products in order to provide both skin coloration and the necessary protection before going into the sun. This idea has already been implemented in various self-tanning formulations on the market.

We do strongly believe, however, that even the incorporation of an UVB sunscreen in a self-tanning product will not provide the UV protection expected by the consumer, since such products are not generally applied just before sun exposure, but rather several hours if not a whole day before going to the beach, at which time the sunscreen will have no effect whatsoever.

The proper labelling of self-tanning products with a cautionary statement clearly stating to the consumer that the coloration that develops on the skin will not, contrary to natural UV-induced pigmentation, provide any sun protection, is in our opinion the best defense against product misuse.

Consumers using self-tanning products to improve their skin coloration at the beach should apply them between 3 and 24 hours before going to the beach, and apply the proper UV protection (at least SPF 15) immediately before exposure to the sun.

It is reasonable to exepct that, because of the great commercial success of self-tanning products, we shall see many new innovative formulae on the market, since we do believe significant improvements will be made to existing products. For example, the development of the skin coloration process should be made shorter, to provide the consumer with a more immediate idea of how he or she will look.

Products will be developed specifically for the face, since we have found that the skin on the face does not react to the same degree as the skin of other parts of the body. Self-tanning products for the face should be more emollient and contain higher concentrations of DHA.

We do believe that the use of self-tanning products represents the most reasonable alternative for the health-conscious consumer who has finally understood that excessive exposure to the sun will result at best in the acceleration of the premature aging process, if not the formation of cancerous lesions on the skin.

Since a sun-tanned appearance is currently taken to be a sign of wealth and well-being, and may be for some time to come, it is reasonable to expect that self-tanning products will continue to be popular and that they will be developed still further.

REFERENCES

1. McKeever MA, Penetration of DHA in human skin. Estée Lauder R & D, Internal Report IS-95-48, May 1995.

2. Ostrovskaya A, Rosalia AD, Landa PA, Maes D, Stability of dihydroxyacetone in self tanning cosmetic products. Presented at the Annual Meeting of the Society of Cosmetic Chemists, New York, December 1996.

3. Muizzuddin N, Marenus K, Maes D, UVA and UVB photoprotective effects of melanoids formed with DHA and skin. Poster presented at the American Academy of Dermatology Meeting, San Francisco, March 1997.

13

Masks and astringents/toners

Myra O Barker

INTRODUCTION

Worldwide use of skin care products continues to grow, and sales remain strong, driven by basic demographic and economic trends. As the so-called 'baby-boom' generation of consumers born after World War II continues to age, skin care products are expected to continue to grow in popularity as consumers seek to postpone the visible signs of skin aging. In addition, as disposable incomes rise in formerly less-developed economies, and as capitalist systems partially or fully supplant managed economies in formerly communist states, luxury items such as skin care products should be expected to see sustained sales increases. As manufacturers of these products forecast continued robust markets worldwide, they have been expanding their research and development efforts directed toward improved skin care product formulations. Skin cleansers and moisturizers, discussed in Chapter 10, have been the focus of much of the research and development activity of the 1990s. However, masks and astringents/toners, the other popular categories of facial skin care products, have benefited from new technology and new ingredients as well, though to a somewhat lesser extent.

Masks and other types of cosmetic exfoliants are widely sold for both adolescent and adult skin, for home and salon use. Astringents, toners and skin fresheners are also popular in both the teenage and adult user groups. Both product types can be formulated as convenient delivery systems for anti-acne and other active therapeutic ingredients, as well as for hydrating agents, botanicals, hydroxy acids, and other cosmetic functional ingredients. Both masks and astringents/toners are usually sold as part of a skin care product system or regimen in the prestige market, but are often sold as speciality stand-alone products in the mass market. In 1993, US sales for toners and astringents totaled $171 million, with mask sales totaling $50 million. While masks have expanded from general-use facial products to products for the hair, body and specialized areas such as the lips, toners and astringents have largely remained confined to general facial use, although a few products marketed for acne control may also be recommended for use on the chest, upper back and shoulders to reduce surface sebum and treat localized acne lesions.

MASKS

History

Mud baths and mud packs, said to 'detoxify', relieve stress or treat skin diseases, have a long history of use in various cultures. Mud baths are part of the repertory of most well-known spas even today. Masks have also been part of the standard beauty routine in many ancient and modern cultures. A 1972 expedition to study archeological and ethnological relics of the civilization of Etruria discovered linseed flour used in the preparation of beauty masks, and it is believed that the writings of Ovid refer to specialized flours used for such purposes as emolliency in mask formulas.[1]

Facial masks

Masks formulated for facial use generally fall into four major categories:

- clay-based masks, usually designed to dry on the skin's surface;
- polymer-based masks, often based upon polyvinyl alcohol, which harden to a flexible film upon drying and are usually designed to be peeled off the face;
- dual-purpose mask/scrubs, designed for vigorous exfoliation;
- therapeutic masks, which can be any of the above types of products, but are primarily designed as a delivery system for one or more active ingredients.

In addition to the four principal mask types, there are masks consisting of rigid sheets of a dried matrix, usually collagen, which may be plasticized with water or solutions of other materials and applied to the face, and masks consisting of cloth strips impregnated with active materials that are moistened prior to application, or cloth strips soaked in a solution of materials designed to be delivered to facial or body skin after the skin is wrapped with the saturated cloth strips. These latter types are largely confined to salon or spa use, since self-application at home is difficult.

Other types of mask include homemade or commercially prepared 'mud packs', and yoghurt-based, fruit-based, egg-based and peelable wax-based masks. The popularity of 'natural' cosmetics in recent years has led to a proliferation of such products, and of books and magazine articles explaining how to formulate them at home from such 'ingredients' as bananas, eggs, cucumbers, honey, oatmeal and buttermilk. Unfortunately, these books and magazine articles rarely instruct users about the necessity for preserving such concoctions if they are to be stored for later use. At the opposite end of the spectrum from these 'natural' masks, a Japanese company's American subsidiary has recently marketed a mask for unclogging pores based on the cyanoacrylate type of 'sticky slide' popularized by Kligman[2] for removing impacted material from follicles for therapeutic or analytical purposes.

Masks are intended to improve the skin's surface texture and appearance by removing loose corneocytes, dissolving or adsorbing surface sebum, causing an apparent reduction in the size of external follicular orifices, and are also designed to leave a pleasant 'stimulated' feel by stimulating cutaneous microcirculation. Improvements in surface texture may be readily demonstrated by a variety of techniques, including computer color-enhanced shadowing of corneocytes removed from the skin surface, as demonstrated in Figure 13.1. Corneocyte removal may be demonstrated by the use of D-Squames (CuDerm Corporation, Dallas, TX) as seen in Figure 13.2, or by controlled rinsing followed by cell counting,[3] among other methods.

Many mask formulas, particularly those containing physical abrasive agents, may also double as scrubs, with instructions for use often suggesting that the user allow the mask to dry, then apply water to re-wet the product and scrub with a gentle fingertip motion or a soft brush prior to removing the product with a facial cleanser or by rinsing with water.

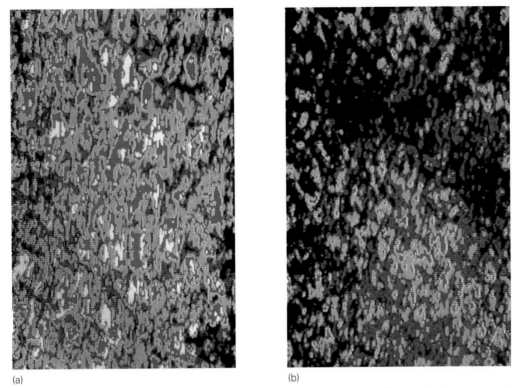

(a)   (b)

Figure 13.1 Photomicroscopy of D-Squames taken before (a) and after (b) masking of skin. Computerized pseudo-color is used to represent the gray scale produced by shadowing of corneocytes, with white representing the largest clumps of corneocytes or the deepest shadowing, followed by red and green, with blue representing background color or little shadowing due to corneocytes.

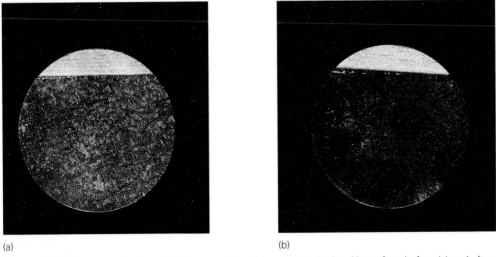

(a)   (b)

Figure 13.2 Macroscopic view of D-Squames taken from extremely dry skin surface before (a) and after (b) mask treatment.

Many masks are intended for once- or twice-weekly use, although they are often used more frequently by women and adolescents with oily skin. Masks intended for salon or spa use are designed to be used on a less-frequent basis.

Mask ingredients

Popular featured ingredients for facial mask formulas include mineral salts, botanical oils and extracts, menthol, magnesium sulfate, zinc sulfate, oatmeal, rice bran, aloe vera, and both α- and β-hydroxy acids used as exfoliants or antiacne agents. In addition, proteolytic enzymes are enjoying new popularity as mask ingredients for their exfoliant properties, and some companies are employing ingredients that inhibit naturally occurring enzymes in the skin such as those that cleave collagen and elastin molecules in the dermis.[4] Many physical exfoliating agents, including polyethylene granules or beads, and natural exfoliating scrub materials such as ground walnut shells or corn meal, are used in masks and scrubs. Such formulations utilizing naturally occurring scrubbing materials present a challenge to the cosmetic chemist, because these materials have a high bioburden and must be well preserved to assure an adequate shelf life, taking into account both the type and numbers of contaminating microorganisms typical to the scrubbing agents chosen. Recent patents disclose a gel mask containing polyethylene beads preferably of a diameter of 100–500 μm,[5] a scrub product utilizing wax capsules containing protease, lipase and muramidase enzymes,[6] ornithine derivative-coated microspheres of vinylidene chloride/acrylonitrile copolymer as exfoliants,[7] and gel spheres of β-1,3-diglucan as scrubbing agents.[8] A substantial effort has been devoted in recent years toward providing scrub agents with controlled particle size and shape to control the degree of exfoliation and irritation. In mask formulations containing scrubbing agents such agents are normally present at concentrations ranging from less than 5% to over 60%. Acne treatment masks may contain salicylic acid, benzoyl peroxide or sulfur, all of which would be considered over-the-counter drug products in the USA.[9] Other mask products containing α-hydroxy acids for exfoliation may be positioned similarly in the marketplace, but are not regulated as drugs.

New products in the mask/scrub category

New mask/scrub products introduced in recent years include a lipophilic gel that is claimed to stimulate the skin's natural renewal process, and a mask containing α-hydroxy acids and a complex of glucooligosaccharides of beetroot and corn sugars, said to preserve the barrier qualities of the stratum corneum. Preservative-free masks have been introduced into the German market, in common with trends toward preservative-free moisturizers in Germany. A Japanese company has introduced a sebum-clearing mask containing a lipophilic resin, silica powder to adsorb sebum, and botanical extracts said to contribute astringency and control of sebum flow. An American manufacturer has recently introduced a mask containing zinc oxide, salicylic acid, sulfur and camphor to treat oily skin.

Usage of masks in dermatology

A recent review of masks in dermatology suggests they are useful in the treatment of seborrhea, seborrheic dermatitis, acne, psoriasis, eczema, mycoses and other skin conditions. Heated masks can be used to stimulate cutaneous microcirculation, to deliver actives such as sulfur compounds, and to provide vasodilation. Masks containing sulfur are said to be particularly useful for their keratoplastic and keratolytic activity, treating blackheads and comedones, reducing seborrhea, and exerting antiseptic, antifungal and antiparasitic activity. Vitamins and steroids may be delivered via masks. Seaweed-based masks contain carotenoids, phytosterols, lipid-linked polysaccharides, and other active compounds. Arsenical and iron–arsenical muds are said to be useful in the treatment of chronic eczema, lichen planus, acne and psoriasis.[10]

Efficacy studies of masks and scrubs

A recent Japanese study by Nakahira, Nakata and Konishi compared the scrubbing/cleansing efficacy of various vehicles with and without abrasive agents such as 5% polyethylene granules. Makeup residue (either an oil-based or a cake-type foundation) was more effectively removed from a matrix simulating the skin surface when 5% polyethylene granules were included in either a foam- or cream-based cleanser compared with a control cleanser of the same type without granules. Scrub ingredients frequently used in the Japanese market include natural plant materials such as the endocarp of apricot and almond seeds, walnut, birch bark powder, and fibers derived from sunflowers or palm trees. The authors developed a spherical particulate compound made of hydrogenated jojoba oil for cosmetic scrubs, which they believe is superior to the cellulose beads, silica particles and polyethylene beads often used in scrubs. The authors urge that exfoliating particles should be selected by size and shape for the desired degree of abrasiveness.[11]

A nonionic, oil-in-water scrub cream containing polyethylene granules of irregular shape, sized 100–200 µm was evaluated by the Swedish researchers Lodén and Bengtsson. Transepidermal water loss (TEWL) and blood flow measurements showed that a single 30-second scrub treatment was equivalent to 2.4–2.9 tape strippings. A visual assessment of scrubbed skin showed that scrubbing was the equivalent of about three tape strippings. Profilometry of scrubbed skin demonstrated a more pronounced microprofile. The authors suggest that this could represent removal of loose corneocytes from the 'valleys' of the skin surface.[12]

Marks et al[13] studied an abrasive agent (aluminium oxide particles) in normal and photoaged skin and compared it with topical tretinoin (0.05%). Over a 3-day study period, the abrasive was found to increase the desquamation rate significantly and to increase epidermal thickness and the epidermal labeling index compared with white soft paraffin or no treatment. Over an 8-week period, the abrasive treatment was found to significantly increase cutaneous blood flow measured by the laser–Doppler flowmeter, whereas tretinoin treatment showed only a trend in this direction but not a statistically significant increase. Both abrasive-treated and tretinoin-treated skin sites were increased in thickness over 8 weeks, but the abrasive-treated sites showed a greater increase. Measurement of skin extensibility showed that only in the abrasive-treated site was the force needed for 30% skin extension increased.

A similar study was conducted by Bergfeld and co-workers,[14] who compared the effects of a topical abrasive agent (a loofah sponge) and an α-hydroxy acid exfoliating product, containing 50% nonbuffered glycolic acid, pH 1.2, on photoaged skin of the hands. They found that the glycolic acid product was far more effective than the topical abrasive agent in reducing overall photodamage scores as well as wrinkling and texture abnormalities. There was also a positive trend toward more even skin color and toward a reduction in hyperpigmentation and skin laxity after glycolic acid treatment, while mechanical abrasion led to no significant change in overall severity, texture or wrinkling. Neither glycolic acid treatment nor mechanical abrasion resulted in any significant change in telangiectasia or pore size. Though cutaneous reactions to glycolic acid treatment were limited to mild erythema, peeling and dryness, as well as some inflammation at the site of application, significantly less irritation was seen in skin treated with the mechanical exfoliant.

An efficacy study conducted by an American mask manufacturer is said to demonstrate that sebum secretion is reduced by 40% for six hours following product use, with pore size reduced by 50%.[15]

Lorraine Kligman and her co-workers compared the action of such 'peeling agents' as lactic, glycolic and salicylic acids, as well as a product containing the hydroxy acids, with retinoic acid 0.05% on the skin of female Skh-hairless-1 albino mice treated with ultraviolet radiation. Though retinoic acid treatment produced the typical deep, elastosis-free repair zone in UV-irradiated mouse skin, with deposition of new collagen, other treatments produced at most a shallow, focal zone of repair. The authors concluded that hydroxy acids are not comparable to tretinoin for treatment of photodamage.[16]

Adverse reactions to mask products

Adverse reactions seen to facial masks usually are limited to contact irritancy, but contact allergy to individual ingredients is also possible, as well as irritant folliculitis or 'pustulogenicity'. Frictional melanosis from lengthy rubbing of the skin with nylon towelling or plastic sponge has been reported;[17] it is suggested that Asian skin may be more susceptible than Caucasian skin to this effect.[11] In 1991–1994, the last years for which US Food and Drug Administration (FDA) statistics on reported adverse reactions are available, masks accounted for 2.68 reports per million units sold. For the sake of comparison, moisturizers accounted for 11.75 reports per million units sold.[18]

Body and hair masks

Body masks include both the clay-based and cloth-strip products discussed earlier, as well as wax-based masks, popular in salons for softening and moisturizing the hands, and specialized products such as exfoliating lip masks, which can contain mild physical abrasives or chemical exfoliants such as hydroxy acids. Salon products and spa products can also include traditional 'mud baths' incorporating various naturally occurring or added minerals. Hair masks are periodically popular for scalp treatment or deep conditioning of hair; they can be clay-based with botanical or conditioning additives,[19] or can include other natural polymeric materials and additives such as marine algae.[20]

Rheology of cosmetic clays and mask products

Though peelable masks based on polyvinyl alcohol or other polymers are periodically popular, traditional clay-based masks remain the principal types in both the home-use and the salon or spa markets. An understanding of the functionality of clay-based masks is dependent on knowledge of the chemical structure and rheologic properties of cosmetic clays. Smectite clays are a family of naturally occurring clays that can be swollen by addition of water to form flowable dispersions. Bentonite and hectorite clays are the predominant forms of the smectite clay family used in cosmetic products. Smectite clays have a triple platelet structure, with two tetrahedral silicon dioxide layers enclosing a single layer of aluminium or magnesium oxide in an octahedral form. These three-layer structures are themselves layered, with water between the layers comprising the clay structure.[21] Opaque dispersions of clays with water and various additives are highly thixotropic. Thixotropic materials are those that thin markedly upon shearing but regain their original viscosity as their structure reforms over time. When mask products containing clays are dispensed from a typical tube package with a small dispensing orifice, they may thin markedly, but regain much of their original viscous mud-like properties after application to the facial skin. In addition, many masks are designed to lose water through evaporation once applied to the facial surface, hardening substantially in the process. However, some clay-based masks are designed to remain moist on the skin surface, particularly those designed for dry skin. In this case, plasticizers and humectants may be added to prevent hardening of the clay ingredients. In a typical mask formulation, clays may be employed at a concentration between 15% and 50%, along with additives such glycerol or urea, botanicals, preservatives, and sometimes color and fragrance.[22,23]

Use of hydroxy acids and other chemical exfoliants in masks

The tremendous success of hydroxy acid products in markets throughout the world during the 1990s has led to a proliferation of product types based on these ingredients. Although most of the extensive literature on the safety and efficacy of these products deals with hydroxy acids in moisturizers and other emulsions, the known exfoliating activity of the hydroxy acids has inevitably led to their use in exfoliating products such as masks and toners. Many such products have been introduced in recent years, including traditional clay-based and peelable masks, scrub creams, toners and other astringents. Concentrations of hydroxy acid are usually 10% or less.

Although lactic and glycolic acids are still widely used in cosmetic products, mixed fruit acids, long-chain and cyclic acids, and esters of hydroxy acids are all encountering increasing use. Recent products have used glycolic esters and lactones, decanoic and octanoic acids, gluconolactone, and cystamine bis-lactamide in addition to or in place of lactic or glycolic acids. Finally, salicylic acid, a β-hydroxy acid, is enjoying renewed popularity in various cosmetic product types.

The mechanism of action of hydroxy acids is not well understood. It has been claimed that they function as antioxidants, that they exert a plasticizing effect on the stratum corneum,[24] that they stimulate cell proliferation and/or cell turnover,[25] and that they interfere with cell adhesion,[26] but no specific receptors for hydroxy acids have been located

in the skin.[27] Although skin penetration of α-hydroxy acids has been studied, virtually all such studies to date have utilized emulsion vehicles.[28] One bioavailability assay suggests that aqueous solutions compare poorly with traditional emulsions when the bioavailability of α-hydroxy acids from these vehicles is compared,[29] suggesting that utilization of hydroxy acids in toners poses special formulation challenges.

TONERS

Product nomenclature and functional purpose

Product nomenclature in the toner category can be confusing at best. In various world markets, marketing names for products in this category can include toner, astringent, skin freshener, skin lotion, pore lotion, and other terms. From one manufacturer to another, from one product to another, and from one country to another, nomenclature follows no consistent pattern. In particular, the product name should not be taken to indicate strength of the formula or denote the presence of any particular ingredient. In the USA, astringents are categorized as over-the-counter drugs by the FDA,[30] but the name 'astringent' is often used in a cosmetic context, particularly for older products introduced into the market years before the drug monograph establishing the astringent category was published.

Astringents/toners/fresheners are often marketed and used as a 'second cleansing step', particularly when sold as part of a product regimen with a cold cream or water-in-oil emulsion cleansing cream. They can also be important in cleansing the skin of residue from use of anhydrous foundation makeups, which are typically incompletely removed by facial cleansers. However, they have additional uses in removing excess surface sebaceous secretions, providing a mild exfoliating action, providing a stimulated or cooling sensation to the skin's surface, and acting as an aqueous or hydroalcoholic delivery vehicle for active or cosmetically important ingredients.

Typical product formulations may be alcohol-based or non-alcoholic clear or tinted solutions, though light emulsions are popular in Asian markets. Various types of denatured ethanol are used in astringents, toners and fresheners, depending on regulations covering the use of denaturants, which vary from country to country. Isopropanol and propylene glycol were occasionally used years ago, but now are out of favor. Specialized astringent/toner/freshener types such as anti-acne or botanically based products may occasionally require other solvents or cosolvents, depending on the solubility of their featured ingredients. There are pronounced formulation trends in the category, with non-alcoholic product types becoming more popular in the United States and Japan, and botanical types on the increase in Europe and the USA. In Japan, women use two types of toners – the first tightens and tones skin and exerts an astringent effect on pore openings, and the second adds moisture and is often used over makeup. This second type is often referred to as a lotion, and may be presented as a light emulsion with various lipidic ingredients.

Astringent, toner and freshener ingredients

Witch hazel distillate, also known for labeling purposes as hamamelis water USP in the USA or as *Hamamelis virginiana* in Europe, is a monographed over-the-counter astringent ingredient in the USA. A botanical extract prepared from the twigs, bark and leaves of the *Hamamelis virginiana* plant,[31] witch hazel is a complex essence containing hamamelitannin (an astringent, ribofuranose compound), gallic acid (an astringent compound from hydrolysis of tannin), volatile oils with antiseptic properties, and other ingredients. Witch hazel may be used in formulating skin toners and fresheners at a concentration of approxi-

mately 2%. Solutions of witch hazel itself are frequently sold in mass-market outlets for use as an astringent or toner. Other botanical extracts with high tannin content are recommended for astringency in products marketed for combination and oily skin, whereas alcohol-free toners containing honey, aloe vera, glycerin, sorbitol and comfrey as a natural source of allantoin are recommended for dry skin.[32] One of the most popular mass-market oily-skin cleanser/antiseptic toners in the USA market contains 48% alcohol by volume (SD 40B), camphor, clove oil and peppermint. Sodium PCA, glycerol, sodium hyaluronate, sorbitol and other humectant or moisturizing agents may be used in toners. Mixed fruit acids and specific α-hydroxy acids are used in some products. Vitamins and antioxidants are also currently popular. Anti-irritants used in toners and fresheners include imidazole compounds, antioxidants, polymeric compounds and miscellaneous hydroxy compounds. Cooling materials of various chemical classes can be used. Salicylic acid, found in many toners and skin fresheners, is used as keratolytic/exfoliating agent, and is also a monographed over-the-counter drug anti-acne agent.[9] Astringent drug products[30] are drug products applied to the skin or mucous membranes for a local and limited protein coagulant effect, according to the FDA monograph governing the sale of such products in the USA. Active ingredients permitted by the monograph are aluminium acetate, 0.13–0.5%, aluminium sulfate, 46–63%, and hamamelis water USP.

New products in the toner/astringent category

Recent toner, freshener, and astringent product introductions feature botanical extracts from juniper berry, citrus, witch hazel, rose water, camphor, aloe vera, calendula, clove, peppermint and eucalyptus. α-Hydroxy acids and salicylic acid are also popular. In the Japanese market, collagen, hyaluronic acid, royal jelly and ceramides are popular new freshening lotion ingredients. A recent US patent discloses the use of extensions, plant-derived hydroxyproline-rich glycoproteins that can be incorporated into toners as substitutes for animal collagen.[33] Astringent lotions based on the astringent ingredient glycyrrhizic acid zinc are disclosed in another recent patent.[34] A plant native to Korea, China and Japan, *Sanguisorba*, produces a root extract widely used in Asian cosmetics for its astringent effect.[35] It is said to offer antimicrobial and anti-inflammatory effects as well, and to function much like superoxide dismutase as an antioxidant. A recent patent[36] covers the use of butylene oxide-based ethers and propylene oxide-based ethers in skin toners.

Use of astringents and toners in dermatology

The use of astringents and toners in dermatology has primarily been limited to their anti-acne properties, although some also function as mild antiseptic agents suitable for mild or limited bacterial infections of the skin surface. The FDA, in their astringent drug monograph,[30] limits astringent drug use to situations requiring 'a local and limited protein coagulant effect', such as styptic effects to control minor bleeding. It should be remembered, however, that such products, whether called astringents, toners, fresheners, skin lotions or by any of their other names, have utility in treating patients with seborrhea or mild acne, and leave the skin feeling clean and refreshed. As such, their cosmetic acceptability assures patient compliance when compared with traditional drug vehicles that lack aesthetic characteristics preferred by patients.

Adverse reactions to toners, fresheners and astringents

Adverse reactions to these product categories are most likely to consist of transient contact irritation, but contact allergy is possible, especially with more pharmacologically complex products such as those containing multiple botanical extracts and penetration enhancers.[37] It is important when formulating with higher concentrations of alcohol or other solvents to avoid destruction or disruption of lipids in the cutaneous barrier. Acetone, representative of solvents used in some products of this type in the past, has been shown to disrupt the cutaneous barrier and stimulate cytokine production in mouse epidermis,[38] leading to epidermal hyperplasia.[39] FDA statistics for the years 1991–1994 show 7.07 reported adverse reactions to toners and fresheners per million units sold[18] – a low rate compared with other skin care product categories.

SUMMARY

Masks and astringents/toners are important skin care products. They serve to exfoliate, adsorb or dissolve sebum, and leave skin with a clean, fresh feeling and a smooth texture. They can be formulated as cosmetically acceptable vehicles for anti-acne and other drugs. Each has a place, not only in cosmetology, but in dermatology as well.

ACKNOWLEDGEMENTS

The author is grateful to John Schiltz, PhD, Mary Kay Holding Corporation, for providing Figures 13.1 and 13.2, and Cecilia Armas-Benavides, Mary Kay Holding Corporation, for research assistance.

REFERENCES

1. Rovesti P, On the trail of lost cosmetics – Etruria. *Dragoco Report* 1976; **10**: 215–26.
2. Mills O, Kligman A, The follicular biopsy. *Dermatologica* 1983; **167**: 57–63.
3. Nicholls S, Marks R, Novel technique for the

estimation of intracorneal cohesion in vivo. *Br J Dermatol* 1977; **96**: 595–602.

4. Idson B, Treatment cosmetics overview. *Drug Cosmet Ind* 1995; November: 38–43.

5. Marion C, Louvet N, Patent EP688561-A1 (to L'Oreal SA), 1995.

6. Patent JP8073344-A (to Kanebo Ltd), 1996.

7. Philippe M, Bordier T, Patent EP738710-A1 (to L'Oreal SA), 1996.

8. Patent JP6321718-A (to Noevir KK), 1994.

9. Topical acne drug products for over-the-counter human use; Tentative final monograph, Federal Register **50**, No. 10:2172, January 15, 1985.

10. Di Grazia G, Usefulness of masks in dermatology. *J Appl Cosmetol* 1992; **10**: 49–52.

11. Nakahira C, Nakata S, Konishi H, Scrub cosmetics. *Cosmet Toiletries* 1986; **101**: 41–7.

12. Lodén M, Bengtsson A, Mechanical removal of the superficial portion of the stratum corneum by a scrub cream: methods for the objective assessment of the effects. *J Soc Cosmet Chem* 1990; **41**: 111–21.

13. Marks R, Hill S, Barton S, The effects of an abrasive agent on normal skin and on photoaged skin in comparison with topical tretinoin. *Br J Dermatol* 1990; **123**: 457–66.

14. Bergfeld W, Tung R, Vidimos A et al, Improving the cosmetic appearance of photoaged skin with glycolic acid. *J Am Acad Dermatol* 1997; **36**: 1011–13.

15. Clinique product alert (Deep Cleansing Emergency Mask), January 22, 1996.

16. Kligman L, Sapadin A, Peeling agents and irritants, unlike tretinoin, do not stimulate collagen synthesis in the photoaged hairless mouse. *Arch Dermatol Res* 1996; **288**: 615–20.

17. Hayakawa R, *J Jap Cosmet Sci Soc* 1986; **10**: 26.

18. Office of Cosmetics and Colors, Division of Program and Enforcement Policy, Participation status report for cosmetic voluntary registration program, Food and Drug Administration, 1995.

19. Anonymous, Hair mask formulary. *Cosmetics and Toiletries* 1996; **111**: 96.

20. Anonymous, Algae hair mask treatment formulary. *Cosmetics and Toiletries* 1993; **108**: 134.

21. Clarke M, Rheological additives. In: *Rheological Properties of Cosmetics and Toiletries* (Laba D, ed). New York: Marcel Dekker, 1993:55–152.

22. Gaffney M, Beauty masks. In: *Cosmetics: Science and Technology*, 2nd edn, Vol 1 (Balsam M, Sagarin E, eds). New York: Wiley, 1972:307–15.

23. Anonymous, Face mask formulary. *Cosmetics and Toiletries* 1993; **108**: 125.

24. Takahashi M et al, The influence of hydroxy acids on the rheological properties of stratum corneum. *J Soc Cosmet Chem* 1985; **36**: 177–87.

25. Smith W, Hydroxyacids and skin aging. *Cosmet Toiletries* 1994; **109**: 41–8.

26. Cosmetic Ingredient Review, *Scientific Literature Review on Glycolic and Lactic Acids, Their Common Salts, and Their Simple Esters.* Washington, DC: The Cosmetic, Toiletry, and Frangrance Association, 1995.

27. Smith W, Hydroxy acids and skin aging. *Soap/Cosmetics/Chemical Specialties* 1993; September: 54–76.

28. Hood H, Robl M, Kraeling M, Bronaugh R, *In Vitro Percutaneous Absorption of Cosmetic Ingredients After Repeated Application of an Alpha Hydroxy Acid In Vivo.* Washington, DC: Food and Drug Administration, 1996.

29. Ohta M, Ramachandran C, Weiner N, Influence of formulation type on the deposition of glycolic acid and glycerol in hairless mouse skin following topical in vivo application. *J Soc Cosmet Chem* 1996; **47**: 97–107.

30. Skin protectant drug products for over-the-counter human use; Astringent drug products; Final rule, Federal Register, October 21, 1993.

31. Wenninger J, McEwen G (eds), *International Cosmetic Ingredient Dictionary*, Vol 2. Washington, DC: The Cosmetic, Toiletry, and Fragrance Association, 1995.

32. Dweck A, Natural extracts and herbal oils: concentrated benefits for the skin. *Cosmet Toiletries* 1992; **107**: 89–98.

33. Wolf B, Tietjen M, Patent US5443855-A (to Revlon), 1995.

34. Patent JP7149787-A (to Toyo Beauty), 1995.

35. Lee O, Kang H, Han S, Oriental herbs in cosmetics. *Cosmet Toiletries* 1997; **112**: 57–64.

36. Smith H, Patent US5133967 (to Dow Chemical), 1992.

37. Pittz E, Skin barrier function and use of cosmetics. *Cosmet Toiletries* 1984; **99**: 30–5.

38. Wood L, Jackson S, Elias P et al, Cutaneous barrier perturbation stimulates cytokine production

in the epidermis of mice. *J Clin Invest* 1992; **90:** 482–7.

39. Denda M, Wood L, Emami S et al, The epidermal hyperplasia associated with repeated barrier disruption by acetone treatment or tape stripping cannot be attributed to increased water loss. *Arch Dermatol Res* 1996; **288:** 230–8.

PART FIVE

COSMETOLOGY FOR SPECIAL LOCATIONS

14

Ancillary skin care products

Zoe Diana Draelos

INTRODUCTION

Ancillary skin care encompasses products designed to supplement the basic cleansing and moisturizing of the skin. Frequently, they are recommended as part of a skin care routine by a beauty consultant or esthetician, and may be utilized in the home or spa setting. Ancillary skin care products include astringents, exfoliants, facial scrubs, epidermabrasion implements and face masks.

ASTRINGENTS

Astringents are liquids applied to the face with a cotton ball following cleansing. They comprise a broad category of formulations known by many labels: toners, clarifying lotions, controlling lotions, protection tonics, skin fresheners, toning lotions, T-zone tonics, etc. Originally, astringents were developed to remove alkaline soap scum from the face following cleansing with lye-based soaps and high-mineral-content well water. The development of synthetic detergents and public water systems has greatly decreased the amount of post-washing residue. A new use for astringents was found when cleansing creams became a preferred method of removing facial cosmetics and environmental dirt. The astringent then became an effective product for removing the oily residue left behind following cleansing cream use.

Astringent formulations are presently available for all skin types (oily, normal, dry, sensitive), with a variety of uses. Oily-skin astringents contain a high concentration of alcohols, water, and fragrance functioning to remove any sebum left behind following cleansing, to produce a clean feeling, and possibly deliver some treatment product to the face. For example, 2% salicylic acid, witch hazel or resorcinol may be added for a keratolytic and drying effect on the skin of acne patients. Clays, starches or synthetic polymers may be added to absorb sebum and minimize the appearance of facial oil. Astringents for normal skin are generally formulated to give the skin a clean, fresh feeling without much dryness. Products formulated for dry or sensitive skin are alcohol-free and are based on propylene glycol. These formulations are designed to remove oily residue from cleansing products or makeup removers while functioning as a humectant moisturizer. Soothing agents may also be added, such as allantoin, guaiazulene and Quaternium-19.[1]

EXFOLIANTS

Exfoliants are liquids applied to the face following cleansing, and incorporate keratolytic agents designed to hasten stratum corneum desquamation. They are similar in formulation to oily-skin astringents, with the addition of substances such as witch hazel, salicylic acid, lactic acid, malic acid, citric acid and/or glycolic acid.

Currently, the most popular exfoliant additives are the α-hydroxy acids for their ability to produce epidermal and dermal changes. The epidermal changes are immediate, and occur at the junction of the stratum corneum and stratum granulosum. They consist of a reduction in the thickness of the hyperkeratotic stratum corneum due to decreased corneocyte adhesion.[2] The dermal effects, which are delayed, consist of increased glycosaminoglycan synthesis.[3] The natural acidic pH of glycolic acid is sometimes buffered for facial application with phosphoric acid and monosodium phosphate or neutralized with sodium hydroxide.[4] The pH of the exfoliant solution is important, since minimal desquamation occurs at pH levels above 6. It appears that a pH of 3 produces the most effective epidermal renewal.[5]

FACIAL SCRUBS

Facial scrubs are mechanical exfoliants employing abrasive scrubbing granules in a cleansing base to enhance corneocyte desquamation. The scrubbing substance may be polyethylene beads, aluminium oxide particles, ground fruit pits or sodium tetraborate decahydrate granules.[6] Sibley et al[7] consider abrasive scrubbing creams to be effective in controlling excess sebum and removing desquamating tissue. However, these can cause epithelial damage if used too vigorously. This view is held by Mills and Kligman,[6] who noted that the products produced peeling and erythema without a reduction in comedones. Aluminium oxide particles and ground fruit pits provide the most abrasive scrub, followed by polyethylene beads, which are softer. Sodium tetraborate decahydrate

granules dissolve during use, providing the least abrasive scrub.

EPIDERMABRASION IMPLEMENTS

Another method of abrasive scrubbing has been labeled epidermabrasion by Durr and Orentreich,[8] who examined the use of a nonwoven polyester fiber web sponge. They and others have concluded that physical–mechanical exfoliation with the nonwoven polyester fiber web sponge was valuable in the removal of keratin excrescences and trapped hairs in pilosebaceous ducts.[9] Other epidermabrasion implements include rubber puffs, sea sponges and loofahs. The texture of the material rubbed over the face and the amount of pressure applied determine the amount of stratum corneum removed. Certainly, these implements can cause epidermal damage if used with vigor.

FACE MASKS

Face masks are applied to the skin for therapeutic and/or esthetic purposes as prepackaged home-use products or in custom salon products. There are four basic mask types: wax, vinyl or rubber, hydrocolloid, and earth.

Wax masks

Wax masks are popular among women for their warm, esthetically pleasing feel. They are composed of beeswax or, more commonly, paraffin wax to which petroleum jelly and cetyl or stearyl alcohols have been added to provide a soft, pliable material for facial application with a soft brush. The wax is heated and sometimes applied directly to the face or at other times applied over a thin gauze cloth draped over the face. Gauze is used to enable the facial technician to remove the wax in one piece.[10]

Wax face masks temporarily impede transepidermal water loss. This effect is limited only to the time the mask is in direct contact with the face, unless a suitable occlusive moisturizer is applied immediately following mask removal.

Vinyl and rubber masks

Vinyl and rubber masks are popular for home use, since they are easily applied and removed. Vinyl masks are based on film-forming substances such as polyvinyl alcohol or vinyl acetate, while rubber masks are usually based on latex. They are premixed and squeezed from a tube or pouch onto the palm and applied with the fingertips to the face. Upon evaporation of the vehicle, a thin flexible vinyl or rubber film remains behind on the face. The mask is generally left in contact with the skin for 10–30 minutes, and is then removed in one sheet by loosening it at the edges.

Vinyl and rubber masks are appropriate for all skin types. The evaporation of the vehicle from the wet mask creates a cooling sensation, and the shrinking of the mask with drying may give the impression that the skin is actually tightening. These masks can temporarily impede transepidermal water loss while they are in contact with the skin.

Hydrocolloid masks

Hydrocolloid masks are used both in professional salons and at home. Hydrocolloids are substances, such as oatmeal, that are of high molecular weight and thus interfere with transepidermal water loss. These masks are formulated from gums and humectants, and enjoy tremendous popularity since many specialty ingredients are easily incorporated into their formulation. They are marketed in sealed pouches in the form of dry ingredients that must be mixed with warm water prior to application. The resulting paste is then applied to the face with the hands and allowed to dry.[11]

Hydrocolloid masks leave the skin feeling smooth, and create the sense of tightening as the water evaporates and the mask dries. Temporary moisturization can occur while the mask is on the skin. Specialty additives such as honey, almond oil, zinc oxide, sulfur, avocado, witch hazel, etc. may be used to customize the mask.

Earth-based masks

Earth-based masks, also known as paste masks or mud packs, are formulated of absorbent clays such as bentonite, kaolin or china clay. The clays produce an astringent effect on the skin, making these masks most appropriate for oily-complected patients. The astringent effect of the mask can be enhanced through the addition of other substances, such as magnesium, zinc oxide, salicylic acid, etc.

REFERENCES

1. Wilkinson JB, Moore RJ, Astringents and skin toners. In: *Harry's Cosmeticology*, 7th edn. New York: Chemical Publishing, 1982:74–81.
2. Dietre CM, Griffin TD, Murphy GF et al, Effects of alpha-hydroxy acids on photoaged skin. *J Am Acad Dermatol* 1996; **34**: 187–95.
3. Van Scott JE, Yu RJ, Hyperkeratinization, corneocyte cohesion and alpha hydroxy acids. *J Am Acad Dermatol* 1984; **11**: 867–79.
4. Yu RJ, Van Scott EJ, Alpha-hydroxy acids: science and therapeutic use. *Cosmet Dermat Suppl* October 1994: 12–20.
5. Smith WP, Hydroxy acids and skin aging. *Cosmet Toiletries* 1994; **109**: 41–8.
6. Mills OH, Kligman AM, Evaluation of abrasives in acne therapy. *Cutis* 1979; **23**: 704–5.
7. Sibley MJ, Browne RK, Kitzmiller KW, Abradant cleansing aids for acne vulgaris. *Cutis* 1974; **14**: 269–74.
8. Durr NP, Orentreich N, Epidermabrasion for acne. *Cutis* 1976; **17**: 604–8.
9. Mackenzie A, Use of But-Puf and mild cleansing bar in acne. *Cutis* 1977; **20**: 170–1.
10. Gerson J, *Milady's Standard Textbook for Professional Estheticians*. Buffalo, NY: Milady, 1992:240–2.
11. Draelos ZD, *Cosmetics in Dermatology*. Edinburgh: Churchill Livingstone, 1995:213.

15

Topical deodorants

Daniel Lambert

INTRODUCTION

From the beginning of time, people have sought to dispel unpleasant body odours. In the absence of good hygiene, the use of strong-smelling perfumes was fashionable to mask bad odours. In recent years, thanks to progress in biochemical research, deodorants now give better results.

Cosmetic deodorants are preparations that modify, reduce, remove or prevent the development of body odours, or act on all these factors at the same time.

The sweat that comes from the eccrine, apocrine and apo-eccrine sudoral glands is odourless. However, under the action of saprophyte bacteria living on the skin surface, an enzymatic degradation appears, producing caproic, caprylic, isovaleric and butyric acids, together with mercaptans, amines, indoles and other metabolites. This flora is responsible for unpleasant odours called bromidrosis.

According to Seitz and Richardson,[1] there are three types of deodorants:

- deodorant fragrances, which generally act by modifying odour;
- odour-removing or odour-reducing ingredients;
- odour-preventing substances, such as antimicrobiol agents and antiperspirant salts.

DEODORANT FRAGRANCES

The most popular deodorant method until modern times was the use of fragrances to mask body odours.

In the middle ages, perfumes and bathing were the methods usually used, but the price of soap and the lack of bathing facilities could explain the lack of personal hygiene. After this period, several methods were used to modify foul odours.

Odour-masking substances

Odour masking consists of adding a pleasant fragrance to the bad odour, thus providing competition between the two in which the pleasant odour attenuates and complements the bad one. The malodorous components are left out of the fragrance, and the combined effect of the deodorant fragrance and body odours gives a pleasant result.

For odour masking, a mixture may show a stronger intensity (hyperaddition), the same intensity (complete addition) or a lower intensity (hypoaddition) than the sum of the components. The most common observation is hypoaddition. Regardless of the effects on intensity, the odour-masking effect works primarily by modifying the character of the bad odour.

Reodorants

Certain terpenes (e.g. α-ionone, α-methylionone, citral, geranyl formate and geranyl acetate) have been found to enhance the odour-masking effects of other compounds in deodorant formulations for the mouth. These materials have been called 'reodorants'. However, odour-masking fragrances such as flower oils alone may give rise to unpleasant sensations. To circumvent this, the use of reodorants in a concentration of 10–2000 parts per million is recommended. These substances should volatize competitively with whatever odour may be present, and must act at low concentrations.[2]

Odour counteraction

In this, two or more odours are mixed and give a combined odour intensity that is less than that of either of the individual components.[3] Here again, the resulting odour must overcome the primary ones to obtain a pleasant smell.

This new odour has been further subclassified as a compromise odour (less than the stronger odour) or compensation odour (less than both foul odours). Odour compromise is by far the most common.[1] Success in the art of chemists and manufacturers of perfumes consist in obtaining this compromise to obtain stable and commercially viable products.

Odour desensitization

Some materials may temporarily deactivate nasal sensory receptors, and they act as deodorants. In this way, isolates from flavanoid plants can produce a real deodorant activity. This results from a complex mechanism involving clathrating, addition and neutralization reactions with the active ingredients of malodorous sources in addition to biological reactions in human beings, such as inhibition of olfactory receptors. More research is required into these subtle effects.

Biochemical effects

Deodorant components show a significant capacity to inhibit lipoxidase (lipoxygenase).[4,5] A lipoxidase can catalyse the hydroperoxidation of polyunsaturated fatty acids and esters of linoleic acid containing the pentadienyl group, which are present in the epidermis.

The hydroperoxides that could be generated by the action of lipoxidase on epidermal linoleates are known to decompose or undergo further oxidation to short- and medium-chain aldehydes, ketones and acids, most of which have strong, unpleasant odours.[6] According to Osberghaus,[7] the potential oxidation of unsaturated compounds on the skin should be involved in odour development. These purely chemical procedures can be reproduced.

Antimicrobial fragrances

Sturm[8] has described 'deosafe' fragrances that not only reduce the perception of odour with odour masking but also stop odour development through antimicrobial action. However, according to Morris et al,[9] the best anitmicrobial fragrance chemical is 100–1000 times less effective than the most common antimicrobial soap. This kind of soap represents the first step towards elementary body hygiene, which removes a large quantity of bad odours.

It appears that the most successful applications of antimicrobial fragrances would probably be with products that are intended to be left on the skin.

ODOUR REDUCTION AND ODOUR REMOVAL

Control by good skin hygiene

Simple daily bathing with soap and water reduces the tendency of perspiration to develop offensive odours.

Good skin hygiene can reduce the total number of bacteria on the cutaneous surface, but can also remove a lot of odorous substances, no matter what their origin. Elimination of maceration and all bacterial decomposition represents a fundamental step in eliminating bad odours.

Odour removal

One of the earliest chemical deodorant ingredients was sodium bicarbonate. In 1946 Lamb[10] recommended a bicarbonate-based deodorant for general use and for treatment of severe bromidrosis. This author suggested a mechanism of action in which part of the deodorizing action of sodium bicarbonate is to chemically neutralize odiferous short-chain fatty acids in the axilla.

Sodium and potassium bicarbonates are still in use as deodorant ingredients, and are the basis of several recent patents. The formulation of bicarbonates into a stick deodorant form is difficult because of problems of solubility, compatibility, stability and commercial presentation. The best results are obtained with suspension in acrosol products.

There are other deodorant ingredients that may also exhibit a chemical odour-removal effect. Among these are zinc glycinate, zinc carbonate, and magnesium or lanthanum oxides, hydroxides or carbonates.

Adsorption or absorption

An odour absorbant is a substance that captures and then retains odour molecules in its interior. An odour adsorbant only retains odour molecules on its surface.

Odour-adsorbing deodorant ingredients include aluminium and potassium double sulphate, 2-naphtholic acid dibutylamide and isonanoyl-2-methylpiperidide. Zinc or magnesium salts of polycarboxylic acids have an odour-absorbing action by trapping the small molecules that are responsible for the bad odours in their crystal lattices.

With ion-exchange powder, deodorization is an adsorptive effect. However, the powders alone wash off with perspiration. Odour-absorbing deodorant ingredients have a more effective action.

Among odour-absorbing deodorants there are ion-exchange resins (Amberlite), a complex mixture with tea extract as its basis (Phytoneutral), and numerous natural essential oils: lavender, cedar, lavendin, rosemary and lemon essences. The active agents include linolanol, geraniol and sentatol, among others.

PREVENTION OF ODOUR DEVELOPMENT

Chemical antimicrobial agents and antitranspirant substances can prevent odour development.

Antimicrobial agents

The bacteria responsible for axillary odour are Gram-positive micrococci and lipophilic diphtheroids. The main substrate for the odour-causing bacterial action is apocrine and probably apo-eccrine sweat. The micrococci are thought to produce a sweaty acid odour and the lipophilic diphtheroids a pungent acrid odour.[11] Elimination of decomposing bacteria can prevent bromhidrosis.

In the past some deodorant manufacturers used antibiotics such as neomycin. However, side-effects have led to its removal from deodorant products.

The early ingredients used for deodorants included aluminium chloride, boric acid, benzoic acid, chloroamine-T, chlorothymol, formaldehyde, hexamine, oxyquinoline sulphate, sodium perborate, zinc salicylate, zinc sulphocarbonate, zinc sulphide and zinc peroxide. All these materials were claimed to have deodorizing and/or antimicrobial properties.[12] However, some of them were described as generating various skin irritations. A good product should be well tolerated.

Later products with cresylic acid were more effective as odour-masking agents than those with antimicrobial ingredients.

Since 1950, a number of successful antimicrobial ingredients have been developed. The first was hexachlorophene, but the toxic symptoms that were observed in rats, monkeys and premature infants led the US Food and Drug Administration to ban hexachlorophene in soaps, cosmetics and drugs.

Together with undecylenic acid byproducts, the most popular antiseptics used are salicylamides, polyhalides, carbanilides, and quaternary ammonium compounds. Quaternary ammonium compounds are colourless, odourless, antiseptic salts, which are often incorporated in water-based deodorants. The most frequently used are cetylpyridinium, trimethylpyrimidine and benzalkonium salts. These cationic substances are incompatible with anionic products (soap, lauryl sulphates, etc.), and after washing careful rinsing is necessary before using this type of deodorant.

A dual antibacterial action and trapping of decomposition products is realized by copper and zinc metal chelators. These block bacterial metabolism and absorb the decomposing waste present in sweat. Antioxidants such as butylhydroxyanisole (BHA), butylhydroxytoluene (BHT) and tocopherols act depending on the amount of oxygen present. They stop bacterial metabolism, and therefore the production of rancid lipids is prevented.

Cetoglutaric acid maintains an acid pH in the sweat, and melanic acid eliminates the action of the enzymes responsible for disagreeable fermentations.

Two compounds are generally used today as antiseptics: triclocarban and triclosan.

Triclocarban

Triclocarban (3,4,4'-trichlorocarbanilide, TCC) is effective against Gram-positive organisms, including odour-causing bacteria, usually at a concentration of 0.5–1.5%, depending on the molecular weight. The antibacterial action of triclocarban is similar to that of several other membrane-active compounds. Once adsorbed, however, such compounds can exhibit specific effects on the plasma membrane of the cell.[13]

These specific effects include uncoupling of proton translocation, increase in both H^+ and Cl^- permeability,[14] and inhibition of the cell's ability to accumulate isoleucine by active transport.

Triclosan

Triclosan (2,4,4'-trichloro-2'-hydroxydiphenyl ether) is effective against Gram-positive and Gram-negative bacteria, and has found application in deodorants, bar soaps and other deodorant products. Here the levels of use of triclosan are lower than those of triclocarban. As with triclocarban, the primary site of action of triclosan is the cell membrane. At low bacteriostatic concentrations, the action on the membrane interferes with the uptake of amino acids, uracil and other nutrients from the medium. At higher bactericidal concentrations, the membrane lesions lead to leakage of cellular contents and the death of the cell.[15] To avoid irritation, these products should be washed off abundantly with water.

Antiperspirant salts

For a long time, the most frequently used substances were tannin, formol, hexamine and glutaraldehyde. Today, aluminium salts are used in the making of cosmetics.

These salts can combine with keratin fibrils, and form a deposit in the sudoral channel lumen. This deposit is responsible for a functional and temporary regulation of the sudoral secretion. Moreover, they transform volatile short-chain fatty acids into nonvolatile and odourless metallic salts. They also block the development of bacteria.

The aluminium salts most used in cosmetics are the acetate, acetotartrate, benzoate, boroformate, borotartrate, bromhydrate, citrate, gluconate, glucolate and salicylate. But the most popular and best known is aluminium chlorohydrate (ACH).

Aluminium and zirconium salts used together are very efficient, but unfortunately too irritating to the skin. The best activity is obtained with the hexahydrated chloride of aluminium at 20–25% in absolute ethanol.

Today the best results are found with aluminium salt derivatives in solution in absolute ethanol. This antiperspirant product appears more effective than all the deodorant factors used alone.

Continual efforts are being made to develop new antimicrobial agents for use in cosmetic deodorant products:

- deodorants containing propylene glycol;
- creams with hydrogen peroxide;
- alkenylidene bisphenols;
- alkylsalicylanilides and halosalicylanilides;
- prenylamine, bicyclic oxazolidines, thiocarbamates, tocopherol and Zylene.[5]

Today, the use of aerosols is diminishing, but gels in the form of a deodorant stick can be found in plastic bottles with screw-on caps. Liquid deodorants are sold in vaporizers, atomizers, roll-ons and bottles with a moisturized wad. Creams, soaps and tablets are more commonly used than powder and impregnated sachets. The newest products are presented in the form of microparticulates whose collagen envelope slowly disintegrates under the action of sweat bacteria.

CONCLUSIONS

This chapter has covered three major mechanisms of action for deodorant ingredients:

odour modification, reduction and prevention.

Today, three types of deodorants are the most effective:

- antibacterial substances;
- antiperspirant inhibitors of sweat such as aluminium salts;
- physico-chemical adsorbers of nauseous odours.

The best deodorant should associate these three qualities.

An efficient treatment of hyperhidrosis and bromhidrosis should involve the use of active antiperspirants (aluminium salts, iontophoresis, etc.) to block the activity of the sudoral glands, after which a subtle and light perfume (neither aggressive nor irritating) should be added according to individual preference.

REFERENCES

1. Seitz EP Jr, Richardson DI, Deodorant ingredients. In: *Antiperspirants and Deodorants* (Laten, J, Selger C, eds). New York: Marcel Dekker, 1989:345–78.
2. Linfield WM, Casoly RE, Noel DR, Studies in the development of antibacterial surfactants II. Performance of germicidal and deodorant soaps. *J Am Oil Chem Soc* 1960; **37**: 251–4.
3. Buckenmayer RH, Odor control. In: *Kirk–Othmer Encyclopedia of Chemical Technology*, 34th edn, Vol 16. New York: Wiley-Interscience, 1981:297.
4. Cain WS, Drexier M, Scope and evaluation of odor counteraction and masking. *Ann NY Acad Sci* 1974; **237**: 427–39.
5. Regos J, Zak O, Solf R et al, Antimicrobial spectrum of triclosan, a broad spectrum antimicrobial agent for topical application. II. Comparison with some other antimicrobial agents. *Dermatologica* 1979; **158**: 72–9.
6. Sonntag NOV, Reactions of fats and fatty acids. In: *Balley's Industrial Oil and Fat Products*, 4th edn, Vol 1 (Swern D, ed). New York: Wiley-Interscience, 1979:140.
7. Osberghaus R, Nonmicrobicidal deodorizing agents. *Cosmet Toiletries* 1980; **95**: 48–50.
8. Sturm W, Deosafe fragrances: fragrances with

deodorizing properties. *Cosmet Toiletries* 1979; **94:** 35–48.

9. Morris JA, Khettry A, Seltz EW, Antimicrobial activity of aroma chemicals and essential oils. *J Am Oil Chem Soc* 1979; **56:** 595–603.

10. Lamb JH, Sodium bicarbonate: an excellent deodorant. *J Invest Dermatol* 1946; **7:** 131–3.

11. Shehadeh N, Kligman AM, The bacteria responsible for axillary odor, II. *J Invest Dermatol* 1963; **41:** 3.

12. Chilson F, Deodorants. In: *Modern cosmetics, Drug and Cosmetic Industry.* New York, 1934:167–77.

13. Hamilton WA, Membrane active antibacterial compounds. *Biochem J* 1970; **118:** 46P–47P.

14. Hamilton WA, Jeacocke RE, The ion specific increases in membrane permeability with a group of membrane active antibacterial agents. *Biochem J* 1972; **127:** 56P-57P.

15. Regos J, Hitz HR, Investigations on the mode of action of triclosan, a broad spectrum antimicrobial agent. *Zentralbl Baktirol Hyg I Abt Orig A* 1974; **226:** 390–401.

16

Hair care

Rodney Dawber

NORMAL HAIR

The feel of natural, healthy hair is firm and soft, whilst it is easy to disentangle when wet or dry (Figure 16.1). When it is in a clean state it has a glossy, non-greasy appearance given by the sebum taken up by the hair. The general purpose of hair care products is mainly to restore the natural beauty of hair, giving it lightness, volume, spring and control, together with suppleness, softness and sheen.[1]

The above is essentially aesthetic in its definition, and many individuals with dry or greasy hair would not consider themselves as abnormal in the sense of needing 'treatment'.[1] The concept of 'normal' hair in the cosmetic sense is thus a very broad one; it is inevitably subjective, depending on personal, professional, social and cultural factors.

Apart from the specific components to be described in individual sections of this chapter, the main cosmetic range used for normal hair is shampoos.[2]

Shampoos[2,3]

A shampoo may be defined as a suitable detergent for washing hair that leaves the hair in good condition. Original[4] shampoos were used solely for cleansing hair, but their range of function has extended in recent years to include conditioning, and the treatment of some hair and scalp diseases. In principle, to wash hair, a shampoo must remove sebum, since it is the latter that attracts dirt and other particulate matter. The polar group of a detergent achieves this by displacing oil from the hair surface. The evaluation of shampoo

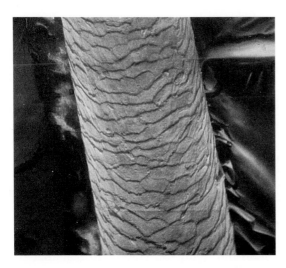

Figure 16.1 Normal hair at the root end before any weathering has taken place (scanning electron micrograph).

detergency is difficult and complicated. The consumer tends to equate detergency with foaming; in Western society few shampoos sell unless they possess good foaming power. In the evaluation of detergents as shampoos, no single criterion can be used, though instrumental methods have been devised. Efficacy can be based only on the subjective impression of the consumer. The factors taken into consideration include:

- ease of distribution of shampoo over the hair;
- lathering power;
- ease of rinsing and combing of wet hair;
- lustre of hair;
- speed of drying;
- ease of combing and setting.

Safety is of paramount importance.

Shampoo formulations

These vary enormously, but the essential ingredients can be resolved into a few groups: water, detergent and some fatty material. Soap shampoos are made from vegetable or animal fats, and remove dirt and grease as efficiently as detergents; however, a scum forms with hard water, and the trend has therefore been increasingly towards detergents as the principal washing ingredient. Detergents are synthetic petroleum products, and form no hard water scum.

Shampoos contain

- principal surfactants for detergency and foaming power;
- secondary surfactants to improve and 'condition' hair;
- additives that both complete the formulation and add 'special' effects – whatever the claims of some manufacturers, most special additives end up down the sink!

In general, cosmetic shampoos can be dry (powder types), liquid, solid cream, aerosol or oily. Anti-dandruff, 'medicated' and scalp treatment shampoos contain antiseptics and active agents such as coal- and wood-tar frac-

tions. Clear liquid shampoos are the most popular, including 'cleansing' types, sold for treating greasy hair, and 'cosmetic' types having good conditioning action and popular among women with dry or 'normal' hair. The modern two-in-one formulations now dominate world markets.[2]

Shampoo safety

Shampoos obviously must be non-toxic, and at concentrations used by the consumer that irritate neither skin nor eyes. New shampoo formulations are tested extensively prior to marketing, particularly to assess their propensity to cause eye irritation, scarring and corneal opacities. Skin irritation is not usually encountered from shampoos that have low eye irritancy potential. Eye safety is assessed by the technique known as the Draize test. This animal test has proved to be efficacious and necessary to satisfy the requirements of government bodies, although the cosmetic and pharmaceutical industry is constantly attempting to define satisfactory in vitro substitutes. In the Draize test standard solutions of shampoo are instilled into the conjunctival sac of an albino rabbit. In general, the eye irritancy of detergents is greatest with cationics, followed by anionics, and least with nonionics. Factors that may vary this include surface activity, pH, wetting power, foaming power, and wetting and foaming together.

DRY HAIR[5]

When sebaceous secretion is insufficient, the scalp appears taut and dry, and the hair becomes dull looking and brittle to the touch. This is known as 'dry' hair, and it has physiological causes. When hair is traumatized by over-vigorous mechanical or chemical treatments, it also ends up with the appellation 'dry'. This happens to hair that is often wound too tightly on curlers, to hair that is highly bleached, and to hair treated with alkaline permanent wave lotions or shampoos with excessive detergency power. Or, it can

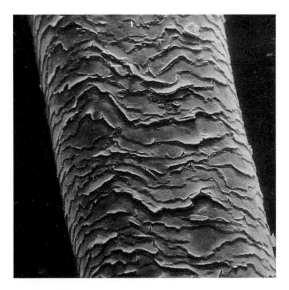

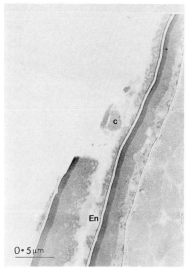

Figure 16.2 Early cuticular breakage and weathering (scanning electron micrograph).

Figure 16.3 Early cuticular weathering; surface cell breaking off (silver methenamine stain). En, endocuticle; C, cortex.

occur when brushing is too frequent or excessive; hot blow-drying intensifies the drying effect to an extent determined by its frequency.

Dry hair is prone to tangles. Combing enhances hair shaft damage and the appearance of split ends, cuticle cells become fragile and break off (Figures 16.2 and 16.3). A further factor in the frailty of hair is weathering. This term covers the cumulative effect of climatic exposure, namely sunlight, air pollutants, wind, seawater and spindrift, or chlorinated water of swimming pools. The prevailing inducer of damage is sunlight, which, apart from bleaching brown hair and yellowing blond hair, causes photo-oxidative splitting of cystine linkages, initiates free radicals detrimental to the protein matrix, and increases the porosity of the cuticle. Degrading weathering processes are enhanced by ambient humidity. The physico-chemical changes are more pronounced on bleached, waved (Figure 16.4) or dyed hair, but intact hair itself is more sensitive to cosmetic handling. The alterations are not restricted to surface properties – tactile, frictional, glossy, etc. – tensile strength has been shown to decrease progressively with increasing exposure. It is not a matter of inadequate

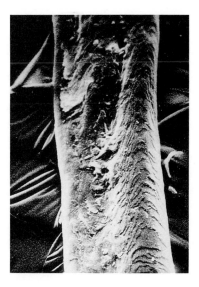

Figure 16.4 Severe exaggerated 'weathering' following bleaching and waving over-treatment (scanning electron micrograph).

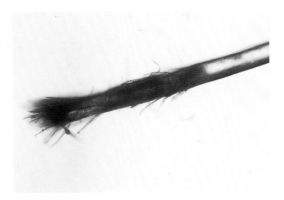

Figure 16.5 Hair breakage of extrinsic (cosmetic) type (light micrograph).

sebum level, but of an alteration in fibre texture.

All these physico-chemical or chemical alterations can be defined, and may be measured according to the following characteristics:

- loss of sheen;
- more brittleness to the touch, with a loosening of cuticle scales and increase in the friction coefficient;
- increased porosity, with subsequent increase in drying time;
- lower disruption point, with the hair breaking more easily (Figure 16.5) as a result of the disruption of certain linkages providing fibre cohesion (e.g. cystine and salt linkages, hydrogen bonds);
- decrease in sulphur content;
- degradation in polypeptide chains, leading to the elimination of oligoproteins etc.

Whether it originates from a physiological lack of sebum, mechanical or chemical over-processing, or environmental factors, the result is the same: what is generally, and rather vaguely, known as 'dry hair', 'weakened hair' or 'damaged hair'.

Basic compounds

The causes and effects of dryness in hair are reasonably well known. It is extremely difficult to remove the causes. There are virtually no compounds known that are capable of restoring normal size and function to malfunctioning or underactive sebaceous glands. It is the task of the cosmetic chemist to limit the degradation brought about by overactive hair products. It is of equal importance that proper application techniques be observed. Another objective is to reduce damage resulting from handling abuse by providing suitably lubricating or scale tightening products that ease brushing and combing. It is easier to tackle the consequences, preventing them if possible using the following principles. Since there is a deficiency in fatty compounds, it is useful to try to fix fatty compounds to the hair fibre. Substances naturally existing in sebum should be preferentially used, so as to remedy any natural deficiency. To offset the modification in polypeptide chains, hair should be given back the amino acids and microelements it has lost. Treating dry hair is, in fact, restoring the chemical components it has lost. But treatment will be more effective if these products are fixed to the fibre by a chemical or physico-chemical process, so as to avoid elimination by rinsing. With different formulation bases, this goal is sometimes attained.

Recent research has made progress in seeking to reconstitute disrupted linkages, restore protein chains, and replace disrupted chemical linkages by new ones that are different but equally strong.

The main chemical compounds used in formulating hair care products specifically designed to treat dry hair are the following.

Organic acids

The acids are acetic, lactic, malic, citric, tartaric, adipic, etc. Lay people traditionally know the virtues of rinsing with lemon juice or vinegar! They are useful for several reasons. After washing hair with soap, hair looks dull. This is due to its having been given an alkaline treatment and to its being more or less saturated with insoluble lime soaps. The acid rinse brings the epidermal pH and the 'hair pH' back to a normal level. It also dissolves the soap and through the fatty acids released, gives back its normal feel and sheen to the hair. After bleaching, an acid rinse precipitates proteins and thus prevents the elimination of amino acids or oligoproteins resulting from the fibre degradation. Many hair products intended for the treatment of dry hair contain a fairly high proportion of organic acids.

Fatty compounds and derivatives

The generally accepted composition of 'hair' sebum is free unsaturated fatty acids (20%), free saturated fatty acids (10%), triglycerides (30%), fatty esters other than triglycerides (20%), cholesterol, pure or combined (5%), and squalene (15%), and giving back to hair the lacking fatty elements seems to be a logical, though unproven, step. The most frequently used products belong to a number of categories:

- fatty acids: oleic, stearic, behenic, ricinoleic, linoleic and linolenic (vitamin F) acids;
- fatty alcohols: lauryl, myristyl, oleyl, cetyl and stearyl alcohols;
- natural triglycerides: almond, castor, peanut, avocado, corn, olive, monoi and karite oils;
- natural waxes, such as beeswax, spermaceti and jojoba oil;
- fatty esters like the stearates or oleates of glycol or glycerol and isopropyl fatty esters;
- oxyethylenated or oxypropylenated derivatives of waxes, alcohols and fatty acids;
- partially sulphated fatty alcohols;
- lanolin and its derivatives (see below);
- other animal waxes, e.g. mink oil, containing 75% unsaturated esters, of which 20% is an unusual C_{16} unsaturated acid (palmitoleic acid), which is also present in sebum;
- phospholipids, especially lecithins, mixtures of phosphatides extracted from egg yolk or soybean; among these extracts are egg oil and the hexane extract of spray-dried egg yolk;
- fatty acyl lactylate salts such as sodium isostearoyl lactylate.

Lanolin is an animal wax of complex composition. It contains a great number of saturated fatty acids and virtually no unsaturated fatty acids. These fatty acids are esterified either by fatty alcohols or by cyclic alcohols (containing the cyclopentanophenanthrene ring, etc.). Lanolin also contains fatty alcohols and non-esterified sterols. It contains neither squalene nor triglycerides. It is sometimes used, pure, in the formulation of hair care products, but, more frequently, extracts or derivatives are employed: liquid or waxy lanolin, resulting from the separation of esters with a relatively low molecular weight and those with a high molecular weight, hydrogenated lanolin, oxyethylenated derivatives, isopropyl esters of lanolin, acetylated lanolin, lanolin alcohols, etc.

Vitamins

Vitamins, mostly from those of groups A and B, can be provided by miscellaneous extracts. Wheat germ, separated out during the milling process, is also favoured: it contains liposoluble or hydrosoluble vitamins, auxin, agents promoting the development of yeasts, diastases, microelements, fatty acids, phosphatides, amino acids and sugars. It is especially rich in group E vitamins, in particular α-tocopherol, which is useful because it is involved in the regulation of oxidoreductive phenomena and may facilitate irrigation of the scalp by the blood.

Protein derivatives

Protein molecules are too large to penetrate the hair and fix onto hair keratin. They can be used either in the form of partial hydrolysates, a peptide mix, or amino acids resulting from total hydrolysis. Extracts or hydrolysates of keratins (cow horn, hoof, horsehair, wool or hair), silk proteins, collagen, gelatin, casein, isinglass, protamines from fish milt, etc. are used. Sometimes use is made of their condensation products with fatty acids.

Cation-active surfactants

Natural hair can be regarded as an amphoteric gel possessing basic and acidic groups with nearly equal and inverse strengths. A slight predominance of acid groups suffices to give hair the nature of an anionic resin. This occurs in the case of damaged hair, especially bleached hair, which becomes very rich in free acid groups as a result of cystine-linkage disruption and oxidation. These groups are sulphonic acids, which are strong acids that give the hair surface a strongly anionic valence. Intense exposure to sun can lead to this kind of transformation through the action of ultraviolet light on the cystine linkage, increasing hair sensitivity.

The cation-active derivatives are surfactants with a hydrophilic cationic group carrying one or two lipophilic hydrocarbon fatty chains. When a cation-active compound comes into contact with a damaged hair possessing numerous anionic sites, an electrochemical bonding between the negatively charged fibre and the positively charged cationic site of the cation-active substance can take place. Cation-active compounds are substantive for the keratin fibre. Because of their polarity, they can neutralize and eliminate the discrepancy in electrical charge between different hairs.

Basically, the action of a cation-active surfactant entails fixing a monomolecular film to the hair through electrochemical bonding. Immediately, even very damaged hair is given a pleasant, soft feel and excellent combability, because the film is composed of a fatty chain, which provides lubrication, reduces fibre friction, and minimizes the abrasive effects of combing and brushing. These qualities are most dramatic on wet hair. The lubricant contribution, however, is less noticeable on dry hair, where 'weighing down' should be avoided.

There are many cation-active substances. Depending on the type of anion or cation, their properties (detergent, emulsifying, conditioning and adsorption) can be varied. The longer-fatty chain compounds, such as the stearyls, are far more effective conditioners than the shorter fatty compounds, such as the lauryls. This category includes the following:

- quaternary ammonium salts with one or two fatty chains, such as the stearyl (or oleyl) dimethylbenzylammonium, lauryl pyridinium, and distearyldimethylammonium salts;
- fatty amines, such as stearyldimethylamine;
- ethoxylated fatty amines, quaternized or non-quaternized, such as Quaternium 52;
- α- or β-fatty amino acids, such as alkyldimethylglycines and alkyldimethyl-β–alanines;
- quaternized sugars or derivatives, such as quaternized gluconic amino amides, such as Quaternium 22;
- quaternized or non-quaternized amino amides of fatty acids, such as stearoylaminopropyldimethylamine (e.g. Quaterniums 61, 62, 63 and 70) or the amides of lanolin acid (e.g. Quaternium 33) or mink-oil fatty acids (e.g. Quaternium 26);
- amine oxides.

These are particularly useful in the form of anion–cation complexes produced by reacting a cation-active compound with an anion-active compound. For example, if ammonium oleate is mixed with a fatty amine in stoichiometric proportions, the result is an anion–cation complex: the oleate of the fatty amine. When a hydroalcoholic solution of the amine oleate is applied to a bleached hair, the following is thought to occur:

1. The free acid groups in the hair keratin are stronger than, and displace, the oleic acid and fix the fatty cationic chain by electrovalent bonding.

2. The released fatty acid can fix itself to the hair by adsorption.
3. Thus, the hair is treated both by anion–cation exchange (as occurs with a cation-active product) and by adsorption (as with fatty compounds).

Cationic polymers

Cation-active surfactants are the ideal compounds to normalize the hair surface, protect damaged areas, smooth out scales, impart softness, and facilitate disentangling, combing and brushing. But they do not improve hair texture. Moreover, the use of these compounds has certain limitations. Some are not well tolerated by the eye; but the main drawback is that most of them are incompatible with the major anionic surfactants used in formulating shampoos. Hence a new category of cation-active compounds was developed that are equally substantive for hair and able to sheathe the surface with a continuous film and thus impart body, texture and firmness. These are the cationic polymers, in which the substantive cationic poles are no longer attached to a fatty chain, as they are in cationic surfactants, but rather are grafted or integrated into a polymeric structure. Cationic polymers are a breakthrough in conditioner formulation given their specific properties and the compatiblity shown by many with the most commonly used anionic surfactants. They are also revolutionary in the way in which they protect weakened or fragile hair against external attack. The first polymer used was a cellulose resin called 'Polymer JR' (Polyquaternium 10*), introduced in an anionic shampoo in 1972. It was obtained by quaternization of trimethylamine by the product resulting from the reaction of hydroxyethylcellulose with epichlorhydrin. The average molecular weight of this type of resin lies between 250 000 and 600 000.

Subsequently, many cationic polymers have been patented, marketed and used in formulating dry hair treatment products. The main categories of interest to cosmetic chemists are as follows.

Cationic celluloses and starches

Examples of these polymers are: Resin JR 30 M.125, 400 (Union Carbide), Jaguar C 13 S (Celanese) and Cosmedia Guar C261 (Henkel), which are reaction products from guar gum, epichlorhydrin and trimethylamine; and Celquat L 200 (National Starch), which is a copolymer (Polyquaternium 4*) of hydroxyethylcellulose with diallyldimethylammonium chloride (Polyquaternium 4*). These polymers generally have much lower molecular weight (between 1000 and 20 000). Examples are Mirapol A-15 (Miranol) (Polyquaternium 2), with $A = (CH_2)_3NHCONH(CH_2)_3$ and $B = CH_2CH_2OCH_2CH_2$, and Onamer-M (Millmaster Onyx Corp) (Polyquaternium 1*), with $A = B = CH_2CH=CHCH_2$ and triethanolamine endings.

Cationic silicones

An example is Amodimethicone (Dow Corning), which is available as an emulsion containing cationic silicone, together with tallow trimethylammonium and an oxyethylenated alkylphenol.

Quaternized protein hydrolysates

These are cation-active surfactants in which the anion is a carboxylate belonging to the polypeptide chain of a partially hydrolysed protein. The preceding compounds were polycations, generally with halide or methylsulphate as counterions (anions), whereas these are polyanions with benzalkonium, alkyltrimethylammonium or quaternized amido amines as cation partners. A feature of these modified hydrolysates is reinforced substantivity for the hair fibre.

GREASY HAIR[6]

To the dermatologists, the term 'seborrhoea' (Figure 16.6) refers to hypersecretion by seba-

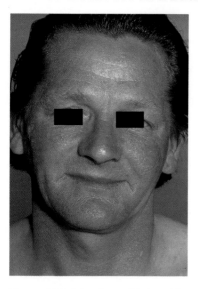

Figure 16.6 Seborrhoea of hair and face.

ceous glands. Frequently, it is restricted to the scalp, which acquires an oily appearance and generates 'greasy' hair. It is often associated with excessive secretion by the sweat glands of the scalp. The physiological mechanisms of seborrhoea are fairly well understood, but the process leading to the appearance of greasy hair is much more complicated. The perception of a seborrhoeic condition is rather subjective – often more rheological than quantitative in nature – and is the result of a series of alterations that can vary greatly from one subject to the next. The unpleasant cosmetic consequences of seborrhoea are many. The hair rapidly becomes greasy and sticks in clumps. Hairstyles do not last long after being set, since the excess sebum weighs the hair down. Dust accumulates on greasy hair, causing it to get dirty very quickly. The sebum may undergo peroxidative transformation and acquire a disagreeable odour. These are the cosmetic defects for which cosmetologists try to find remedies.

Causes

Basically, there is the sebaceous gland, and the pilosebaceous duct, the part of the hair follicle into which the gland secretions are discharged. These secretions are composed of triglycerides (60%), wax esters of fatty acids and long-chain fatty alcohols (20–25%), and squalene (15%), which is the element characterizing human sebum and is very rarely found in the animal kingdom.

The sebaceous cells disintegrate (holocrine secretion) and release this sterile mixture of lipids into the pilosebaceous duct, already containing some protein and lipid residue, and inhabited as well by microorganisms belonging to the normal skin flora, i.e. *Pityrosporum ovale*, *Staphylococcus epidermidis* and *Propionibacterium acnes*. The population is mainly engaged in enzymatic activity, directed towards the triglycerides, which the microbial lipases hydrolyse progressively, releasing fatty acids. Once excreted onto the surface, the modified sebum mixes with another type of lipid emanating from the epidermal cells – free cholesterol and cholesterol esters and glycerides.

Although the sebaceous-gland concentrations on the scalp are as great as those on the forehead (400–900/cm²) and the composition of the lipids synthesized is identical, there are marked differences in the kinetics of sebum replacement following shampooing. The sebum recovery process is much slower on the scalp – no doubt because of the lower capacity of the follicular reservoir, up to 80% of whose volume can be taken up by the hair shaft.

On the basis of subjective evaluation, some authors suggest that repeated use of excessively detergent shampoos can accelerate this process; the sebeceous gland is said to react to the 'insult' caused by excess secretion. Specific studies, particularly those using precise measurements taken with an adapted Lipometer, have proved that this hypothesis is unfounded. Even after daily shampooing, there is no evidence of change in the sebum excretion rate. The kinetics of sebum replacement on the scalp remain unaffected by shampoo frequency.

The kinetics of sebum replacement on the hair are rather different, varying greatly according to the kind of shampoo and the treatment applied. Sebum does not spread spontaneously over the hair; it does not move by capillary action along the hair shaft, but by a passive process, migrating by direct contact of hair with scalp. Running a comb or brush or the fingers through the hair speeds up its migration. The root of the hair, in close proximity to the scalp, is generally affected more rapidly by this mechanical transfer.

The state of greasy hair is a complex phenomenon related only in part to the quantity of sebum secreted by the sebaceous gland. Study of lipids from the scalp and the hair reveals that this modification results from considerable chemical transformations taking place during the days following a shampoo:

1. Enzymatic hydrolysis of triglycerides, releasing mostly saturated-chain fatty acids.
2. Formation of insoluble calcium salts from fatty acids with a high melting point and calcium ions provided by hard water.

In addition to these rheological changes in the sebum, which can range from a more or less liquid oil to a waxy solid, other factors must be taken into consideration: the importance of the hair surface condition and implantation, the influence of the corneocyte state of the scalp, as well as that of environmental factors on the regulation of excretion and casual level of sebum, etc. This brief insight shows how elusive the nature of the sebum recovery mechanism can be. The fact that a number of factors are involved indicates that many different approaches to combat greasy hair may be considered.

Antigrease agents

There does not yet exist a product that, applied locally, can cure acute seborrhoea.

Only relatively toxic compounds with many restrictions on their use can bring about a significant reduction of sebaceous gland secretion when given systemically. The anti-androgens, or 13-*cis*-retinoic acid, a derivative of vitamin A, are examples of such agents. It is, however, possible to formulate good products to treat milder cases of seborrhoea cosmetically. Antiseborrhoea agents recommended for mild cases should theoretically possess the following characteristics:

- be non-toxic;
- eliminate excess sebum without excessive detergent action or drying – this excludes shampoos with high detergent power and solvents that are too active in removing grease;
- stop itching;
- possess adequate bactericidal and fungicidal properties;
- contain elements inducing a return to normal, regulated biosynthesis of keratin and normal desquamation.

The prevalent compounds in cosmetic treatments for greasy hair are the following.

Sulphur and sulphur derivatives

Elemental sulphur has long been considered the specific remedy for seborrhoea, either in the form of solutions of octahedral sulphur in carbon disulphide or as a colloidal dispersion. It possesses many advantages (antiparasitic, anti-itching, keratolytic, keratoplastic, vasomotor, oxidoreductive, and other qualities). However, it is now thought that sulphur should be used with caution because of its excessive drying effect and irritancy.

Interesting results have been obtained using mineral or organic derivatives of sulphur, which are gentler; their drawback is an unpleasant odour, which is difficult to overcome. Examples are polythionic acids and their alkaline salts, quaternary ammonium polythionates, and mercaptocarboxylic acids in the form of the acid, related esters or amides.

Among the inorganic sulphur derivatives is selenium disulphide. This is still frequently used, especially in cases of greasy dandruff and seborrhoeic dermatitis. Its mode of action and effectiveness remain controversial. It has been shown that it increases the volume of the sebaceous glands and stimulates the production of sebum excreted by reducing the level of bacterial hydrolysis. A study of shampoos containing selenium disulphide showed a 20% decrease in free fatty acids and a 160% increase in triglycerides. Although it is efficient in treating dandruff, it appears to aggravate the problem of sebum recovery, provoke irritation, and be unattractive for use as a cosmetic.

Sulphur-containing amino acids and thioethers

Sulphur-containing amino acids such as cysteine and methionine are known to play an important part in the keratinization process. Therefore, it was considered logical to investigate their action on seborrhoea and on the hair production process, through local applications. Methionine, the esters (methyl or benzyl ester) of *N*-acetylmethionine and especially cysteine, so fundamental in the biosynthesis of keratin and in the maturation of the hair structure, have been tested. However, it is hard to develop cosmetic formulation based on cysteine or related thiols because of the inherent drawbacks of this kind of reducing agent. They are unstable and highly sensitive to oxidation. They have unpleasant odours that are difficult to mask. There is also a risk of cutaneous intolerance. Investigations were therefore designed to find appropriate protecting groups without these unwanted secondary effects, but still capable of releasing the biologically active compound in situ.

This approach has produced molecules that may prove useful in reducing the level of sebaceous excretion. A number of active compounds have been selected following local application in tests on animals in which sebor-rhoea has been induced by a diet lacking in biotin or by androgen supplementation:

- *S*-carboxymethyl-, *S*-benzhydryl- and *S*-trityl-cysteine;
- 4-thiazolidine carboxylic acid;
- thialysine (*S*-β-aminoethylcysteine);
- *N*-acetylhomocysteine thiolactone;
- thioethers derived from cysteamine, glutathione and pyridoxine;
- *N,N*-sebacoyl dimethionine;
- thiolanediol and oxidation derivatives.

Certain mechanisms of action have been elucidated. Thus the salts of 2-benzylthiothylamine have inhibition properties vis-à-vis bacterial lipases. They have also been shown to act on lipid synthesis by selectively blocking an enzymatic step leading to triglyceride formation.

Tars

Tars are remarkable and unique in that they yield promising results when used to treat cases of seborrhoea, dandruff, and dry scalp. For years, they have been held to be the best treatment for a number of chronic disorders: psoriasis, eczema, and atopic dermatitis.

They are obtained either by carbonizing coal – coal tar being a by-product – or certain kinds of wood, resulting in pine tar oil, cade (juniper) oil, cedar and birch oil, etc. Whatever the origin of tars, their composition is always extremely complex: they contain polyphenols, high-molecular-weight acids and alcohols, esters, ketones, waxes and hydrocarbons. They show antiseptic, anti-itching and astringent properties. They measurably slow down cell proliferation.

There have been many studies on coal tar, given its dermatological applications. Its composition varies according to the geographic origin of the coal and the distillation temperature. Crude tar is often purified by fractional distillation or extraction. It is available in the form of an extract, a solution or a distillate. There was some concern that coal tar when applied topically may cause tumours, as suggested by some animal studies. Among the hundreds of substances it contains, some (in particular the polynuclear hydrocarbons produced in high-temperature furnaces) have been suspected of presenting a carcinogenic risk. A panel of US Food and Drug Administration experts investigated the matter and, after having gone through the epidemiological data, concluded that coal tar preparations were safe for topical application – at least in shampoo formulations.

Substances retarding sebum recovery

Another approach to slowing down sebum uptake by hair consists of depositing an oleophobic film on the surface of the hair. For this kind of physico-chemical treatment, perfluorinated fatty acids or acrylic resins have been proposed for use. Being both hydrophobic and lipophobic, these compounds, used in low concentrations, can retard sebum transfer from scalp to hair.

Grease absorbers: rheology modifiers

Proteins such as gelatin or casein, in addition to finely divided starches and silicas, have been used to absorb sebum and give it a more waxy consistency in order to make the seborrhoeic state less obvious. They are reasonably effective and satisfactory, but they leave hair looking dull.

Products for greasy hair

Different types of formulations have been developed for treating greasy hair. Lotions would seem to be the most effective in initiating action and modifying the regreasing process. They are applied preferably at the root: active ingredients are deposited on the scalp or along the hair shaft, and, being left there, can be active over lengths of time. As liquids or more or less fluid gels, these lotions are formulated for daily use or as after-shampoo lotions.

- Lotions for daily use have a higher alcohol content (40–50%) for quicker drying and to dissolve a portion of the sebum to be desorbed onto the towel during the drying process. In general, they contain a small amount of anionic polymer to lend greater volume to the hair.
- After-shampoo lotions have a lower alcohol content. They usually contain gums or hydrocolloids to act as absorbers and to help in setting the hairstyle. Lotions for reinforcing hairstyle hold and duration also include specific resins.
- Hydroalcoholic gels are an interesting variant; their consistency makes localized application on the greasy roots and scalp possible and makes dosage by an appropriate device easy. The gels liquefy when lightly rubbed in after application; this creates a sensation of freshness and lightness. Good results have also been achieved with gels in which a gelling polymer is associated with non-ionic polymers, acting as sebum absorbers and simultaneously 'unsticking' the hair from the scalp. The swelling imparted to the root retards sebum uptake, renders styling easier, and favours longer-lasting hairstyle retention and volume.
- Antigrease compounds can also be incorporated into hair rinses, though it is difficult to obtain effective action during the brief time lapse before rinsing and to ensure adequate substantivity so as to avoid eliminating active agents when rinsing. To overcome this difficulty while still rinsing with water, gelling emulsions have been developed. Their viscosity is favourable for distribution throughout the hair and for good penetration. The treatment is left to act for a period of time and then rinsed out. These emulsions contain clays, plant extracts, proteins and/or resins (polymers) to strengthen the hair. A small amount of surfactant is often included to favour emulsification and ensure proper rinsing.
- Dry shampoos are based on associations of sebum-absorbing substances (starches, clays and vegetable powders). They help to reduce greasy deposits without wetting the

hair, and therefore do not require setting and drying. Their main failing is that they tend to leave hair dull.

- More recently, a new approach has been developed to treat seborrhoea of the scalp, based on the observation that, by carefully selecting the surfactants, it is possible to formulate shampoos for regular use that greatly influence the scalp condition and the kinetics of hair regreasing.

The surface state of a scalp with seborrhoea is often highly disturbed, heterogeneous, weakened, and highly sensitive to physical (massage, etc.) or physico-chemical demands made upon it. It must be treated with great caution and gentleness. However, hygiene products for greasy hair must have sufficient detergent strength to eliminate greasy deposits on hair and the abundant dirt they trap. Shampoos are therefore crucial, and their formulation comes under very close scrutiny.

It has been found that the regular use of certain surfactants, in particular non-ionic derivatives of polyglycerol, which have good foaming and detergent properties, leads to progressive and marked lengthening of the hair regreasing process without requiring any additional treatment or antigrease ingredient. This improvement probably arises from a gradual return to a normal scalp state, as the disappearance of itching in affected subjects would seem to indicate. They probably act upon the hair surface as well.

HAIR STYLING/SHAPERS

Permanent waving[3,7]

Permanent waving has been defined as the process of changing the shape of the hair so that the new shape persists through several shampoos. During the last 70 years, increasing knowledge of keratin chemistry has enabled semipermanent chemical methods to be developed. Whatever the process used, three stages are involved in hair waving:

1. physical or chemical softening of the hair;
2. reshaping;
3. hardening of fibres to retain reshaped position.

Softening

Water can extend the hydrogen bonds between adjacent polypeptides in the keratin molecule, allowing temporary reshaping to be carried out – exposure to high humidity or rewetting immediately reverses the process. To obtain a more durable effect from water, steam may be used; this, in a limited way, disrupts disulphide bonds. Heat and steam alone are rarely acceptable to modern women, because their effects are temporary and the treatment is uncomfortable. Heat can be more effectively utilized in conjunction with ammonium hydroxide and potassium bisulphite or triethanolamine as agents to reduce disulphide bonds; great skill is involved in this process, since failure to judge the time of application of chemicals and heat may cause severe damage. Chemical heat pads are still rarely used, for example, utilizing heat produced from an exothermic reaction (e.g. that between quicklime and water).

Since 1945, cold wave processes utilizing substituted thiosulphates, i.e. thioglycolates, have largely superceded hot waving. Thioglycolates are potent reducers of disulphide bonds in the keratin molecule. A typical cold waving solution contains thioglycolic acid plus ammonia or monoethanolamine.

Acid permanent waves have recently become popular for salon use. They contain glyceryl monothioglycolate and produce a softer curl, and can be used on damaged and bleached hair. Their disadvantage is the high frequency of sensitization in hairdressers using the product and, occasionally, sensitization of the client.

Reshaping

The type of rollers or curlers used to reshape the softened hair depends on the training of the hairdresser and the fashion desired. The degree of curl or tightness of the permanent wave depends both on the diameter of the roller and the size of the strand wound round the roller. Increasing the time of exposure to the perming solution up to 20 minutes increases the curl, but longer times do not lead to a further increase. The strength of the solution used depends on the hair type, texture and previous bleaching. Home permanent waves are weaker and cannot achieve the same degree of curl. 'Tepid' waving involves using a weaker thioglycolate solution plus warm air. Neutralization is carried out initially with the curlers in place and again after they have been carefully removed. The reshaping stage is thus a great test of hairdressing skill and experience.

Hardening (neutralizing or setting)

In general, this process involves a reversal of the softening (reduction) stages:

$$2 -SH \xrightarrow{\text{oxidation}} -S-S-$$

It is important to note that complete reversal to pre-softened 'strength' cannot occur, since many free –SH groups may not be in a position for oxidation to be effective, for example

$$2 -SH \rightarrow -S-C-S- \quad (C = carbon)$$
$$2 -SH \rightarrow -S-Ba-S- \quad (Ba = barium)$$

Atmospheric oxidation may efficiently neutralize the waving process. This method is slow, and rollers must be left in position for several hours overnight. Chemical oxidation is now the rule. Hairdressers generally use hydrogen peroxide, whilst most solutions for home use contain sodium perborate or percarbonate (UK) or sodium or potassium bromate (USA). This is why hair is 'lighter' after permanent waving. Some neutralizers contain shellac, which may react with alcohol groups to cause hair discoloration.

Practical procedures

Hot waving

This is almost never used. The procedure is as follows:

1. shampooing;
2. hair divided and rollers or curlers applied under slight tension;
3. waving solution applied;
4. heating.

Heating varies according to the solution used or the type of wave required. Electric rollers or exothermic reactive chemicals may be used. The latter allow free head movement during the waving. The skill of this procedure lies in good hair sectioning, judging the right amount of solution, correct winding tension and appropriate steaming time.

Cold waving

This also involves initial shampooing, hair division into locks, moistening with waving lotion and application of croquignole curlers. Further solution may then be applied. The softening time is 10–20 minutes. Occasionally, mild heat is included, using exothermic chemicals or the natural heat from the head by enclosing the scalp in a plastic bag. These may add to the comfort of the process. Rinsing then takes place, followed by neutralization with the oxidizing solution for up to 10 minutes. After removing the curlers, further 'hardening' solution is usually applied. 'Loose' curl waves last for no more than a few weeks, but 'tight' curl styles may persist for 4–12 months.

Hair straighteners

In principle, the methods used to straighten hair are similar to those used in permanent waving. The practice is almost exclusively used to straighten negroid hair.

Pomades

These are mostly used by men with relatively short hair. They are greasy and act by 'plastering' hair into position.

Hot comb methods

Shampooing is carried out and the hair is towelled dry; oil is then applied, e.g. petroleum jelly or liquid paraffin, which act as heat-transferring agents. Heat pressing with hot combing is then used (64–127 °C), causing breakage and reforming of disulphide bonds, allowing the hair to be moulded straight. Structural damage (and breakage) of hair is common with this process, and scarring alopecia may occur as a result of hot waxes entering the follicles. Sweating and rain reverse this procedure.

Cold methods

The chemical methods employed utilize alkaline reducing agents (caustics), thioglycolates, ammonium carbonate or sodium bisulphite. Caustic soda preparations are usually creams, and require the application of protective scalp oil or wax. They are combed through the hair and left for 15–20 minutes; the hair is combed and straightened again, then rinsed and neutralized. These preparations are limited to salon use because of their potential to cause irritant dermatitis and damage the hair. Thioglycolate creams are the commonest agents used; the cream is applied liberally to the hair, which is then combed until it is straight. The cream is then washed off and a neutralizer (oxidizing agent) applied. Other straighteners ('relaxers') do not contain thioglycolates; examples of these are sodium bisulphite and ammonium carbonate, acidic ethylene glycol and 1,3-propylene glycol. Bisulphite straighteners are suitable for home use in combination with alkaline stabilizers.

HAIR SETTING LOTIONS AND SPRAYS

Setting lotions have changed considerably in recent years. The traditional semiliquid gels based on water-soluble gums (e.g. tragacanth, karaya and acasia) have been replaced by various synthetic polymers in a bewildering array of forms – aerosol foams and sprays, liquids and gels. Most are based on polyvinylpyrrolidone (PVP) in a gelled aqueous solution, and given an attractive glossy, non-greasy appearance. Some preparations incorporate other ingredients to condition or to add antistatic action, lustre or sheen.

Setting lotion and spray formulations are considered safe, after early reports of foreign body granulomatous inflammation had been questioned and not supported by further cases. Hair sprays were incriminated as a possible cause of peripilar casts, but this was not confirmed by later work. However, there is now grave concern about the damage to the ozone layer from the chlorofluorocarbon propellants.

METHYLOLATED COMPOUNDS

Many cosmetic preparations, by their action on the keratin molecule, irreversibly weaken the hair. Cosmetic scientists have produced chemicals that attempt to combat this problem. The formulations contain methylolated compounds of varying strengths, depending on the type of hair under treatment and the solubility of the compound. Most preparations containing alkylated methylol compounds have greater stability and release very little formaldehyde.

CONDITIONERS[2-4]

Dry hair lacks gloss and lustre and is difficult to style. This results from natural weathering, and is worsened by chemical and physical processes applied to the hair. Conditioners comprise fatty acids and alcohols, natural triglycerides (e.g. almond, avocado, corn and olive oils), waxes (e.g. beeswax), jojoba oil, mink oil, lanolin, phospholipids (e.g. egg yolk and soya bean), vitamins A, B and E, protein hydrolysates of silk, collagen, keratin (horn and hoof), gelatin, and cationic polymers. Conditioners are available in a variety of forms, and are widely used. They provide lubrication and gloss, and render the hair easier to comb and style. The most commonly used are creams and emulsions applied for a few minutes after washing and then rinsed off. Deep conditioners are left on for up to 30 minutes, often with damp heat. Fluids, gels and aerosol foams have become popular recently, and aid styling. Hair oils are traditional conditioners. Men use brilliantines, greases or oils to leave the hair glossy and sleek.

REFERENCES

1. Zviak C, Bouillon C, Hair treatment and hair care products. In: *The Science of Hair Care* (Zviak C, ed). New York: Marcel Dekker, 1986:87–144.

2. Dawber RPR, *Shampoos – Scientific Basis and Clinical Aspects.* London: Royal Society of Medicine Press, 1996.

3. O'Donoghue MN, Hair care products. In: *Disorders of Hair Growth* (Olsen EA, ed). New York: McGraw-Hill, 1994:375–88.

4. Rushton H, Gummer CL, Flash H, 2-in-1 shampoo technology. State of the art shampoo and conditioner in one. *Skin Pharm* 1994; **7:** 78–83.

5. Zviak C, Bouillon C, Hair care – dry hair. In: *The Science of Hair Care* (Zviak C, ed). New York: Marcel Dekker, 1986:115–38.

6. Zviak C, Bouillon C, Seborrhoiec conditions (greasy hair). In: *The Science of Hair Care* (Zviak C, ed). New York: Marcel Dekker, 1986:98–109.

7. Wickett RR, Permanent waving and straightening of hair. *Cutis* 1987; **39:** 496–500.

17

Isolated dandruff

Caroline Cardin

DANDRUFF (PITYRIASIS CAPITIS)

Pityriasis capitis is a near-physiological scaling of the scalp, which may or may not be associated with seborrhea. Dandruff, commonly known as pityriasis simplex or furfuracea,[1] is a cosmetic affliction of adolescence and adult life, and is relatively rare and mild in children.[2,3] Its peak incidence and severity, reached at the age of about 20 years, becomes less frequent after 50 years.[2] The age incidence suggests that an androgenic influence may be important and that the level of sebaceous activity may be a factor. However, gross seborrhea may occur without pityriasis, and commonly severe pityriasis may be present without clinically apparent excessive sebaceous activity.[2,3] About 50% of the world's population are afflicted to some degree.[2] The severity and prevalence of the disease may be dependent on the availability of antidandruff therapies, and hair shampoo frequency.

CLINICAL FEATURES

Dandruff has the clinical feature of small white or gray scales that accumulate on the surface of the scalp in localized patches or more diffusely (Figure 17.1). After removal with shampooing, new scales form within 4–7 days. The detachment of the flakes from the scalp can cause aesthetically unpleasant deposits on the collar and shoulder. In seborrhea patients, the scales are greasy and yellowish in color (Figure 17.2). They accumulate in adherent mounds on the scalp, and underlying inflammatory changes are evident.

PATHOLOGY

The stratum corneum of the normal scalp consists of 25–35 fully keratinized and closely

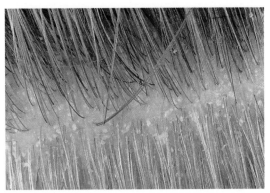

Figure 17.1 Pityriasis simplex.

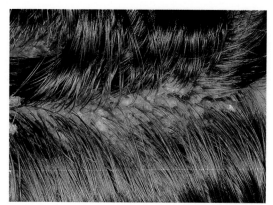

Figure 17.2 Seborrheic dermatitis.

adherent cell layers. In dandruff, there are usually fewer than 10 layers of cells in irregular disposition, often with parakeratotic and irregularly arranged cells, with deep crevices being apparent. Autoradiographic studies show a high labeling index of the basal layer of the epidermis and an accelerated stratum corneum transit time of 3–4 days.[2] In seborrheic dermatitis, the stratum corneum is mildly acanthotic with focal parakeratosis. Spongiosis with serum and leukocyte infiltrate occurs in the paraketarotic lamellae. Early to late lesions with a mild polymorphonuclear leukocytic infiltrate in the upper dermis or in the epidermis are observed. In subacute or chronic stages of seborrheic dermatitis, the epidermis appears increasingly acanthotic, while spongiosis is minimal.[4]

ETIOLOGY

The microbial origin of pityriasis capitis involving yeasts/fungi of the genus *Malassezia*, currently considered synonymous with *Pityrosporum*, has been proposed since the 19th century.[1,2,5–8] Recently, the genus *Malassezia* has been extensively studied for morphological ultrastructural, physiological and molecular biological differences, and

seven species have been identified:[7,8] *M. furfur* (*Pityrosporum ovale*), *M. pachydermatis*, *M. sympodialis*, *M. globosa*, *M. otusa*, *M. restricta* and *M. slooffiae*. The pathogenic role of *P. ovale* as the principal causative agent of dandruff[2,5,6,9] and its association with disease severity have been reported.[10] The role of the four newly identified *Malassezia* species (*M. globosa*, *M. otusa*, *M. restricta* and *M. slooffiae*) in pityriasis has not been established.[7,8]

The etiology of seborrheic dermatitis and dandruff was argued for many years. Different schools of thought debated whether *Pityrosporum* yeasts were of primary etiologic significance or were a secondary phenomenon, with epidermal hyperproliferation as the primary pathology.[11] Effective therapies in seborrheic dermatitis and dandruff have been linked to antipityrosporal activity. With the introduction of new effective antifungal drugs, the primary pityrosporal etiology for dandruff has been strengthened. In addition, the recent discovery that human epidermal cells themselves make and secrete the components necessary for activation of the alternative complement pathways appears to provide an explanation for how human skin is ordinarily able to avoid colonization by molds and other organisms. It also helps clarify the mechanisms underlying clinical and laboratory findings seen in chronic mucocutaneous candidiasis, dandruff and psoriasis.[12]

ANTIDANDRUFF ACTIVES AND MODES OF ACTION OF ACTIVES

Several topical agents identified in the last several decades have proven to be successful therapies for the treatment of pityriasis capitis. These agents include pyrithione zinc,[13–22] selenium sulfide,[13,23–27] salicylic acid,[13] sulfur,[13] coal tar,[13] hydrocortisone[13] and ketoconazole.[20,21,24–26,28–34] The consistent mode of action of most of the actives is their antifungal activity against *P. ovale*. In vitro fungistatic and fungicidal activities of ketoconazole,[14,35–38] zinc pyrithione[36] and selenium disulfide[36] have demonstrated extremely low MICs against specimens isolated from patients with dandruff and seborrheic dermatitis using *P. ovale* as the marker organism. Coal tar[15] was also demonstrated to possess activity against 54 *M. furfur* strains isolated from patients with dandruff, seborrheic dermatitis and pityriasis versicolor. Other agents, such as itraconazole, bifonazole, climbazole, fluconazole, clotrimazole, dithranol and liquor carbonis, also have the ability to inhibit *P. ovale*.[36,38] Salicylic acid, sulfur and liquor carbonis possess exfoliative qualities expected to improve the appearance of scaling, while the antimitotic effect of topical corticosteroids and coal tars might also be involved in reducing the hyperproliferation associated with dandruff scaling.

THERAPIES AND EFFICACY

Pityriasis in its milder presentations is an exaggerated physiological process. The objective of treatment is to control the disease at the lowest possible cost and inconvenience to the patient.[2] Since the 1960s, various shampoos, conditioners and treatment products have been marketed as over-the-counter or prescription products for the treatment of seborrheic dermatitis and dandruff. Many of these products not only treat the scalp, but can also provide hair grooming needs for cleansing and conditioning hair.

Pyrithione zinc (PTZ) shampoo and conditioning rinse-off products have been marketed since the 1960s. This category of antidandruff products has been approved for over-the-counter use for the treatment of dandruff and seborrheic dermatitis at levels of 0.3–2% PTZ in rinse-off products[13] and 0.1–0.25% PTZ in leave-on products.[13,19] The efficacy of these products has been demonstrated in many clinical trials.[13,16–19] The relative antidandruff efficacy of a 1% PTZ-containing shampoo has been compared with 1% and 2% ketoconazole shampoos.[20,21] In a 364-patient, 6-week, randomized, double-

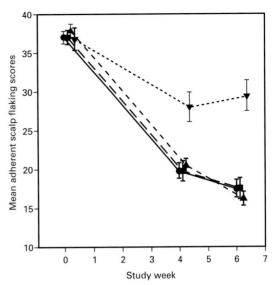

Figure 17.3 Mean adherent scalp flaking scores for 1% PTZ versus 2% ketoconazole shampoos:[20] ●, 1% PTZ (regimen I); ■, 1% PTZ (regimen II); ▲, 2% ketoconazole; ▼, placebo.

blind, parallel group study,[20] three groups of 112 patients were assigned a 1% PTZ shampoo, or a 1% PTZ shampoo with a different use regimen, or a 2% ketoconazole shampoo; and a fourth group of 28 patients was assigned to a placebo shampoo. The antidandruff efficacy of the two 1% PTZ shampoos, regardless of the use regimen, was found to be comparable to the 2% ketoconazole shampoo. All three active treatments were significantly more efficacious than the placebo shampoo (Figure 17.3). In a small 60-patient, 8-week, randomized, double-blind, parallel group study,[26] a 1% ketoconazole shampoo was found to be more efficacious than a 1% PTZ shampoo after 6 and 8 weeks of therapy in a subpopulation of patients with severe dandruff. A small, 4-week, unblinded, open study[22] reported marked decreases in scaling, seborrhea, erythema, and the burning and itching of the scalp of seborrheic dermatitis patients treated with either a 1% PTZ or a 1% econazole shampoo. The 1% econazole shampoo was assessed to be slightly better than the 1% PTZ shampoo.

Selenium sulfide has been approved for over-the-counter use for the treatment of dandruff and seborrheic dermatitis at levels of 0.6% (micronized form)[23] and 1%.[13] A recent report of the comparative efficacy of a 1% selenium sulfide shampoo versus a 2% ketoconazole shampoo[24] suggests that the 1% selenium sulfide shampoo is more effective than the 2% ketoconazole shampoo after 4 weeks of therapy. In this large, 350-patient, 6-week, double-blind, randomized parallel group trial,[24] two groups of 150 patients, with moderate to severe dandruff or seborrheic dermatitis, were randomly assigned to 1% selenium sulfide shampoo or 2% ketoconazole shampoo; and one group of 50 patients was randomly assigned to placebo shampoo. Adherent scalp flaking scores were assessed at baseline, and weeks 2, 4 and 6. Both the 1% selenium sulfide shampoo and the 2% ketoconazole shampoo were significantly more efficacious than the placebo shampoo at all treatment time points. While the efficacy of these shampoos was comparable at week 2, the 1% seleniun sulfide shampoo was found to be significantly more effective at reducing adherent scalp flaking in comparison with the 2% ketoconazole shampoo after 4 and 6 weeks of therapy (Figure 17.4). The superior efficacy associated with the 1% selenium sulfide shampoo may be a function of the shampoo frequency. When the hair was shampooed 3 times weekly, patients using the 1% selenium sulfide shampoo had significantly better improvement than patients using the 2% ketoconazole shampoo. When the shampoo frequency was comparable at 2 times per week, the efficacy of the two active products was comparable.

In a 7-week study,[25] 246 patients with moderate to severe seborrheic dermatitis and dandruff used either a 2% ketoconazole shampoo, a 2.5% selenium sulfide shampoo or a placebo shampoo, twice weekly for 4 weeks. Both active shampoos produced signif-

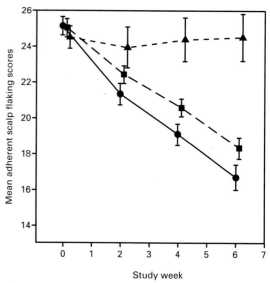

Figure 17.4 Mean adherent scalp flaking scores for 1% selenium sulfide versus 2% ketoconazole shampoos:[24] ●, 1% selenium sulfide; ■, 2% ketoconazole; ▲, placebo.

icant improvement in total adherent dandruff scores relative to the placebo shampoo. The 2% ketoconazole shampoo was found to be significantly better than the 2.5% selenium shampoo after 1 week, but not after 2 and 4 weeks of therapy. Assessments of the reduction in yeast cell counts paralleled the adherent flaking results, with the ketoconazole and selenium sulfide shampoos having significantly reduced yeast cell counts relative to placebo treatment. Following the active treatment phase, 103 patients who responded to treatment entered the regression phase, where they used a non-medicated shampoo for an additional 3 weeks. A progressive increase in adherent and loose dandruff scores and an increase in the percentage of patients with yeast colonization were noted, indicating relapse on cessation of therapy.

In a 4-week, double-blind study,[26] 102 patients with moderate to severe dandruff were shampooed at the test facility with either a 2% ketoconazole shampoo, a 2.5% selenium sulfide shampoo or a placebo shampoo, twice weekly for 4 weeks. Adherent scaling and yeast organism density were assessed pre-treatment and at 2 and 4 weeks post-treatment. The 2% ketoconazole shampoo was comparable to the 2.5% selenium sulfide shampoo in flaking reduction scores, and both active shampoos were significantly more effective than the placebo shampoo. The mean yeast count reduction scores paralleled the flake reduction efficacy measures, with the 2% ketoconazole and 2.5% selenium sulfide shampoos producing a significantly higher reduction in yeast density than the placebo shampoo.

In a small (8 patients on selenium sulfide and 15 patients on miconazole nitrate treatment), parallel group study,[28] the antidandruff efficacy of a 2.5% selenium disulfide shampoo was compared with a 2% miconazole nitrate shampoo. Miconazole nitrate was found to possess antidandruff activity equivalent to selenium disulfide. The endpoint for efficacy determination was clinical assessment of disease severity supplemented by cytodiagnosis of exfoliated scalp epidermal cells by smear examination.

Ketoconazole, an imidazole antimycotic agent, has been used orally for the treatment of mycoses. This agent has demonstrated in vitro and in vivo activity against *P. ovale*, an organism known to play an important role in the etiology of seborrheic dermatitis.[14,28,35-38] Several large antidandruff efficacy studies have demonstrated its efficacy topically in the control of pityriasis capitis and seborrheic dermatitis.[20,21,24-26,28-34] Ketoconazole has been approved for topical over-the-counter and prescription use of 1% and 2% respectively in shampoos.

In a 4-week, double-blind, placebo-controlled study,[29] 2 respective groups of 19 (a total of 38) *P. ovale* culture-positive patients were treated with a 2% ketoconazole or placebo shampoo, twice weekly for 4 weeks. A significant reduction in the severity of disease involvement was observed in 89% of patients treated with ketoconazole shampoo versus 44% of patients treated with placebo sham-

poo. In a 4-week open study,[30] 30 patients with scalp seborrheic dermatitis were treated with a 2% ketoconazole gel. Efficacy was assessed by clinical signs (erythema and flaking) and subjective assessment of scalp itch. At week 4, all patients showed improvement. No clinical signs or symptoms of seborrheic dermatitis were observed in 80% of the patients. An additional 16.6% of the patients had a good response to treatment, while 3.3% had a satisfactory response. Remission of disease lasted from 2 to 12 weeks following the cessation of therapy.

A large, double-blind, 7-month, multicenter trial[31] demonstrated that 2% ketoconazole shampoo was highly effective in the treatment and prophylaxis of seborrheic dermatitis. In this trial, 575 patients, with moderate to severe seborrheic dermatitis and dandruff of the scalp, were treated with the 2% ketozonazole shampoo twice weekly for 2–4 weeks. An excellent response was produced in 88% of the patients, and 312 patients who responded to the 2% ketoconazole treatment continued into a prophylactic phase lasting 6 months. Patients were instructed to use either the 2% ketoconazole shampoo once weekly or once every other week; or the placebo shampoo only once weekly. A total of 47% of the patients in the placebo group experienced a relapse of disease compared with 31% in the group treated with 2% ketoconazole once every other week and 19% in the group treated with 2% ketoconazole once weekly.

In a 6-week, double-blind, placebo-controlled trial,[32] 28 and 24 patients respectively, with moderate dandruff or seborrheic dermatitis, shampooed twice weekly with either a 2% ketoconazole shampoo or a placebo shampoo for 4 weeks. Clinical assessments (adherent and loose dandruff flaking, irritation and itching) were conducted at days 15 and 29. Patients treated with the 2% ketoconazole shampoo had a significant reduction in flaking at both days 15 and 29, in comparison with the placebo shampoo. At the completion of the treatment phase, 16 and 15 patients respectively from the ketoconazole and placebo groups with complete or excellent clearance of disease were enrolled in a 2-week study, where they were treated with a non-medicated commercial shampoo, and examined for relapse of their dandruff symptoms. The mean relapse times were 15.2 versus 11.3 days for the ketoconazole and placebo shampoos.

In a 4-week, double-blind, placebo-controlled trial,[33] 176 patients applied a 1% ketoconazole or placebo shampoo for a period of 4 weeks. Good or excellent results were observed in 74% and 80% of the patients treated with 1% ketoconazole versus 20% and 23% of patients on placebo shampoo after 2 and 4 weeks respectively. In a double-blind, two-week, randomized parallel group comparison study,[34] three respective groups of 24, 30 and 24 moderate dandruff sufferers were treated once daily with 0%, 0.5% or 1.0% ketoconazole shampoo for two weeks. Colorimetric measures (Chroma C*) of flake density, as well as *P. ovale* density, were assessed pre- and post-treatment. The 1% ketoconazole shampoo group had significantly higher flake reduction activity than the 0.5% ketoconazole and the placebo shampoo group. In addition, the 0.5% ketoconazole shampoo was significantly more effective at reducing flaking in comparison with the placebo shampoo. A dose–response relationship was noted in the flake density reduction versus the level of ketoconazole present in the shampoos. After 2 weeks of treatment, the *P. ovale* density was reduced by more than 85% in the patients, regardless of treatment. This lack of difference observed in the *P. ovale* density suggests that this methodology may not be sensitive enough to reveal differences between active and placebo products. In addition to topical application, oral ketoconazole has been shown to improve patients with scalp psoriasis in a randomized, double-blind, placebo-controlled study.[39]

Coal tar, approved for over-the-counter treatment of dandruff, seborrheic dermatitis and psoriasis at levels of 0.5–5% (tar equivalent),[13] reduces the number and size of epidermal cells, and decreases epidermal proliferation and dermal infiltrates. Coal-tar-containing shampoo and treatment products have been marketed for decades.

Salicylic acid, approved for over-the-counter treatment of dandruff, seborrheic dermatitis and psoriasis at concentrations of 1.8–3%,[13] is an exfoliative agent that loosens the scales, enabling them to be washed away. Sulfur is approved for over-the-counter treatment of dandruff at levels of 2–5%. Combinations of salicylic acid and sulfur have not been approved for over-the-counter use in the USA.[13] The effectiveness of 2% sulfur and 2% salicylic acid either alone or in combination in a shampoo were assessed in a double-blind, parallel controlled study[40] using scaling and corneocyte counts as the endpoints for efficacy. A total of 48 patients with moderate to severe dandruff were shampooed twice weekly at the study site for 5 weeks. At weekly intervals, scalp flaking and corneocyte counts were assessed. Significantly greater and earlier reductions in the degree of scaling and corneocyte counts were observed in patients treated with the formula containing 2% sulfur and 2% salicylic acid versus the individual ingredients.

EFFICACY MEASURES (DERMATOLOGIC AND MICROBIOLOGIC)

The primary efficacy measure of antidandruff activity in pityriasis capitis trials is adherent scalp flaking severity. This assessment is generally based on an 11-point flaking scale ranging from 0 to 1 (very light scaling) to 8 to 10 (severe scaling),[13,21,25,26,29–33] or from 0 (no scaling) to 10 (very heavy scaling).[13,16,18,20,24] The scalp is divided into six[13,21,25,26,29–33] or eight[13,16,18,20,24] anatomic sites, and the adherent flaking density is scored after parting the hair at each anatomic site multiple times. The adherent flaking score from each site is then summed across sites (giving a total of 60 or 80) for the primary efficacy measure. An alternative method, the colorimetric method (Chroma C*), called squamometry, is used to assess the amount of flakes obtained on D-Square tapes collected from the most severely affected area pre-treatment and the same area post-treatment to assess flaking density changes resulting from treatment.[34] Corneocyte counting is another method for assessing flaking changes. These latter two methods are not used in the conduct of current clinical studies. In addition to the adherent scalp flaking scores, assessment of loose dandruff, global involvement in the disease process, and subjective assessment of itch and dandruff severity serve as secondary efficacy measures. Another secondary, but extremely important, efficacy endpoint is the assessment of *P. ovale* or yeast cell density.[25,26,34] Microbiological specimens obtained from the scalp pre- and post-treatment from the same site with the highest flaking severity pre-treatment are smeared onto a slide and stained to highlight the yeast organisms. The slides are assessed for yeast cell density under oil-immersion light microscopy, and are scored based on a 4-point scale ranging from 0 (no yeast cells observed) to 3 (>10 yeast cells per oil immersion field).[41]

REFERENCES

1. Dawber RPR, *Shampoos – Scientific Basis and Clinical Aspects.* London: Royal Society of Medicine Press, 1996.

2. Dawber RPR, Isolated dandruff. In: *Cosmetic Dermatology*, 1st edn (Baran R, Maibach HI, eds). London: Martin Dunitz, 1994:133–7.

3. Broberg A. *Pityrosporum ovale* in healthy children, infantile seborrheic dermatitis and atopic dermatitis. *Acta Derma Venereol Suppl. (Stockh)* 1995; **191**: 1–47.

4. Orfanos CE, Frost Ph, Seborrheic dermatitis, scalp psoriasis and hair. In: *Hair and Hair Diseases* (Orfanos CE, Happle R, eds). Berlin: Springer-Verlag, 1990:641–62.

5. Saint-Leger D, The history of dandruff in history. A homage to Raymond Sabouraud. *Ann Dermatol Venereol* 1990; **117**: 23–7.

6. Shuster S, The aetiology of dandruff and the mode of action of therapeutic agents. *Br J Dermatol* 1984; **111**: 235–42.

7. Guillot J, Gueho E, Lesourd M et al, Identification of *Malessezias* species. *J Mycol Med* 1996; **6**: 103–10.

8. Gueho E, Midgley G, Guillot J, The genus *Malassezia* with description. *Antonie van Leeuwenhoek* 1996; **69**: 337–55.

9. Leyden JJ, Kligman AM, Dandruff cause and treatment. *Cosmetics and Toiletries* 1979; **94**: 3.

10. Leyden JJ, McGinley KJ, Kligman AM, Role of microorganisms in dandruff. *Arch Dermatol* 1976; **112**: 333.

11. McGrath J, Murhy GM, The control of seborrheic dermatitis and dandruff by antipityrosporal drugs. *Drugs* 1991; **41**: 178–84.

12. Rosenberg EW, Noah PW, Skinner RB, Psoriasis is a visible manifestation of the skin's defense against micro-organisms. *J Dermatol* 1994; **21**: 375–81.

13. Dandruff, seborrheic dermatitis and psoriasis drug products for over-the-counter human use; final monograph. *Federal Register* 1991; **56**: 63 554–69.

14. Richardson MD, Shankland GS, Enhanced phagocytosis and intracellular killing of *Pityrosporum ovale* by human neutrophils after exposure to ketoconazole is correlated to changes of the yeast cell surface. *Mycoses* 1991; **34**: 29–33.

15. Nenoff P, Haistein UF, Fielder A, The antifungal activity of a coal tar gel in *Malassezia furfur* in vitro. *Dermatology* 1995; **191**: 311–14.

16. Marks R, Pearse AD, Walker AP, The effects of a shampoo containing pyrithione zinc on the control of dandruff. *Br J Dermatol* 1985; **112**: 415–22.

17. Rappaport MA, A randomized controlled clinical trial of four anti-dandruff shampoos. *J Int Med Res* 1981; **9**: 152–6.

18. Cardin CW, Amon RB, Hanifin JM et al, The antidandruff efficacy of Head and Shoulders rinse-in shampoo (1% zinc pyrithione) and Head and Shoulders shampoo (1% zinc pyrithione) with Head and Shoulders conditioning rinse (0.3% zinc pyrithione) versus Merit shampoo

with Merit Moisture Rinse. *Nishinon J Dermatol* 1990; **52:** 1208–16 (in Japanese).

19. Dandruff, seborrheic dermatitis and psoriasis drug products for over-the-counter human use. *Federal Register* 1982; **47:** 54 664–6.

20. Billheimer WL, Bryant PB, Murray KP et al, Results of clinical trial comparing 1% pyrithione zinc and 2% ketoconazole shampoos. *Cosmet Dermatol* 1996; **9:** 34–9.

21. Cauwenbergh G, *International Experience with Ketoconazole Shampoo in the Treatment of Seborrheic Dermatitis and Dandruff.* London: Royal Society of Medicine Services, 1988.

22. Rigoni C, Toffolo P, Cantu A et al, 1% econazole hair-shampoo in the treatment of pityriasis capitis; a comparative study versus zinc-pyrithione shampoo. *G Ital Dermatol Venereol* 1989; **124:** 117–20.

23. Dandruff, seborrheic dermatitis and psoriasis drug products for over-the-counter human use; amendment to the monograph. *Federal Register* 1994; **59:** 4000–1.

24. Neumann PB, Coffindaffer TW, Cothran PE et al, Clinical investigation comparing 1% selenium sulfide and 2% ketoconazole shampoos for dandruff control. *Cosmet Dermatol* 1996; **9:** 20–6.

25. Danby FW, Maddin WS, Margesson LJ et al, A randomized, double-blind, placebo-controlled trial of ketoconazole 2% shampoo versus selenium sulfide 2.5% shampoo in the treatment of moderate to severe dandruff. *J Am Acad Dermatol* 1993; **29:** 1008–12.

26. Hickman JG, Nizoral (ketoconazole) shampoo therapy in seborrheic dermatitis. *J Int Postgrad Med* 1990; **2:** 14–17.

27. Sheth RA, A comparison of miconazole nitrate and selenium disulfide as antidandruff agents. *Int J Dermatol* 1983; **22:** 123–5.

28. Ive FA, An overview of experience with ketoconazole shampoo. *Br J Clin Pract* 1991; **45:** 279–84.

29. Faergemann J, Treatment of seborrheic dermatitis of the scalp with ketoconazole shampoo. *Acta Derma Venerol (Stockh)* 1990; **70:** 171–2.

30. Zecevic R, Toskic-Radojicic M, Mijailovic B, Therapy of dysseborrheic dermatitis with ketoconazole. *Vojnosanit Pregl* 1993; **50:** 61–3.

31. Peter RU, Richarz-Bathauer U, Successful treatment and prophylaxis of scalp seborrheic dermatitis and dandruff with 2% ketoconazole shampoo: results of a multicenter, double-blind, placebo-controlled trial. *Br J Dermatol* 1995; **132:** 441–5.

32. Berger R, Mills OH, Jones EL et al, Double-blind, placebo-controlled trial of ketoconazole 2% shampoo in the treatment of moderate to severe dandruff. *Adv Ther* 1990; **7:** 247–56.

33. Go IH, Wientjens DP, Koster M, A double-blind trial of 1% ketoconazole shampoo versus placebo in the treatment of dandruff. *Mycoses* 1992; **35:** 103–5.

34. Arrese JE, Pierard-Franchimont C, De Doncker P et al, Effect of ketoconazole-medicated shampoos on squamometry and *Malassezia ovalis* load in pityriasis capitis. *Cutis* 1996; **58:** 235–7.

35. Van-Cutsem J, Van-Gervan F, Fransen J et al, The in-vitro antifungal activity of ketoconazole, zinc pyrithione, and selenium sulfide against *Pityrosporosis* in guinea pigs. *J Am Acad Dermatol* 1990; **22:** 993–8.

36. Nenoff P, Haustein UF, Effect of anti-seborrhea substances against *Pityrosporum ovale* in vitro. *Hautarzt* 1994; **45:** 464–7.

37. Faergemann J, Borgers M, The effect of ketoconazole and itraconazole on the filamentous form of *Pityrosporum ovale*. *Acta Derma Venereol (Stockh)* 1990; **70:** 172–6.

38. Schmidt A, Ruhl-Horster B, In vitro susceptibility of *Malassezia furfur* against azole compounds. *Mycoses* 1996; **39:** 309–12.

39. Farr PM, Krause LB, Marks JM, Response of scalp psoriasis to oral ketoconazole. *Lancet* 1985; **ii:** 921–2.

40. Leyden JJ, McGinley KJ, Mills OH, Effects of sulfur and salicylic acid in a shampoo base in the treatment of dandruff: a double-blind study using corneocyte counts and clinical grading. *Cutis* 1987; **39:** 557–61.

41. Skinner RB, Noah PW, Taylor RM et al, Double-blind treatment of seborrheic dermatitis with 2% ketoconazole cream. *J Am Acad Dermatol* 1985; **12:** 852–6.

18

Facial and body hair

Rodney Dawber

HAIR REMOVERS[1]

The terms 'epilation' and 'depilation' have varied in their exact definition over the years. It is more convenient to define the exact process used, or the principle behind it, under the general term 'hair removers'. Superfluous hair may be masked by bleaching or removed by a variety of methods, such as plucking, waxing, shaving, chemical processes and electrolysis – only the latter is permanent. No method is entirely satisfactory, and the one adopted will depend on personal preference and the character, area and amount of hair growth.

Bleaching

This is widely used for hair, particular on the upper lip and the arms. It is painless, and when repeated often inflicts sufficient damage to cause hair breakage. However, bleached hair can look very obvious against dark skin. Some individuals develop an irritant reaction to bleach; it is therefore advisable to carry out a preliminary test – if irritation occurs within 30–60 minutes, the peroxide strength and duration of application should be reduced.

Shaving

This is unacceptable to some women as being too 'masculine'; however, the majority are happy to shave axillary and leg hair. Modern bathing costumes are very brief, and require the wearer to shave the inner thighs and even part of the pubic region. In these sites it is common to experience folliculitis during regrowth, sometimes also due to infection with *Staphylococcus aureus*.

Waxing

This is one of the oldest methods known. Typically, the wax is preheated, applied to the area to be treated, allowed to cool, and then stripped off, taking the embedded hair with it. Some 'cold' waxes are available that act in the same way. Glucose and zinc oxide waxing has the advantage of lasting up to several weeks before a repeat is required. Only relatively long hair can be treated in this way. Some women find it painful and irritating. It is more often used by beauticians than in the home.

Plucking

This is really satisfactory only for individual or small groups or scattered coarse hairs. It is useful for sparse nipple or abdominal hair. It is usually done with tweezers. As with waxing, it requires to be treated only every few weeks.

Chemical hair removers

These are now widely used for superfluous hair removal from most sites, including the face. Their use on the face is limited by their irritancy potential. Sulphides and stannites, widely used in the past, have now been largely superceded by substituted mercaptans. Sulphides were unsatisfactory – both because of skin irritancy and because of their odour (hydrogen sulphide), generated particularly when the preparation was washed off; however, strontium sulphide preparations are still available. Substituted mercaptans form the basis of virtually all modern chemical depilatory preparations. They are slower in action than sulphides, but are safe enough for facial use if necessary. Thioglycolates are used in a concentration of 2–4%, and typically act within 5–15 minutes. Of the thioglycolates, the calcium salt is most favoured, since it is the least irritant – the pH is maintained by an excess of calcium hydroxide, which also acts to prevent the excess alkalinity known to irritate skin. Attempts to formulate products that accelerate the rather slow thioglycolate action have not been particularly successful. Modern preparations are available in foam, cream, liquid and aerosol forms, the choice being made according to personal preference. Since thioglycolates attack keratin, not specifically hair, they may have adverse effects on the epidermis if manufacturers' recommendations are not adhered to; it is generally suggested that a small test site should first be treated in order to prevent more extensive irritant reactions in susceptible individuals.

Electrolysis

All the above methods are temporary, the only practical permanent procedure being 'electrolysis'. This involves passing a fine wire needle into the hair follicle and destroying the bulb with an electric current passed along it – the hair is loosened and plucked from each treated follicle. Disposable needles should be used to prevent transmission of infection. Either a galvanic or modified high-frequency electric current is used. Galvanic electrolysis is slower, but destroys more follicles in one treatment. High-frequency current (electrocoagulation) is quicker, but more regrowth is seen with this method. Relatively cheap, battery-operated machines have been developed for home use. These have all the disadvantages and potential hazards of those used by electrolysists, with the added problem of an amateur operator.

The limitations of electrolysis in skilled hands are those of cost and time; even the best operators can only deal with 25–100 hairs per sitting, and hair regrows in up to 40% of the follicles treated. Shaving a few days prior to electrolysis increases the number of hairs in anagen, and these are more easily destroyed. In general, electrolysis is mostly used for localized, coarse facial hair, and alternative methods are employed for excess hair on other body sites. Apart from regrowth of hair, the problems that can occur with this mode of hair removal include discomfort during treatment, perifollicular inflammation and scarring (Figure 18.1), punctate hyperpigmentation and, rarely, bacterial infection.

In a controlled investigation carried out to compare the results of electrolysis with those of diathermy, permanent destruction of the hairs could be achieved by either method, and the time required for the total destruction of all hair roots in a given area was the same; but the diameter of hairs regrowing after diathermy was possibly greater than that of hairs regrowing after electrolysis. The results of depilation depend on the skill and dexterity of the operator. In countries such as Britain, in which a Diploma in Medical Electrolysis exists, patients should wherever possible be referred to technicians who have obtained this certification of their proficiency.

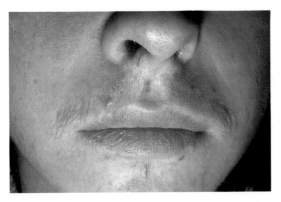

Figure 18.1 Hirsutism of the upper lip and chin: some follicular damage and inflammation (temporary) is evident, due to electrolysis.

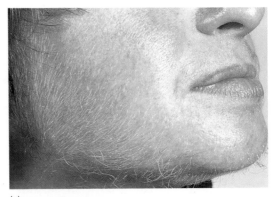

(a)

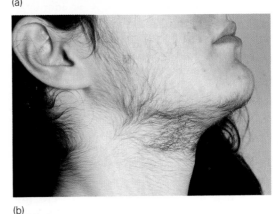

(b)

In the USA, the American Electrolysis Association regulates professional standards. A variety of laser methods for permanent hair destruction are currently under investigation – the author feels that the current advertising claims of great success remain somewhat premature.

Perception of hirsuties is by definition subjective, and women present with a wide variation of severity (Figure 18.2). Both the severity of the hirsuties and the degree of acceptance are dependent on racial, cultural and social factors. Even the criteria for the definition of hirsuties used by physicians vary widely. In order to solve this issue, different groups have evolved different grading schemes for hair growth. The method of Ferriman and Gallwey, which has become the standard grading system, has defined hirsuties purely on quantitative grounds. Other physicians have examined women complaining of hirsuties and compared them with controls; they have demonstrated that there is a considerable overlap in the grades of hirsuties between those women who consider themselves to be hirsute and control women. Hair

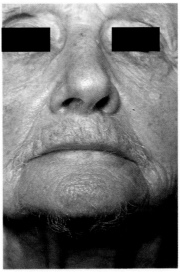

(c)

Figure 18.2 Degrees of hirsutism in 'normal' women, with no specific cause found: (a) downy type; (b) coarse hirsutism; (c) post-menopausal hirsutism.

on the face, chest or upper back is a good discriminating factor between hirsute women and controls with similar hair growth scores.

Hair is second only to skin colour as a feature of racial difference. Facial and body hair is less commonly seen on the Mongoloid, Negroid and American Indian races than on Caucasians. Even amongst Caucasians there are differences; hair growth is heavier on those of Mediterranean than those of Nordic ancestry.

The pattern of hair growth in hirsuties within different racial groups is identical; however, different criteria have made the determination of the comparative incidence and severity within these groups difficult to assess. One study of a random population stated how many women considered themselves to be hirsute; 400 selected students were examined, 60% of whom were Welsh; 9% were considered by both the women and investigator to be hirsute and 4% were considered to be disfigured by their facial hair growth. This investigation also included studies of hair growth in women who were not complaining of hirsuties. These studies have been rigorously performed, and confirm ethnic variations in density of hair growth. It is important to the definition of hirsuties that a sizeable proportion of normal women have some terminal hairs on their faces, breasts or lower abdomen.

In hirsutism, one role of society is to determine the threshold level for normality, and this is now determined by the media. Women receive a barrage of advertisements for cosmetics that are based on the premise that only a woman with a hairless body can be both normal and healthy.

There have been few studies on the psychological status of hirsute women. One study concluded, on the basis of a small sample of patients studied within a psychoanalytic framework, that many suffered reactive psychic disturbances. Another small controlled study revealed increased levels of anxiety.

Another approach to the psychological aspect of hirsuties has been to implicate 'stress' as an aetiological factor for hirsuties. It has been stated that: 'Lack of peace of mind appears at the core of the problem. It is believed to be both a cause and result of hirsutism.' This view has been endorsed many times.

REFERENCES

1. Dawber RPR, Van Neste D, *Hair and Scalp Disorders*. London: Martin Dunitz, 1995:164–7.

19

Eye make-up

Anne-Marie Orecchioni

INTRODUCTION

Since ancient times eye make-up preparations have been used in order to modify or accentuate the appearance of the eyes by use of suitably chosen colorants. Modern eye preparations include the following main categories:[1]

- mascara;
- eye-shadows;
- eyeliners;
- eyebrow make-up;
- eye creams;
- eye make-up removers.

Each of these plays a particular part, and all must be easy to apply, reasonably permanent when applied, and, of course, neither irritant nor toxic. For most of them, colouring agents are the major constituents,[2] but the formulations still vary widely. However, those products used near the area of the eyes can be divided into three main categories:

- those used to enhance the appearance of the eyelashes – mascaras;
- those used to colour, for cosmetic appeal, the eyelids and the orbital areas of the eyes – eye-shadows, eyeliners and eyebrow make-up;
- those used to reduce the dryness of the thin-skinned eye area or to remove eye make-up – eye creams and eye make-up removers.

All the products entering into the composition of these cosmetics must be used in a highly purified form, and must be chosen according to appropriate national or international legislation (e.g. French[3] or European[4]). Such legislation can be very strict, particularly regarding colorants and preservatives. Thus the former must appear on the list of those authorized for preparations to be applied to the areas of the eyes. They must be insoluble in water.[2] They are, for the most part, inorganic pigments. The most common consist of metallic oxides: iron or chromium oxides (in the case of the latter, either hydrated or anhydrous), ultramarine pigments, aluminium lakes, white pigments such as titanium or zinc oxides, nacreous pigments such as titanium dioxide-coated micas, bismuth oxychloride to produce a pearlescent effect, and sometimes finely powdered metal such as aluminium to give a metallic appearance. Preservatives used must also be selected from those on the appropriate register, and authorized concentration limits must be respected. As a general rule, only pure, non-irritating and non-toxic raw materials should be used. The harmlessness of each component must be established.[5] About 400 substances are prohibited from use in the production of cosmetics and toiletries, and there are restrictions on the use of many other ingredients. In addition to these general primary protective measures, user instructions should indicate that misuse may be harmful, and all ingredients capable of inducing an allergic reaction should be indicated on the packaging. Finally, evaluation of products is essential during production and after packaging. Safety, sensory, physicochemical and microbiological analysis of preparations must be performed in order to guarantee constant quality.[5,6]

ENHANCEMENT OF EYELASH APPEARANCE: MASCARAS

Definition

Mascaras are generally black-pigmented preparations for application to the eyelashes to darken them and increase their apparent length. The brightness and expressiveness of the eyes are enhanced because the whiteness of the whites of the eyes is intensified. Colour selection is wide, but black, brown or blue are commonly seen.[1,2,7]

Mascara was previously applied from a cake, using a wetted brush. This presentation has almost disappeared because it is unhygienic. The modern presentation is a cream contained in a cylindrical tube filled by an automatic applicator. Sometimes, to produce a lengthening effect for the lashes, nylon fibres are added to the cream.

Composition

The basic ingredients are various, and the 'magic mixture' is composed of the following:

- *Oils:* petrolatum or petrolatum distillate whose physical properties and stability are of great value.

- *Silicon oils* improve water resistance.
- *Waxes:* microcrystalline wax or ozokerite, complex mixtures of hydrocarbons in order to stiffen the preparation; beeswax, whose plasticity facilitates the application of the preparation; carnauba or candellila wax form a water-repellent film and give lustre; lanolin and derivatives give lubricating and adhering power.
- *Stearic acid and oleic acid soaps* are widely used as emulsification aids.
- *Polymers* such as cellulose derivatives, acrylic polymers and vinyl polymers are used in order to control viscosity, and also for their binding, thickening and emulsifying power. They are employed not only as flow materials but also as pigment dispersants. Low-molecular-weight polyethylene can be used in combination with oils or fatty esters to provide gels.[1,2,6]
- *Preservatives.*
- *Pigments.*

Formulation and procedure

Cream mascaras are prepared by milling the pigments into a vanishing-cream base or by use of a suitable oil-soluble dye, in this case with the aid of a suitable wetting agent to lower the surface tension in order that the colour will adhere to the applicator. To avoid smudging, these preparations generally include a little castor oil. For instance, the following mascara composition is found in the cosmetic formulatory of Laboratoires Gattefossé (France):[8]

Formula

(1)	poly(ethylene glycol) PEG-8b	
	beeswax ester	8%
	glyceryl tribehenate	1.5%
	castor oil	2%
(2)	demineralized water	53.20%
	Carbomer 934	0.30%
	triethanolamine	0.60%

(3) black pigments   7%
     talc   19%
     tri-isostearin PEG ester   19%
(4) vinylpyrrolidone–
     dimethylaminoethyl methacrylate
     copolymer   7%
     preservatives   QS

Procedure

The carbomer is dispersed in demineralized water and left to stand. The oily mixture (1) and the water mixture (2) are then heated at 75°C, and (2) is poured into (1) under stirring to obtain a cream. The colorants (3), after milling, are added together with the copolymer and the preservatives (4) in the cream base. Stirring is maintained while cooling at room temperature.[8]

There is a colourless 'mascara' on the market. The raw materials are quite different from those used in a traditional mascara. The product contains a hydroalcoholic medium thickened by a polymeric gellant, and of course has no colorant. It can be used for swimming without smudges. This product contradicts the definition of a mascara as a cosmetic for colouring the eyelashes. It is used in order to condition lashes without the problems due to colorants.[9,10]

Controls

Physicochemical controls
- Aspect, colour, spreadability and drying period must be evaluated.
- The amount of preservatives must be determined.

Microbiological analysis – The products should remain free of microbial contamination, and they must be tested for the possible presence of bacteria.

Evaluation of eye irritation – This must be done by in vivo tests and by developing alternatives to animal tests.[5,7]

COLORATION OF EYELIDS AND ORBITAL AREA

Products employed to colour the eyelids and the orbital area include eye-shadows, eyeliners and eyebrow make-up.

EYE-SHADOWS

Definition

Eye-shadows are preparations applied to the eyelids in order to produce an 'attractive moist-looking background' for the eyes. They may be manufactured in the form of creams, sticks or powders, but the most popular form is a pressed powder cake in a thin plated steel or aluminium pan with a great variety of shapes and sizes. The product is applied to the eyelids with a soft dry brush or a foam-tipped applicator.[2,11,12]

Raw materials

Talc – The basis of a pressed eye-shadow is talc (hydrated magnesium silicate), because of its covering power and for its slip and smoothness. It must be free of asbestos and heavy metals. A proportion of 15–50% or more is useful.[1,11,13]

Kaolin (hydrated aluminium silicate), titanium dioxide, chalk (calcium carbonate) or potato starch – These are used for their covering power, and also because they contribute to the density of the tablet or aid in the compressing of the cake. The percentages entering in the formulation are lower than that of talc – generally 2–8%.

Metallic soaps – These are essential for the adhesion of the powder to the eyelids. The best is zinc stearate. It imparts smoothness to the cake. Magnesium stearate is also used, but it is not as smooth or as adhesive as the zinc compound. The percentages used depend on whether a matt or pearlescent product is desired: they range from 2% to 7%.[12,13]

Binders – These are necessary for the stability of the pressed cake, preventing it from flaking or dusting. Non-aqueous binders are commonly used from 4% to 6%, but higher percentages are necessary when pearlescent pigments are incorporated in significant amounts. The most widely used binders are lanolin and derivatives, mineral oils, isopropyl stearate and isopropyl isostearate. In addition to providing this stabilizing power, binders are used as pigment dispersing agents.[11,12]

Pigments and preservatives – These are suitably chosen as described above.

Modern raw materials are now available to formulators. An example is sericite, which is a talc substitute. This product is a natural powdered mica (aluminium potassium silicate) that gives exceptional smoothness.[14] Better pigments such as micronized titanium dioxide are also now available. For instance, titanium dioxide coated with volatile silicone, giving a smooth product and avoiding a 'chalky' appearance, is now used instead of common titanium dioxide.[14] Polymeric microspheres of poly(methylmethacrylate) can be used in pressed powders to give a lubricating effect that promotes the easy spreading of pigments.[14]

Formulation and procedure

Formula
The following formulation represents the prototype of an eye-shadow cake:[13]

(1)	talc	60%
	zinc stearate	2.5%
	kaolin	4.5%
(2)	iorganic pigments	10%
	titanium dioxide coated mica	15%
	preservatives	0.5%
(3)	lanolin	2%
	isopropyl stearate	4.5%
	carnauba wax	1%

Procedure
The ingredients of (1) are mixed together until homogeneous. The ground part (2) is added and well mixed with (1). A spray of heated part (3) is dispersed into this mixture. The final sample is pressed into godets.

Controls

Physicochemical controls – Aspect, colour, hardness, release and stability of the cake must be evaluated. For instance, no cracking should appear when the pressed tablet is dropped 30 cm onto the floor.

Microbiological analysis – general tests must be employed in order to detect possible contamination.

Evaluation of eye irritation – This must be done as described above.

EYELINERS

Definition

Eyeliners are cosmetic preparations for use on the eyelids, close to the eyelashes, to accentuate the expressiveness of the eyes. They are available in liquid and pencil form, and are generally harmonized with the shade of the mascara. The product must be formulated in such a way that it can be applied in a thin precise line, will not cake and will be water-resistant.[2,7]

Raw materials

The basic component is a polymeric material that is a water-thickening agent. Among these the most common are magnesium aluminium silicate (veegum), poly(vinylpyrrolidone) (PVP), acrylic derivatives and cellulose derivatives. The other components are pigments and preservatives.

Formulation and procedure

Formula

The following is a classical formula:[13]

(1)	veegum	2.5%
	water	75.5%
(2)	poly(vinylpyrrolidone)	2%
	water	10%
(3)	pigments	10%
	preservatives	QS

Procedure

Veegum is slowly poured into water (1) with stirring at maximum available shear. The PVP is dissolved in warm water (2) and added to (1) until homogeneous; (3) is then added and mixed until fully dispersed and uniform.[13]

In this formula the magnesium aluminium silicate provides thickening and pigment suspension while ensuring smooth application properties.

Controls

Physicochemical controls – Aspect, colour, spreadability and smoothness must be evaluated.

Microbiological analysis – Because of their high water content, these products are easily contaminated with bacteria that grow in water, and so they must include preservatives, usually parabens. The latter must be evaluated.

Evaluation of eye irritation – The presence of parabens could induce allergic reaction in paraben-sensitive individuals. Some users may experience contact irritancy, and it is absolutely necessary to evaluate the possibility of adverse reactions. Katon CG[15] is the strongest contact allergen, and this preservative is not encouraged for prolonged skin contact.

EYEBROW MAKE-UP

Definition

Eyebrow make-up is used in order to correct an abnormal structure of the eyebrows or their loss from disease, trauma or other conditions. An eyebrow pencil can be used to draw absent eyebrows. A natural appearance can be created by drawing short strokes rather than a straight line, as was the fashion in the 1930s when eyebrows were plucked.

Raw materials

Eyebrow pencils are formed by mixing pigments, generally iron oxides, waxes (synthetic or natural) and oils. The mass obtained after homogenization is extruded into a pencil-lead form and encased in wood or extruded into rods placed in a plastic holder.

Formulation and procedure

Formula

An eyebrow pencil is generally made up of the following:[6]

• beeswax	9%
• synthetic wax	22%
• hydrogenated glycerides	13.5%
• paraffin oil	4%
• lanolin	3%
• iron oxides	48.2%
• preservatives	QS

Procedure

The waxes and oils are melted down to a clear mass, to which iron oxides are added. The pigment–wax mass is then homogenized in a colloid mill. The finished mass is then extruded in a pencil form.[6]

Controls

Physicochemical controls – Aspect, colour, consistency and hardness are evaluated. The amount of preservatives is determined.

Microbiological analysis – This is performed as described previously.

Evaluation of eye irritation – This is done by the usual methods.

MODERN EYE PREPARATIONS

Eyelash cosmetics are widely used, and patients with problems can find suitable products. Special eyelash cosmetics are available for contact lens wearers and allergic patients. Patients with permanent eyelash loss may use eyeliner tattooing. The tattooing is practiced by ophthalmologists, dermatologists or plastic surgeons because the intradermal insertion of pigments is involved. Of course, the pigments chosen are of low allergenic potential, and the tattooing should be done in a very thin line. This permanent eyeliner does not concern the average patient.[7]

EYE CREAMS AND EYE MAKE-UP REMOVERS

These products technically cannot be considered as eye make-up, but because they are used on the thin-skinned eye area, they are regarded as eye cosmetics.

EYE CREAMS

Definition

These are generally water-in-oil emulsions. Their purpose is to reduce dryness by lubricating the eye area or to provide an adherent base over which eye-shadow can be applied. The products are usually applied with the fingertips.

Formulation and procedure

A classical formulation with some active ingredients such as bisabolol and panthenol is described below.

Formula

This is as follows:

(1)	glyceryl monostearate	5%
	stearic acid	1%
	cetyl alcohol	2%
	beeswax	6%
	perhydrosqualene	4%
	isopropyl stearate	7%
	bisabolol	0.2%
	antioxidants	QS
(2)	propylene glycol	5%
	panthenol	1.5%
	preservatives	QS
	water	ad 100%

Procedure

This emulsion is manufactured in the usual manner of emulsions: the oil phase (1) and the water phase (2) are heated separately to 75°C, then mixed under stirring and cooled. The products are packaged in plastic jars of tubes.

Controls

Physicochemical controls – Aspect, odour, colour, pH and stability are evaluated – the latter by measuring droplet size and viscosity.

Microbiological evaluation – Microbiological contamination is always possible because of the high water content. Preservatives must be evaluated, and no contamination must be observed.

Eye irritation – The evaluation is done using the same methods as described previously.

EYE MAKE-UP REMOVERS

It is necessary to remove eye make-up, and a variety of eye make-up removers have been formulated. The most popular forms are creams, lotions and remover pads. Their composition must be compatible with the delicate skin of the eyelids and of the orbital area.[6]

Formulation and procedure

The basic components of eye make-up removers are oils and mild detergents.

Formula

The following formula is an example of a lotion:[6]

- methyl hydroxycellulose   1.8%
- propylene glycol   5%
- sodium myristyl ether sulphate   5%
- polyethoxylated hydrogenated
  castor oil   5%
- preservatives   QS
- water   ad 100%

Procedure

The cellulose and preservatives are steeped in water. The remaining ingredients are added, and the mixture is gently stirred until homogenous. The lotion is then bottled.

Controls

Physicochemical controls – Aspect, colour and viscosity must be controlled. The amount of preservatives must be evaluated.

Microbiological evaluation – The high water content means that special attention must be paid to prevent bacterial contamination.

Evaluation of eye irritation – This is performed using the classical tests.

CONCLUSIONS

Despite the precautions taken in the choice of raw materials and those used during the manufacturing process, and the constant analytical control during production and after packaging, some accidents may occur because of actions of the consumer. For instance, in the case of mascara, the applicator is inserted in the tube after use, providing numerous opportunities to inoculate bacteria into the latter. It is prudent to discard a mascara tube after two or three months, and above all not lend the mascara to other persons. If an eyeliner is of a pencil type, resharpening will decrease contamination by removing the exposed part.[7] Soft contact lens wearers must use products specially made for them. Finally, in order to reduce the possibility of injuries due to accidental misuse, user instructions must warn of the potential for such misuse. Nevertheless, an unforseeable risk will always remain, however much manufacturers adopt good laboratory practice and good manufacturing practice.

REFERENCES

1. Janousek A, Rouges, blushers and eye cosmetics. In: *Poucher's Perfumes, Cosmetics and Soaps*, Vol 3, 9th edn. London: Chapman and Hall, 1993: 308–34.
2. Schlossman ML, Application of colour cosmetics. *Cosmet Toiletries* 1985; **100**(5): 33–8.
3. Loi du 10 Juillet 1975, *Journal Officiel de la Républice Française*, 11 Juillet 1975.
4. EEC Directives for Cosmetic Substances 76/768/EEC, 27 July 1976, *Official Gazette of the EEC* L 262/169, 27 September 1976; including the Adaptation Directive, 8 May 1996, *Official Gazette of the EEC* L 192, 1 June 1996.
5. Whittman JH, *Cosmetic Safety. A Primer for Cosmetic Scientists.* New York: Marcel Dekker, 1987.
6. Umbach W, *Cosmetics and Toiletries, Development, Production and Use.* Chichester: Ellis Horwood, 1991.
7. Kececioglu Draelos Z, *Cosmetics in Dermatology.* New York: Churchill Livingstone, 1990.
8. Anonymous, Make up formulary. *Cosmet Toiletries* 1989; **104**(7): 76–80.
9. Anonymous, *Cosmet Toiletries* 1988; **103**(8): 19.
10. Kapadia YM, Use of polymers in eye make up. *Cosmet Toiletries* 1984; **99**(6): 53–6.
11. Fox C, Color in cosmetics. *Cosmet Toiletries* 1996; **111**(3): 35–53.
12. Rutkin P, Eye makeup. In: *The Chemistry and Manufacture of Cosmetics*, Vol 4 (de Navarre MG,

ed). Orlando, FL: Florida Continental Press, 1975:709–40.

13. Flick EW, *Cosmetic and Toiletry Formulations*, 2nd edn. Noyes, 1989:137–65.

14. Grizzo S, New talc substitutes for decorative cosmetics. *Cosmet Toiletries* 1992; **107**(4): 39–43.

15. Fox C, Technically speaking. *Cosmet Toiletries* 1990; **105**(7): 29–32.

20

Nail varnish formulation

Douglas Schoon

INTRODUCTION

It is easy to underestimate the level of sophistication found in modern nail care products. Nail varnishes are certainly no exception. To their credit, these products have enjoyed great success for over the last 70 years. Much of that success is due to the constant evolution of this product category, as well as the consumer's desire to coat their nail plates with a wide range of beautiful colors.

Nail varnish is also called enamel, lacquer or polish. The varnish may be clear, opaque or shaded with color. On the surface varnishes may seem to be nothing more than a paint-like coating for the nail plates. However, nail varnish chemistry is actually much more complex. In its simplest form, a nail varnish is defined as a strong film coating created by evaporation of a volatile solvent component. However, the coating must withstand severe abuse without losing color, gloss or adhesion. Luckily, a clever formulator has a wide range of raw materials from which to choose, and through proper ingredient selection these properties can be greatly enhanced. Still, the cosmetic appearance and durability of the final product are not the only considerations when choosing ingredients. Regulatory agencies and consumer perception also play important roles. For these and other reasons, it is instructive to examine each ingredient type to gain a better understanding of these useful cosmetics.

NAIL VARNISH BASICS

A typical varnish formulation consists of seven basic types of ingredients:

1. film formers
2. film modifiers
3. plasticizers
4. solvents/diluents
5. viscosity modifiers
6. stabilizers
7. coloration additives.

Each of these contributes to the quality of the final product. If proper ingredient selections are made and correctly balanced, the varnish will be easy to apply and remove, quick-drying, waterproof, glossy, chip- and scratch-resistant, and flexible, and will adhere well to the natural nail plate. Ideally, by today's standards, a properly applied coating should remain cosmetically attractive and intact for five days to a week. Also, the varnish coating must have a low potential for toxicity and adverse skin reactions.

FILM FORMERS

The role of the film former is to create a continuous coating over the nail plate. The coating material of choice is an organic polymer called nitrocellulose (cellulose nitrate). This was the first natural polymer to be successfully modified by chemical manipulation, and was first produced commercially in 1860. Nitrocellulose was created by treating cellulose with a mixture of nitric and sulfuric acids. Originally, it was used was in high explosives. As a dry powder, nitrocellulose is highly unstable and sensitive to light, heat, atmospheric moisture and oxygen, as well as alkaline pH. Its polymeric structure is easily disrupted, which may lead to yellowing and viscosity breakdown. This highly sensitive material must be transported in a polar organic solvent, usually ethanol or isopropanol, to prevent explosive detonation. For example, cellulose nitrate motion picture film has, through spontaneous combustion, caused major fires in film repositories. Because the explosive potential is much higher for highly nitrated derivatives (trinitrates), these grades are avoided in commercial nail varnish. Formulators can choose from several viscosities and grades of the lesser nitrated materials and use them alone or in synergistic blends.

Other non-nitrated cellulosic materials are also used with varying degrees of success, namely cellulose acetate and derivatives. Polyurethanes, polyamides and polyesters have also been utilized. However, none can match the toughness and surface hardness of nitrocellulose. Also, nitrocellulose blends superbly with colored pigments, producing bright and vibrant colors. Still, nitrocellulose has several disadvantages that drive formulators to constantly seek alternate materials. The surfaces produced by this polymer have low gloss, and the films are brittle and adhere poorly to the nail plate. Upon evaporation, nitrocellulose films shrink excessively, which leads to poor adhesion. Until an advanced film former is discovered, most formulators will continue to rely on film modifiers to overcome these serious drawbacks.

FILM MODIFIERS

The purpose of a film modifier is to favorably offset some deficiencies of the primary film former. Specifically, film modifiers are used to improve adhesion and gloss. The most commonly used modifier is toluenesulfonamide/formaldehyde resin (TSFR). This resin dramatically improves nail plate adhesion while producing water-resistant, glossy surfaces with improved flexibility. This resin's most significant drawback is that a small number of users have reported sensitization.

Many alternate modifiers have been tried, including toluenesulfonamide/epoxy resin,[1] polyester sucrose benzoate, polyesters,[2] acrylic ester oligomers, SAIB (sucrose acetate isobutyrate), arylsulfonyl urethanes,[3] etc. None has replaced TSFR, despite the certain amount of controversy surrounding this important ingredient (see 'Formaldehyde controversy' below). Some newer types of formulations succeed without secondary film modifiers. At least one company now claims to have eliminated the need for such modifiers by replacing them with proprietary plasticizing systems (personal communication from Robert Sandowitz, Revlon R&D, 1996).

PLASTICIZERS

Plasticizers are chemical flexibilizers for polymer films. Nitrocellulose must be heated to 53°C before it begins to soften, which explains why it is brittle at room temperature. Plasticizers offer a useful way to improve the strength of nitrocellulose films. They reportedly increase separation between the cellulose links, as well as increasing the rate of solvent evaporation.[4] Plasticizers provide unique benefits. Film modifiers counterbalance the negative aspects of nitrocellulose, whereas plasticizers alter the properties of the entire film. When used judiciously, they have profound, positive effects on film flexibility. They may also improve adhesion and gloss. There are dozens of useful plasticizers, but not all are suitable for nail varnish. A plasticizer must be compatible and remain in solution without negatively affecting viscosity, consistency, flow or shelf-life. It must not readily escape from the film through migration or volatilization. Finally, it must be dermatologically innocuous.

Excessive loads of plasticizer create films that are flimsy and exhibit poor adhesion. Conversely, insufficiently plasticized films have low durability. Dibutyl phthalate (b.p. 342°C) and camphor (b.p. 96°C) are the most common examples of low-molecular-weight, high boiling point plasticizers. Dibutyl phthalate is a very aggressive plasticizer for nitrocellulose, but it is a suspected skin sensitizer. Other examples of plasticizers are castor oil, glyceryl tribenzoate, acetyl tribenzoate citrate, PPG-2 dibenzoate, glycerol, citrate esters, triacetin and a polymeric plasticizer called NEPLAST (a polyether–urethane).[5]

SOLVENTS/DILUENTS

Nail varnish solvents give these products their characteristic odor. Although many consider the vapors to be unpleasant, solvents are vital to varnishes. Solvents dissolve the solid, film-forming polymers, and, upon evaporation, deposit them on the nail plate. Besides their strong characteristic odors, solvents are often highly flammable. The most commonly used solvents are alkyl esters (ethyl, amyl and n-butyl acetate) and glycol ethers (propylene glycol monomethyl ether). Since each solvent has a different boiling point and evaporation rate, a skillful formulator can balance several solvents to achieve the desired drying time. Good solvents are those that easily dissolve solid ingredients and lower viscosity or improve brushability. Even though they are not solvents for nitrocellulose, aliphatic alcohols such as ethanol, isopropanol and butanol are very useful in varnishes. These ingredients couple synergistically through hydrogen bonding with esters to increase the overall solubility and flow of the system. For this reason, alphatic alcohols are called 'coupling agents'.

Diluents are usually non-polar compounds that are also non-solvents for nitrocellulose. They are used in lesser amounts than solvent ingredients. Primarily, diluents help to regulate evaporation rates and stabilize viscosity. Uneven or overly rapid evaporation may affect the surface gloss, color and clarity, especially in humid conditions. A great advantage of diluents is that they may be added in controlled amounts without reducing the viscosity.

Toluene is the most important example of a nail varnish diluent. A high-quality product may contain as much as 25% toluene. This diluent has been used since the 1930s without any significant problems. However, because of the California Proposition 65, *Safe Water and Toxic Enforcement (Act) of 1986*,[6] toluene has become the focus of numerous questions and studies. Proposition 65 was mainly designed to protect drinking water in the state from trace levels of contaminants – not to regulate cosmetic ingredients. However, a 'bounty hunter' clause in this regulation made it very lucrative for individuals and groups to seek out any and all violators. Problems first began for toluene when California listed it as potential reproductive toxicant.[7] Soon after passage of the Proposition, a self-proclaimed environmental group formed and quickly threatened court action against nail varnish manufacturers and resellers. Rather than engage in a court battle, retail companies signed agreements to cease the use of toluene and sell only 'toluene-free' nail varnish. However, the professional nail industry, under the guidance of the Nail Manufacturer's Council (NMC), challenged the lawsuit and proved to the State of California that the average salon was about 1000 times below the NOEL (No Observable Effects Level) (personal communication from Jim Nordstrom, President, NMC). As a result of the study, professional nail varnish manufacturers retained the right to continue using toluene, with the assurance that nail technician exposure was far below OSHA safe levels of exposure. Even so, most companies are scurrying to develop toluene-free formulas that are comparable to toluene-containing varnishes. Retail marketers have swayed public opinion with 'toluene-free' claims to the point that public concerns and irrational fears will probably force change.

VISCOSITY MODIFIERS

Ideally, a nail varnish should have a gel-like consistency to help keep pigments suspended. However, a thinner more brushable liquid will produce better and more uniform films. Luckily, both consistencies are possible in systems that display thixotropic behavior. This strange effect is achieved quite nicely in modern nail varnishes. Thixotropic systems become thinner as they are mixed and brushed. When at rest, a thixotropic liquid will reform a semigel structure. Examples of substances used to create this useful effect are cationic modified montmorillonite clays that are approximated by the formula $(Al,Mg)_2$ $4SiO_2(OH)_2 \cdot nH_2O$. Treating these clays with quaternary ammonium compounds will render them organophilic. Stearalkonium hectorite is the most frequently used of these clays. The main disadvantage of clay additives is that they lower surface gloss. This can be offset by the addition of various polymers, i.e. acrylate copolymers and nylon. These additives improve gloss, as well as toughness and scratch resistance.

COLORATION ADDITIVES

Unless the nail varnish is clear and colorless, additives must be used to alter the opacity and shade. In theory, these color additives must have very low or no lead content, as well as being FDA certified or approved colors. Occasionally, smaller manufacturers will risk using non-approved colorants (e.g. 'day-glo' colors) to satisfy faddish demands of younger consumers. However, for the most part, these regulations are adhered to closely. Of course, coloration additives must have relatively high light fastness. Colorants should also be non-soluble pigments, to prevent staining of the nail plate. The most frequently used technique is to create a 'pigment lake'. Typically, a lake is formed by precipitating a particular pigment with aluminium hydroxide to form a salt complex. Some examples of these colorants are D&C Red No. 7 Calcium Lake and D&C Yellow No. 5 Zirconium Lake. Pastel shades are achieved by the addition of titanium dioxide (TiO_2). Ferric ferrocyanide (Prussian blue) is used in small amounts to enhance blues and alter other shades. In order to achieve complete pigment dispersion and suspension, high-energy ball or roll mills must be used. The advantage of using sophisticated blending equipment is that nail varnishes can give full coverage, while using only 2% dry colorant or less.

Pearlescent pigments continue to be highly desirable commodities in modern varnishes. Guanine, derived from scales of Atlantic herring and other fish, is prized for its low density (reduced settling) and soft luster. However, adverse skin reactions to this ingredient have been reported.[8] Bismuth oxychloride and mica coated with TiO_2 and other colorants are used to create the many beautiful iridescent shades. More complete information on approved colorants can be obtained from the *CTFA International Handbook*.[9]

OTHER ADDITIVES

A variety of highly specialized additives are known to those skilled in the art of nail varnish formulation. Even tiny amounts of many of these special additives can give dramatic differences in performance. Some examples are surfactants to improve wetting and adhesion and organic acids to stabilize colorants. However, some additives serve no function other than to increase consumer appeal (e.g. proteins, minerals and vitamins).

BASE AND TOP COATS

Base coats are applied to the nail plate before application of the nail varnish. They are usually of similar composition to varnish, but with some alterations. Many additives improve adhesion (e.g. TSFR), but excessive levels reduce gloss and scratch resistance. Since surface characteristics are less important for base coats, formulators may use higher levels of these adhesion promoters to dramatically improve retention and coating toughness. Also, base coats that contain no colorants act as a protective antistain barrier between the nail plate and shaded varnish.

The opposite is also true. Top coats utilize higher levels of ingredients that maximize surface gloss and hardness. Certain additives (e.g. nitrocellulose) improve gloss and shine, but reduce nail plate adhesion. However, they still have excellent adhesion between coats when applied over wet varnish. Often, the top coat contains special UV-absorbing materials to help protect the underlying colorants from photoinitiated decolorization. Other cellulosic materials, (e.g. cellulose acetate butyrate) may also be used.

It should be pointed out that not all top coats are evaporative coatings. Some are UV-cured acrylate oligomer blends.[10] These protect the varnish, but have several important drawbacks. Acrylated oligomers have a greater tendency to cause adverse skin reactions. They shrink considerably, and may cause wrinkling in certain shades and/or slower-drying formulations. Finally, UV-cured top coats are very difficult to remove with solvents, and must be filed away with abrasive boards. Several products are marketed as UV top coats and sold with UV lamps, even though they are evaporative coatings. The warmth of the UV lamps accelerates evaporation and hardening. These evaporative coatings are easy to distinguish from true UV-cured top coats by their dramatically differing solubility in solvents: the false UV top coats are easily removed with ketones or alkyl esters.

FORMALDEHYDE CONTROVERSY

The FDA allows the use of up to 5% formaldehyde in nail hardeners. In exchange, the FDA requires warning labels on nail care products with greater than 0.5% free formaldehyde, as well as 'nail shields which restrict application . . .'.[11] Not only are these requirements frequently ignored, but formaldehyde-containing nail hardeners are sold to the public on a national level without listing formaldehyde as an ingredient. It is suspected that formaldehyde crosslinks proteins in the nail plate. The result is an increase in surface hardness and decreased flexibility, which the user misinterprets as improved strength. This creates a special problem. Users see noticeable 'improvements' after several uses, which encourages regular application. After months of continued use, nail hardeners may eventually increase nail plate hardness and rigidity to the point that brittleness becomes obvious. Users remember the early success of the hardener, and usually respond to the brittleness by increasing the frequency of application. This leads to further crosslinking and nail plates may end up in a worse condition than before they resorted to nail hardeners. Onycholysis and abnormal growth of the hyponychium are common end results of prolonged formaldehyde overexposure.

This may also explain the controversy over the use of TSFR, which contains low levels of formaldehyde. Typically, TSFR is used at levels of 10–15% by weight. These levels produce nail varnishes with about 1500 ppm formaldehyde,[12] which is a small amount considering the FDA allows up to 50 000 ppm formaldehyde in nail hardeners. With such widespread use of formaldehyde, it is difficult to determine what impact these trace levels have on creating new allergic reactions. Since formaldehyde is a sensitizer, many adverse skin reactions presently attributed to TSFR may be a result of previous repeated exposure to nail hardeners and subsequent sensitization. Therefore residual levels found in nail varnish are likely to affect only those with previously existing sensitivities.

NEW DEVELOPMENTS

Until recently, most nail varnish research was focused on faster drying times, improved durability and adhesion. However, nail varnishes that improve nail plate heath are presently the hottest topics of interest for consumers. So, there is a tremendous economic incentive for manufacturers to discover ingredients that provide demonstrable benefits to the nail plate. Improved nail plate toughness and solutions for yellow, dry, brittle and splitting nails would be enormously beneficial. The obvious first step toward this goal is the development of water-based nail varnishes. Within a few years, these will undoubtedly be commercially available. Once these products are on a parity with organic solvent technology, they are sure to supplant all present-day formulations. When successful water-based technologies exist, it will be possible to incorporate a wider variety of additives, which may eventually lead to the Holy Grail of nail varnishes – one that truly prevents or helps treat common nail pathologies.

REFERENCES

1. Mallavarapu L, US Patent 4,996,284 (1991).
2. Schlossman ML, US Patent 4,301,046 (to Tevco) (1981).
3. Lecaheur M, Mutterer J, Wimmer E, French Patent 9202486 (1992).
4. Schlossman ML, Nail cosmetics. *Cosmetics and Toiletries* 1986; **101**: 24.
5. Schlossman ML, Advances in nail enamel technology. *J Soc Cosmet Chem* 1992; **43**: 331–7.
6. California Environmental Protection Agency, Office of Environmental Health Hazard Assessment Proposition 65 Implementation, Sacramento, CA.
7. Donald JM, Hooper K, Hopenhayen-Rich, Reproductive and development toxicity of toluene: a review. California Department of Health Services, Health Hazard Assessment Division, Sacramento, CA.
8. Stritzler C, Dermatitis in the face caused by guanine in pearly nail lacquer. *Arch Dermatol* 1958; **78**: 252.
9. CTFA, *International Color Handbook*. Washington, DC: Cosmetics, Toiletries and Fragrance Association, 1992.
10. Schoon D, Nail polish chemistry. In: *Nail Structure and Product Chemistry*. Albany, NY: Milady/Delmar Publishing, 1996:45–62.
11. FDA, *Cosmetic Handbook*, June 1989.
12. Nater IP, de Groot AC, Liem DH, *Unwanted Effects of Cosmetics and Drugs Used in Dermatology*, 2nd edn. New York: Elsevier, 1985.

21

Cosmetology for normal nails

Robert Baran, Douglas Schoon

INTRODUCTION

The nail has been decorated since time began. As it has evolved from the primaeval claw, the nail's aggressive and working uses have become less important than its aesthetic value. The application of cosmetics to the nail represents an attempt to enhance its beauty, and the widespread use of cosmetics often results in unwanted reactions to them.

The nail is a convex, hard, horny plate covering the dorsal aspect of the tip of the fingers and toes (Figure 21.1). Its appearance is determined by the integrity of the terminal bony phalanx and the paronychium, i.e. matrix, nail bed and hyponychium, and nail folds.

The nail plate, produced by the matrix, grows from a pocket-like invagination of the epidermis, and adheres firmly to both the nail bed and the undersurface of the proximal nail fold, which, at its free border, forms the cuticle that seals the nail pocket.

The most distal part of the matrix, the whitish semicircular lunula, is not covered by the proximal nail fold. Juxtaposed with the lunula, the pink nail bed epithelium is made of parallel longitudinal rete ridges and subepithelial capillaries running longitudinally at different levels.

Adjacent to the nail bed, the hyponychium, an extension of the epidermis under the nail plate, marks the point at which the nail separates from the underlying tissue.

There is little space between the nail and the distal bony phalanx, but it is occupied by non-keratinizing nail epithelium and highly vascular mesenchyme containing glomus organs.

The following should be borne in mind:

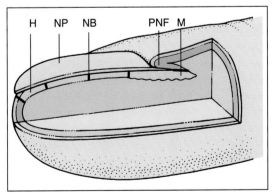

Figure 21.1 Anatomy of the nail aparatus: M, matrix; NB, nail bed; H, hyponychium; NP, nail plate; PNF, proximal nail fold. (After Dr E Haneke.)

- The proximal matrix forms the surface of the nail plate, and the distal matrix forms its inferior part. It is therefore possible to locate initiating pathology by a thorough examination of the nail.

- Fingernails grow at a rate of 0.1 mm a day; toenails grow much more slowly (it takes 12–18 months to replace a large toenail).

The nail has a functional role. It protects the nail bed and provides counter pressure for the pulp, which is essential for tactile sensations involving the fingers. The nail can act as a weapon and as a tool for scratching, scraping or gripping small objects. Finally, the nail enhances the appearance of the fingers.

Nail beauty depends on three main factors:

- the shape of the nail
- its decoration
- its texture.

CARE AND ADORNMENT OF NORMAL NAILS

The shape of the nail

The shape of the nail depends on proportion and contour. The ratio of length to breadth of the nail is critical to its aesthetic appeal, and the two dimensions should be approximately equal,[1] at least on the thumb. When the 'magic' ratio differs from the ideal, the nail is less attractive (Figure 21.2). Polish adds little in cosmetic improvement to a broad, short fingernail.

In the past, attractive nails were oval in shape, but nowadays there is a tendency to cut the tip more or less squarely (Figure 21.3), although the basic nail shape may be round or pointed.

Length creates the impression of thin, tapered and graceful fingers. When too long, however, they may become unsightly. Excessive length may even interfere with the efficiency of hand performance. In addition, a long nail may act as a lever and facilitate the rupture of the nail plate–nail bed attachment, a condition called onycholysis.

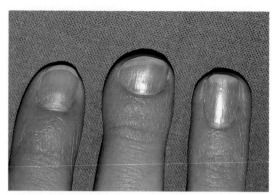

Figure 21.2 The racquet nail of the middle finger is less attractive than the nail exhibiting the ideal ratio.

The decoration of the nail

For nails of equal length and corresponding contour, a painted nail is usually considered more attractive (Figure 21.4). Renewed interest has recently been given to sculptured artificial nails. Diamonds or emeralds have even been fixed into elongated nails, and intricate jewellery attached to the free edge (Figure

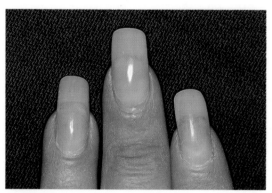

Figure 21.3 There is a tendency to cut the tips of the nails more squarely.

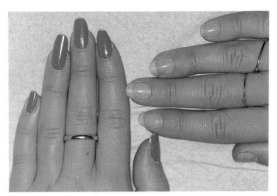

Figure 21.4 Painted nails are more attractive than plain nails.

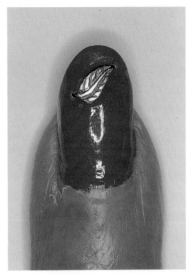

Figure 21.5 Intricate jewellery attached to the free top extremity of the nail.

21.5). The art of the jeweller has also been engaged to form artificial nails. Thus preformed nails in gold or gold plate may be decorated with precious stone insets.

A more likely decoration is called nail art (Figure 21.6) – painted designs that are airbrushed onto the surface of the finished nail or fashioned with stencils and fine brushes, but this is considered faddish and not part of the mainstream nail technician's daily routine. Holograms, Chagalling, abstracts and graffiti are the latest inspirations for nail artists.[2]

total of unwanted responses to cosmetic procedures. In addition, a sound knowledge of nail cosmetics as well as the way in which instruments are used for manicures and nail care is essential for proper care.

The texture of the nail

The condition of the nail may be a function of its aesthetic appeal. The nail may be softened, or, more frequently, rendered brittle. The brittle nail is vulnerable to single or multiple longitudinal splitting and horizontal splitting into layers (onychoschizia) (Figure 21.7) or less often to transverse breaking (Figure 21.8). Nail fragility requires different kinds of treatment. The wide variety of techniques employed in treating brittle nails can occasionally be responsible for some adverse reactions, and these must be added to the

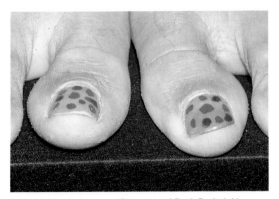

Figure 21.6 Nail art. (Courtesy of Dr A Batistini.)

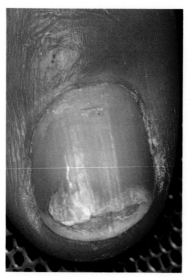

Figure 21.7 Onychoschizia (splitting into layers).

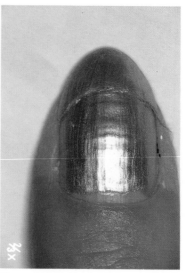

Figure 21.8 Complete transverse breaking.

Items for nail care[3]

Clippers – These are slightly curved, jaw-like blades operated by a spring mechanism for severing the free edge of the nail plate. They are available in many sizes.

Scissors – These have slightly curved blades for cutting soft, thin, flexible nail plates. Blades with blunted ends minimize injury to soft tissue.

Emery board – A flat, disposable, 'paperboard' wand, coated with emery powder, can be used to shape, file down in length or smooth off sharp, rough portions of the free edge of the nail.

Nail file – This is an elongated board made of wood or foam covered with abrasives that vary in grit depending on the intended use. The grit is a determination of how many abrasive particles there are per cubic centimetre. Low-grit boards (60–120 grits) are for quickly removing the layers of the artificial nail. Medium-grit boards (120–800) are for smoothing and shaping both artificial and natural nails.

Blocks – These are similar to files, but usually take the form of a larger, rectangular foam block that fits comfortably into the hand. Files and blocks are the most widely used types of abrasives.

Metal-particle file – Fine metallic particles are electroplated on a metal wand; this lasts indefinitely, and has the delicacy, speed and efficiency of an emery board.

Acrylic nippers – These are designed specifically to chip back the acrylic at the base of the nail in preparation for a fill.

Cobalt-steel fibreglass shears – These are fine, but strong, scissors that bear up well against thick fibreglass while maintaining a sharp cutting edge.

Cuticle pusher – A polished, metallic probe with various-shaped ends can be used for separating the cuticle edge from the nail plate and loosening cuticle remnants. The probe has rounded edges to minimize injury to soft tissue.

Orange stick – This is a reed-like wooden or flexible pencil-shaped plastic implement that is used like the cuticle pusher, but is less likely to cause injury to the nail fold. It was originally fabricated from orange wood.

Cuticle trimmer (Figure 21.9) – Tiny, clipper-jawed scissors are used for cutting frayed cuticle. Recently, a curette-like V-shaped blade, mounted in a plastic handle has been introduced to efficiently shave down this tissue.

Nail buffer – Chamois or similar fabric, usually padded and mounted on a convenient holding device, is used for polishing the nail plate. It is used in conjunction with mild pumice-type abrasive creams or waxes to produce a high lustre to the nail surface. Many types of nail buffers are coated with three different abrasive materials (called three-way buffers). These are used stepwise, from fine (# 1) to the finest surface (# 3), to smooth out ridges and impart ultrahigh gloss without the use of buffing oils, waxes or creams.

Nail whitener – This is a pencil-like device with a white clay (kaolin) core used to deposit colour on the undersurface of the free edge of the nail.

Disinfectant container – This should be large enough to hold a disinfectant solution in which items to be sanitized are immersed.

Pedicures

Pedicures demand a special set of implements because of the size and thickness of toenails. The toenail cutter works with a squeeze-grip action.

Toiletries and cosmetics

Nail enamel solvents – Solvents containing acetone and/or ethyl acetate or similar compounds are used to rapidly soften and solubilize nail enamel, oils and waxes for quick and easy cleansing.

Cuticle and nail creams and lotions – Oil-in-water emulsion preparations aid in softening the keratin of nail plate and contiguous skin. This is achieved initially by the addition of water, and subsequently by the reduction in evaporation into the environment of the tissues' inherent moisture.

Cuticle removers – These are lotions or gels containing approximately 0.4% sodium or potassium hydroxide. They are applied to the proximal edge of the nail plate in the vicinity of the cuticular ridge to eliminate the remnants of cuticle that adhere to the nail plate as it grows outward. The lotion is left in place

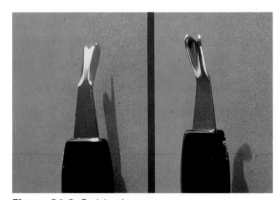

Figure 21.9 Cuticle trimmer.

for approximately 1–3 minutes and then washed off. Creams containing low levels of α-hydroxy acids (AHA) are also used as cuticle removers. These usually contain 1–5% lactic acid (pH 3–3.7). Besides their ability to soften and remove cuticle, daily use virtually eliminates hangnails and new growth of excess cuticle.

Base coats, top coats and nail enamel – (See also Chapter 20). These three cosmetic products have similar basic formulas. They consist of a film former, such as nitrocellulose, a thermoplastic resin (e.g. toluenesulfonamide/ formaldehyde) for gloss and adhesion, and a plasticizer (e.g. dibutyl phthalate) for flexibility; these are incorporated in an acetate and ketone solvent. Thickening agents or flow modifiers and UV absorbers may or may not be added. Polishes also vary in the solvent blends used, which greatly affects drying time and surface appearance. Therefore the quantities of the basic ingredients vary with the desired performance of the different products. For example, when a base coat is applied, good adhesion or bonding to the nail plate and the superimposed enamel is accentuated at the price of gloss; with a top coat, which is applied over the nail enamel, the gloss factor is dominant.

Film drying accelerant – There are silicone oil blends and silicone/water oil-in-water emulsions. The latter work best. Film drying accelerant is sprayed or brushed over freshly applied enamel to give rapid protection from minor environmental insults while the enamel sets.

REACTIONS TO NAIL COSMETIC PROCEDURES

Reactions to nail cosmetic procedures may be divided into two main categories:

- reactions to cosmetics applied to the nail;
- nail instrument damage.

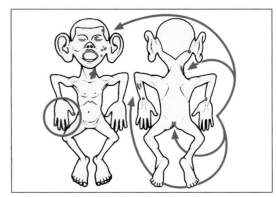

Figure 21.10 Distribution of nail varnish ectopic dermatitis. (After G Bonu.)

Reactions to cosmetics applied to the nail

Cosmetics may produce reactions both at the site of application to the nail area and secondarily elsewhere as the fingernails act as a reservoir for small amounts of cosmetic preparations that can be transferred by the hand to other areas of skin.

Nail polish
Nail polish dermatitis
Nail polish dermatitis of allergic origin can appear on any part of the body accessible to the nails (Figure 21.10), but usually with no signs in the nail apparatus. Exceptions, however, may exist – mainly in the periungual area[4] (Figure 21.11). The eyelids (Figure 21.12), the lower half of the face, the sides of the neck, and the upper chest are the most commonly affected areas.[5,6] In addition to ectopic dermatitis, allergic airborn contact dermatitis caused by nail polish ingredients should be suspected when lesions on the face, neck and ears are symmetrical.[7] The allergen in nail enamels is usually thermoplastic resin. Diagnostic skin patch testing with nail enamel should be performed without occlusive cover-

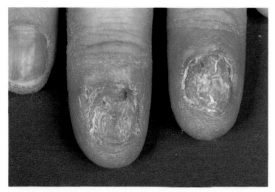

Figure 21.11 Rechallenge of nail varnish onto two fingers only, showing severe local dermatitis. (Courtesy of Dr R Staughton.)

ing, or with dry enamel films to avoid false-positive reactions from the solvent.

Thermoplastic resin is the main culprit,[8-11] but when the nail polish is completely dry it is only a weak allergen.[12] However, nail polish that has completely dried on the fingernails contains water-soluble components that reach the skin during extensive but transient contact.[13] These substances are *p*- and *o*-toluenesulfonamide, dibutyl phthalate and three constituents of toluenesulfonamide–formalde-

hyde resin (TSFR), which is the basic material of almost all nail polishes sold worldwide.

Some cosmetic manufacturers have reformulated their nail polish so that it does not contain TSFR or toluene, because the latter was added to the list of chemicals for which California's Proposition 65 requires a warning label. Toluene is suspected of causing birth defects and cancer. However, the Nail Manufacturers Council's study indicates that nail technicians can be confident provided that they cap all products tightly after each use and make sure their salon has adequate ventilation. Levels of exposure in nail salons indicate that technicians are exposed to levels that are approximately 1000 times below the US Federal safe limit set by the Occupational Safety and Health Administration (OSHA).[14]

Polishes using TSFR contain approximately 1500 ppm free formaldehyde. 'Formaldehyde-free' polishes contain approximately 5–10 ppm free formaldehyde. They are made in the same manufacturing facilities, using the same kettles and lines. This low-level contamination is unavoidably carried over from the TSFR products. Dry films have probably between 500–1000 ppm.

Nickel mixing-balls put into bottles of nail polish to maintain a liquid state may cause distant reactions and/or isolated onycholysis (personal written communication from B Magnusson, 1972). For patch testing, several nail lacquers should be used as they come from the bottle, but should be allowed to dry for 15 minutes, since the solvents and diluents may cause false-positive reactions.

The following substances should be included in a test battery:

- TSFR (10% petrolatum)
- nickel (0.5% petrolatum) DMG spot test for nickel
- glyceryl phthalate resin (polymer resin) 10% petrolatum
- pearly material – guanine powder (pure)
- formaldehyde (1–2% in aqua)

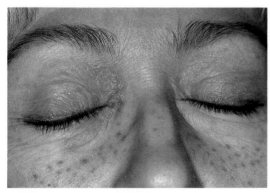

Figure 21.12 Eyelid dermatitis.

- colophony (resin) 10% or 20% petrolatum[15]
- drometrizole (Tunuvin P) 1% to 5% petrolatum
- nickel (0.5% petrolatum)

Several companies are responding to the fears of TSFR by marketing TSFR-free polishes. They may contain glycerophthalic polyester resin (Phase), 4-methylbenzene sulfonamide–epoxy resin (Clinique), phthalic polyester resin (Shiseido), polyester saturated hydroxylated resin (Deborah), and glyceryl tribenzoate (Revlon).[16] Unfortunately, some of these and related 'hypoallergenic' resins[17] and methyl acrylate[18] have already produced distant contact dermatitis. Most of these new resins do not chip and peel as often as the previous alkyd resin, but most manufacturers are now developing water-based nail polish for marketing reasons.

Contact urticaria

Recurrent urticaria involving the same area as contact dermatitis plus the distal phalanx of the fingers has been reported with isomorphic response to nail polish testing, immediately after simple contact.[19]

Nail plate staining

Nail staining from the use of deeper shades of red and brown nail enamel is most commonly yellow-orange in colour[20] (Figure 21.13). Typically, it begins near the cuticle, extends to the top of the nail, and becomes progressively darker from base to tip. With the leaching out of the varnish, the dyes (D & C Red Nos 6, 7 and 34; FD & C Yellow No. 5 Lake) generally penetrate into the nail too deeply to be removed.

The staining can be significantly avoided by the application of a base coat prior to the use of the offending nail enamel.

Fingernail discoloration can be produced by chloroxine, an active ingredient in a shampoo used for control of seborrhoeic dermatitis.[21] Chloroxine is known to be highly

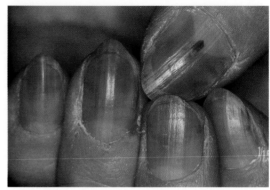

Figure 21.13 Yellow-orange nail-plate staining. (Courtesy of A Tosti.)

reactive to metals, and since iron oxides are commonly used as pigments in women's cosmetics, it is likely that the discoloration is caused by the reaction between chloroxine and some pigment-containing cosmetic.

Patients undergoing therapy with minocycline may develop discoloration of the nails.[22] The drug is often prescribed over long periods – for example in the treatment of acne vulgaris. Analysis of the nail clippings from minocycline-treated women showed a large amount of iron concentrated only in discoloured areas of the nail plate. The discoloration did not occur in women who did not paint their nails, nor did it occur in men. These nail clippings were free of significant amounts of iron. Iron is frequently present in nail polish, where iron oxides may be employed in the colouring agents, and has also been demonstrated in the upper strates of nail plates that have been subjected to frequent applications of the nail polish. It appears that there is a relationship between the presence of iron and the use of nail polish in the aetiology of the discoloration produced by minocycline.

Nail discoloration may also result from the combined effect of nail varnish and dermato-

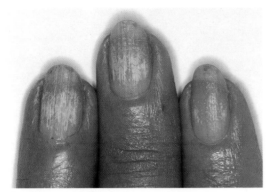

Figure 21.14 'Granulation' of nail keratin.

logical treatment containing either resorcinol or resorcinol monoacetate. The contribution of the lacquer has been narrowed down to its content of nitrocellulose.[23]

Nail keratin granulation

Injury to the nail from nail lacquers is rare. However 'granulations' of nail keratin (Figure 21.14), presenting as superficial friability,[24] can sometimes be observed. In these cases individuals continually apply fresh coats of enamel over old ones for periods of weeks. It is also reported to result from poor formulation of the product. Nail keratin granulation may be avoided by following a 5–7-day nail care schedule, including a few days with the nails free of cosmetic agents.[3]

Nail polish removers

Nail enamel removers usually need to be applied only weekly. They contain acetone and/or butyl or ethyl acetate, methyl ethyl ketone or similar compounds. These organic solvents dehydrate the nail plate and decrease corneocyte adhesion, contributing to brittleness.[25] The latest acetone-based polish removers contain significant amounts of water (17%) and/or conditioners for skin to reduce

tissue damage, making them the preferred solvents for polish removal.

They dissolve nitrocellulose and remove lipids from the nail plate. Oils are sometimes added to prevent excessive drying of the nail. Old nail enamel or buffer waxes are thoroughly removed with a cotton ball saturated with nail enamel remover, but this may cause inflammation of the paronychial area when the remover solution is left in contact with the skin. Rarely, irritant and allergic contact dermatitis, blistering, onycholysis and brittleness may occur. Ingredients may be tested in an open patch test:

- acetone (10% olive oil) or dimethyl ketone
- ethyl acetate (10% petrolatum)
- *n*-butyl acetate (25% olive oil)
- methyl ethyl ketone (MEK).

Nail polish removers also represent a fire hazard, and may cause systemic toxicity when inhaled excessively or accidentally swallowed.

Cuticle removers and softeners

Cuticle removers contain 2–5% sodium or potassium hydroxide, a primary irritant, or α-hydroxy acids pH 3–3.5 in a liquid, gel or cream base, with substances such as propylene glycol or glycerol added as humectants. They are designed to destroy keratin by attacking the disulphide bonds of cystine. After the nails have been soaked in soapy water, cuticle removers are applied and left in place for approximately 10 minutes before being washed off. The softened cuticle is usually pushed back from the nail by rubbing it gently with an orange stick covered with cotton.

The fibrous cuticular ridge should not be removed with cuticle nippers, although a V-shaped curette may sometimes be used to shave down this tissue.

Cuticle softeners contain substances such as quaternary ammonium compounds or urea. They are used as emollient creams to maintain a soft cuticle.

Triethanolamine may act as a sensitizing agent (5% in petroleum for patch testing),

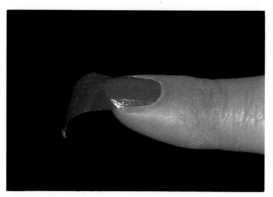

Figure 21.15 Stick-on nail dressing.

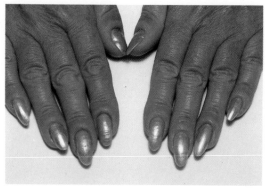

Figure 21.16 Onycholysis due to overzealous manicure.

but all the reactions to the other ingredients
are of irritant type.

Stick-on nail dressings

'Stick-on nail dressings' (press-on nail polish,
synthetic nail covers) are thin, coloured synthetic films (Figure 21.15) with an adhesive
that fixes them firmly to the nail. Pathological
changes[26] of traumatic origin are said to be
produced in nails by the occlusive nature of
the film. In fact, they can be attributed to a
temporary overhydration of the nail plate.
When the enhancements are removed, the
plate feels very weak and thin because of the
increased moisture content. These changes
can vary considerably in intensity from patient
to patient. Mild paronychia inflammation and
broken nails are the usual complaints. In
some instances it takes a year for the nail to
return to normal.

Artificial nails

These are discussed in Chapter 22.

Instrument nail damage

The most important adverse nail and skin
reactions to nail cosmetic practices are

trauma and infection, *the latter being common to
that observed with artificial nails.*

Traumatic injuries from using nail files,
wooden or plastic orange sticks, metal or
porcelain spatulas may cause not only infection but also onycholysis (Figure 21.16) and
Beau's lines or transverse white streaks from
over-zealous manicuring. It is therefore wise
to use orange sticks covered with cotton wool.
Almost without exception, nail technicians
remove too much of the natural nail plate
with coarse abrasives and powered Dremel-
type drills. This can lead to a variety of ail-
ments and increase the likelihood of allergic
reactions to uncured liquid monomers and
additives.

Ideally, it may not be advisable to cut or
clip the nail, since this produces a shearing
action that weakens the natural layered structure and promotes fracturing and splitting. In
fact, this is usually due to unsharp tools. The
cutters use blades which need to be changed

often. It may sometimes be better to shape the fingernail with an emery board, filing from the sides of the nail toward the centre.

The subungual space of the hand is heavily colonized with microorganisms. It is well known that contaminated instruments may lead to acute bacterial or chronic *Candida* paronychia and onycholysis. Over-filing the nail plate with coarse abrasives or heavy handed filing techniques with even the mildest buffing block can disrupt the thin tissue seal that holds the plate to the bed and lead to onycholysis associated with *Candida.*

Acrylic nail extensions also favour *Candida* nail bed infection[27] and increase bacterial carriage versus natural nails,[28] particularly of Gram-negative bacteria. *Staphylococcus aureus* and *epidermidis* are not uncommon beneath the nails, and it seems almost impossible to get the bacteria out of this area despite surgical scrubs.[29] In contrast to fresh nail polish worn on short healthy nails,[30] chipped nail polish is a known potential reservoir for bacterial growth on natural nails.[29] In addition, bacterial carriage is higher in subjects with artificial nails than in those with natural nails.[31] Serious eye infections have also been reported following *Pseudomonas* involvement in the nail apparatus,[32] as has subacute bacterial endocarditis after nail trauma.[33]

Warts can affect mainly the periungual area, but transmission of herpes simplex, hepatitis B and AIDS (HIV) seem to be virtually impossible through nail services.[34]

Infectious complications can be avoided with effective sanitary practices.

Sanitary practices

Sanitation

This is low-level cleansing, in which some microorganisms, such as household germs, are destroyed significantly enough to be considered safe by public health standards. The simple act of wiping an object with soap and water is a method of sanitation.

Disinfection

This is the elimination of most microorganisms, except bacterial spores, on a surface. Only hard, non-porous surfaces can be disinfected. Wooden cuticle sticks and files, which cannot be sanitized, should be disposed of after use, or put aside for one specific client only. Patrons may be asked to bring their own clippers, but doing so means a loss of all control over these devices.

Bacterial infection of the plate's upper surface between the nail plate and artificial enhancement or polish coating has several common causes – mainly improper preparation of the surface before coating. Therefore nails should be cleansed and decontaminated with a disinfectant solution such as Scrub Fresh, which contains isopropanol, acetone and five antibacterial/antifungal ingredients.

The California State Board of Cosmetology requires that all non-electrical instruments with a sharp point or edge capable of piercing the skin and drawing blood be disinfected by cleaning them with soap and water and immersing them in a closed container of 70% isopropanol for at least 10 minutes.

The trend is toward recommending an Environmental Protection Agency registered, hospital level disinfectant. This is also the standard recommended by the Nail Manufacturer's Council (NMC).

Sterilization

This is the elimination of living organisms, including viruses, bacteria and bacterial spores, from a surface. The dry heat temperature in an electric glass bead sterilizer reaches 246°C, and is said to kill these organisms on implements in 10 seconds, but only clean metal implements should be inserted into the well of the sterilizer. These sterilizers are actually ineffective in the salon.

Glutaraldehyde or ethanol 90% (effective against herpes) and sodium hypochlorite are good alternatives if the instruments are fully submerged in the solution for a minimum of 10 minutes.

In fact, some authorities think paradoxically that sterilization is not to be recommended in salons, claiming that it is unnecessary and often involves the use of substances that are far too toxic for salon use.[34]

In conclusion, misuse of nail instruments is potentially far more damaging to the nail than are many cosmetic preparations.

REFERENCES

1. Alkiewicz J, Pfister R, *Atlas der Nagelkrankheiten.* Stuttgart: Schatthauer-Verlag, 1976.
2. Hill S, What's new in nail art? *Nails Magazine* October 1991; 96–110.
3. Brauer E, Baran R, Cosmetics: the care and adornment of the nail. In: *Diseases of the Nails and their Management,* 2nd edn (Baran R, Dawber RPR, eds). Oxford: Blackwell, 1994:285–96.
4. Liden C, Berg M, Färm G, Wrangsjö K, Nail varnish allergy with far-reaching consequences. *Br J Dermatol* 1993; **123:** 57–62.
5. Calnan CD, Sarkany J, Studies in contact dermatitis: nail varnish. *Trans St John's Hosp Dermatol Soc* 1958; **40:** 1–11.
6. Schorr WF, Nail polish allergy. *Dermatol Allergy* 1981; **4:** 23.
7. Dooms-Goossens E, Contact dermatitis caused by airborn agents. *J Am Acad Dermatol* 1986; **15:** 1–18.
8. Tosti A, Guerra L, Vincenzi C et al, Contract sensitization caused by toluene sulfonamideformaldehyde resin in women who use nail cosmetics. *Am J Contact Dermatitis* 1993; **4:** 150–3.
9. Hausen BM, Nagellack-Allergie. *Z Hautkr* 1994; **69:** 252–62.
10. Anonide A, Usiglio D, Pestarino A, Massone L, Frequency of positivity to nail varnish allergens. Study of eighty women. *G Ital Dermatol Venereol* 1995; **130:** 13–16.
11. De Groot AC, Weyland JW, Nater JP, *Unwanted Effects of Cosmetics and Drugs used in Dermatology,* 3rd edn. Amsterdam: Elsevier, 1993:524–9.
12. Fisher AA, *Contact Dermatitis.* Philadelphia: Lea & Febiger, 1986.
13. Hausen BM, Milbrodt M, Koenig WA, The allergens of nail polish. *Contact Dermatitis* 1995; **33:** 157–64.
14. Schoon D, The truth about toluene. *Nails Magazine* November 1994; 76.
15. Cronin E, *Contact Dermatitis.* Edinburgh: Churchill Livingstone, 1980:150–7.
16. Giorgini S, Brusi C, Francalanci S et al, Prevention of allergic contact dermatitis from nail varnishes and hardeners. *Contact Dermatitis* 1994; **31:** 325.
17. Shaw S, A case of contact dermatitis from hypoallergenic nail varnish. *Contact Dermatitis* 1989; **20:** 385.
18. Kanerva L, Lauerma A, Jolanki R, Estlander T, Methyl acrylate: a new sensitizer in nail lacquer. *Contact Dermatitis* 1995; **33:** 203–4.
19. Bonu G, Zina G, Reazione da contatto morfologicamente inconsueta. *Minerva Dermatol* 1959; **33:** 507–9.
20. Calnan CD, Reactions to artificial colouring materials. *J Soc Cosmet Chem* 1987; **18:** 215–23.
21. Cortese TA, Capitrol shampoo, nail discoloration. *The Schoch Letter* 1981; **31:** item 154.
22. Gordon G, Sparano BM, Iatropulos MJ, Hyperpigmentation of the skin associated with minocycline therapy. *Arch Dermatol* 1985; **121:** 618–23.
23. Loveman AB, Fliegelman MT, Discoloration of the nails. Concomitant use of nail lacquer with resocinol or resorcinol acetati as a cause. *Arch Dermatol* 1955; **72:** 153–6.
24. Baran R, Pathology induced by the application of cosmetics to the nail. In: *Principles of Cosmetics for the Dermatologist* (Frost, P, Horowitz SN, eds). St Louis: Mosby, 1982:181–4.
25. Kechijian P, Nail polish removers. Are they harmful? *Semin Dermatol* 1991; **10:** 26–8.
26. Samman PD, Onychia due to synthetic coverings. Experimental studies. *Trans St John's Hosp Dermatol Soc* 1961; **46:** 68–73.
27. Symonds J, O'Dell CA, Candida nail bed infection and cosmetic acrylic nail extension – a potential source of hospital infection? *J Hosp Infect* 1993; **23:** 243–7.
28. Pottinger J, Burns S, Manske C, Bacterial carriage by artificial versus natural nails. *Can J Infect Control* 1991; **6:** 52.
29. Wynd CA, Samstag DE, Lapp AM, Bacterial carriage on the fingernails or OR nurses. *AORN J* 1994; **60:** 796–805.
30. Baumgardner CA, Maragos CS, Walz JA, Larson

E, Effects of nail polish on microbial growth of fingernails. *AORN J* 1993; **58:** 84–8.

31. Senay H, Acrylic nails and transmission of infection can. *J Infect Control* 1991; **6:** 52.

32. Parker AV, Cohen EJ, Arentsen JJ, Pseudomas corneal ulcers after artificial fingernails injuries. *Am J Ophthalmol* 1989; **107:** 548–9.

33. Aderka D, Bacterial endocarditis following nail trauma. *Arch Intern Med* 1988; **148:** 752–4.

34. Schoon D, *Milady's Nail Structure and Product Chemistry*. Albany, NY: Milady/Delmar Publishing, 1996.

22

Cosmetics for abnormal and pathological nails

Robert Baran, Douglas Schoon

'It is a mistake for the physician to view a patient's complaint of unattractive nails as too
trivial for medical consideration.'

Earle Brauer, MD

INTRODUCTION

Medical or surgical nail disorders can sometimes be camouflaged by cosmetic nail techniques. This, however, covers up the
underlying process, and proper diagnosis and
therapy are therefore essential to correct the
underlying condition.[1]

There are limits to the use of cosmetics,
such as acrylic chemicals, in some at-risk
patients: those who have had a reaction to
acrylics in the past, for example, or individuals with circulatory disorders, particularly with
scarring or ulceration around the fingertip.
Any bacterial or fungal infection should be
treated before applying acrylic nails.
Individuals whose hands are in water for long
periods will have difficulty keeping on acrylic
nails. Psoriasis produces an isomorphic reaction,[2] so acrylic nails should be avoided in persons affected by this condition, since just
nicking a cuticle may provoke a Koebner reaction. Lichen planus and lupus erythematosus
may also precipitate this type of reaction.
Even if the condition is minor or temporary
(while waiting for hangnails to heal or onycholysis to grow out, for example), it is prudent not to use acrylics. This will avoid
medico-legal problems.[3] For the same reasons,
a UV light-cured acrylic should never be used

in people who are taking photosensitizing
medications, or who are affected by photodermatitis.

SCULPTURED ARTIFICIAL NAILS

These form 70% of the market for false nails,
and have become popular for two main reasons:

- they may be used to increase the length and
  the hardness of a normal nail or to deco-
  rate it with ornaments and jewels;
- they can attractively replace a deteriorated
  nail plate, one reduced by onychophagia,
  affected by splitting for example, or one
  that is simply broken – acrylics can even
  cosmetically correct ski-jump nails or the
  unsightly racket nails.

Sculpturing is performed in salons, but kits
are available for home use as a set containing:

- a metallized paperboard template, placed
  on the natural nail surface to frame the new
  nail;
- a liquid ethyl or isobutyl methacrylate
  monomer, which may be combined with
  hydroquinone;
- a powdered poly(methyl methacrylate) or
  poly(ethyl methacrylate) polymer (or a

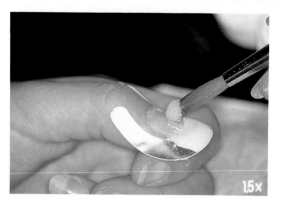

Figure 22.1 Metallized paper board template for sculptured artificial nails.

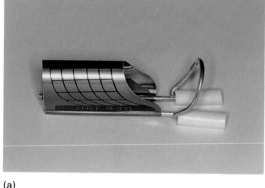

(a)

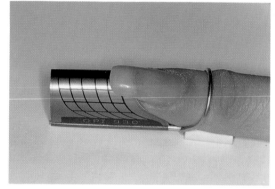

(b)

Figure 22.2 (a,b) Teflon templates for sculptured artificial nails.

copolymer of both methacrylates) with benzoyl peroxide as an initiator;

• a stabilizer such as resorcinol, eugenol, thymol or (most commonly) hydroquine (HQ) or methyl ethyl hydroquinone (MEHQ);

• *N,N*-dimethyl-*p*-toluidine to catalyse the production of free radicals from benzoyl peroxide in the polymer powder;

• plasticizers such as tricresyl or phthalate phosphate;

• solvents;

• dyes.

In salons, metallized nail forms (Figure 22.1) and Mylar-coated nail forms predominate over reusable Teflon nail forms (Figure 22.2).

The nail is first thoroughly cleansed, soaped, brushed and painted with antiseptic and antifungal solutions. The nail is frequently dried with a diethyl ether-based nail dehydrator and primed with methacrylic acid/solvent, blended before application. 'Primer' works like a double-sided tape. It sticks to the nail and to the acrylic, providing the necessary adhesion for both surfaces. Primers contain an acid called an 'adhesion promoter'. Methacrylic acid is one kind of adhesion promoter, while various others are used in non-methacrylate acid primers. The former will dry chalky-white, while the latter will dry shiny. Non-methacrylic acid primers are adhesive promoters in a solvent base, and are less likely to burn the soft tissue.

Using a paper or Teflon nail form, the natural nail is painted with a fresh acrylic mixture that hardens at room temperature. The prosthetic nail is enlarged by repeated applications. The sculptured nail can be filed and manicured to shape, and, as the nail grows out, further applications of acrylic are added every few weeks to fill in the surface defect at the lunula. They may be used alone or over a tip.

A clear acrylic for sculptured nails may be used on the natural nail plate over the nail bed area so that the natural pink colour shows through, while a white acrylic is used distally for the nail plate's free edge. This combination perfectly simulates a natural nail, and enamel need not to be used. Pink-coloured powders are also often used to hide visible defects in the nail bed and plate.

Allergic reactions

These may occur 2–4 months, and even as long as 16 months, after the first application.[5] The first indication is an itch in the nail bed. Paronychia, which is usually present in allergic reactions, is associated with excruciating pain in the nail area, and sometimes with paraesthesia. The nail bed is dry, thickened (Figure 22.3), and there is usually onycholysis (Figure 22.4). The natural nail plate becomes thinner (Figure 22.5), split, and sometimes discoloured. It takes several months for the nails to return to normal. Permanent nail loss (Figure 22.6) is exceptional, as is intractable

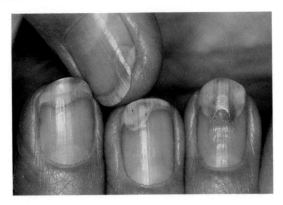

Figure 22.4 Onycholysis due to sculptured artificial nails.

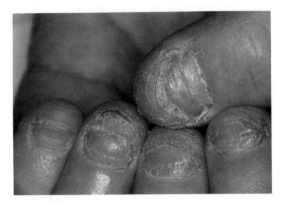

Figure 22.5 Thinning of the nail plate after use of sculptured artificial nails.

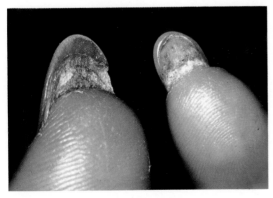

Figure 22.3 Nail bed and hyponychium thickening from sculptured artificial nails.

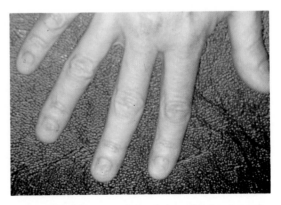

Figure 22.6 Permanent loss of the nails due to sculptured artificial nails. (Courtesy of A Fisher.)

prolonged paraesthesia.[6–8] Distant allergic contact dermatitis may affect the face and the eyelids,[9] and is probably caused by touching the face with the hands. Filings contain lots of unreacted monomer, since it takes up to 48 hours for the enhancement to fully cure, especially if the technician uses the product too wet (which most do). The filings and trace monomer on the hands can certainly cause these problems. Technicians should be instructed to wash their hands before touching the face or eye area. Usually, the area involved is the chin, where technicians tend to rest their faces in their hands. Also, they should be warned to avoid contact with the dust of freshly applied product and to avoid using the product wet. Unreacted UV gel in the dusts and filings can do the same. In this case, technicians should be told to change the bulbs in their lights three times per year and to apply thinner, multiple coats of products, rather than thicker coats, which are more difficult to cure. Although sensitization to butylhydroxytoluene is possible, gels use acrylated oligomers and monomers. Acrylates are many times more likely to cause sensitization than methacrylates or stabilizers.

Patch testing to identify reactions to sculptured artificial nails

Allergic patients react strongly to the acrylic liquid monomer[10] (1–5% monomer in petrolatum or olive oil). In the series of 11 patients of Koppula et al,[10] 0.1% ethyl acrylate in petrolatum detected 91% of the acrylate-allergic artificial nail users. These authors proposed the following five chemicals be used as screens: ethyl acrylate, 2-hydroxyethyl acrylate, ethylene glycol dimethacrylate, ethyl cyanoacrylate and triethylene glycol diacrylate. The pattern of acrylate crossreactivity among the most frequently positive acrylates suggests that a functional group that is a carboxyethyl side group may be requisite for allergic contact dermatitis to acrylates.

The powder contains ethyl methacrylate homopolymer or ethyl/methyl metacrylate copolymer, but also small amounts of monomeric methyl methacrylate monomer and ethyl methacrylate. This explains why the powder may in some cases provoke an allergic patch test reaction.[11,12]

Since there are no real monomer-free acrylic resins, an adaptable nail prosthesis made of silicone rubber is an alternative. This 'thimble-shaped' finger cover takes nail polish well[13,14] (Figure 22.7).

Non-allergic reactions

With continued wear of the sculptured nails, the edges become loose. These must be clipped and then rebuilt to prevent development of an environment prone to bacterial and, beneath the nail plate, candidal infection. In fact, this is a result of improper application and maintenance.

Failure to undergo filing every two weeks will result in creation of a lever arm that pre-

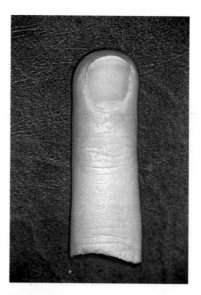

Figure 22.7 Adaptable nail prosthesis made of silicone rubber.

disposes to traumatic onycholysis or damage to the natural nail.

Onycholysis[15] is very common with nail extensions that are too long (lever effect). It has also been said that the bond between the sculptured and the natural nail is stronger than the adhesion between the nail plate and the nail bed. There is no evidence that occlusive prosthetic nail interferes with the nail's normal vapour exchange. Irritant reactions to monomers are possible. These are manifested as a thickening of the nail bed's keratin layer, which can sometimes cause the entire nail bed to thicken with or without onycholysis. Still, without question, the overwhelming majority of cases result from physical trauma or abuse.

Damage to the natural nail is not unusual after two to four months of wear of a sculptured nail. If it becomes yellow or crumbly, this means that the product was applied and maintained incorrectly. Therefore, instead of wearing prosthetic nails for no more than three consecutive months with one-month intervals before resuming applications,[16] the dermatologist should find a better-qualified nail technician. The problem may well not be the acrylic nail materials but rather the thinning of the nail due to over-filing with heavy abrasives. Primer (methacrylic acid) is a strong irritant, which may produce third-degree burns. Primer is hazardous if one floods the cuticles, neglects to wash-up spills immediately, or ignores an individual complaining of burning. One must rinse any area immediately with water when the client says it is burning. Primer can permeate the plate and soak the nail bed if the nails are too thin. Soap or baking soda, used with water, are excellent neutralizers. If primer gets in the eye, the eye should be flushed with water for at least 15 minutes, making sure that all traces of the chemical have been rinsed, and poison control should be called. There is a general tendency to disregard manufacturers' instructions and warnings, which causes the majority of disorders. Encouraging individuals to remove the product every three months may worsen the situation.

Removing sculptured artificial nails

The use of acetone-free nail polish remover on painted nails is not necessarily desirable. The alternative solvents, especially methyl ethyl ketone, have higher orders of toxicity and can damage the polymer surface. Butylhydroxytoluene has caused a non-allergic contact urticaria.[17]

Reports have been published of severe and even fatal cases following ingestion or inhalation of acetonitrile-containing acrylic nail removers, because the acetonitrile is metabolized into cyanide.[18–20] Nitroethane poisoning from artificial fingernail remover has led to cyanosis and 39% methaemoglobinemia.[21]

Ethyl methacrylate monomer and polymer nails and the photobonded variety may produce severe and prolonged paresthesia, even without associated allergic dermatitis.[3] Unfortunately, the product the patient was using could have contained methyl methacrylate monomer.

GEL SYSTEMS: GEL NAILS

The word gel applies to the form of the product – not the product itself. Gel system products are premixed and either acrylic-based (14% of the market) or cyanoacrylate-based (1% or less of the market).[12]

Their virtual lack of odour makes gels popular in full-service beauty salons.

The gel market encompasses three different technologies. In all three, the nail is primed when required, then the gel is brushed on the nail, like nail polish, and cured with either UV or visible light, or with a brush-on, dropper-applied or spray catalyst.

UV light-cured gels are perhaps the best known of the three systems. These gels contain urethanes and (meth)acrylate compounds, a photoinitiator, anti-yellowing agents and a UV light unit. The gel remains in a semi-liquid form until cured in a photobonding box. The proportion of resins to monomers determines the gel consistency. When the gel is exposed to light of an appropriate wavelength, polymerization occurs, resulting in hardening of the gel. UV gels never use external catalysts and often do not use primers.

Visible light systems work in a similar fashion. They are composed of either urethane acrylate or urethane methacrylate.

No-light cyanoacrylate gels use a spray or a brush-on or dropper-applied activator. In spray-setting gels, a chemical initiator replaces the photoinitiator, since UV lights and primer are never used with cynoacrylate gels.

Gels are not meant to replace liquid and powder systems, wraps or other services. They are occasionally used as 'caps' over the natural nails of persons who do not want nail extensions but have trouble growing their own nails because of chipping, cracking or peeling. Capping with fabric adds greater strength. In fact, this overlay is identical to traditional wraps.

Individuals with distal fissure or men who bite their nails may want more attractive hands, but shy away from liquid and powder systems. A gel-capped nail can look completely natural, and the smooth hard finish will make the nail more resistant to chewing and picking.

Gels can also be used as tip overlays for individuals who want natural tips. Some companies provide a thicker gel designed for building and sculpting nail extensions. Some gels may also be used over polish, making it impervious to clipping, wearing and fading away.

Coloured gels

Coloured gels are sometimes recommended to persons who do not often change polish colour. They are noted for easy application, high shine and durability. However, if nail infection or onycholysis occurs, the permanently coloured gel makes detection nearly impossible. These gels are adapted to UV light systems.

Removing gels

Usually gels must be removed every three or four months because a large percentage of enhancement may contain uncured oligomer.

The best way to remove UV gels is to let the nails grow out or to grind them off with heavy abrasives for patients who develop an allergic reaction. Acetone will have no effect on UV gels. This is a serious disadvantage that gel promoters wish to conceal, and is one of the major reasons why they are not healthier for the nail.

Adverse reactions

Gel enhancement products shrink by up to 20%, resulting in lifting, tip cracking and other types of service breakdown. As effects of excessive shrinkage, clients may comment that the enhancement feels tight on the nail bed. Other symptoms include throbbing or warmth below the nail plate. This may lead to tender, sore fingertips.

Adverse nail reaction with even nail loss[22] and paresthesia from photobonded acrylate have been observed.[23] In patients wearing photobonded acrylic nails who had perionychial and subungual eczema, Hemmer et al[24] have patch tested 'hypoallergenic' commercial products. The omission of irritant methacrylic acid in UV-curable gels does not reduce the high sensitizing potential of new acrylates. In contrast to the manufacturers' declaration, all 'hypoallergenic' products continue to include acrylate functional monomers, and therefore continue to cause allergic sensitization. Gels and acrylics, being chemically distinct entities, will not necessarily cross-react.[12,22]

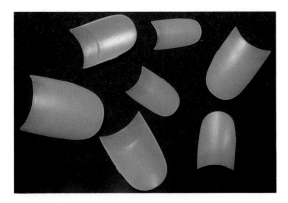

Figure 22.8 Preformed plastic nail 'tips'.

PREFORMED ARTIFICIAL NAILS

Plastic press-on nails are preformed and glued to the nail (Figure 22.8). They are packaged in several shapes and sizes to conform to normal nail plate configurations. They are used as full nails or nail tips, fixed with a special adhesive supplied with the kit. Preformed nails in gold plate (Figure 22.9) may be used in the same way as plastic nails. The application of preformed prosthetic nails is limited by the need for some normal nail to be present for attachment. Some manufacturers recommend that they do not remain on for one or two days at a time. Artificial tips are the primary application of prosthetic nails. Most nail technicians feel it is too time-consuming to sculpt nails. Therefore they use acrylic tips and overlays (Figure 22.10).

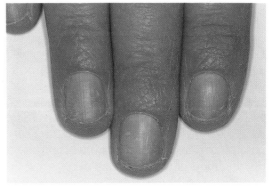

(a)

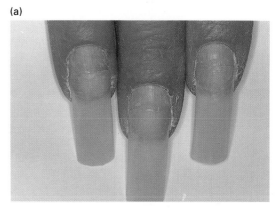

(b)

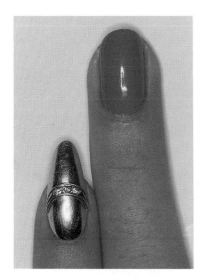

Figure 22.9 Preformed nail in gold plate.

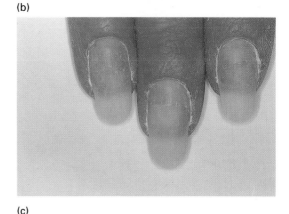

(c)

Figure 22.10 (a–c) Different stages for shaping the tips of nails.

Before the introduction of cyanoacrylate instant glue, daily insults to the nails caused the preformed plastic nails to loosen. Preformed nails remaining in place for more than three to four days have sometimes caused onycholysis and nail surface damage. In some cases, allergic changes may be indistinguishable from dermatitis caused by formaldehyde nail hardeners. Ectopic allergic or irritant contact dermatitis may affect the face and eyelids[25] and large areas of the trunk,[26] and disappears with removal of the cause.

Allergic onychia and paronychia due to cyanoacrylate nail preparations require some comment.[9,27] After about three months, painful paronychia, onychia, dystrophy and discoloration of the nails may become apparent and last for several months (Figure 22.11). Eyelid dermatitis disappears with removal of the allergen.

Shelley and Shelley[28] reported an isolated chronic allergic contact dermatitis simulating a small plaque of parapsoriasis due to an allergic reaction to cyanoacrylate adhesive used on the fingernails.

Interestingly, patients react far more often on patch testing to the adhesive than to the plastic nails. Suggested allergens for patch testing are

- *p*-t-butyl phenol resin (1% petrolatum)[28-30]
- tricresyl ethyl phthalate (5% petrolatum)
- cyanoacrylate adhesives (10% petrolatum)
- other adhesives (5% methyl ethyl ketone)
- methyl ethyl hydroquinone
- artificial nail itself

Most cyanoacrylate adhesive formulations contain hydroquinone. Therefore most investigators perform patch testing not only with cyanoacrylate glue or nail preparations as such, but also with hydroquinone and acrylic monomer.

NAIL MENDING AND WRAPPING

The purpose of nail mending is to create a splint for a partially fractured nail plate (Figure 22.12) or one longitudinal split

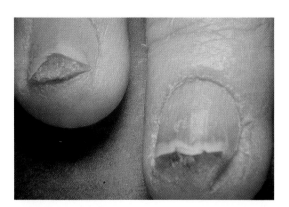

Figure 22.11 Dystrophic nails with subungual hyperkeratosis due to preformed plastic nails. (Courtesy of P Lazar.)

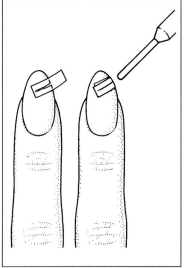

Figure 22.12 Nail mending.

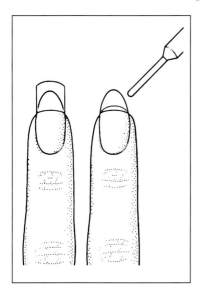

Figure 22.13 Nail wrapping.

extending the full length of the nail. The split is first bonded with cyanoacrylate glue, then the nail is painted with fibred clear nail polish. A piece of wrap fabric is cut and shaped to fit over the nail surface. This is then embedded in polish of high solid content, and several coats are applied.

In nail wrapping, the free edge of the nail should be long enough to be splinted with paper, silk, linen, plastic film or fibreglass and fixed with cyanoacrylate glue (Figure 22.13). The activator of cyanoacrylate wraps acts much as a catalyst to harden wrap adhesive. The most important ingredient in cyanoacrylate catalysts is *N,N*-dimethyl-*p*-toluidine (DMPT). Methaemoglobinaemia with resultant cyanosis may follow its ingestion.[31] DMPT is typically 0.5% of the formulation and hydroquinone approximately 0.001%. It is present in all but one type of catalyst. The ethyl acetate and trichloroethane that set the gel do not promote curing, but are merely sol-

vents. Silk wraps are sheer and very thin. Linen is thicker and offers increased strength, but inhibits cyanoacrylate penetration to the nail, thus lowering adhesion. Fibreglass is the newest wrap, combining many benefits of both silk and linen.

Most fibreglass systems consist of three basic elements.[32]

- a resin, or adhesive composed of cyanoacrylate; resins polymerize from moisture in the air or in the natural nail's surface, forming the hard nail coating that is both the base and top coats of the nail wrap;
- fibreglass mesh;
- an activator or catalyst that cuts the hardening time to seconds.

See above for patch testing of patients sensitized to cyanoacrylate.

NAIL HARDENERS

Some products are just modified nail enamels containing, among their ingredients, nylon fibres, acrylate resin and hydrolysed proteins. They function as a base coat. Others may contain up to 5% formaldehyde tissue fixative, but are designed in the USA to be applied only to the free edge of the nail while the skin is shielded.[33] Formaldehyde permanently alters the structure of the nail plate by crosslinking the keratin, which leads to embrittlement since the crosslink density rises over time with continued regular use. Formaldehyde increases the hardness of the nail plate, but it also lowers flexibility and increases strength, resulting in an imbalance called brittleness. The property that people really want is toughness. This is a favourable balance between strength and flexibility.

Nail changes caused by formaldehyde preparation may be bluish (Figure 22.14), then turn red, with intense throbbing pain.[34] Resolving haemorrhages produce reddish-rust or yellow discoloration of the nail. Formaldehyde can also be responsible for paronychia, onycholysis (Figure 22.15), sub-

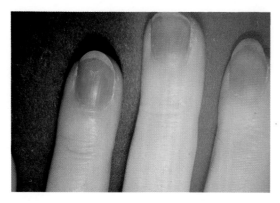

Figure 22.14 Formaldehyde acute reaction. (Courtesy of P Lazar.)

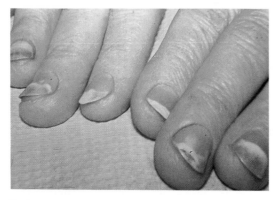

Figure 22.15 Long-standing onycholysis due to formaldehyde.

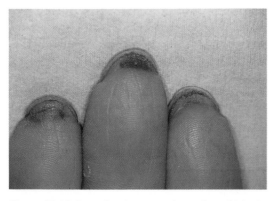

Figure 22.16 Pterygium inversum due to formaldehyde.

ungual hyperkeratosis and dryness of the fingertips, but nail shedding is uncommon. Pterygium inversum[35] (Figure 22.16) has been observed, sometimes accompanied by severe pain necessitating systemic corticosteroids.[33]

Isolated onycholysis and ectopic contact dermatitis, even associated with haemorrhages of the lips in nail biters,[36] have been reported. Airborne contact dermatitis of the face may also be seen.

Formaldehyde (1–2% in water) should be used for patch testing, but caution is necessary in interpreting the reactions, because the agent also acts as an irritant.

Quaternium-15 and 2-bromo-2-nitro-propane-1,3-diol are both formaldehyde releasers.

Alternatives to formaldehyde hardeners are aluminium chloride (5% in water), tannin and nail creams with a low water (30%) and high lipid content for minimizing nail fragility. Alternative nail hardeners consist of polyesters, acrylics and polyamides. These nail hardeners are essentially a modification of clear nail enamel with different solvents and resin concentration. They are the first coat of enamel applied to clean nail plate, functioning as a base coat to allow better adhesion of the coloured nail plate.[16]

OVERALL RISK

Precise figures are not available for the number of adverse reactions related to the use of nail cosmetics. Nevertheless, according to the United States manufacturer's file, the risk is low. According to the US Food and Drug Administration pilot study tabulating complaints received directly from consumers, the risk is medium.[37,38] Finally, there is a third source of information, namely the National Electronics Injuries Surveillance System (NEISS).[39]

REFERENCES

1. Barnett JM, Scher RK, Nail cosmetics. *Int J Dermatol* 1992; **31**: 675–81.

2. Fisher AA, Baran R, Occupational nail disorders with a reference to Koebner's phenomenon. *Am J Contact Dermatitis* 1992; **3**: 16–23.

3. Baran R, Schibli H, Permanent paresthesia to sculptured nails. A distressing problem. *Dermatol Clin* 1990; **8**: 138–41.

4. Engasser P, Cosmetics and contact dermatitis. *Dermatol Clin* 1991; **9**: 69–80.

5. Marks JC, Bishop ME, Willis WF, Allergic contact dermatitis to sculptured nails. *Arch Dermatol* 1979; **115**: 100.

6. Fisher AA, Permanent loss of fingernails from sensitization and reaction to acrylic in a preparation designed to make artificial nails. *J Dermatol Surg Oncol* 1980; **6**: 70–6.

7. Fisher AA, Baran R, Adverse reactions to acrylate sculptured nails with particular reference to prolonged paresthesia. *Am J Contact Dermatitis* 1991; **2**: 38–42.

8. Freeman S, Lee MS, Gudmundsen K, Adverse contact reactions to sculptured acrylic nails: 4 cases – reports and a literature review. *Contact Dermatitis* 1995; **33**: 381–5.

9. Fitzgerald DA, Enolish JSC, Widespread contact dermatitis from sculptured nails. *Contact Dermatitis* 1994; **30**: 118.

10. Koppula SV, Fellman JH, Storrs FJ, Screening allergens for acrylate dermatitis associated with artificial nails. *Am J Contact Dermatitis* 1995; **6**: 78–85.

11. Lane CW, Kost LB, Sensitivity to artificial nails. *Arch Dermatol* 1956; **74**: 671–2.

12. Kanerva L, Lauerma A, Estlandeer T et al, Occupational allergic contact dermatitis caused by photobonded sculptured nails and a review on (meth)acrylates in nail cosmetics. *Am J Contact Dermatitis* 1996; **7**: 1–9.

13. Pillet J, The aesthetic hand prosthesis. *Orthop Clin North Am* 1981; **12**: 961–9.

14. Beasley RW, de Beze G, Prosthetic substitution for fingernails. *Hand Clin* 1990; **6**: 105–12.

15. Goodwin P, Onycholysis due to acrylic nail applications. *Clin Exp Dermatol* 1976; **1**: 1991–2.

16. Draelos ZK, *Cosmetics in Dermatology*, 2nd edn. Edinburgh: Churchill Livingstone, 1995.

17. Schubert HJ, Lindner K, Prater E, Kontaktallergie im Nagelstudio. *Z Hautkr* 1992; **67**: 1067–9.

18. Turchen SG, Monaguerra AS, Whitney C, Severe cyanide poisoning from the ingestion of an acetonitrile containing cosmetic. *Am J Emerg Med* 1991; **9**: 264–7.

19. Caravati EM, Litovitz TL, Pediatric cyanide intoxication and death from an acetonitrile containing cosmetic. *J Am Med Assoc* 1988; **260**: 3470–3.

20. Rainey PM, Roberts WL, Diagnosis and misdiagnosis of poisoning with cyanide precursor acetonitrile: nail polish remover or nail glue remover? *Am J Emerg Med* 1993; **11**: 104–8.

21. Hornfeldt CS, Rab WH, Nitroethane poisoning from an artificial remover. *J Tox Clin Toxicol* 1994; **32**: 321–4.

22. Halgmüller T, Hemmer W, Kusak I et al, Loss of fingernails due to persisting allergic contact dermatitis in an artificial nail designer. *J Allergy Clin Immunol* 1995; **95**: 250.

23. Fischer AA, Adverse nail reactions and paresthesia from photobonded acrylate sculptured nails. *Cutis* 1990; **45**: 293–4.

24. Hemmer W, Focke M, Wantke F et al, Allergic contact dermatitis to artificial fingernails prepared from UV light-cured acrylates. *J Am Acad Dermatol* 1996; **35**: 377–80.

25. Calnan CD, Cyanoacrylate dermatitis. *Contact Dermatitis* 1970; **5**: 165–6.

26. Fitzgerald DA, Bhaggoe R, English JSC, Contact sensitivity to acyanoacrylate nail-adhesive withe dermatitis at remote sites. *Contact Dermatitis* 1995; **32**: 175–6.

27. Shelley ED, Shelley WB, Nail dystrophy and periungual dermatitis due to cyanoacrylate glue sensitivity. *J Am Acad Dermatol* 1988; **19**: 574–5.

28. Shelley ED, Shelley WV, Chronic dermatitis simulating small-plaque parapsoriasis due to cyanoacrylate adhesive used on fingernails. *J Am Med Assoc* 1984; **252**: 2455–6.

29. Burrows D, Rycroft RJG, Contact dermatitis from PTBP and tricresyl ethyl phthalate in a plastic resin. *Contact Dermatitis* 1981; **7**: 336–7.

30. Pigatto PD, Giacchetti A, Altomare GF, Unusual sensitization to cyanoacrylate ester. *Contact Dermatitis* 1986; **14**: 193.

31. Potter JL et al, Methemoglobinemia due to ingestion of *N,N*-dimethyl-*p*-toluidine, a component used in the fabrication of artificial finger nails. *Ann Emerg Med* 1988; **17:** 1098–100.

32. Hill S, The fiberglass option: natural look, supernatural strength. *Nails Mag* August 1990; 44–52.

33. Norton LA, Common and uncommon reactions to formaldehyde-containing nail hardeners. *Semin Dermatol* 1991; **10:** 29–33.

34. Lazar P, Reactions to nail hardeners. *Arch Dermatol* 1966; **94:** 446–8.

35. Daly BM, Johnson M, Pterygium inversum inguis due to nail fortifier. *Contact Dermatitis* 1986; **15:** 256–7.

36. Hüldin DH, Hemorrhages of the lips secondary to nail hardeners. *Cutis* 1968; **4:** 708.

37. Nater JP, de Groot AC, Liem DH, *Unwanted Effects of Cosmetics and Drugs used in Dermatology*, 2nd edn. New York: Elsevier, 1985.

38. de Groot AC, Bruynzeel DP, Bos JD et al, The allergens in cosmetics. *Arch Dermatol* 1988; **124:** 1525–9.

39. Brauer E, Baran R, Cosmetics: The care and adornment of the nail. In: *Diseases of the Nails and their Management*, 2nd edn (Baran R, Dawber RPR, eds). Oxford: Blackwell, 1994:285–96.

23

Efficacy of moisturizers assessed through bioengineering techniques

Whitney Hannon, Howard I Maibach

INTRODUCTION

Moisturizers are a major portion of the skin care industry, yet relatively little has been published on their efficacy. With the increasing usage and refinement of non-invasive bioengineering techniques, better study designs and an increasingly sophisticated understanding of the mechanisms leading to dry skin, a more objective, scientifically rigorous and specific approach to the design of moisturizers is being achieved. However, much progress remains to be made in all of these areas: instrumentation, design of experiments, and stratum corneum pathophysiology.

This chapter introduces the reader to the basic science behind hydration of the stratum corneum (SC), or, as some authors[1] have argued, 'dehydration', and discusses theories on the action of moisturizers and the bioengineering techniques that can be used to objectively assess these actions. Lastly we review the literature on the efficacy of a single application of moisturizer to normal skin using indirect electrical bioengineering techniques.

DRY SKIN

Moisturizers by the simplest definition are topical substances whose primary action is to prevent or treat dry skin. Since dry skin has a wide range of etiologies[2,3] (Table 23.1), many substances could be considered moisturizers.

DEFINITIONS

The medical literature is confusing in its use of the term moisturizer, because there is no consensus on definitions. Table 23.2 gives a flavor of the confusion. For a thorough discussion on this topic one should refer to the review by Gabard.[4]

In this chapter, the definitions used will be those suggested by Gabard.[4] For example, a moisturizer will be defined as an emulsion-containing active substance applied to the skin

Table 23.1 Causes of dry skin	
Exogenous	Exposure to extremes of climate (cold, heat, wind, dryness), exposure to chemicals (detergents, solvents), excessive washing, various therapies (e.g. retinoids), UV radiation, mechanical abrasion
Endogenous: Non-pathologic	Fragile skin, senile skin, minor dry skin (xerosis vulgaris)
Pathologic	Ichthyoses, chronic eczema, psoriasis, atopic dermatitis

Table 23.2 Definitions	
Term	**Examples of definitions from the literature**
Moisturizer	• Any water-miscible material externally applied that hydrates the skin[4] • A product that actively increases water content of skin[5] • A product that effects SC already formed[6] • A product that is applied to the skin (and not the compounds contained in that product) – mostly an emulsion containing or an active substance such as a lotion, a cream, an ointment or bath oil with the purpose of rehydrating the skin, of regenerating a dry rough and/or scaly surface due to xerosis, irritation or other cause[4] • Compounds imparting water-bearing properties to cream[7] • Materials impairing the evaporation of water from the cream after application to the skin[4]
Humectant	• Compounds imparting water-binding properties to creams[8] • Compounds that attract moisture to the skin[9] • Compounds that will attract water to the surface, but the source of water is transepidermal water, not water from the atmosphere[10] • Compounds in which the source of attracted water is dependent on relative ambient humidity[11]
Emollient	• Softeners, occlusive moisturizers that help hydrate the skin by occluding the surface and conserving water in the SC[5] • A material that imparts a smooth, soft feeling to the skin but increases water content passively by occluding the surface[4] • Creams containing moisturizers[4] • Systems that smooth the roughed surface of the SC but usually do not show any effect on TEWL unless applied in great quantities[10] • Cosmetic ingredients or mixtures that help to maintain the soft, smooth and pliable appearance of the skin[12]
Keratolytics	• Protein-denaturing agents where actual lysis of SC occurs[6]
α-Hydroxy acids	• Substances that reduce abnormal cohesion between cells, determine the quality of SC at its formation; some have primarily hydroscopic properties and could be considered moisturizers but most could not; good for treating xerosis due to ichthyosis[6]
Hygroscopic	• Descriptive of substances that absorb water from the atmosphere[12]

with the purpose of rehydration or regeneration of a dry, rough and/or scaly surface due to xerosis, irritation or another cause. Examples of moisturizers are lotions, creams, ointments and bath oils. Under Gabard's definition, moisturizers are the total product, not the separate active compounds contained within the product. Humectants are compounds or materials that bind and/or attract water to the stratum corneum or any emulsion that contains these compounds. Emollients will not be considered as separate entities.

SKIN HYDRATION

The stratum corneum (SC) is the primary structure mediating water exchange or flux between the internal and external environments. This exchange is a process that depends on the difference between the water concentration in the epidermis and that in the outside environment, as well as on the water-holding/releasing properties of the substances making up the stratum corneum. Water concentration C and flux J are two separate measures of SC hydration, which are related through a modification of Fick's law, which describes passive diffusion from the highly hydrated tissues through the SC:[4,13]

$$J = K_m D \frac{dC}{dx}$$

In this equation, J is the flux of water in flow per unit area (mol/cm^2/h), K_m is the partition coefficient (concentration in membrane/

concentration in solution), D is the diffusion coefficient of water (cm^2/h), which itself depends on water content, dC is the change in water concentration across the SC (mol/cm^2) and dX is the distance across the SC (cm); dC/dX is referred to as the water concentration gradient.

There are limitations to this modified version of Fick's law.[14] For example, it only applies to the steady-state transport of low-molecular-weight substances. Accumulation and binding of substances in the SC and metabolism are not accounted for, and some external agents such as detergents can alter the permeability constant of SC during penetration.[14] In addition, we are gaining an appreciation for the complex ultrastructure of the membrane and the biochemical and physical nature of its interactions with water.[15] An example of this complexity is that water exists in at least three different binding states:[16] tightly bound water (water bound to polar groups of lipids and proteins); bound water (water attached via hydrogen bonds, which are able to exchange protons and thus account for the electrical properties observable in hydrated skin); and intermediate water (water that is closer to the liquid state but does not have the rotational properties of free water[17]). The state that predominates varies depending on the concentration of water in the SC; in general, the higher the SC water content, the greater the proportion of intermediate water.[18] Lastly, we must consider that the external environment can also affect flux. For example, in vivo water flux can be altered by changes in skin temperature and by ambient relative humidity.[13]

Another way to visualize the steady state of water content in the SC is to consider three factors:

- water exchanged with the outside environment – this can be water absorbed from the environment, defined as percutaneous absorption (PA), or water lost to the environment, defined as transepidermal water loss, TEWL (note that TEWL and PA are directly linked[19]);
- water within the corneum – this water can be extracellular or intracellular, and bound or unbound to protein;
- water exchanged with the free water in the deeper levels of the epidermis and dermis.

RELATIONSHIP BETWEEN TEWL AND WATER CONTENT

The relationship between TEWL and SC water content is complex,[20,21] and at times may seem paradoxical if one takes an overly simplistic view. TEWL and SC water content can be directly or indirectly proportional, depending on the clinical situation.[22] Both TEWL and water content should be measured in order to obtain a clear picture of the hydration status of the SC.

WATER-HOLDING SUBSTANCES

Adequate hydration depends on the presence of an intrinsic mixture of hydroscopic water-soluble materials or natural moisturizing factors (NMFs), which appear to be enveloped in cell membrane lipids. Important components of this mixture include the sodium or potassium salt of 5-pyrrolidone-2-carboxylic acid (PCA), sodium lactate, urea, ions (chloride, potassium and sodium), lactates, citrates and formates, amino acids, and unidentified substances.

ACTION OF MOISTURIZERS

Moisturizers appear to act at various locations within this system.[19] Since they are applied externally to the SC, it is theorized that they increase water content by (1) increasing the percutaneous absorption of water and/or (2) by reducing TEWL. The percutaneous absorption of water could theoretically be increased

(1) by substances capable of holding water (humectants), which can increase the water concentration at the surface, thus favoring an inward gradient (but this has not been conclusively shown experimentally[23]), or (2) by creating a hydrophobic barrier that reduces the TEWL so that water builds up under the surface, also leading to an inward gradient of reabsorption,[24] or (3) a combination of the two. Another mechanism that is becoming increasingly understood is that topical substances are absorbed into the SC and may directly or indirectly influence the water-exchange properties of the intrinsic proteins/lipids within the SC.[20] Research in this area is needed,[16] since water itself cannot restore the skin if the NMF are absent.[23]

Note that this is a complex, delicately balanced system posed to maintain homeostatic levels of hydration – that is to say, neither too

Table 23.3 Common humectants

Category	Examples	Properties	Notes
NMF	PCA	Synthesized from glutamic acid in epidermis	Hydrating at 3–5%
	Urea		Best at concentrations below 10%. Keratolytic over 10% concentration; useful in states of hyperkeratosis such as ichthyosis, keratosis pilaris, Darier's disease and severe dry skin)[25] but may not be tolerated well even at low concentrations on children and on the face due to stinging; does not cause sensitization
	Lactic acid	Part of α-hydroxy family; useful in states of hyperkeratosis such as ichthyosis, keratosis pilaris, Darier's disease and severe dry skin	Best at concentrations of 5–10%. May cause some irritation and stinging, but not sensitizing
Polyols	Glycerol	Excellent hydrating ability	Best at concentrations of <10%? Keratolytic at high concentrations (>40%); useful in states of hyperkeratosis such as ichthyosis, keratosis pilaris, Darier's disease and severe dry skin; can be an irritant, and occasionally causes causes contact dermatitis
	Sorbitol	Moderate hydrating ability	
	Propylene glycol	Good hydrating ability at low concentrations (below 10%); one of the common solvents for topical steroids[25]	
Macro-molecules	Glycosamino-glycans (hyaluronic acid, chondroitin sulfate)	Found in ground substance of all connective tissue	
	Collagen	Structural proteins of connective tissue	Used in denatured or hydrolyzed form. Further hydrolysis turns it into gelatin
	Elastin	Structural protein of connective tissue	Used in denatured or hydrolyzed form
	DNA	Hydroscopic because of numerous phosphate groups	Used in denatured and partially hydrolyzed form
Liposomes	Niosomes	Phospholipids are replaced by synthetic non-ionic amphiphilic lipids	

Table 23.4 Emollients or filmogenic compounds

Category	Example	Properties
Hydrocarbons	Petrolatum	No water, so no need for preservatives; penetrates intercellular epithelium; heavy, so may not be esthetically pleasing[25]
	Paraffin	
	Perhydrosqualene	
	Mineral oil	No water, no need for preservatives
Silicones		Inert, pulverized into small particles, added to products to give 'slip'; lubricates, protects, water-repellent; not absorbed topically; no allergenicity or comedogenicity[25]
Natural lipids polyesters: oils, acids and fatty acid esters		Integrate with proteins of SC; long chain is less comedogenic because of molecular size
	Capric/caprylic triglyceraldehydes	Short-chain acid; can be comedogenic
	Coconut oil	Short-chain acid; can be comedogenic
	Linoleic acid C18:2ω-6	Precursor of ω-6 fatty acids; essential fatty acid, present in six types of ceramides in man (which account for 40% of intracellular lipids), oils rich in polyunsaturated fatty acids (PUFAs), ω-6 or ω-3 fatty acids
	γ-Linoleic acid C20: 3ω-6	Essential fatty acid, precursor of prostaglandin PG1, rich in PUFAs
	Arachidonic acid C20: 4ω-6	Essential fatty acid, precursor of prostaglandin PG2, rich in PUFAs
	α-Linoleic acid C18:3 ω-6	Precursor of ω-3 fatty acids, rich in PUFAs
	Eicosapentaenoic acid (C20:5, ω-3)	Precursor of prostaglandin 3, rich in PUFAs
	Fish oil	Rich in prostaglandins, animal-derived oils
	Evening primrose	Rich in prostaglandins, plant-derived oils
	Borage	Rich in prostaglandins, plant-derived oils
	Grape seed oil	Rich in prostaglandins, plant-derived oils
	Sorbitol oleate	Synthesized unsaturated fatty acid esters; comedogenic because of interaction with SC
	Lanolin linoleate	Synthesized unsaturated fatty acid esters; comedogenic because of interaction with SC
Fatty alcohols	Cetyl	
	Stearic	
	Palmitic	
Low-molecular-weight ethers/esters	Isopropyl myristate	Comedogenic, must keep concentration below 2%; may have preservative action
	Isopropyl stearate	Comedogenic, must keep concentration below 2%; may have preservative action
Waxes	Fatty acid esters	
	Beeswax	Usually no adverse reactions
	Synthetic beeswax	Usually no adverse reactions
	Cholesterol	Polycyclic alcohol; usually no adverse reactions
	Lanolin	Complex mixture of esters, polyesters, high-molecular-weight alcohols and fatty acids secreted by sebaceous glands of sheep; has both occlusive and humectant properties; can be mixed with up to twice weight of water without separation; esters of lanolin can be comedogenic[25]

much water nor too little, since both would be devastating for the organism. Moisturizers by definition interfere with this system, and combined with presence of SC pathology, they have the potential to throw the system out of balance and could ironically lead to the exact situation they are trying to avoid, namely water depletion.

COMPOSITION OF MOISTURIZERS

A variety of moisturizers exist, but at the most basic level these can be divided into three categories based on their theorized mode of action:

1. humectants or 'water-providing substances';
2. occlusive agents;
3. substances with both properties.

Humectants may or may not be absorbed, depending on their molecular weight. Higher-molecular-weight substances are less easily absorbed. Common humectants found in moisturizers are listed in Table 23.3.

Predominantly occlusive creams, also known as emollient creams are divided into

1. oil-in-water (O/W);
2. water-in-oil (W/O);
3. combinations of the two, or triple-phase preparations.

When applied, the water evaporates leaving a film, so the component of the oil phase is also known as the filmogenic component (Table 23.4).

Many moisturizers contain additional ingredients for practical, hygienic or esthetic purposes. For example, emollients contain emulsifiers to keep the phases uniformly mixed, and commercial preparations contain preservatives and often fragrances.

Note also that the composition of a moisturizer is more complex that simply the sum of its independent ingredients. Interactions may occur between water-binding substances,[26] and theoretically also between any of the other ingredients.

VARIABLE FORMS OF COSMETIC MOISTURIZERS

The major cosmetic products used as moisturizers or emollients are creams, lotions and bath oils.[5] Hand lotions are typically stearate-based, and are combined with non-ionic surfactants to make thin occlusive films to protect from environmental insult.[5] Bath oils are used if there is generalized dryness over the body, and are divided into[5]

1. dispersing types;
2. floating types;
3. beads.

Dispersing types are composed of mineral oils combined with emulsifying agents. Floating types form a film on water and coat the skin upon exiting the bath. They are composed of mineral oil modified by oils such as isopropyl myristate or oleyl alcohol. Beads are composed of free-floating detergent with oil coating the surface. These components separate during the bath, forming a surface film.

OVERVIEW OF IN VIVO BIOENGINEERING TECHNIQUES FOR THE ASSESSMENT OF MOISTURIZER EFFICACY

A variety of bioengineering techniques have been used to assess the efficacy of moisturizers on the human SC. These techniques can be divided into measurements of skin surface contour:

- desquamation;
- mechanical properties;
- indirect electrical properties;
- direct electrical properties;
- TEWL;
- skin imaging;
- optical techniques.

The tables in the Appendix to this chapter give details of the techniques, some of the researchers involved in the development of the technology, names of different machines, variables measured, principles behind the technologies, and their respective advantages and disadvantages.

Many authors have reviewed and compared these technologies. Marks[27] took a unique approach by using an arbitrary scale to compare the reproducibility, sensitivity, directness of measurement, capability for quantitation, standardization, and cheapness, ease and convenience.

IN VIVO ELECTRICAL BIOENGINEERING TECHNIQUES

This chapter focuses on electrical bioengineering methods, since they have been the

Table 23.5 Variables affecting TEWL[31]

Variable affecting TEWL	Specific source of error	Suggestions to minimize effect
Instrument-related variables	Zeroing	Zero only if necessary after warm-up period
	Measuring	Minimize time that probe is on skin
	Zero drift	Minimize humidity and temperature changes
	Surface plane	Standing person will act like a 'chimney' due to increased convection of air close to surface; minimize by placing measuring surface horizontally and applying probe parallel to this surface
	Contact pressure	Use constant, light pressure
	Use of probe protective covers	Be aware of variables introduced by probe covers
	Intra- and interinstrumental variability	Check calibration of instrument periodically
	Calibration	Calibrate regularly according to manufacturer's specifications
	Accuracy	Evaporimeter may underestimate TEWL at high evaporation rates
Environment-related variables	Air convection	Use draft shield
	Ambient air temperature	Control for room temperature (recommend 22°C) since TEWL may double at 30°C
	Ambient air humidity	Control for this complex variable (ideal is a relative humidity of 40%); record measurement
	Seasonal variation	Publications should state time of year; control for air temperature and humidity
	Direct light	Will heat up object; do not measure under light sources or windows with direct sunlight
Individual related variables	Sweating	Maintain ambient temperature below 20°C; subject should have 15–20 min premeasurement rest in climate-controlled room; control emotional sweating by performing 'dummy' measurements to put subject at ease
	Skin surface temperature	Measure and report; equilibrate subject to room
	Anatomical sites	Baseline TEWL varies depending on anatomical site; should state site of measurement
	Intra- and interindividual variations	Baseline TEWL is stable personal characteristic (does not vary depending on sex, race); elderly people may have decreased TEWL, and premature infants may have increased TEWL – otherwise TEWL stable with age

most common and convenient ways of quantifying the nature of the water in the SC. There are three main groups of electrical techniques which are useful:

1. machines that measure TEWL or evaporimeters;
2. machines that indirectly measure the water content through impedance, capacitance or conductance;
3. devices that can directly measure the water content in the SC.

Each method has its respective advantages and disadvantages, and thus measurement using several different techniques simultaneously gives useful data for comparison.[28]

MEASUREMENT OF TEWL

Total evaporative water loss (or transepidermal water loss TEWL) is an important parameter to study in assessing the efficacy of moisturizers. Its value varies in a complex manner depending on the clinical state,[22] the time course after moisturizer application[4] and the type of moisturizer. Two machines can measure TEWL: the Evaporimeter and the Tewameter. Their efficacy has been compared.[29]

Guidelines for TEWL measurements exist in order to allow comparisons between studies and to minimize errors.[30] Pinnagoda reviewed the sources of error in TEWL measurements, and his conclusions are summarized in Table 23.5.[30]

INDIRECT MEASUREMENTS

Measurements of impedance

Skin changes its electrical properties depending on the hydration state. This is thought to be due to at least three factors:

1. large structural components such as keratin chains and the embedding matrix protein have dipolar movements and are made more movable by water;
2. ions within and outside cells can react to applied electrical current and move with it;
3. water molecules themselves can form a continuous network of hydrogen bonds, allowing exchange between H_3O^+ and OH^- ions.[18]

The first bioengineers utilizing these convenient electrical changes with hydration measured impedance. Impedance is defined as the total electrical opposition to the flow of an alternating current.[18] The formula for impedance is

$$X = \sqrt{\left[R^2 + \left(\frac{1}{2\pi f C} \right)^2 \right]}$$

where f is the frequency of the applied current, R is resistance and C is capacitance.[11] Skin impedance falls as the skin becomes more hydrated.

Though impedance is the simplest parameter to obtain technically, it yields results that are difficult to interpret because impedance varies with season, circumstances and electrode paste used.[18] For example, at low frequencies the impedance is high and necessitates contact with a liquid junction. Liquid junctions or so-called 'wet electrodes' had the disadvantage that they directly affected the hydration state, were occlusive and required about 20 minutes in contact with the skin to make a measurement. Impedance has therefore largely been replaced by other electrical parameters, such as capacitance or conductance, that can be measured with fewer technical drawbacks.

Measurements of conductance

As frequency increases, the impedance drops, and this can be measured with a dry electrode, which interferes less with skin hydration. However, early investigators found it impossible to measure R and C simultaneously at the high frequencies that were technically preferable. In the early 1980s, researchers overcame this difficulty by measuring resistance *R*, conductance (the reciprocal of the resistance; that is, $1/R$) or capacitance *C* separately at high frequencies. Conductance behaves similarly to capacitance in a first approximation.[18] One of the first machines developed in this category was the Skicon-200 (skin surface hygrometer, IBS Ltd, Japan) by Masuda and associates,[32] which measures conductance to a single fixed high-frequency current (3.5 MHz).

The fixed high-frequency conductance method has some disadvantages, however. For example, the depth of SC is not well defined; agents other than water, dermal irritants and probe pressure can influence readings; the probe is still somewhat occlusive; and measuring only one frequency is oversimplistic and leads to an unacceptably high rate of false positives and negatives.[33] In addition, a direct relationship between the recorded conductance and the actual water content cannot be made in vivo. To make optimal skin conductance measurements, an electroconductive underlying wet medium is required and the high frequency current must propagate for at least 5 mm into the skin.[18]

Later, the Corneometer was developed (Courage and Khazaka, Cologne, Germany), which was capable of measuring capacitance with a low-frequency current. One disadvantage of capacitance is that it appears to be more susceptible to qualitative changes in SC. For example, capacitance is disproportionately low on the palmoplantar skin – possibly because palmoplantar SC is functionally inferior as a skin barrier membrane.[18] Another disadvantage is that capacitance is a less sensitive parameter for skin surface hydration in normal skin than conductance, and therefore some authors prefer to only use conductance in vivo.[18] However, though capacitance has poor sensitivity for hydration processes in normal skin, its sensitivity to changes in extremely dry skin have been reported to be better than conductance.[18,34]

A debate exists as to the relative merits of the two technologies, conductance versus capacitance. For example, the Skicon instrument is claimed to be more sensitive to dynamic water sorption and desorption than the Corneometer, and thus to be more suited for evaluating moisturizers.[18] However, in a first approximation, they are both capable of evaluating moisturizers in a consistent, comparable, reproducible manner as evidenced by a study[35] in which the ranking of the efficacy of seven moisturizers was the same for conductance and capacitance techniques.

STUDIES ON THE EFFICACY OF MOISTURIZERS USING TEWL AND ELECTRICAL BIOENGINEERING TECHNIQUES: ANALYSIS OF STUDY DESIGN AND SUMMARY OF RESULTS

Ideal study to assess efficacy

The ideal study must consider the following potential confounding variables when making measurements with indirect electrical techniques: anatomic skin area used for testing, external environmental factors, seasonal influences, sex and age.[36] In addition, comparisons between studies are easier if standard designs to evaluate the efficacy of moisturizers are agreed upon. Barel has proposed a study design for the evaluation of the short-term effects of moisturizers that takes into account most of these factors, described in Table 23.6.[36]

Studies to assess the efficacy of moisturizers using electrical bioengineering techniques

Gabard[4] has a useful classification for studies on the efficacy of moisturizers, in which he divides the studies into five main groups

1. single application to normal skin;
2. multiple application of moisturizers over time to normal skin;

Table 23.6 Recommended study design for moisturizer efficacy studies	
Category	**Description**
Location	Volar forearm or anterior lower leg
Design	Double-blind with contralateral, randomly assigned comparison of treated versus untreated areas
Methods of application	Gently rub hydrated product into test area
Concentration	$1–2$ mg/cm^2
Size of test area	4 cm $\times$ 4 cm
Measurements	
Baseline	Reading 10–30 min before application of product
Following application	Readings on treated and untreated area every 10–15 min
Total duration	60–180 min

3. moisturizer applied to experimentally irritated skin (one large irritant insult);
4. moisturizer applied to experimentally irritated skin (mild irritant applied repeatedly over time);
5. clinical studies in which moisturizer was applied to groups of patients with various conditions.

Studies on the effect of TEWL after a single application of moisturizer on normal skin

Blichmann characterized the effect of a single application of moisturizer on normal skin into two phases based on TEWL: the evaporation phase and the lipidization phase.[4,37] The evaporation phase lasts about 10–15 minutes, and is characterized by a sharp increase in TEWL followed by a gradual decrease to baseline, a phenomenon thought to be due to evaporation of the water in the applied product and temperature adjustment. The larger the TEWL, the more water the product contains.[4,38–40] If products are wiped off then there is an increase in TEWL that is *directly* proportional to the amount of water in a product.[4,38–41] Of course, in the case of water-free-petrolatum, in which there is no water, there is no evaporation phase.[38,42]

The lipidization phase comes next, and lasts up to several hours. It is characterized by an increase in SC water content, but no change or a decrease in the TEWL detected in comparison to a control area. Whether there is no change or a decrease in TEWL depends on the type of moisturizer applied. The greater the lipid content, the greater is the decrease in TEWL.[4,37,38,42] This phase is thought to be characterized by a slow clearing of the nonvolatile emulsion lipid components. If products are wiped off during this phase, an increase in TEWL is observed that is *inversely* related to the water content of the product, presumably due to more build-up of water under a more occlusive product. This increased TEWL returns to basal levels after 10–15 minutes.[38]

Studies on capacitance, conductance and impedance after single application of moisturizing materials to normal skin

Table 23.7 summarizes the studies that used indirect bioelectrical techniques to assess the efficacy of a single application of moisturizer to normal skin. In normal skin, the capacitance ratio (moisturizer-treated-skin capacitance/untreated-skin capacitance) and time course vary, depending on the type of moisturizer. In addition, electrical readings are not always proportional to the water present, depending on the substance. For these

Table 23.7 Summary of studies on normal skin with single application of moisturizer

Author (year)	No. of patients	Females	Age range (years)	Skin disease; instructions before experiment	Variables measured	Materials tested	Application location	Amount applied	Size of area	Treated versus untreated sites compared?	Contralateral side used?	Baseline taken?	Measurement frequency and duration
Serban (1983)[52]	27	n.s.	21–57 (mean 40.5)	Healthy, 20 had dry skin; 7 no c/o dryness	Skin capacitance	Anhydrous petroleum	Inner forearm	5 µl	3.8 cm²	No	No	Yes (1 h before)	At 10 min; two subjects measured at short intervals up to 10 min
Batt (1988)[46]	5	n.s.	18–35	Healthy	Impedance	15% glycerol, double-blind	Inner forearm	0.05 ml per 20 cm²		No	Yes	Yes	0, 2.5, 10, 15, 20, 25, 30, 40, 50, 60, 90, 120 min
Blichmann (1988)[41]	10	7	30–47	No comment on skin dx; no moisturizers allowed for 12 h, no hand washing for 1 h	Skicon (conductance); Corneometer (capacitance); TEWL	Distilled water	Flexor; forearm; palm of hand	0.75 ml	2 cm	No	No	Yes	At zero and each min up to 10 min, 60 min
Blichmann (1989)[27]	12	12	45–66	Healthy, hx unknown	TEWL; conductance capacitance; surface lipids; skin surface temperature	Decubal (O/W emulsion)	Flexor; forearm	0.4 ml	6 cm × 18 cm	Yes	Contralateral arm served as control only	Yes, on both arms	3–5, 15, 30, 60, 120, 240 and 360 min
Stender (1989)[50]	8	n.s.	25–40	Healthy; no skin care products during or before study	TEWL; conductance with Skicon; capacitance at 0.1 mm (Corneometer) and Sebumeter	Bath oil (Triton X-45 25 g; paraffin 225 g, purified water 1000 g)	Flexor; forearm skin; full body	5 ml bath oil in 10 l water gives 0.011% emulsified paraffin oil	Full body	Tap-water-only bath first day; bath-oil bath second day	No	Yes on both control and treatment groups	At 0, 5, 10, 15, 20 and 30 min
Loden (1990)[47]	12	12	19–54 (mean 39)	Normal skin; tx with diethyl ether before	Corneometer	Petroleum; glycerol; PCA(glycerol); urea	Volar forearm	20 µl creams; 10 µl petroleum	4 areas (4 cm²)	Yes	Yes, random allocation to sites	Yes	2 h, 6 h
Serup (1992)[35]	26	18	21–58 (mean 36.3)	1 patient with mild psoriasis, 7 with dry skin using moisturizer regularly, 11 using intermittent moisturizers, 7 with normal skin	Conductance; capacitance; scaling with D-squame; lipids	HTH lotion with 10% urea and 5% lactic acid; HTH lotion with 3% urea and 1.5% lactic acid; base HTH with 0% urea and 0% lactic acid; and 4 other moisturizers, which were ranked only	Flexor; forearm	50 µl	25 mm × 45 mm areas, which were covered by medical gauze	Untreated control area, randomized to sites	No	Yes	3 h

Table 23.7 Summary of studies on normal skin with single application of moisturizer (continued)

Author (year)	No. of patients	Females	Age range (years)	Skin disease; instructions before experiment	Variables measured	Materials tested	Application location	Amount applied	Size of area	Treated versus untreated sites compared	Contralateral side used?	Baseline taken?	Measurement frequency and duration
Martinsen (1995)[44]	8	4	26 (±4)	No moisturizers in 48 h; healthy, not otherwise specified	Corneometer; conductance; susceptance; admittance	Distilled water; liposome with 10% phospholipid; O/W emulsion (Spenol)	n.s.	0.1 ml	2.5 cm-diameter circle	Yes, measured untreated site in parallel each min	No	Yes	O/W emulsion 0, 10, 30, 60, 240, 360 min; water and liposome each min for 10 min
Tagami (1980)[49]	7	0	24–39 (mean 30.7)	Healthy volunteers	V, (output voltage of loss resistance detector equal to the reciprocal relation to resistance)	10% urea cream (Urepearl); hydrophilic ointment; petrolatum	Extensor; lower leg	0.02 ml	4 cm²	No	n.s.	Yes	0, 10, 20 and 30 min
Clar (1975)[53]	6	n.s.	n.s.	Healthy, otherwise unspecified; wiped with saline 15 min before measurements	Impedance; distribution parameter; dielectric decrement	10% sodium lactate; liquid paraffin; 2% PCNa in aqueous solution; 2% PCNa in cosmetic prep; 10% PCNa in aqueous solution; base W/O PCNa	Distal forearm	n.s.	n.s.	Yes, randomized application to 5 sites including untreated site	Yes, randomized	Yes	For PCNa 10 min after treatment, 5 min after removal of moisturizer; for sodium lactate and paraffin, tx for 30 min, substance removed, measurements taken
Sasai (1996)[45]	16	n.s.	n.s.	Healthy	Conductance (Skicon) with different probes; capacitance with Corneometer	Water	Whole body, except for scalp, face, hands and feet	Drop of water, on skin for 10 s	n.s.	No	n.s.	Yes	After drop on skin for 10 s, measurements at 0, 30, 60, 90 and 120 s

n.s., not specified.

reasons, we consider the indirect electrical data for each substance separately in the sections that follow.

Water

Many authors have observed that normal skin shows a sudden jump in conductance, admittance and susceptance within seconds after hydration with a water droplet. In the next 30 seconds to 1 minute, there are rapid decreases in conductance, admittance and susceptance to nearly 50% of peak values. During the next minute (2–3 minutes after the water droplet) there is a more gradual return to prehydration levels,[23,43] or to values slightly increased above baseline.[44] Tagami[43] calls this test the sorption–desorption test.

In another study by Blichmann[41] comparing the Skicon and Corneometer, the same time course was observed for capacitance and conductance of normal skin. The Skicon was more sensitive to increases in hydration, presumably because its depth of penetration is very shallow and therefore it is more sensitive to fluctuations in water diffusion. On the other hand, a study of reproducibility showed that the Corneometer is more accurate and is able to measure to a depth of 0.1 mm, the full thickness of the SC in most regions.

Sasai[45] performed a water sorption–desorption test on 16 patients with normal skin to compare (i) a Skicon-200 equipped with a specially designed MT-8C probe (the skin attachment portion is studded with 8 needle-like electrodes) and (ii) a standard flat-surfaced probe. He found that the MT-8C probe recorded statistically significantly higher conductance values compared with the standard probe at baseline and at 30, 60, 90 and 120 seconds. The standard probe, however, had higher conductance values at time zero (10 seconds after water absorption). The MT-8C probe was also noted to have less reproducible results. Though the author concluded that these results show that the MT-8C probe was more sensitive, we are not convinced by the data presented, particularly since no specific mention of controls is given. In fact, these data appear to show the converse: the standard probe is more sensitive, since it records higher conductance values than the MT-SC probe when the skin is maximally hydrated at time zero. If anything, the MT-8C probe appears to be more sensitive to random variation and prone to more errors.

Glycerol (glycerine)

Serban found that glycerol had a higher capacitance than the other substances studied, namely 10% urea and 2% sodium PCA.[28] He also found that the conductance increased with increasing concentrations from 0% to 1.5% to 3.0% to 3.2%, but above 7% (i.e. 10% and 15%) there was little further increase in conductance.[28] Impedance increased for glycerol-containing products for at least 2 hours after application, compared with 10 minutes for pure water and 15 minutes for non-glycerol-containing emulsions.[46]

Loden notes that skin treated with glycerol cream had significantly increased (about 40% relative) capacitance at 2 hours. Capacitance decreased but remained significantly above baseline at 6 hours.[47]

Loden also found that skin treated with glycerol/PCA cream had decreased capacitance when compared with a glycerol-only cream, but the glycerol concentrations used in this study are not stated.[47] Capacitance values remained increased compared with baseline at 2 and 6 hours. However, at 6 hours, capacitance was decreased when compared with the 2-hour values.[47]

Loden reports that washing off pure glycerol or combined glycerol/PCA after 2 hours led to a prompt and significant decrease in capacitance. For pure glycerol, the washed site still had significantly increased capacitance at 6 hours, but the glycerol/PCA was not increased above baseline.[47]

Serban warns, however, that glycerol has some properties that limit its usefulness. For example, under low relative humidity (20%), it loses water, it increases TEWL and therefore could act as a vehicle for water loss at low humidity. In addition, it forms no bond with skin, so it can be easily washed away.[28]

Urea

Serban reports that capacitance for urea demonstrates a biphasic behavior. During the first 2–3 hours, capacitance was decreased. After about 3 hours, it steadily increased.[28] Tagami showed that with urea, capacitance peaked immediately, had a phase of rapid decrease like water and then returned gradually to former levels.[48] Specifically, during the first 30 minutes, V_r (the output voltage of the loss resistance detector, which is a reciprocal relation of resistance) for a 10% urea cream was statistically significantly ($p < 0.01$) increased compared with a hydrophilic cream of unknown composition and petrolatum. At 30 minutes, V_r was still statistically significantly increased ($p < 0.05$). Loden showed a 40% relative increase in capacitance at 2 hours, which decreased, but remained increased over controls, for 6 hours.[47]

In one study by Serup,[35] HTH cream, a cream originally designed by Swanbeck and used for the treatment of ichthyosis and atopic dermatitis, was modified to contain different levels of urea combined with lactic acid. Capacitance and conductance were measured at 3 hours. Vehicle alone (0% urea and 0% lactic acid) versus untreated skin had statistically significant ($p < 0.01$) increased conductance and capacitance. Lotion with 3% urea and 1.5% lactic acid had statistically significantly ($p < 0.01$) increased conductance and capacitance when compared with the vehicle alone. Lotion with 10% urea and 5% lactic acid had statistically significantly increased conductance when compared with 3% urea and 1.5% lactic acid, but no significant difference in capacitance.

Loden found that washing off the unabsorbed parts of a urea cream after 2 hours led to a prompt and significant decrease in capacitance.[47] However, the washed site still had sig-

nificantly increased capacitance above controls for at least 6 hours.[47]

Sodium lactate

Clar found that skin treated with an unquantified amount of sodium lactate for 10 minutes and then rinsed off showed a decrease in alpha-relaxation time and impedance (Z) and a random fluctuation in the dielectric decrement and distribution parameter.

PCNa

Clar[53] studied the following concentrations of the sodium salt of 5-pyrrolidone-2-carboxylic acid (PCNa) in different vehicles: 2% PCNa in aqueous solution, 10% PCNa in aqueous solution, 2% PCNa in a 'cosmetic prep', and cosmetic prep without PCNa, and compared them to an untreated control site. All treatments were randomized to areas of the forearm bilaterally. The actual amounts applied for 10 minutes were not stated. It was found that 5 minutes after the removal of the creams, impedance was decreased on all sites treated with PCNa but not for the controls (cosmetic prep alone or untreated site). The 2% cosmetic prep showed the greatest decrease in impedance (-113 kohm $\pm$ 67 SD), followed by the 10% aqueous prep (-90 kohm $\pm$ 68 SD) and then the 2% aqueous prep (-0.5 kohm $\pm$ 18 SD).

O/W emulsions

Tagami showed that a hydrophilic ointment had a capacitance curve like that for water alone but capacitance values were lower.[48]

Blichmann[37] observed that conductance showed a peak after application analogous to the evaporation curve. The evaporation curve for the O/W emulsion was equal to the control side at 15 minutes, while the conductance leveled off but remained significantly increased in comparison with the contralateral control throughout the 360-minute experiment. Capacitance was significantly increased during the entire 360 minutes, with values holding at a plateau. This showed that conductance was more sensitive to the fluctuations in evaporation phase than capacitance. Both convergance and capacitance were able to distinguish skin in the evaporation phase versus controls.

Martinsen found that after application of Spenol, an O/W emulsion, there was a peak in conductance, admittance and susceptance, which decreased rapidly in the first 10 minutes to a stable level significantly above baseline by 30 minutes.[44]

Liposomes

Martinsen reports that liposomes with 10% phospholipid showed the same conductance, susceptance and admittance behavior as water.[44]

Petrolatum

Tagami reports a lowering of skin impedance after treatment with petrolatum.[48] Initially there was no increase in the capacitance, but gradually there was a slow increase over time.[48,49] Martinsen showed a statistically significant increase in capacitance of about 25% over controls at 2 hours after treatment.[44] By 6 hours, however, there was no difference in capacitance between controls and treated groups.[44]

Martinsen also found that if petrolatum was wiped off at 2 hours, there was no significant change in capacitance.[44]

Liquid paraffin

Clar[53] applied liquid paraffin for 30 minutes, then rinsed it off with water and took measurements at an unspecified time point. She found an increase in impedance Z but a decrease in the dielectric constant and relaxation time and random fluctuations of the distribution parameter. She concluded that the decrease in the dielectric constant showed that paraffin was a highly resistive substance that caused an increase in impedance. Despite the misleading nature of the impedance, the actual effect of paraffin was concluded to be moisturization due to the decrease in the relaxation time.

Stender found no significant difference between capacitance or conductance measurements between arms treated with 0.011% bath oil for 1 second, those treated with immersion in bath-oil water for 5 minutes and 20 minutes, and those treated with tap water (control).[50] For all conditions, the same curve was followed: there was an initial increase in capacitance or conduction after contact with water, followed by a sharp fall in conductance to normal values within 5 minutes.[50]

Summary of studies with single application of moisturizer to normal skin

In summary, there have been few studies using capacitance, conductance, or impedance to assess the efficacy of one application of a moisturizer to normal human skin in vivo. Glycerol, urea and petrolatum are the best studied substances. Lactic acid (sodium lactate), PCNa and paraffin have been less well studied. When substances have been combined, most of these studies have not attempted to separate the effects of each of the components. A well-controlled and detailed time course has not been studied for PCNa, sodium lactate or paraffin.

One application of urea, glycerol or petrolatum is capable of increasing SC hydration for at least several hours: urea for at least 6 hours even if washed off, glycerol for at least 6 hours even if wiped off, and petrolatum for at least 2 hours (but not if it is wiped off).

Studies show conflicting data on whether capacitance is increased or decreased during the first 3 hours after treatment with urea. After 3 hours, there is consensus that conductance/capacitance is increased.

O/W emulsions have an evaporation phase lasting for about 15 minutes, in which there is a peak in the conductance/or capacitance followed by a longer-term plateau of increased capacitance/conductance, which can last for up to 6 hours.

Table 23.8 Problems with studies

Category of problem	Issue	Implications
Materials and methods		
Patient selection	Volunteers	May not be representative of consumer population.
	Histories not clearly stated, age/sex not always stated	Population in unknown; biased population; clinical extrapolation is difficult
Study size	Tends to be small	May not be enough subjects to satisfy study objective
Controls	Often inadequate	Cannot account for changes during experiment
	Most studies only measured on one side, rather than contralateral side	Need to control for variation between different sides of body
	Often not stated whether or not other moisturizer/beauty products were used	Effects may be due to other moisturizers
	Complex mixtures studied, not broken down into parts so that they could be compared and evaluated	Unable to separate effects
	Often studies not blinded, no placebo group	Potential for bias
Materials studied	Materials used or concentrations not always stated	Cannot compare studies easily; moisturizer effects are presumably dose-responsive
	Range of concentration often was not studied	No information on dose-response
Measurements	Not enough time points	Gaps in information about time course
	Often did not assess both TEWL and SC at same time	Cannot make conclusions about hydration state
	Three-prong approach often not used: panelist self-appraisal, expert grader evaluation and relevant instrumental measures[51]	Risk obtaining clinically irrelevant data; risk lack of objectivity
Statistics	Statistics not always used to analyze data	Comparisons have no scientific basis
	If statistics used, p values not always stated	No knowledge of level of significance
General	Not enough studies	No verification of findings
	Few materials studied	Large amount of materials have unknown efficacy
Bioengineering methods		
Manufacturer-dependent	Monofrequency machines used rather than multifrequency approaches	Monofrequency methods more prone to confounding variables, false-negatives and false-positives
Operator-dependent	Potentially improper use of machines	Misleading data
	Some studies have no statement of ambient conditions	Misleading data
Information access	Journals/books not easily accessible; not all sources in Medline; information published in obscure locations or not at all	Missing data
	Conflicts of interest not stated	Unable to quantify sources of bias and therefore control for them
	Proprietary information	Missing data

Pure petrolatum, in contrast, has no water and therefore no evaporation phase, and thus capacitance builds up gradually over time, presumably due to petrolatum's occlusive properties. Its hydrating action also did not last for the full 6 hours, because a single application was absorbed or otherwise reduced and presumably unable to occlude sufficiently.

Paraffin, and presumably any other dielectric substances, can give confusing results if only impedance measurements are relied upon.

Bath oils or liposomes with 10% phospholipids were not as effective as single applications of moisturizer, and showed no statistically significant difference from control treatment with water.

Cosmetic preparations necessitated lower concentrations of PCNa than aqueous solutions in order to achieve a similar decrease in impedance. In other words, the vehicle used is a very important consideration. This observation points to the need to control for the vehicle type (aqueous versus cream) as well as ingredients.

CONCLUSIONS

From this review, it is apparent that the quest to obtain reliable, useful information on the efficacy of moisturizers encounters three main categories of difficulties: problems with the experiments, problems with the measurement technologies, and problems with the availability/accessibility of information. Table 23.8 lists the specific issues in each of these categories, and the implications that these problems could have on the interpretation and validity of the information.

Pressure for improvement emanates from numerous sources: new laws,[16] the courts[33] and the consumer. Future research in this field needs to focus on

1. performing scientifically rigorous studies on a wider range of materials;
2. demanding, developing and using the most relevant/technologically sound bioengineering techniques;
3. obtaining a better understanding of the pathophysiology of dry skin;
4. developing moisturizers that can target and correct specific deficits in the skin without compromising homeostasis.

REFERENCES

1. Borroni G, Zaccone C, Vignati G et al, Dynamic measurements. In: *Bioengineering of the Skin: Water and the Stratum Corneum* (Elsner P, Berardesca E, Maibach HI, eds). Boca Raton, FL: CRC Press, 1994: 217–22.

2. Kligman AM, Grove GL, Studemayer TJ, Some aspects of dry skin and its treatment. In: *Safety and Efficacy of Topical Drugs and Cosmetics* (Kligman AM, Leyden JJ, eds). New York: Grune and Stratton, 1982: 221–38.

3. Black D, Diridollou S, Lagarde JM, Gall Y, Skin care products for normal, dry and greasy skin. In: *Cosmetic Dermatology*, 2nd edn (Baran R, Maibach HI, eds). London: Martin Dunitz, 1998: 125–50.

4. Gabard B, Testing the efficacy of moisturizers. In: *Bioengineering of the Skin: Water and the Stratum Corneum* (Elsner P, Berardesca E, Maibach HI, eds). Boca Raton, FL: CRC Press, 1994: 147–70.

5. Idson B, Moisturizers, emollients and bath oils. In: *Principles of Cosmetics for the Dermatologist* (Frost P, Horwitz SN, eds). St Louis, MO: CV Mosby, 1982: 37–40.

6. Van Scott EJ, Yu RJ, Substances that modify the stratum corneum by modulating its function. In: *Principles of Cosmetics for the Dermatologist* (Frost P, Horwitz SN, eds). St Louis, MO: CV Mosby, 1982: 70–4.

7. Charlet E, *Kosmetik fuer Apotheker*. Stuttgart: Wissenschaftliche Verlagsgesellschaft, 1989: 77.

8. Ummenhofer B, Hautschutz durch Dermatika. In: *Externa Therapie von Hautkrankheiten: Pharmazeutisches and Medizinische Praxis* (Hornstein OP, Nurnberg E, eds). Stuttgart: George Thieme Verlag, 1985: Chap 15.

9. Wilkinson JB, Moore RJ, *Harry's Cosmetology*, 7th edn. New York: Chemical Publishing, 1982: 62.

10. Wehr RF, Krochmal L, Considerations in selecting a moisturizer. *Cutis* 1987; **39:** 512.

11. Idson B, Dry skin: moisturizing and emolliency. *Cosmetics and Toiletries* 1992; **107:** 69.

12. Lazar AP, Lazar P, Dry skin, water and lubrication. Cosmetic and cosmetic surgery in dermatology. *Dermatol Clin* 1991; **9**(1): 45–50.

13. Potts RO, Stratum corneum hydration. Experimental techniques and interpretation of results. *J Soc Cosmet Chem* 1996; **37:** 9–33.

14. Pinnagoda J, Hardware and measuring principles: evaporimeter. In: *Bioengineering of the Skin: Water and the Stratum Corneum* (Elsner P, Berardesca E, Maibach HI, eds). Boca Raton, FL: CRC Press, 1994: 51–8.

15. Warner RR and Lilly NA, Correlation of water content with ultrastructure in the stratum corneum. In: *Bioengineering of the Skin: Water and the Stratum Corneum* (Elsner P, Berardesca E, Maibach HI, eds). Boca Raton, FL: CRC Press, 1994: 3–12.

16. Stab F, Sauermann G, Hoppe U, Evaluation of moisturizers. In: *Bioengineering of the Skin: Skin Surface Imaging and Analysis* (Wilhelm KP, Berardesca E, Maibach HI, eds). Boca Raton, FL: CRC Press, 1997: 315–30.

17. Lévêque J, Water–keratin interactions. In: *Bioengineering of the Skin: Water and the Stratum Corneum* (Elsner P, Berardesca E, Maibach HI, eds). Boca Raton, FL: CRC Press, 1994: 13–22.

18. Tagami H, Hardware and measuring principles: skin conductance. In: *Bioengineering of the Skin: Water and the Stratum Corneum* (Elsner P, Berardesca E, Maibach HI, eds). Boca Raton, FL: CRC Press, 1994: 197–204

19. Rougier A, TEWL and transcutaneous absorption. In: *Bioengineering of the Skin: Water and the Stratum Corneum* (Elsner P, Berardesca E, Maibach HI, eds). Boca Raton, FL: CRC Press, 1994: 103–14.

20. Loden M, Biophysical properties of dry atopic and normal skin with special reference to effects of skin care products. *Acta Derm Venereol (Stockh)* 1995; **192**(Suppl): 1–48.

21. Wilson D, Berardesca E, Maibach HI, In vivo transepidermal water loss and skin surface hydration in assessment of moisturization and soap effects. *Int J Cosmet Sci* 1988; **10:** 201–11.

22. Berardesca E, Maibach HI, Relationship between SC hydration and TEWL in health and disease. *Dermatosen* 1990; **38:** 50–3.

23. Loden M, Lindberg L, Product testing – testing of moisturizers. In: *Bioengineering of the Skin: Water and the Stratum Corneum* (Elsner P, Berardesca E, Maibach HI, eds). Boca Raton, FL: CRC Press, 1994: 275–88.

24. Ryatt KS, Mobayen M, Stevenson JM et al, Methodology to measure the transient effect of occlusion on skin penetration and stratum corneum hydration in vivo. *Br J Dermatol* 1988; **119:** 307–12.

25. O'Donoghue MN, Cosmetics for the physician. In: *Manual of Skin Diseases*, 7th edn (Sauer GC, Hall JC, eds). New York: Lippincott–Raven, 1996.

26. Swanbeck G, Carbamide and other active substances in moisturizers. In: Abstract of paper presented at the Regional Symposium on Rationales behind Moisturizers in Dermatology, Copenhagen, Denmark, June 1989. *Bioeng Skin* 1988: **4:** 383.

27. Marks R, Methods to evaluate the effects of skin surface modifiers. In: *Principles of Cosmetics for the Dermatologist* (Frost P, Horwitz SN, eds). St Louis, MO: CV Mosby, 1982: 50–8.

28. Serban GP, Henry SM, Cotty VF, Marcus AD, In vivo evaluation of skin lotions by electrical capacitance: II. Evaluation of moisturized skin using an improved dry electrode. *J Soc Cosmet Chem* 1981; **32:** 421–35.

29. Barel AO, Clarys P, Comparison of methods for the measurement of transepidermal water loss. In: *Handbook of Non-Invasive Methods and the Skin* (Serup J, Jemec GBE, eds). Boca Raton, FL: CRC Press, 1995: 179–95.

30. Pinnagoda J, Tupker RA, Agner T, Serup J, Guidelines for transepidermal water loss measurement: a report from the standardization group of the European Society of Contact Dermatitis. *Contact Dermatitis* 1990; **22:** 164–78.

31. Pinnagoda J, Standardization of measurements. In: *Bioengineering of the Skin: Water and the Stratum Corneum* (Elsner P, Berardesca E, Maibach HI, eds). Boca Raton, FL: CRC Press, 1994: 59–64.

32. Masuda Y, Nishikawa M, Ichijo B, New methods of measuring capacitance and resistance of very high loss materials at high frequencies. *IEEE Trans Instrum Meas* 1980; **IM-29:** 28–36.

33. Salter DC, Further hardware and measuring approaches for studying water in the stratum corneum. In: *Bioengineering of the Skin: Water and*

the Stratum Corneum (Elsner P, Berardesca E, Maibach HI, eds). Boca Raton, FL: CRC Press, 1994: 205–16.

34. Van Neste D, Comparative study of normal and rough human skin hydration in vivo. *J Dermatol Sci* 1991; **2**: 119–24.

35. Serup J, A three-hour test for rapid comparison of the effects of moisturizers and active constituents (urea). *Acta Derm Venereol (Stockh)* 1992; **117**(Suppl): 29–33.

36. Barel AO, Clarys P, Measurement of epidermal capacitance. In: *Handbook of Non-Invasive Methods and the Skin* (Serup J, Jemec GBE, eds). Boca Raton, FL: CRC Press, 1995: 165–72.

37. Blichmann CW, Serup J, Winther A, Effects of single application of a moisturizer: evaporation of emulsion water, skin surface temperature, electrical conductance, electrical capacitance and skin surface (emulsion) lipids. *Acta Derm Venereol* 1989; **69**: 327–33.

38. Loden M, The increase in skin hydration after application of emollients with different amounts of lipids. *Acta Derm Venereol* 1992; **72**: 327–30.

39. Vincent CM, Fiquet E, Cohen-Letessier A, Marty JP, Evaluation des proprietes hydratantes de la creme hydrophile lipophile (Effadiane). *Nouvelle Dermatol* 1992; **11**: 419.

40. Marty JP, Vincent CM, Fiquet E, Etude des proprietes hydratantes de la creme hydratantes visage Neutrogena. *Realities Ther Derm Venerol* 1992; **15**: 1.

41. Blichmann CW, Serup J, Assessment of skin moisture: measurement of electrical conductance, capacitance and transepidermal water loss. *Acta Derm Venereol* 1988; **68**: 284–90.

42. Rietschel RL, A method to evaluate skin moisturizers in vivo. *J Invest Dermatol* 1978; **70**: 152–5.

43. Tagami H, Kanamaru Y, Inoue K et al, Water sorption–desorption test of the skin in vivo for functional assessment of the stratum corneum. *J Invest Dermatol* 1982; **78**: 425–8.

44. Martinsen OG, Grimnes S, Karlsen J, Electrical methods for skin moisture assessment. *Skin Pharmacol* 1995; **8**: 237–45.

45. Sasai S, Zhen YX, Tagami H, High frequency conductance measurement of the skin surface hydration state of dry skin using a new probe studded with needle-form electrodes (MT-8C). *Skin Res Technol* 1996; **2**: 173–6.

46. Batt MD, Davis WB, Fairhurst E et al, Changes in the physical properties of stratum corneum following treatment with glycerol. *J Soc Cosmet Chem* 1988; **39**: 367–81.

47. Loden M, Lindberg M, The influence of a single application of different moisturizers on the skin capacitance. *Acta Derm Venereol* 1991; **71**: 79–82.

48. Tagami H, Electrical measurements of the water content of the skin surface. Functional analysis of the hydroscopic property and water-holding capacity of the stratum corneum in vivo and technique for assessing moisturizer efficacy. *Cosmetics and Toiletries* 1982; **97**: 39.

49. Tagami H, Masatoshi O, Iwatsuki K et al, Evaluation of the skin surface hydration in vivo by electrical measurement. *J Invest Dermatol* 1980; **75**: 500–7.

50. Stender IM, Blichmann C, Serup J, Effects of oil and water baths on the hydration state of the epidermis. *Clin Exp Dermatol* 1990; **15**: 206–9.

51. Grove GL, Noninvasive methods for assessing moisturizers. In: *Clinical Safety and Efficacy Testing of Cosmetics* (Waggoner C, ed). New York, NY: Marcel Dekker, 1990: 121–48.

52. Serban GP, Henry SM, Cotty VF et al, Electrometric techinque for the in vivo assessment of skin dryness and the effect of chronic treatment with a lotion on the water barrier function of dry skin. *J Soc Cosmet Chem* 1983; **34**: 383–93.

53. Clar EJ, Her CP, Sturelle CG, Skin impedence and moisturization. *J Soc Cosmet Chem* 1975; **26**: 337–53.

APPENDIX: BIOENGINEERING TECHNIQUES FOR ASSESSING MOISTURIZER EFFICACY

References for the Appendix are listed at the end of the tables.

1. Bioengineering techniques for skin surface contour evaluation
2. Bioengineering techniques to measure desquamation
3. Mechanical bioengineering techniques to measure elasticity
4. Mechanical bioengineering techniques measuring elasticity (acting perpendicular to plane of skin surface)
5. Other mechanical bioengineering techniques
6. Indirect electrical bioengineering techniques
7. Direct electrical bioengineering techniques
8. Bioengineering techniques to measure transepidermal water loss (TEWL)
9. Bioengineering techniques to image stratum corneum
10. Optical techniques to characterize skin properties

1. Bioengineering techniques for skin surface contour evaluation. Topography measurements can be used to demonstrate changes in amount of wrinkling and state of SC hydration as noted by attenuation of the relief due to increase in turgor

Technique	Developer/ machines	Parameters measured/ calculated	Principles	Advantages	Disadvantages
Low-power surface magnification[1]	8× lens magnifier	Skin surface contour	Place mineral oil on skin; cover with coverslip; observe skin under low power	Can visualize epidermis, epidermal–dermal junction and papillary dermis. Easy, non-invasive method. Augments naked-eye observation skills	Technique has learning curve. Hard to visualize dry, scaly skin with this technique
Profilometry of skin surface (replicas with mechanical scanning)	Perth-o-Meter (1971),[2] Surfometer (1975),[3] Surfcom (1979),[4] Talysurf (1979),[5] Anaglyphographe (1982)[6]	Skin surface contour; roughness parameters	Cast replica of skin in silicone rubber is measured with a computerized stylus instrument, which produces plots of data. Valley and peak profile of SC flattens with hydration	Replica measurements give absolute data. Can evaluate hydration status	Complex and slow process. The application of silicone rubber may disrupt the surface; fine lines may be effaced when rubber cools; scales may be removed from subject. Needs a smooth even surface (too many hair follicles, scars, tattoos, detergents, skin damage or scaling can increase error). Stylus geometry can introduce errors.[7] Sources of inter-observer variability are high-pass filters, low-pass filters and sampling intervals.[7] Expensive.[8] Profilometry can identify products that decrease amount of wrinkles but does not reveal mechanisms or safety of these products (irritants, for example, decrease wrinkling). Results in 2D only; show topography in one direction only
Profilometry of skin surface (replicas with optical scanning)	Corcuff (1981)[9]	Skin surface contour; roughness parameters; wrinkle quantification	Cast replica of skin in silicone rubber is measured with an optical scanner (laser beam)	Gives absolute data; operating time reduced over mechanical method; non-contact sensor; 3D data possible	Complex and slow process. The application of silicone rubber may disrupt the surface. Needs a smooth, even surface (too many hair follicles, scars, detergents, skin damage or scaling can increase error). Availability is limited due to sophistication

(Contd)

1. Bioengineering techniques for skin surface contour evaluation (continued). Topography measurements can be used to demonstrate changes in amount of wrinkling and state of SC hydration as noted by attenuation of the relief due to increase in turgor

Technique	Developer/ machines	Parameters measured/ calculated	Principles	Advantages	Disadvantages
Photographic densitometry with laser profilometry	Barton (1989);[10] Gormley (1985)[11]	Contour; roughness parameters; wrinkle quantification	Photographic negative of skin taken under standard light (oblique illumination with incident angle of 25°). Shadows formed are scanned microdensitometrically by a computer and gray level assigned. The relief is reconstructed indirectly from gray level and, using appropriate algorithms, slopes and roughness parameters of relief can be calculated	Rapid measurement of skin surface relief without cumbersome equipment.[12] Good for following clinical progression of scaling disorders	Only provides a reconstruction and not an exact image, so smaller features may be overshadowed by larger ones and omitted from analysis.[12] Less sensitive in screening normal volunteers
In vivo image analysis (digital image processing)	Picton (1976);[13] Taylor (1978)[14]	Quantimet;[13] Magiscan[14]	Using video camera, can record skin surface features directly. Signal is digitized using a high-speed analog/digital converter and arranged into an array of picture points. The picture points are introduced into a digital image processor that interfaces with a minicomputer. Filters (mathematical sieves) can be used to enhance detail	More objective, quantifiable images (shape, color), than clinic notes. Interactive; can be queried, altered, analyzed automatically and rapidly in real time. Permanent record; data easily stored. In vivo, direct measurement of surface possible. Good for evaluation of low to moderate dryness	Inconvenient. Technique less useful for very dry skin

2. Bioengineering techniques to measure desquamation[15]

Technique	References	Principles	Advantages	Disadvantages
Squametry of tape strippings	Wolf (1936),[16] Jenkins (1969)[17]	Tape pressed against skin; outermost portion of skin sticks to tape and keeps topographical relationship and desquamation pattern. Tapes are processed. Scales are sized and counted. Samples stained and viewed with microscope	Simple, non-invasive, painless, more reproducible, objective and consistent than traditional grading systems	Need to assure clean conditions. Tapes not necessarily well characterized in terms of component properties. Need to precut tape under clean conditions
Adhesive disc squametry combined with Chromameter (Minolta) and image analysis	D-Square (CuDerm Co, Dallas, TX)	Small transparent adhesive discs are pressed against skin. Corneocytes stained and viewed under microscope, and intensity of stain measured with a chromameter. Quantitative xerosis (based on stain intensity). Image analysis reveals number, thickness and size of squames	Simple, non-invasive, painless. Allows quantitative assessments of xerosis. Eliminates many of difficulties involved with tape and sticky slides because it is specially formulated and readily available. 3 standard sizes. Easy storage and use	Small disc size more prone to sampling error. May need to delipidize skin to remove scales more effectively. Image analysis is expensive/technical luxury[18]
Sticky slide[15]	Goldschmidt (1967), Dermatology Lab and Supply Co	Prepare slide by coating with adhesive solution and allow organic solid to evaporate. Press on skin, leave on skin for a few seconds, remove and process	More reproducible, objective and consistent than traditional clinical grading systems. Quantification/standardization of desquamation possible. More quantitative than skin scraping because fixed area is sampled and loss of material to air currents is more controlled	Prepared slides have limited life due to gradual air oxidation of adhesive surface. Need skill and practice to perform. Need careful storage and handling to prevent contamination
Skin surface biopsy with microscopy	Marks (1971)[19]	Cyanoacrylate glue is spread on a flexible plastic slide and applied firmly to skin for 30 s. 3–5 layers of corneocytes are detached, stained, viewed under microscope, and classified into one of 5 xerosis classifications	Simple, non-invasive, painless. Removes more stratum corneum than pressure-sensitive adhesives	More difficult to standardize. Skill involved

3. Mechanical bioengineering techniques to measure elasticity

Technique	Parameters measured/ calculated	Machines available/ developer	Principles	Advantages	Disadvantages
Extensometry	Material constants	Extensiometer (Thacker 1977)[20]	The arms of two strain gauges are stuck to the skin surface using adhesive tape. By means of a lead screw and carrier, a motor and gear combination moves one arm away from the other at a constant rate, stretching the skin between the tabs. The separation of tabs is measured with a linear variable differential transformer (LVDT) transducer, and the force developed in the skin is measured by strain gauges attached to the reduced sections of the arms. Recoil apparatus can be installed to measure extension–time characteristics of skin when deforming force is removed[21]	Can be hand-held. In vivo measurements possible	Strain gauges are stiff, and may impose frictional forces. Some systems are bulky and not convenient for clinical use
Gas-bearing electrodynamometer (GBE)	Dynamic spring rate (DSR) (analogous to Young's elastic modulus); loss angle (stiffness, softness and compliance)	Hargens (1977)	GBE measures displacement of skin in response to a rapidly oscillating force placed next to its surface. Dynamic stress–strain loop appears on oscilloscope, which can be analyzed. Application of moisturizer to the skin surface results in a decrease in the DSR and a concomitant increase in the loss angle	Good for quantifying stiffness in surface plane of skin, i.e. SC. High degree of correlation between elastic modulus measurements and visual assessments of skin by a trained grader. Sensitive enough to measure changes in SC induced by topically applied agents or mechanical disruption.[22] Can apply small forces. Measurement is direct rather than implied from inference, as is the case with electrical conductivity or sonic propagation	May measure dermal components as well. Changes perceived by trained subjects may not correspond to GBE measurements. Manual stretching of skin can change baseline. Thickness of SC, size and geometric arrangement of corneocytes, and chemical composition differences may influence measurements[22]

(Contd)

3. Mechanical bioengineering techniques to measure elasticity (continued)

Technique	Parameters measured/calculated	Machines available/developer	Principles	Advantages	Disadvantages
Torque meters (disproportional strain measurements)	Torque and phase angle-extensibility (resistance to stretch), viscoelastic properties	Vlasblom (1967);[23] Finlay (1970);[24] twistometre (Leveque, L'Oreal); Dermal torque meter (Dia-stron, Ltd, Andover, UK) Barbenel (1977)[25]	Disc attached to skin with adhesive. Weak, constant torque applied to rotating disc. Movement of disc monitored by rotational sensor. Fixed guard ring delineates area. When distance between disc and guard ring is less than 1 mm, extensibility reflects SC resistance to stretch. Microprocessor computes main parameters. Immediate rotation corresponds to immediate extensibility, followed by slow increase corresponding to 'creeping' or the viscous and plastic skin characteristics	Sensitive in both short- and long-term studies rating hydrating efficacy. Clear correlation between SC extensibility and severity of dryness. Measurements made parallel to skin surface, so effect of links between dermis and hypodermis are minimized. Can be used to describe mechanical changes in skin with aging, sun exposure, and scleroderma.[26] Weibull or extreme-value distribution is more accurate and sensitive than other torsion methods[24]	Standardization not yet complete.[24] Models such as EXP less accurate and sensitive than those based on Weibull distribution
Mechanical impedance	Point impedance	Franke (1950);[27] Von Gierke (1952);[28] Swept-frequency viscoelastometer[28]	Impedance head is mounted on an electromagnetic actuator or shaker, which is driven by a swept sinusoidal voltage. Corrected force and velocity signals are inputed into RMS circuits and then to a log-ratio amplifier to obtain output proportional to log mechanical impedance. Phase angle between force and velocity signals obtained via a phase meter. Phase angle and log-impedance used as vertical drive signals to a multichannel display multiplexor on an XY storage display oscilloscope. Horizontal drive obtained from frequency to voltage converter and log-amplifier. Thus real-time plots of log Z vs log of frequency can be obtained	Can study elastic tissues or viscous parameters in living soft tissue	Technical difficulties still need to be overcome

4. Mechanical bioengineering techniques measuring elasticity (acting perpendicular to plane of skin surface)[30]

Technique	Parameters measured/calculated	Machines available/developer	Principles	Advantages	Disadvantages
Suction chamber (disproportional superficial strain)	Stiffness (distensibility, resilient distensibility); hysteresis); elasticity (relative elastic retraction (RER))	Cutometer (SEM 474 (Courage and Khazaka)	A suction probe (suction chamber = 2 mm with larger optional probes of 4, 6, 8 mm) is applied vertically on the skin with a constant pressure. The amount of skin elevation is measured using an optical system, which measures the decrease in intensity of an infrared beam. The instrument interfaces with an IBM personal computer, and standard software provided allows the storage of data concerning important variables and graphical display of stress-vs-strain and strain-vs-time curves	More useful for cosmetological purposes, which aim to measure mechanical properties of epidermis and papillary dermis	Type of strain measured may be irrelevant to common practice. May still measure mechanical properties of the deeper layers of dermis and subcutis to an unknown extent
Suction chamber (proportional full-thickness strain)	Material constants (stiffness, resilience, distensibility); hysteresis; elasticity (relative elastic retraction (RER))	Grahame (1970),[31] Gniadecka, Serup (Dermaflex A, Denmark)	A suction probe (suction chamber = 10 mm) is placed directly on the skin. An electronic sensor in the probe measures the amount of skin elevation, by measuring the electric capacitance between the skin surface and the electrode placed in the top of the suction chamber. The data are collected and can be visualized. Skin distensibility and hysteresis increase slightly after epidermal moisturizing[32]	Larger probe is more useful for medical and dermatological applications, for example in scleroderma and chronically inflamed skin	Correlation of separate parameters of skin mechanical properties with structural elements of skin not fully elucidated. Must control for numerous biological and environmental variables.[33] Must avoid repeated measurements at same site for at least 1 hour
Levarometry, tonometry	Index of deformability; skin extensibility (skin slackness); biological elasticity	Dikstein (1979, levarometer),[34] Gartstein (1990),[35] Tonometry; Pierard (1980)[36]	The skin is attached (using Perspex disc and double adhesive tape (Dikstein), or cyanoacrylate (Pierard) or vacuum (Gartstein) with (Pierard) or without (Dikstein) a guard ring) to a counterbalanced measuring rod. Different weights can be applied, elevating the skin. For Dikstein's levarometer, the rod is attached to a linear variable differential transformer, and this output is recorded graphically	The method is sensitive and reproducible. Topical applications or environmental conditions probably do not affect measurements.[37] Highly discriminating between old and young skin and old female and old male skin	Not currently commercially available

(Contd)

4. Mechanical bioengineering techniques measuring elasticity (acting perpendicular to plane of skin surface)[30] (continued)

Technique	Parameters measured/ calculated	Machines available/ developer	Principles	Advantages	Disadvantages
Ballistometry[38]	Coefficient of restitution (amount of energy returned to the tissue)	Tosti (1977);[39] Ballistometer	Measurement of a drop impact of a body onto the skin	Non-invasive. Easy to use. No probes attached to skin. Instrument is cheaper than dynamometer. Good for measuring elastic parameters in deeper dermal structures. Can measure differences in elastic modulus between young and old, various body sites and changes after pharmaceutical treatment. Can obtain a lot of data fast	Cannot obtain data on status of stratum corneum, as one can from shear measurement. Gives only an indirect indication of underlying tissue changes
Indentometry[40]	Skin compressibility	Schade (1912) elastometer; Kirk (1949); Tregear (1965); Robertson (1969); Daly (1974); Pierard (1984); Dikstein (1981)	A circular piece of plastic material attached to a weighted metal rod is applied perpendicularly to the skin to indent the skin. The rod is counterbalanced so that the net pressure in the system is a given value. The measuring rod is loaded with specially constructed weights increasing the baseline pressure to the desired level.[34] The rod is attached to a linear variable differential transformer, and the output of the deformation curve can be plotted using various methods	Good for measuring water state of ground substance–elastin network in dermis; most useful in evaluating edematous skin conditions and altered water handling of the dermis	Not the best method to discriminate between old and young skin or female and male skin

5. Other mechanical bioengineering techniques

Technique	Parameters measured/calculated	Machines available/developer	Principles	Advantages	Disadvantages
Coefficient-of-friction devices	Coefficient of friction (oiliness/greasiness)	Rotating wheel (Teflon Newcastle friction meter); resolving ground glass disc; sliding sled, modified viscometer	Friction of human skin in vivo can be measured by determining how much force is required to drag object across skin surface; smoother or drier skin theoretically needs less force	Good for screening topicals for after-feel greasiness.[41] Some machines are portable. Measurements with Newcastle friction meter can correlate with sensory scores of smoothness	Interpretation of differences in frictional properties between products are very complex. Moisturizers can increase friction as a result of increased contact area. Lubricants make skin more slippery
Scratch-resistance test	Hardness		A stylus just visibly scratches skin; measure lowest pressure load	Can reveal underlying defects not seen at first glance	Somewhat invasive
Acoustic spectrometer[42]	Softness, hydration level; energy loss of viscous component of skin; elastic modulus	Tronnier (1952);[43] Potts (1985);[44] Torgalkar (1981)[42]	Vibration device in audible range gives small-amplitude oscillations normal to skin surface with second stylus as comparison. Spectrum analyzer can calculate time for shear waves to travel and degree of amplitude dampening; resonance frequency can be measured. The more SC hydration, the lower the resonance frequency. Energy loss can also be calculated	Can be used as predictive measure. Indirect measure of hydration state. Correlated with subjective assessments of moisturization	Thickness of horny layer, thickness and tension of the skin and nature of underlying tissues can be sources of error
Cohesography	Intracorneal cohesion measurements	Nicholls (1971); Marks (1977)[8]	After hydrating SC, there is a drop in intracorneal cohesion. Drop follows same magnitude as flattening in surface contour, and changes are of same order of magnitude[8]	Able to assess hydrating agents	Not generally commercially available[8]

6. Indirect electrical bioengineering techniques. (The general advantages of these techniques are that they provide easy to measure, continuous data on skin hydration status and are readily available commercially.)

Technique	Machine/developer	Principles	Advantages	Disadvantages
Low-frequency impedance (frequency domain)	Clar (1975)	Impedance drops with increasing hydration. Frequency-domain approaches examine the response of skin to sinusoidal stimulating frequencies	Low frequencies give most informative data about physiological condition of skin overall because charge carriers can travel more time before field reverses[24]	Need liquid junction. Electrodes are occlusive. Long time needed for data collection (>20 min). Agents other than water can lower impedance. Measurements are quantitative rather than qualitative
High-frequency impedance (3.5 MHz) (frequency domain)	Tregear (1965)[45]	Impedance drops with increasing hydration. Impedance decreased with increasing frequency. Higher frequency, more skin penetration	Provide information on deeper levels of skin; can use dry electrodes	Occludes site. Depth of SC not well defined. Agents other than water can affect readings. Pressure of probe and dermal irritants can influence readings. Cannot measure resistance and capacitance separately at high frequencies
Capacitance	Corneometer (Courage and Khazaka, Germany)	Capacitance increases with increasing hydration. The Corneometer uses variable frequencies in the low-frequency range (40–75 Hz); <75 dehydrated skin; 75–90 skin with tendency to dehydrate, >90 normal skin (arbitrary units)[12]	Easy to operate. Highly reproducible.[12,46] Short measuring time (1 s). Economical.[46] Useful for extremely dry scaly skin	Confined to measurement of variation in SC between initial and final states.[12] Poor sensitivity to hydration process taking place in SC of normal skin because optimal range of water content in the SC for the capacitance method is much lower than for high-frequency conductance methods

(Contd)

6. Indirect electrical bioengineering techniques (continued).

Technique	Machine/ developer	Principles	Advantages	Disadvantages
High-frequency microwave (GHz)	Wavetek 1005	Dielectric probe response (DPR)[47] – a percentage based on the probe's response to skin vs a drop of water. A signal swept several MHz around a GHz resonates in a cable. Charged grid contacts skin, water absorbs energy and produces a standing wave shift, detection of which is adjusted to be linearly proportional to hydration level	Detects quantitative differences. Rapid quantitation. Unaffected by topicals. SC probe depth varies. DPR basic unit is useful for comparisons	DPR is not a true hydration percentage
Conductance	Skicon 100, 200 (Masuda, IBS Co, Ltd)	Uses a fixed frequency (3.5 MHz) to measure conductance and capacitance separately	Dry electrodes can be used. Correlates well with water content of superficial and deep SC layers. Suitable to assess the hydration dynamics of the SC induced in the skin. Not affected by electrolyte-rich solutions[48]	Single-frequency approach subject to more error, confounding variables, decreased sensitivity and specificity (increased false-positives and false-negatives) when compared with multifrequency machines.[24] Current must propagate at least 5 mm to obtain reliable values
Impedance (capacitance calculated)	Nova DPM-9003 (Dermal Phase Meter)	Integrates selected measurements at varying frequencies of the applied alternating current. Capacitance is calculated from the signal phase delay using a proprietary chip. Final readout is in arbitrary units related to capacitance	Good for assessing highly hydrated skin due to low variability of readings.[46] Due to monofrequency approach, subject to less error, less confounding variables, and has increased sensitivity and specificity, (less false-positives and false-negatives) when compared with single-frequency machines, handling easy due to small dimensions and low weight	Less sensitive for grading the dry state than the Corneometer.[49] Agents other than water affect measurements

(Contd)

6. Indirect electrical bioengineering techniques (continued).

Technique	Machine/developer	Principles	Advantages	Disadvantages
Impedance (Surface characterizing)	Surface-characterizing impedance monitor (SCIM) (Servo-Med Sweden)	Impedance is dependent on tissue hydration, composition and condition. SCIM measures impedance magnitude and phase at 31 frequencies to 5 selectable depths	Uses the intrinsically more informative multifrequency approach, which is independent of changes in sweat-gland activity, skin temperature, confounding variables. Allows electrical impedance spectroscopy of selected layers	Same disadvantages as with many electrical methods. Must use probe correctly (perpendicular, with correct pressure); wait 5 s between repeating measurements on same site to avoid occlusion. Measurement failures with wet surface, dirt. Must perform measurements under appropriate ambient conditions (<22°C and >60% RH)

7. Direct electrical bioengineering techniques

Technique	Machine/ developer	Principles	Advantages	Disadvantages
Infrared spectroscopy	Infrared spectral photometer (Perkin/Elmer) with FMIR (frustrated multiple internal reflection assessory); Putnam (1972)[50] and Osberghaus (1978)[51]	FMIR accessory is added to sample compartment of the spectrophotometer. Flexor forearm is placed on horizontal germanium crystal so that SC has direct contact with surface of crystal. Ray is reflected in numerous directions on the surfaces between the crystal, air and the skin. The reduction in total inner-reflection and thus IR intensity is used to measure absorption	Gives information on molecular constitution of skin. Under certain conditions, exact quantitative relationship between IR absorption and water concentration in SC[44]	Topical agents may introduce error. Complicated and costly. IR has shallow penetration depth into SC
Photo-acoustic spectroscopy (PAS)	Rosencwaig (1977);[52] Campbell (1979); Simon (1981)	Skin is exposed to IR radiation (heat). Depth of penetration of a periodic heat wave into a solid depends on its frequency. Radiation is absorbed by water in the SC at that depth. The superposition of thermal waves causes periodic temperature/ pressure fluctuations at the surface of the skin, which can be detected as sound by a microphone in a closed photoacoustic cell. Signal produced depends on both optical and thermal properties of a sample	Can quantitatively measure in vivo, and no contact needed between probe and skin; Good for investigation of the horny layer.[53] One of the most depth-sensitive methods	Not readily available. More technical developments needed

(Contd)

7. Direct electrical bioengineering techniques (continued)

Technique	Machine/ developer	Principles	Advantages	Disadvantages
Magnetic resonance spectroscopy (MRS)	Foreman (1970s in vitro); Cuono (1988 in vitro); Klein (1988 in vitro); *Zemtsov* (1989 in vivo)	Same principles as MRI apply except that the magnetic resonance signal is used to construct a magnetic resonance spectroscopic spectrum. MRS spectra can be obtained from protons as well as ^{13}C or ^{31}P. ^{31}P provides information about intercellular pH, tissue turnover rate and tissue bioenergetics (ATP, Pi, phosphocreatine)	Gives information about presence of chemical species as well as environment in which these materials exist and how this is changing over time. Metabolic, functional and structural information is possible. May be able to quantify specific tissue composition of hemoglobin, melanin, elastin, etc	Still experimental. Expensive. Limited availability. MRI images prone to motion artifacts. Underlying tissue may cause data contamination. Not portable
Fourier-transformed infrared spectroscopy (FTIR)	1970s	Beam of polychromatic IR light is shone through a zinc or germanium selenide crystal applied to skin surface. Crystal creates 5–20 reflections, and absorption cycles between crystal and skin. Reflected beam is detected by spectrophotometer, Fourier transform of beam gives IR spectrum with bands of absorption in SC. Ratio of areas of amide I and II bands (peaks) provides relative SC water content. Amide I at 1645 cm^{-1} is overlapped by band of protein-associated water, and thus will change with protein water content, whereas amide II at 1545 cm^{-1} is not influenced by water[12]	In vivo, direct measurement of water. Quantitative, theoretical relationship between measured parameter and water concentration understood	Expensive. Need signal averaging during time when site is occluded, since water content changes during measurements. Depth of penetration can vary with parameters. Bands from interfering substances could obscure amide bands. IR beam is weak (5–20 μm) penetrator. Data only pertain to superficial SC

8. Bioengineering techniques to measure transepidermal water loss (TEWL)[54]

Machine/developer	Principles	Advantages	Disadvantages
Evaporimeter (ServoMed, Sweden)	Probe with two pairs of humidity transducers and thermistor measures the partial water vapour pressure at 2 points (3 and 6 mm) above skin. Rate of evaporation ($g/m^2/h$) calculated from difference in partial water vapor pressure between these points. Probe has surface area 1.13 cm^2. Normal TEWL between 2 and 5 $g/m^2/h$	Can evaluate products whose mode of action is occlusion. Accurate. Convenient to use. Inexpensive to operate[8]	Strictly speaking, does not measure skin hydration. Many factors can affect measurements, and they need careful monitoring. Evaporimeter may underestimate water evaporation rate at high TEWL[54]
Tewameter (Courage-Khazaka Electronic, Germany)	Same principle of measurement as Evaporimeter except sensors are at 3 and 8 mm above skin, and probe has surface area of 0.79 cm^2	More recent design; measures probe temperature and graphs TEWL over time; more complete, somewhat more convenient, less sensitive to air turbulence than Evaporimeter[54]	Strictly speaking, does not measure skin hydration. Many factors can affect measurements, and they need careful monitoring. Newer instrument, so less well studied

9. Bioengineering techniques to image stratum corneum

Technique	Machines/ developer	Principles	Advantages	Disadvantages
High-frequency ultrasound, A mode	Alexander (1979); Muller (1985); machines: DUB20 (Taberna pro medicum, Germany); Dermascan C (Cortex Technology, Denmark)[55]	A (amplitude) mode can measure the thickness of the skin layers. Adaptations to skin need a strongly dampened high-frequency ultrasound detector with very short impulses produced by ceramic or piezoelectric polymer transducers in order to detect as many echoes generated from as many interfaces as possible. The receptors made up of a device protecting against emitter overcharge, a wide-band radiofrequency amplifier, and a detector of radiofrequency signals. Signals are viewed on an oscilloscope	Good for whole-skin visualization. Can differentiate epidermis from dermis in some cases. Can follow aging, sunlight damage, scleroderma, steroid atrophy	Difficult to measure water quantitatively from images. Motion creates artifacts. Encoding process can distort space. Difficult to visualize very thin sites
High-frequency ultrasound, B mode	DUB20 (Taberna pro medicum, Germany); Dermascan C (Cortex Technology, Denmark)[55]	In B (brightness) mode, a succession of signal lines in A mode is acquired and reconstructed into a 2D image. B scans are oriented in the x or y direction	Useful to measure thickness and depth of skin cancers. Appearance of non-echogenic band in upper dermis may be more sensitive marker of aging than skin thickness. Distinguishes skin irritation vs allergic reactions. Ultrasound waves theoretically carry information on elastic properties	Difficult to measure water quantitatively from images. Motion creates artifacts. Encoding process can distort space. Information on how ultrasound waves carry information on skin elastic properties cannot yet be interpreted. More research needed

(Contd)

9. Bioengineering techniques to image stratum corneum (continued)

Technique	Machines/developer	Principles	Advantages	Disadvantages
High-resolution magnetic resonance imaging (MRI)	1987–1988 Hyde,[56] Querleux,[57] Bittoun,[57] (Skin Imaging Modele, France)	Conventional MRI equipment adapted to reduce field of view and pixel size using surface coils. Skin-imaging module to 18 mm × 50 mm (pixel size 70 µm × 300 µm, slice thickness 3 mm in 2D acquisition; 0.7 mm in 3D acquisition). Small surface radiofrequency coil to improve the signal-to-noise ratio. Bittoun made further advances by using the device with a 1.5 T system, obtaining very high-resolution images of normal skin as well as calculations of $T1$ and $T2$[57]	More adapted to visualization of whole skin. Epidermis can be clearly delineated and analyzed to an axial spatial resolution of 35–70 µm. Able to measure water directly and quantitatively in vivo. Can study proton-exchange phenomenon. Repeated measurements over time in vivo	Errors introduced by very short $T2$, chemical shift and partial-volume effect can overestimate epidermal thickness. Artifacts also caused by motion and spatial distortions introduced by encoding. Clinical utility limited by high cost, cumbersome equipment
In vivo confocal microscopy	Petran (1968); New, Corcuff (1993); Tandem Scanning microscope, (Tracor Northern)	A focused spot of light scans the sample. Reflected light in focal plane passes through a pinhole in front of a photomultiple/TV camera detector. Images received are perfectly focused because almost all of the reflected light from above and below the plane in focus is blocked. The Nipkow disc has two thousand pinholes arranged in Archimede spirals, and allows lightening spot scanning and reflected-light formation, which can be collected by a TV camera. After computer processing, a volume representation can be obtained	Excellent axial (spatial) resolution (1 µm). Very good at visualizing SC. Preserves natural tonicity of skin, hydration of cells and contrast of structures. Possible to measure SC thickness in vivo. Sharp focused; allows study for first time of previously elusive stratum lucidum and stratum granulosum. Can visualize RBC in capillaries. Excellent reproducibility. Can work in 4D space (volume and time) at the microscopic level non-invasively	Artifacts caused by motion and spatial distortions introduced by encoding. Present section thickness that can be imaged is limited to 150 µm.[59] Still needs optical improvements to increase signal-to-noise ratio on images of inner epidermis. Optical sectioning is limited by transparency of tissue, scattering and absorption of light in the sample, working distance and numerical aperture of the sample[59]

10. Optical techniques to characterize skin properties

Technique	Variables measured	Machines available/developer	Principles	Advantages	Disadvantages
Ellipsometry	Refractive index	Jasperson (1969)[60]	Monochromatic light passes through a plane polarizer oriented at 45° with respect to the incidence plane. Polarizer output is fed into a photoelastic modulator composed of a piezoelastic crystal oscillating at a particular frequency. Output of the modulator passes through collimater side of ellipsometer to skin of interest. Reflected light goes to telescopic side of spectrometer and is directed through a second polarizer to a photomultiplier tube (PMT). PMT output and reference signal enter a lock-in amplifier, which gives intensity readings for the ellipsometric parameters. A computer program calculates the refractive index	Changes in refractive index can be used to monitor hydration status, effect of moisturizers	Topical agents may cause a change in reflectivity. Very indirect method
Skin critical surface tension (CST)	Critical surface tension, wettability	Jacobi (1949); Schneider (1951); Ginn (1968); El Khyat (1996)[61]	Droplets of standard liquids applied to skin and viewed under microscope. CST can be calculated using Zisman technique	Can quantify surface energy phenomenon resulting from sweat, serum and emulsion application as well as interactions. Can quantify wettability	Requires some skill on the part of the operator

References for appendix

1. Katz HI, Lindholm JS, In: *Handbook of Non-Invasive Methods and the Skin* (Serup J, Jemec GBE, eds). Boca Raton, FL: CRC Press, 1995: 49–55.

2. Kadner H, Bieshold C, *Dermatol Monatsschr* 1971; **157**: 758–9.

3. Marks R, Pearse AD, *Br J Dermatol* 1975; **92**: 651–7.

4. Ishida T, Kashibuchi M, Morita K, Yuasa S, *Cosmetics and Toiletries* 1979; **94**: 39–47.

5. Makki S, Barbenel JC, Agache P, *Acta Derm Venerol (Stockh)* 1979; **59**: 285–91.

6. Aubert L, Brun A, Grollier JF, Leveque JL, *Cosmet Technol Sci* 1982; **3**: 365–70.

7. Connemann BJ, Busche H, Kreusch J, Wolff HH, *Skin Res Technol* 1996; **2**: 40–8.

8. Marks R, In: *Principles of Cosmetics for the Dermatologist* (Frost P, Horwitz SN eds). St Louis, MO: CV Mosby, 1982: 50–8.

9. Corcuff P, de Rigal J, Leveque JL, *Bioeng Skin* 1981; **4**: 16–31.

10. Barton SP, Marshall RJ, Marks R, *Bioeng Skin* 1987; **3**: 93–107.

11. Gormley DE, In: *Proceedings of Bioengineering and the Skin, San Francisco Meeting, September 1985.*

12. Black D, Diridollou S, Lagarde JM, Gall Y, In: *Cosmetic Dermatology*, 2nd edn (Baran R, Maibach HI, eds). London: Martin Dunitz, 1998: 125–50.

13. Picton W, Devitt H, Forgie MA, *Br J Dermatol* 1976; **95**: 341–8.

14. Taylor CJ, Brunt JN, Dixon RN, Gregory PJ, *Pract Metallogr* 1978; **8**: 433.

15. Miller DL, In: *Handbook of Non-Invasive Methods and the Skin* (Serup J, Jemec GBE, eds). Boca Raton, FL: CRC Press, 1995: 149–51.

16. Wolf J, *Z Mikrosk Anat Forsch* 1936; **46**: 170.

17. Jenkins HL, Tresise JA, *J Soc Cosmet Chem* 1969; **20**: 1.

18. Kligman AM, Schatz H, Manning S, Stoudemayer T, In: *Noninvasive Methods for the Quantification of Skin Functions* (Frosch PJ, Kligman AM, eds). New York: Springer-Verlag, 1993: 309–16.

19. Marks R, Dawber RPR, *Br J Dermatol* 1971; **84**: 117–23.

20. Thacker JG, Iachetta FA, Allaire FA et al, *Rev Sci Instrum* 1977; **48**: 181.

21. Gunner CW, Williams EW, Greaves M, Hutton WC, Burlin TE, In: *Bioengineering and the Skin* (Marks R, Payne PA, eds). Boston: MTP Press Limited, 1981: 31–43.

22. Christensen MS, Hargens CW, Nacht S, Gans EH, *J Invest Derm* 1977; **69**: 282–6.

23. Vlasblom DC, Skin elasticity. PhD Thesis, University of Utrecht, 1967.

24. Salter DC, In: *Bioengineering of the Skin: Water and the Stratum Corneum* (Elsner P, Berardesca E, Maibach HI, eds). Boca Raton, FL: CRC Press, 1994: 205–16.

25. Barbenel JC, Evans JH, *J Invest Dermatol* 1977; **69**: 318–20.

26. Lévêque JL, In: *Cosmetic Dermatology*, 2nd edn (Baran R, Maibach HI, eds). London: Martin Dunitz, 1998: Chap 46.

27. Franke EK, *J Appl Physiol* 1950; **3**: 582.

28. Von Gierke HE, Oestreicher HI, Franke EK et al, *J Appl Physiol* 1952; **4**: 886.

29. Thompson DE, Hussein HMG, Perritt RQ. In: *Bioengineering and the Skin* (Marks R, Payne PA, eds). Boston: MTP Press, 1981: 103–13.

30. Wilhelm KP, Cua AB, Maibach HI, In: *Non-Invasive Methods for the Quantification of Skin Functions* (Frosch PJ, Kligman AM, eds). New York: Springer-Verlag, 1993: 191–203.

31. Grahame R, *Clin Sci* 1970; **39**: 223–38.

32. Jemec GBE, Jemec B, Jemec BIE, Serup J, *Plast Reconstruct Surg* 1990; **85**: 100–3.

33. Gniadecka M, Serup J, In: *Handbook of Non-Invasive Methods and the Skin* (Serup J, Jemec GBE, eds). Boca Raton, FL: CRC Press, 1995: 329–34.

34. Dikstein S, Hartzshtark A, In: *Bioengineering and the Skin* (Marks R, Payne PA, eds). Boston: MTP Press, 1981: 45–53.

35. Gartstein V, Elsau WH, In: *Proceeding of the 8th International Symposium on Bioengineering and the Skin, Stresa*, 1990: 70.

36. Pierard GE, *Bioeng Skin Newsl* 1980; **2**: 31.

37. Manny-Aframian V, Dikstein S, In: *Handbook of Non-Invasive Methods and the Skin* (Serup J, Jemec GBE, eds). Boca Raton, FL: CRC Press, 1995: 345–7.

38. Hargens CW, In: *Handbook of Non-Invasive Methods and the Skin* (Serup J, Jemec GBE, eds). Boca Raton, FL: CRC Press, 1995: 359–66.

39. Tosti A, Compagno G, Fazzini ML, Villardita S, *J Invest Dermatol* 1977; **69**: 315–17.

40. Manny-Aframian V, Dikstein S, In: *Handbook of Non-Invasive Methods and the Skin* (Serup J, Jemec GBE, eds). Boca Raton, FL: CRC Press, 1995: 349–52.

41. Nacht S, Close J-A, Yeung D, Gans EG, *J Soc Cosmet Chem* 1981; **32:** 55–65.

42. Torgalkar AM, In: *Bioengineering and the Skin* (Marks R, Payne PA, eds). Boston: MTP Press, 1981: 55–65.

43. Tronnier H, Wagener HH, *Dermatologica* 1952; **104:** 135–51.

44. Potts RO, Christman DA, Buras EM, *J Biomech* 1983; **16:** 362–72.

45. Tregear RT, *Nature* 1965; **205:** 600.

46. Distante F, Berardesca E, In: *Bioengineering of the Skin: Methods and Instrumentation* (Berardesca E, Elsner P, Wilhelm KP, Maibach HI, eds). Boca Raton, FL: CRC Press, 1995: 5–12.

47. Jacques SL, A linear measurement of the water content of the stratum corneum of human skin using a microwave probe. Presented at the 32nd Annual Conference on Engineering in Medicine and Biology, Denver, CO, 1979.

48. Tagami H, In: *Bioengineering of the Skin: Water and the Stratum Corneum* (Elsner P, Berardesca E, Maibach HI, eds). Boca Raton, FL: CRC Press, 1994: 59.

49. Gabard B, Treffel P, In: *Bioengineering of the Skin: Water and the Stratum Corneum* (Elsner P, Berardesca E, Maibach HI, eds). Boca Raton, FL: CRC Press, 1994: 147–70.

50. Putnam NA, *J Soc Cosmet Chem* 1972; **23:** 209–26.

51. Osberghaus R, Glohuber C, van Raay HG, Braig S, *J Soc Cosmet Chem* 1978; **29:** 133–46.

52. Rosencwaig A, Pines E, *J Invest Dermatol* 1977; **69:** 296–8.

53. Kolmel K, Nicolaus A, Giese K, *Bioeng Skin* 1985; **1:** 125–31.

54. Barel AO, Clarys P, In: *Handbook of Non-Invasive Methods and the Skin* (Serup J, Jemec GBE, eds). Boca Raton, FL: CRC Press, 1995: 179–95.

55. El-Gammal S, Auer T, Hoffmann K et al, In: *Non-Invasive Methods for the Quantification of Skin Functions* (Frosch PJ, Kligman AM, eds). New York: Springer-Verlag, 1993: 104–29.

56. Hyde JS, Tesmanowicz H, Kneeland BJ, *Magn Reson Med* 1987; **5:** 449–61.

57. Bittoun J, Saint-James H, Querleux BG, *Radiology* 1990; **176:** 457–60.

58. Querleux B, Yassine MM, Darrasse L et al, *Bioeng Skin* 1988; **4:** 1–14.

59. Corcuff P, Lévêque JL, *Dermatology* 1993; **186:** 50–4.

60. Jasperson SN, Schatterly SE, *Rev Sci Instrum* 1969; **40:** 761.

61. El Khyat A, Mavon A, Leduc M et al, *Skin Res Technol* 1996; **2:** 91–6.

24

Hand and body lotions

F Anthony Simion, Michael S Starch, Pamela S Witt, Judith K Woodford, Keith J Edgett

INTRODUCTION

Skin, the largest organ of the body, plays a critical role as the interface between the human body and the environment. Traditionally, it was thought mainly to have a passive role, being a physical barrier from environmental threats such as low humidity, biological pathogens, UV radiation, physical trauma and environmental pollutants. It has always been recognized as playing a vital role as a sensory organ alerting us to the presence and nature of objects surrounding us, extremes of temperature and noxious chemicals. More recently, its active interactions with the environment have become more appreciated. It is physiologically active, being a key initial immunological barrier as well as being able to metabolize xenobiotics. However, it can only be effective as a barrier if it is intact. Hand and body lotions play a vital role in helping to maintain the integrity and plasticity of the stratum corneum in the face of many outside threats. Furthermore, such lotions provide a crucial benefit to consumers – patients – in improving the feel of their skin and eliminating the negative sensations of dryness and itching associated with dry skin. Beyond this, many consumers regard their skin as an outward reflection of themselves to the world. This is especially true for the face and, to a lesser extent, the hands. When the skin feels and looks good, this cosmetic benefit helps support a person's positive image.

Dermatologists continue to see increasing numbers of patients suffering from dryness and itching, often associated with visible scaling and flaking of their skin. This is due to a variety of reasons. Shifting demographics, specifically the aging population in combination with increased usage of low-humidity central heating and air-conditioning systems, has significantly contributed to the increase in dry-skin complaints. In addition, skin is exposed to household detergents and personal cleansers, which can quickly damage the stratum corneum proteins, extract small hygroscopic molecules and deplete or derange the bilayer structure of key intercellular lipids. This will cause a dramatic decrease in the skin's ability to act as a barrier. Detergent-induced dryness and primary irritation has made dermatitis one of the most common forms of occupational disease in developed countries. Health care workers, hairdressers, and food handlers are especially at risk.[1,2]

During the last 50 years, hand and body moisturizers have been designed to provide relief to dry-skin sufferers by increasing the plasticity of the skin while eliminating skin scaling. There are several mechanisms to achieve this. They include increasing the skin's water content by forming an occlusive barrier or by humecantancy, or by supplementing water with other skin plasticizing materials. Indeed, individual moisturizing ingredients may deliver benefits to the skin by several mechanisms. Today's moisturizers are far superior to those of the past. This is due to new materials that are capable of mimicking the skin's biological moisture-holding mechanisms and the ability to deliver these materials effectively to the skin. Ingredients such as ceramide analogs, amino acids and essential fatty acids, have been successfully incorporated into hand and body lotions. When moisturizers are used regularly, they help to mitigate dry skin. Furthermore, there have been advances in formulating aesthetically superior products that consumers enjoy using, yet maintain their efficacy. The leading hand and body lotion brands in the USA are shown in Table 24.1.

A second role for hand and body moisturizers is as vehicles for active ingredients, including over-the-counter drugs such as sunscreens and cosmetically active compounds such as α-hydroxy acids. As a result of increased awareness regarding the effects of the sun, recent marketplace trends show an increase in the number of hand and body moisturizers that offer sun protection factor (SPF) benefits. Importantly, aesthetically optimized SPF moisturizers are now available that provide consumers with much preferred tactile benefits, such as a non-sticky, non-greasy, and non-oily skin feeling: attributes not traditionally found in sunscreen products.

The efficacy and aesthetics of hand and body lotions depend on several factors. Gross chemical composition is not the only variable affecting both efficacy and skin feel. Most lotions are emulsions – heterogeneous mix-

Table 24.1 Leading hand and body lotions in the USA		
Brand	**Manufacturer**	**Emulsion type**
Jergens	Andrew Jergens Co, Cincinnati, OH	Oil-in-water
Vaseline Intensive Care	Cheseborough–Ponds, Greenwich, CT	Oil-in-water
Lubriderm	Warner–Wellcome, Morris Plains, NJ	Oil-in-water
Eucerin	Beiersdorf, Norwalk, CT	Water-in-oil
Curel	Bausch & Lomb, Rochester, NY	Oil-in-water
Neutrogena	Johnson & Johnson, Los Angeles, CA	Oil-in-water
Sauve	Helene Curtis, Chicago, IL	Oil-in-water
Keri	Bristol-Myers Squibb, New York, NY	Oil-in-water

tures of oil- and water-soluble materials. How ingredients are distributed between the oil and aqueous phases plays a significant role in how they are delivered to and partition into the skin. This in turn affects their moisturizing effects, and the feel of the skin during and after application. To account for these factors, this chapter will discuss the ingredients used in lotions separately from emulsion structure. Assessing the safety and efficacy of lotions will also be discussed.

In conclusion, although many skin characteristics are genetically determined, the environment also has significant effects. These negative effects can be ameliorated by regular use of cosmetic moisturizers. The regular use of moisturizers, a healthy diet, protection from the sun, and regular exercise will contribute to significantly healthier, younger-looking and feeling skin.

INGREDIENTS FOR HAND AND BODY LOTIONS

Overview

As anyone who has looked at the ingredient statement for a typical hand and body lotion can attest, the number and variety of ingredients used in these products can be somewhat intimidating. Consequently, it is clear that an exhaustive review of these ingredients is beyond the scope of this chapter. However, this chapter will attempt to cover the major categories of ingredients, organized according to their function in the product.

Before we begin the review of specific ingredients, a few general comments about ingredient disclosure may be helpful. In the USA, manufacturers of cosmetic products are required to provide a complete disclosure of the ingredients used in their products. This requirement was established for the purpose of allowing consumers to monitor ingredients used. Package labeling guidelines require the listing of ingredients in descending order of weight per cent. One exception is for ingredi-

ents used at levels of 1% or less. Such minor ingredients can be listed in any order. Since many of the ingredients used in hand and body lotions are complex or ill-defined chemical entities, a standard nomenclature has been developed by the Cosmetics, Toiletries, and Fragrance Association (CTFA). Under CTFA guidelines, manufacturers are obliged to use the assigned 'International Cosmetic Ingredient' (INCI) name for all ingredients used in their products. Information about these ingredients, manufacturers and chemical structures are compiled in the CTFA *International Cosmetic Ingredient Dictionary*, which is a highly recommended source of cosmetic formulators.

Ingredient classes

Water

This ingredient can be found at the beginning of nearly all ingredient statements for hand and body lotions, since it typically makes up 70% or more of the formula. Water has two important functions in a hand and body lotion. First, it is the vehicle by which many other ingredients are delivered to the skin. Secondly, water can be viewed as an active ingredient in the sense that it hydrates the skin for a short time, usually less than 15 minutes, before evaporating. Although the CTFA does not recognize the use of any particular type of water (e.g. 'purified water') for the purpose of ingredient labeling, most manufacturers do use softened, or demineralized, water in their products to avoid any interactions between calcium and magnesium ions and other components in the formula.

Emollients

An emollient can be defined as an ingredient that softens the stratum corneum and has a soothing effect when applied to the skin. Emollients used in hand and body lotions are generally oily materials that help plasticize dry skin either by direct interaction with the stratum corneum or by providing an occlusive barrier that traps water from the underlying skin strata.

Historically, lanolin was one of the first emollients used widely by the industry. It is a by-product of wool processing, which yields a complex mixture of semisolid oils. This provides a strong occlusive effect when applied to skin, and may also directly plastize the stratum corneum. Lanolin, its constituents and derivatives are still used in some hand and body lotions, but have largely been replaced by other emollients because of its reported sensitization potential. These adverse reactions may be due to the presence of low levels of alkane-α,β-diols and alkane-α,ω-diols.[3] Purified lanolins have recently become available.

Two of the most common emollients used today are mineral oil and petrolatum, which are hydrocarbon-based materials derived from petroleum. Petrolatum, in particular, resembles lanolin in its physical characteristics and its occlusive effect on the skin. Ghadially et al[4] showed that, in addition to forming an occlusive barrier, petrolatum penetrates into the intercellular lipids of the stratum corneum. Kligman[5] reported that petrolatum was very effective at reducing observable skin dryness and preventing its reappearance. Mineral oil is less occlusive, but has better spreading properties and is generally believed to have a less greasy feel on the skin compared with petrolatum.

Silicones are a class of synthetic polymers that are also widely used in hand and body lotions. Most silicones are used for their good spreading and detackifying properties as well as their emolliency. Common examples are dimethicone and cyclomethicone.

Another class of emollients comprises triglycerides, which are derived from animal or vegetable oils. These oils are usually named according to the original source (e.g. sunflower seed oil). Triglycerides have the additional advantage over other emollient oils in that they are sources of essential fatty acids (EFAs) for the skin. Essential fatty acids are unsaturated fatty acids that cannot be synthe-sized by the body yet are required for maintaining the stratum corneum barrier function. Experiments have shown that when EFAs are withheld from rats' diet, their skin becomes scaly and its water barrier function is compromised.[6] Healthy skin can be restored by topical application of triglycerides which are rich in EFAs. Similar results were observed in human patients whose lipid intake had been reduced due to stomach surgery.[7]

The use of unsaturated triglycerides in a hand and body lotion can create problems due to the susceptibility of these oils to oxidation, producing discoloration and off-odors over time. To prevent this oxidation, antioxidants such as tocopherol (vitamin E), BHA or BHT are often added to the formula.

Triglycerides may be processed to provide a large variety of other emollient ingredients. Hydrolysis of triglycerides yields diglycerides, monoglycerides and fatty acids. Glycerides are used not only for emolliency, but also for their ability to stabilize the lotion by emulsification (see the section on physical structure). Examples of glycerides are glyceryl stearate (monoglyceride), glyceryl dilaurate (diglyceride) and palm oil glyceride (mixed glycerides). Fatty acids are also processed to produce fatty esters. Numerous types of fatty esters are used in hand and body lotions. Some common examples are isopropyl myristate, isopropyl palmitate, octyl hydroxystearate and cetyl palmitate.

Humectants

Humectants are water-soluble organic compounds, typically polyhydric alcohols, that have an affinity for water. The most common humectant is glycerin (glycerol), but others include sorbitol, propylene glycol, dipropylene glycol and butylene glycol. Until recently, it was believed that these ingredients helped to moisturize the skin simply by binding additional water in the stratum corneum, plasticizing it and retarding the rate of evaporation. However, recently, two alternate mechanisms by which glycerin may moisturize have been proposed. Froebe, Matti and their colleagues showed that glycerin at low humidity can prevent the transition of intercellular lipids within the stratum corneum from the liquid crystal to the gel phase.[8,9] This effect may be responsible for the improvement in barrier function observed when glycerin (and possibly other humectants) is applied to the skin. Rawlings et al[10] showed that glycerin is able to promote normal desquamation by enhancing the activity of the proteases that degrade desmosomes. It is likely that all three mechanisms occur in the stratum corneum simultaneously.

Emulsifiers

These are ingredients that are used to stabilize hand and body lotions by retarding the natural tendency of oils and aqueous phases to separate. Figure 24.1 shows that the emulsifier included in the left-hand sample prevents the separation of the oil (dyed blue) and the aqueous phases. Many types of emulsifiers are used, and it is quite common for a hand and

body lotion to include three or more emulsifiers to provide the desired stability. Mono- and diglycerides derived from natural fats and oils have already been mentioned, but fatty acids, especially stearic acid, are also effective emulsifiers when converted to soaps (i.e. neutralized to their sodium or triethanolamine salts). Fatty alcohols, also derived from triglycerides, are widely used as emulsifiers and viscosity builders. Examples include cetyl alcohol (C_{16}), stearyl alcohol (C_{18}), and cetearyl alcohol (a mixture of cetyl and stearyl alcohols). Ethoxylated fatty alcohols are another large group of emulsifiers used in hand and body lotions. Examples include ceteareth-20 and steareth-2.

Water-soluble polymers

To provide additional emulsion stability and contribute to the desired consistency of a hand and body lotion, these high-molecular-weight polymers are often used to increase the viscosity of the formula. There are several natural polysaccharides that are used for this purpose, such as xanthan gum. However, these natural polymers have been largely supplanted by synthetic polymers, the most common being the carbomers. These are polyacrylates that provide a strong thickening effect when the acid groups along the chain are neutralized to salts using a base such as sodium hydroxide.

Minor components
Preservatives and fragrances

Although they make up a very small percentage of the total formula, these ingredients are of concern to dermatologists since they cause most of the adverse reactions from lotions that require medical attention. Many consumers prefer unfragranced products. This has prompted some manufacturers to offer fragrance-free product variants. Other manufacturers include various botanical extracts that technically are not fragrances, yet still include many of the same chemicals found in

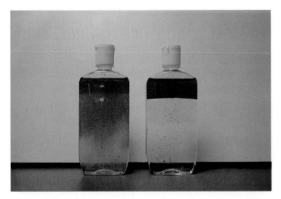

Figure 24.1 Emulsifiers reduce the rate at which the oil and aqueous phases separate. The left-hand bottle contains an emulsifier with the oil and aqueous phases, whereas the right-hand bottle contains no emulsifier. After mixing, the system on the left separates more slowly.

certain fragrances. These are often called 'unscented'.

Preservatives are included in hand and body lotions to prevent the growth of bacteria and molds. Most hand and body lotions contain a high percentage of water, which makes them a good growth medium for these microorganisms. Contamination during manufacture or subsequent use by consumers can lead to rapid growth and spoilage of the product. Further, if the growth of pathogenic bacteria such as *Pseudomonas* is not prevented, serious health consequences could result if the contaminated hand and body lotion is applied in such a way as to introduce these pathogens into an open cut or the eyes.

Given the need to prevent growth of microorganisms in their products, manufacturers use a variety of biocides in sufficient concentration to provide a self-sterilizing effect. In other words, the preservative system is designed and tested to withstand multiple contaminations. Any microorganisms introduced into the product are killed, generally within 24-48 hours. These biocides are most often used in various combinations to provide effective preservation against a broad spectrum of bacteria and molds.

The following is a list of the most commonly used biocides in hand and body lotions:

- DMDM hydantoin
- diazolidinyl urea
- imidazolidinyl urea
- Quaternium-15
- parabens (esters of *p*-hydroxybenzoic acid) – the most common are methyl paraben and propyl paraben, but other esters are also used
- methyldibromoglutaronitrile
- methylchloroisothiazolinone/methylisothiazolinone (Kathon CG)
- phenoxyethanol
- iodopropynyl butylcarbamate

Skin care additives

Many lotions have cosmetic materials added at low levels for marketing purposes, i.e. to influence consumers to buy the product. In these cases the moisturization benefits that consumers require are delivered by the vehicle. However, in the last few years, additives have been identified that improve the appearance and feel of the skin over the vehicle alone. These include α-hydroxy acids, retinol and ceramide analogs.[11,12] Imokawa et al have shown that applying synthetic ceramide analogs effectively and rapidly moisturize the skin.[12] This result is not unexpected as ceramides are a vital constituent of the stratum corneum intracellular lipid barrier. Reduced levels of ceramide are observed in atopic and damaged skin.[13,14] Elias and his colleagues have shown that adding ceramides with other key lipids will restore the stratum corneum barrier to water loss.[15]

The ability of creams containing 8% glycolic or lactic acid to reduce some of the visible signs of photoaging after 22 weeks of treatment was reported by Stiller et al.[11] They reported a improvement in observer-scored global photodamage on the forearms compared with a vehicle control. Panelists also reported a self-assessed improvement.

PHYSICAL STRUCTURE OF HAND AND BODY LOTIONS

Overview

Most hand and body lotions are emulsions, which can be defined as mixtures of mutually insoluble materials that are stabilized against separation. The insoluble ingredients are dispersed in the vehicle (usually water) and can form tiny droplets or particles that scatter light strongly. This gives these products their characteristic opaque, white appearance (see Figure 24.2). Addition of titanium dioxide will also give the product a white appearance. Some hand and body lotions are not emul-

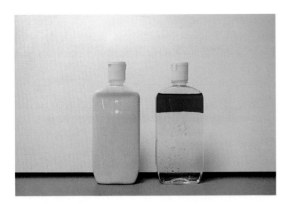

Figure 24.2 Emulsions are opaque systems compared with an unemulsified two-phase oil/water system.

sions, but consist entirely of an oil phase. Examples include petrolatum and 'baby oil', i.e. mineral oil.

Hand and body lotions can be further characterized as being one of two emulsion types. The first type of emulsion, which is by far the most common, is referred to as an oil-in-water emulsion, often abbreviated 'o/w'. This type of emulsion consists of tiny droplets of oils or waxes dispersed in water. The second type of emulsion takes the opposite form: droplets of water dispersed in a mixture of oils. This is referred to as a water-in-oil, or 'w/o', emulsion. In addition to the binary (o/w or w/o) emulsions, there are more complicated tertiary emulsions, which will be discussed briefly at the end of this section.

Oil-in-water (o/w) emulsions

This is the typical form of emulsion used in hand and body lotions. The water-insoluble ingredients (oils) are the emollients, which are typically used in the range of 5–25% of the total formula, and the fragrance. Water together with all of the soluble ingredients (e.g. humectants) form a solution into which the water-insoluble ingredients are dispersed.

In the o/w emulsion, the emulsifiers have two important functions. First, the emulsifiers act at the interface between the oil and water phases to reduce the energy required to produce a fine dispersion of the oil ingredients into the water. In a typical o/w emulsion, the particle size of the dispersed oils is about $10 \ \mu m$ (10^{-5} m), which is much too small to observe without the aid of a microscope. The second function of the emulsifiers is to stabilize the emulsion, retarding the natural tendency of the oils to separate from the water phase of the formula. Emulsifiers stabilize the formula by coating each oil droplet and preventing it from coalescing with other oil droplets and thereby growing in size. Preventing growth in droplet size is critical for stabilizing an emulsion. The appearance of large droplets would compromise the lotion's smooth texture and appearance.

In terms of aesthetics, o/w hand and body lotions can range from very 'light' (low oil content) to heavy (high oil content). The skin feel of the product during rub-in and after drying is affected not only by the amount of oil, but also the composition of the emollient oils used in the formula. For example, if the oil phase is composed mainly of mineral oil, the lotion will generally provide an 'oily' feel on the skin, while the use of emollients like lanolin or petrolatum gives a heavier 'greasy' skin feel.

Oil-in-water emulsions may be better able to deliver water-soluble materials to the skin. Sah et al[16] showed enhanced delivery of lactic acid to the skin from an o/w emulsion compared with an w/o emulsion that had a similar composition. A tertiary w/o/w emulsion (see below) showed an intermediate rate of delivery.

Water-in-oil (w/o) emulsions

This type of emulsion is much less common than the o/w type for several reasons. The most important reason is probably aesthetics. In order to have enough emollient oil to surround the water, a relatively large percentage of oil is required, usually in excess of 25%. Thus it is very difficult to formulate a w/o hand and body lotion with a light skin feel. Another reason why w/o emulsions are not common is they are more expensive to manufacture. Oils are more expensive than water, and increasing the oil content will increase formula cost. Additionally, in order to produce and stabilize w/o emulsions, special emulsifiers are necessary: these generally cost more than o/w emulsifiers.

Complex emulsions

In addition to the binary emulsion systems already discussed, there are more complicated emulsions that have been developed for use in personal care products. One such system is the w/o/w emulsion, where a water phase is first dispersed and stabilized into an oil phase, and this w/o emulsion is in turn dispersed into a second water phase. The purpose of this elaborate emulsion structure is to protect water-soluble ingredients: these are sequestered inside the oil phase, where they will not come into contact with other ingredients in the second water phase that may degrade them. Examples of ingredients that might require such protection are biological materials such as enzymes.

ASSESSING MOISTURIZER EFFICACY

Overview

The primary use of hand and body moisturizers is to alleviate skin dryness and prevent its return, especially on the legs, arms and hands. Measuring these effects is therefore a primary objective for assessing moisturizer efficacy. Clinical methods have been developed that quantify dry skin or its absence via visual scoring by a trained observer and by using biophysical measurements of the skin. However, clinical efficacy alone is not sufficient to make a product commercially successful. To appeal to consumers, the lotion must be both efficacious and aesthetically pleasing, i.e. pleasantly scented (or unscented) and have acceptable tactile characteristics during and immediately after application.

Clinical evaluation of moisturizer efficacy

Clinical evaluation is a key component in the measurement of moisturizer efficacy. The visual assessment of skin dryness is a direct link to the perceivable benefits of 'moisturization' that consumers readily recognize: these include skin flaking and scaling, fine dry lines, rough texture, ashiness and skin cracking. Figure 24.3 shows the different levels of skin dryness observed in clinical studies. In many studies, visual assessments are supplemented with instrumental measures of skin hydration, surface topography or elasticity. These instrumental measurements are more easily standardized than observer assessments, and provide objective assessments of cosmetic treatment effects.

The majority of cosmetic clinical studies utilize either the Kligman regression protocol[5] or a modified version[17–20] to measure the relief of dry skin following lotion application. Typically, these studies start out with dry skin, which is treated for an extended period, followed by a short regression phase during which product usage is discontinued. Kligman originally studied the effect of ingredients and products on the lower legs of 10–30 female panelists (see Figure 24.4). These dry-skin sites were treated with an ingredient or lotion twice daily for up to three weeks. The visual dryness was assessed prior to treatment (baseline) and at the end of each week. Panelists started with dry skin, and the improvement in dryness from baseline was the measure of moisturization efficacy, or the relief of dryness.

The prevention of the return of dryness is measured during the regression phase immediately following the treatment period. A slow

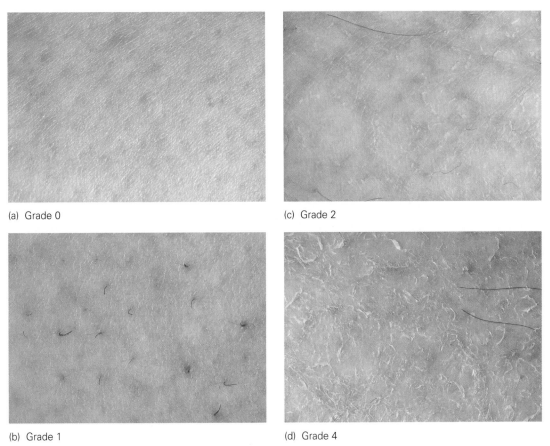

(a) Grade 0   (c) Grade 2

(b) Grade 1   (d) Grade 4

Figure 24.3 Different levels of skin dryness observed in a moisturization study, utilizing a 0, . . . , 4 scoring scale.

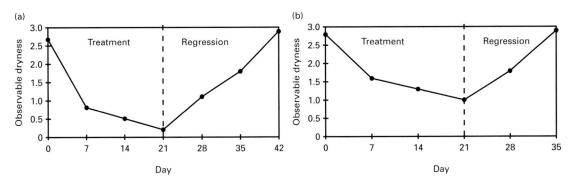

Figure 24.4 Petrolatum is more effective than lanolin in alleviating dry skin and preventing its return.
(a) Effect of petrolatum on dry skin. (b) Effects of lanolin on dry skin. The Kligman regression test[5] was used: test material is applied to the lower leg daily for 3 weeks; after treatment stops, the legs are followed until the skin's condition regresses to its original level of dryness. Regression takes longer for petrolatum than for lanolin.

return to baseline is indicative of an efficacious product with lasting effects. Figure 24.4 shows the data obtained by Kligman for two cosmetic moisturizing ingredients: petrolatum and lanolin. The data clearly demonstrate efficacy during the treatment and regression phases. During the regression, persistent moisturizing effects are demonstrated – 21 days after the last treatment with petrolatum, but only 14 days for lanolin. Using the regression test, Kligman showed that hydrophobic oils, such as mineral oil or olive oil, alone had little ability to alleviate dry skin. The efficacy of these oils was enhanced when they were formulated with hydrophilic materials into cold creams. Kligman's data suggested that the moisturizer's composition could have a greater influence on its efficacy than the number of applications (dosage). He demonstrated a large range in the ability of ingredients to alleviate dryness, but increasing the dosage had limited effects especially beyond four applications a day.

The Kligman regression protocol has been modified by several groups to meet different assessment needs. Boisits et al[18] applied more rigorous conditions to reduce the experimental variability and increase test sensitivity. The most notable modifications include

- conducting the test only if the temperature and humidity were below 45°F (7°C) and 40% respectively;
- washing test sites with Ivory soap prior to lotion application to increase the propensity of the skin to dry out;
- requiring leg shaving no more than two times a week and no later than 30 hours before an observation.

Biosits et al claimed that the refined methodology allows for better differentiation between products.

Another modification has been dubbed the mini-regression. Prall et al[17] reported a regression study conducted using a 4-day treatment followed by a 6-day regression phase. The protocol was similar to Kligman's method, since

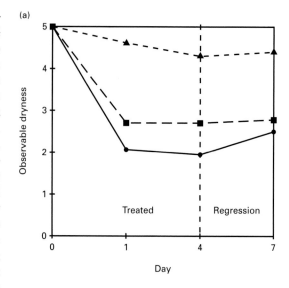

(a)

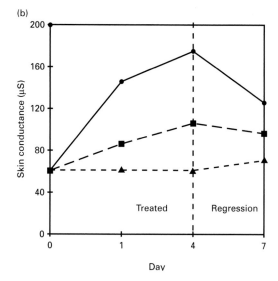

(b)

Figure 24.5 Effect of two lotions on skin dryness as assessed by a mini-regression test. (a) Effect of products on observable dryness. (b) Effect of products on skin conductance. ●, product A; ■, product B; ▲, untreated. (Data from Grove et al.[20])

the applications were conducted twice daily, with a dose of approximately 2 mg/cm². Product efficacy differences were determined during regression in the following descending order of efficacy: 5% lactic acid lotion > o/w lotion > placebo. Grove et al[17] utilized the same mini-regression time frame to examine the efficacy of marketed moisturizers. Clear differences between each of the two products and between the treated sites and the untreated site were observed (Figure 24.5). In this study, skin conductance was used to confirm the observer-scored dryness.

In a similar study of moisturizers containing glycerin, Appa et al[21] utilized a 7-day treatment period followed by a 7-day regression. These investigators demonstrated that moisturizer efficacy increased with the concentration of glycerin. A plateau was reached, with a 25% glycerin lotion being similar in efficacy to a 40% glycerin cream. These results could also relate to the ability of the products to deliver glycerin into the skin, or to the effect of ancillary ingredients.

A third adaptation of the regression test utilizes the lower arms – either the volar or dorsal aspect. Prall et al[17] used a mini-regression design to compare the performance of two lotions on the legs using a controlled lotion dosage, with performance on the outer aspect of the arms using ad-libitum dosage. They concluded that either method accurately predicted the directional efficacy of the lotions. Grove[19] originally used the mini-regression methodology to examine lotion efficacy on the volar forearm using the instrumental method of skin conductance to evaluate performance.

The regression phase of the clinical evaluation may be used to examine the persistence of moisturization efficacy when skin is stressed by winter weather or washing with soap. A more direct approach to measure the prevention of dry skin was developed by Highley et al.[22] In the Highley hand wash protocol, the analysis begins with non-dry, healthy skin. The panelists wash their hands with bar soap for 1 minute, 5 times a day for up to 4 days. One hand remains otherwise untreated, while lotion is applied to the other hand after the first four washes each day. The dryness of the hands are assessed by a trained observer

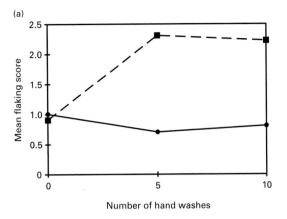

(a)

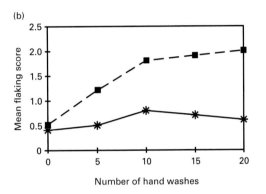

(b)

Figure 24.6 Ability of petrolatum (a) and lotion (b) to prevent the induction of skin flaking by repeated washing with soap: ●, petrolatum; ✶, lotion; ■, no treatment. (Data from Simion et al.[62])

before the first wash of the study (baseline) and approximately one hour after the last (fifth) wash each day. Results show that ingredients such as petrolatum and commercial lotions can prevent the induction of dry skin, which can be considerable on the untreated hand (Figure 24.6 and Table 24.2). By determining the difference between the treated and untreated hands, more than one product or ingredient can be compared. Although panels as small as 5 have been used, it is more usual to use panels of 10 or more to enable the data to be statistically analyzed.

Hannuksela and Kinnunen[23] performed a

Table 24.2 The ability of ingredients to prevent the induction of skin dryness due to repeated hand washings with soap (data from Highley et al[22])

Ingredient	Ability to prevent dryness (the higher the score the more effective the ingredient)
Petrolatum	54
Mineral oil	49
Glycerin (25% aqueous solution)	34
Sorbitol (25% aqueous solution)	14
Propylene glycol (25% aqueous solution)	−1

similar study using 1-minute washes with dish-washing liquid, twice a day, on the arms over a 7-day period. The authors evaluated cleanser-induced irritation using transepidermal water loss (TEWL) as a measure of stratum corneum integrity and laser–doppler flowmetry to assess blood flow. They demonstrated that moisturizer application could prevent surfactant-induced skin damage and accelerate repair compared with no treatment, but were unable to differentiate between products. The ability of moisturizers to prevent detergent-induced skin dryness has important public-health implications. Dermatitis is a leading occupational disease, and professions that involve frequent hand washing are at particular risk. Frequent, effective moisturization may provide a significant preventative benefit.

Instrumental evaluations of moisturizer efficacy

Instrumental evaluation of skin condition is often used to supplement visual assessments in clinical moisturization protocols.[17,19,23] They provide an objective method to evaluate a specific skin parameter. For example, conductance is used as a measure of skin hydration, and TEWL is a measure of stratum corneum barrier function. However, a single bioinstrumental parameter should not be used alone as a measure of moisturization. Instruments measure a defined physical parameter, which may not always correlate with moisturization

or skin condition. For instance, hydrophobic materials such as petrolatum, silicones and mineral oil, which can be effective moisturizers, reduce skin conductance immediately after application. This contradicts the usual interpretation of this parameter, which correlates increased conductance with moisturization. Instead, the bioinstrumental measurement should be used to support observer scoring, and, if possible, multiple bioinstrumental measures should be used simultaneously.

Several bioinstrumental methods will be briefly reviewed in this chapter. More thorough reviews of bioinstrumentation are available in the literature.[24–28]

Measuring water content of the skin

Several methods have been developed. The most frequently used is the indirect method of measuring the electrical properties of the skin.[25,29–31] More direct methods such as nuclear magnetic resonance (NMR) and near-infrared spectroscopy are currently under development.

The three most common instruments for measuring electrical skin properties are the Skicon, which measures skin conductance, and the Corneometer and Nova Dermal Phase Meter, which measure skin capacitance. These parameters have been shown to strongly correlate to each other in moisturizer studies ($r^2 = 0.92$).[32] In theory, conductance and capacitance are expected to increase with hydration level owing to the higher dielectric constant of water compared with other skin

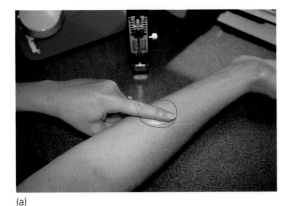

(a)

(b)

Figure 24.8 Expert panel testing of lotions. (a) Product application. (b) Prototypical results for the sensory profile of two lotions: ●, lotion A; ▨, lotion B.

Claims made for moisturizers

Modern hand and body moisturizers have been developed to meet the varied needs of today's consumers. These products span the range from lightweight lotions designed to provide a pampering feeling for normal skin to heavy, greasy creams formulated to relieve severely dry skin. The manufacturers of these products make many claims concerning product efficacy. Some of the common descriptors found on hand and body lotion packaging are listed in Table 24.3.

Any claim that is made on these packages must be supportable by the manufacturer. If the label is found to be false, the product is considered to be misbranded under Section 601 of the US Federal Food, Drug and Cosmetic Act (FDC). A deceptive act or practice, i.e. false claim, is also illegal under Section 5 of the Federal Trade Commission Act (FTC). The cosmetic industry is largely self-regulated by the National Advertising Division (NAD) of the Council of Better Business Bureaus, through which competitors or outside agencies can challenge claims made in advertising. In deciding whether a claim has been adequately substantiated, the NAD assesses three types of support: rationale, subjective or consumer data, and objective, clinical data.[40] The manufacturer will use a combination of the test methods reviewed earlier in this section to provide the necessary support.

Table 24.3 Common descriptors of moisturizer efficacy used in advertising		
Action of moisturizer	**Description of skin**	**Other claims**
Controls dry skin	Severe dry skin	Long-lasting relief
Heals dry skin	Extra dry skin	Fast relief
Protects dry skin	Over-dry skin	Penetrates skin
Relieves dry skin	Rough, dry skin	Soft, smooth, healthy skin
Ends dry skin	Normal to dry skin	Lasts up to 'x' hours

THE TOXICOLOGY OF HAND AND BODY LOTIONS

Overview

Although cosmetic hand and body lotions are leave-on products, they have a low rate of adverse reactions in normal usage. Adams and Maibach[41] reported that cosmetics caused 5.4% of the contact dermatitis cases studied by the North American Contact Dermatitis Group from 1979 to 1983. Hand and body lotions were probably a small group within this total, based on the type of product and body site of reactions. This is supported by more recent data from the US Food and Drug Administration (FDA). They reported that for the years 1991–1994, hand and body lotions caused approximately three 'possible allergic or other serious irritation' reactions for the first million units distributed. In contrast, facial moisturizers caused six reactions for the first million units distributed, and bath soaps caused 45. This indicates that the hand and body lotions developed and sold by leading US manufacturers deliver their benefits with little risk to consumers. However, even with minimal rates of adverse reactions, some consumers do experience reactions. This section will review the types of adverse reactions experienced by consumers, the materials that may cause the reactions, and how industry tests for them.

Most adverse reactions to hand and body lotions experienced by consumers are forms of primary dermal or sensory irritation. These are usually dependent on three factors:

- the lotion's composition;
- the condition of consumers' skin;
- how consumers use the product.

Lotion composition

The first point appears self-evident. If a product does not contain any potential irritants then it is unlikely to cause irritation. Lotion manufacturers strive to market non-irritating and non-sensitizing products.

However, the addition of beneficial ingredients to lotions can cause adverse reactions. Such ingredients include sunscreens and α-hydroxy acids (AHAs), which may cause sensory irritation such as facial stinging or burning in about 15% of the population. Preservatives such as Quaternium 15 can potentially cause sensitization, but are required in order to prevent microbiological contamination of products. Such contamination, especially by *Pseudomonas*, could pose a greater threat to a larger number of consumers. Novel delivery systems, skin protectants and anti-irritants have been used to reduce adverse reactions by limiting the release of or penetration into the skin of potential allergens or irritants. Responsible manufacturers seek to minimize these risks for lotions that consumers essentially regard as being 'risk-free', while maximizing the benefits to their consumers.

Role of consumers' skin condition

Most hand and body moisturizers are well tolerated by the general population, as evidenced by the low adverse-reaction rate reported by the FDA. However, there are groups of consumers who respond adversely to a product or ingredient more readily than the general population. There are several different reasons for this phenomenon. People with a damaged stratum corneum barrier due to pre-existing trauma or pathology may be more reactive, especially to marginal or cumulative irritants. This group, which includes people with atopic dermatitis, is discussed in more detail later in this chapter.

A subset of the population experiences sensory irritation (stinging or burning) when they apply lactic acid or sunscreens to their facial skin. This sensory irritation is distinct from detergent-induced irritation. This conclusion is based on the observations that sodium lauryl sulfate, an irritating surfactant, does not cause stinging,[42] but stingers to lactic acid demonstrate a wide range of irritation responses to lauryl sulfate.[43]

Finally, people with a known allergy must avoid exposure to the allergen. Listing the ingredients in all cosmetic and over-the-counter drug products sold in the USA facilitates this process. If there are any questions, especially about a fragrance component, the lotion manufacturer can be contacted. The names of the contact persons for each major US manufacturer are listed in the 'CTFA on Call' book. This is distributed annually to all members of the American Academy of Dermatology.

How consumers use the product

Usually consumers do not misuse hand and body lotions in such a way that they harm themselves. Most lotions are relatively mild to the eyes and are not usually toxic when ingested. However, it is advisable to contact the manufacturer or Poison Control Center in case of a question.

Predicting adverse skin effects

Primary dermal irritation

Erythema occurs when the concentration of an irritant and the time and conditions of skin exposure exceed critical threshold levels. Redness is usually localized to the exposure site. It may occur rapidly after the first exposure to an acute irritant or after several applications of a weaker or cumulative irritant. Diagnostically, irritation is frequently differentiated from sensitization reactions by factors such as

- the composition and dose of the product;
- if the response occurs after the first usage;
- its rapid onset after usage;
- the type and spreading of the reaction.

Lotion manufacturers routinely probe for this type of information when consumers complain concerning an adverse reaction, and may utilize a dermatologist to diagnose or follow up as appropriate. Ingredients that could cause primary irritation in lotions are anionic or cationic surfactants used as emulsifiers.

A sensitive method to assess and differentiate lotions based on their primary dermal irritation potential is the 21-day cumulative irritation test (21-day Cum).[44] Panelists are randomly selected from a general population. The product is applied under an occlusive patch for 24 hours. The patch is removed, and the site is evaluated for irritation using a 0, . . . , 3 scale. This process is repeated for 21 consecutive days, with patches remaining in place over the weekend. The cumulative irritation score in a panel of 10–25 subjects is a measure of primary irritation potential. The mean cumulative score per panelist for most lotions is low – less than 5 out of a possible 63. Subsequently, Berger and Bowman[45] developed a 14-day modification of this test. They demonstrated similar product trends at 14 and 21 days, but with less damage and tape reaction.

An alternative method utilizes the induction phase of the human repeated-insult patch test (HRIPT) as a measure of irritation potential. Although this test's primary purpose is to identify sensitizing ingredients or products, it begins with an induction phase. The induction phase can be used to assess primary irritation potential of lotions. During induction, usually more than 100 panelists are occlusively patched with the product for 24–48 hours over a three-week period. Since the irritation response is assessed before a new patch is applied to the test site, this methodology resembles the 21-day cumulative irritation test. The Draize modification, in which patches are applied for 48 hours and are removed shortly before scoring and repatching, is especially appropriate, since it does not give the skin time to recover. After the induction phase, the panel is rested. Two weeks later, panelists are challenged by patching with the product at the original and at a naive site.

Damaged skin may be more readily irritated than 'normal' skin. This has been confirmed epidemiologically for occupations that involve repeated hand washings, such as nurses and kitchen workers; they have significantly higher rates of hand dermatitis than those who do not do 'wet' work (e.g. clerical workers).[46] Atopy also increases the risks of occupational dermatitis. Such effects can be modeled. For instance, Freeman and Maibach[47] showed a greater TEWL response on skin repatched with lauryl sulfate two weeks after the initial insult, even though the skin appeared normal. This suggested that there was a level of subclinical or 'invisible dermatitis' still present at the cellular level. Indeed, Kligman[48] reported that patching with 0.5% lauryl sulfate can cause spongiosis even though the skin's surface appears normal.[48] Typically, subclinical levels of skin damage are caused by cold winter weather, repeated exposure to detergent solutions (i.e. 'wet' work), or physical microtrauma. Recently, it has been suggested that the use of ancillary cosmetic or cleansing products can cause subthreshold levels of irritation. Subsequent application of a second product such as a lotion may elevate the irritation above the threshold, resulting in observable irritation.[49]

To examine the role of the stratum corneum in preventing irritation, Frosch and Kligman[50] developed a model. The stratum corneum is mechanically damaged by scratching with a needle, and then is occlusively patched for three consecutive days. They showed that damaging the stratum corneum barrier reduced the concentration of water soluble compounds required to cause irritation: 10-fold for sodium lauryl sulfate to 50-fold for nickel salts. The threshold concentration to cause irritation by lipophilic irritants such as triclosan or fatty acids was reduced less than 6-fold by this method.

The final approach to assess the irritation potential of a product on a vulnerable group is to have individuals from that group (e.g. atopics or lactic acid stingers) use the product under exaggerated conditions.

Sensory irritation

This type of irritation is more common than many people realize. It may cover several different mechanisms, such as subclinical irritation, and low-level contact urticaria, as well as effects like lactic acid stinging. Frosch and Kligman[42] examined many ingredients for their potential to cause facial stinging; they showed that 5% lactic acid and sunscreens such as PABA had the potential to cause facial stinging in approximately 15% of the population. It is unclear what the rate of reaction would be on other parts of the body. Undoubtedly, it would be lower. More recently, Christensen and Kligman[51] showed that damaging the skin by repeated facial washing with soap will enhance the stinging response. Low levels of cinnamic aldehyde (0.01%) have been used to cause tingling in chewing gum. At higher concentrations, it can produce visible contact urticaria and, with repeated exposure, sensitization.

Sensitization

Delayed (type IV) contact hypersensitivity

Typically, dermatologists are most familiar with this type of adverse reaction. From 1979 to 1983, the North American Contact Dermatitis Group (NACDG) reported that 60% of adverse reactions to cosmetic products observed by the group were allergic in nature.[41] This differs from epidemiological data that indicate that most adverse reactions are due to irritation.[52] This difference may reflect the greater intensity and duration of allergic reactions that would require medical intervention. The leading allergens identified by the NACDG found in cosmetics are fragrances and preservatives (Table 24.4).

Sensitization to ingredients may occur more readily on damaged or irritated skin. Previously, the parabens had developed a reputation as potential sensitizers. However, this may be due to their use to preserve medicants for dermatitic skin. The parabens will penetrate the damaged stratum corneum more readily and be more available to induce

Table 24.4 Ingredients that are the principal causes of sensitization reactions in cosmetics (data from Adams and Maibach[41])

Ingredient	Number of positive reactions (total = 379)	
Fragrance	161	
Preservative	149	
Lanolin and derivatives	29	
Sunscreen	20	

Fragrance component	**Number of positive reactions (total = 161)**	
Unspecified	67	
Cinnamic aldehyde or alcohol	23	
Eugenol and isoeugenol	15	
Hydroxycitronellal	11	
Musk ambrette	11	

Preservative component	**Number of positive reactions (total = 149)**	
Quaternium 15	65	
Imidazolidinyl urea	21	
Parabens (unspecified)	19	
Formaldehyde	16	
Sorbic acid	6	

Data from later NACDG studies

Cosmetic ingredient	Percent positive reactions (US: 1985–1989)[60]	Percent positive reactions (US: 1984–1985)[61]
Quaternium 15	6.2	6.7
Diazolidinyl urea (in petrolatum)	1.4	Not reported
Imidazolidinyl urea (in petrolatum)	1.5	Not reported
Cinnamic alcohol	4.8	2.7
Cinnamic aldehyde	3.1	5.9
Lanolin alcohols	1.5	1.2

sensitization reactions.[53] Recent epidemiological data have shown the parabens to have a relatively low sensitization rate compared with other preservatives.

Preservatives Lotion manufacturers prefer to avoid potential allergens by excluding them from products. When this is not possible, such as in selecting effective preservatives, the least sensitizing product that ensures microbiological integrity is utilized. The preservatives frequently used in US products are listed in the ingredients section in this chapter.

Fragrances There is a fragrance industry organization, RIFM (Research Institute for

Fragrance Materials), that evaluates the safety of individual components. It recommends if a component should not be used and if there is a maximum usage level. Most major US manufacturers follow these or even more stringent guidelines.

Sensitization testing

After reviewing the proposed ingredients for potential allergens, lotion manufacturers utilize the HRIPT to confirm experimentally that the products do not sensitize. This testing involves occlusively patching a panel of over 100 individuals from the general population with a lotion for up to three weeks. After a two-week rest period, the panelists are challenged with a 24–48-hour patch, and the response is evaluated.[54] If the responses at challenge are greater than during the induction phase, are long-lasting (increasing in the 48 hours after patch removal) or spread beyond the patch site, there is a possible sensitization that should be investigated further. The sensitivity of the test can be enhanced by pre-damaging the stratum corneum with sodium lauryl sulfate.[55] This method, known as the maximization test, is not often used, as it gives many false-positive results.

Acnegenesis and comedogenesis

These two terms are frequently used interchangeably, although they likely represent different biological events. Acnegenesis is the occurrence of breakouts, blackheads and whiteheads – especially on the face but also on the back. Frequently, there is a strong inflammatory component that is not observed in comedogenesis. Inflammation is due to *Propionibacterium acnes* proliferation and the body's immune response to this. Lesions seem to appear rapidly, although formation of the initial hyperkeratotic plug may occur subclinically over a longer period.

Comedogenesis was originally the term given to the formation of large hyperkeratotic impactions due to exposure to chlorinated hydrocarbons. Such exposure can result from industrial accidents such as in Searveso, Italy. These comedones do not have an inflammatory component, are larger and develop more slowly than facial acne.

The interchangeably of the terms arose from two factors. The first is mechanistic – both events involve the formation of hyperkeratotic plugs. Secondly, the models for assessing comedone formation – the rabbit ear test and comedone formation on the human back – are more convenient than for acnegenesis.[56,57] This enables many products and ingredients to be readily assessed and claims to be made that a product is non-comedogenic. Comedogenic materials include branched and unsaturated fatty acids and esters.

However, combining these ingredients into products may modify their comedogenic potential. In contrast, the test method for acnegenicity requires a panel of at least 40 normal and acne-prone subjects to use a product on their faces for at least six weeks. A non-acnegenic product will not significantly increase the level of acne over this test period.[58] This is a more expensive test than patching, since only one product can be tested by each panelist at one time.

Contact urticaria

Clinically defined contact urticaria is often characterized by the rapid formation of wheals or flares – frequently within an hour of exposure to a causative agent. This can be caused through either an immunological or a non-immunological pathway. However, the exact molecular and cellular mechanisms are not well understood.

Potential urticants that may occur in cosmetic products include the preservative benzoic acid and fragrance components (cinnamic aldehyde and balsam of Peru). It should be stressed that the incidences of reaction to these ingredients are not known, so their epidemiological importance is not clear. At lower concentrations, many urticants can produce sensory irritation (especially itching or tingling), without observable clinical signs. von Krogh and Maibach[59] proposed a cascade of increasing rigorous testing for contact urticaria. It must be stressed that this testing (especially invasive scratch or prick testing) should be carried out by an experienced physician who has resuscitation apparatus readily available.

Photoreactions

The interaction of UV radiation with certain ingredients can cause chemical changes that produce irritation or allergic reactions. Usually, products are tested only if they contain ingredients that absorb UV light. These include sunscreens and fragrances, although fragrance ingredients that cause photoallergy and phototoxicity have been identified by RIFM and are not used by most lotion manufacturers. Predictive test methods involve application of the test material to the skin, then exposure to UV radiation. A parallel site has the product applied, but is not exposed to UV light. This accounts for normal irritation or sensitization.

Use testing to assess adverse reactions

It is apparent from the discussion above that there are many causes of adverse reactions that consumers describe as 'irritation'. In normal usage, any of these reactions may occur. The reaction rate depends not only on the product's composition and the consumer's skin condition, but also on how the product is used. This last factor can only be determined when a consumer uses a product. Thus the best way of assessing how a product effects a population is to analyze data from a usage test on target consumers. Such tests require a panel size of 75 or more, since the adverse reaction rate is low. For those panelists who do experience an adverse reaction, follow-up is appropriate. This may include a questionnaire to better understand the symptoms and their causes, and in a few cases diagnostic testing. Diagnostic tests include exaggerated usage such as the repeated open application test (ROAT).[63] For contact urticaria, von Krogh and Maibach[59] suggested a cascade of open application on normal skin, then slightly affected skin, followed by open then occlusive patching on slightly or previously affected skin. Whealing or erythema and edema indicate contact urticaria. If indicated, diagnostic patch testing for suspected allergic reactions should be run. All the diagnostic testing should be run by a dermatologist experienced in these issues.

Eye irritation

Accidental exposure of hand and body lotions to the eyes does occur, since a sizable minor-ity of consumers use these products on their faces. As with skin irritation, pre-marketing safety assessment has two major steps. First, there is a review of the ingredients' toxicological profiles – is this ingredient an eye irritant, and at what concentration will it be used? Secondly, there is testing. Traditionally, the Draize test in rabbits has been used to assess irritation potential. Recently, this has been supplemented and in many cases superseded by predictive in vitro methods. These include the chorioallantoic membrane vascular assay (CAMVA) in hen's eggs, which models damage to the conjunctiva, and the bovine corneal opacity and permeability test (BCOP), which models corneal damage. Cell culture is also used. Human test methods such as direct eye instillation under the direction of an ophthalmologist may be used, but these are more common for facial care products.

REFERENCES

1. Wall LM, Gebauer KA, Occupational skin disease in Western Australia. *Contact Dermatitis* 1991; **24**: 101–5.
2. Halkier-Sorensen L, Notified occupational skin diseases in Denmark. *Contact Dermatitis* 1996; **35**(Suppl 1): 1–35.
3. Takano S, Yamanaka M, Okamoto K, Saito F, Allergens of lanolin: parts I and II. *J Soc Cosmet Chem* 1983; **34**: 99–125.
4. Ghadially R, Halkier-Sorensen L, Elias PM, Effects of petrolatum on stratum corneum structure and function. *J Am Acad Dermatol* 1992; **26**: 387–96.
5. Kligman AM, Regression method for assessing the efficacy of moisturizers. *Cosmetics and Toiletries* 1978; **93**: 27–35.
6. Elias PM, Brown BE, Ziboh VA, The permeability barrier in essential fatty acid deficiency: evidence for a direct role for linoelic acid in barrier function. *J Invest Dermatol* 1980; **74**: 230–3.
7. Prottey C, Hartop PJ, Press M, Correction of the cutaneous manifestations of essential acid deficiency in man by application of sunflower seed oil to the skin. *J Invest Dermatol* 1975; **64**: 228–34.

8. Froebe CL, Simion FA, Ohlmeyer H et al, Prevention of stratum corneum lipid phase transition in vitro by glycerol – an alternative mechanism for skin moisturization. *J Soc Cosmet Chem* 1990; **41**: 51–65.

9. Mattai J, Froebe CL, Rhein LD et al, Prevention of model stratum corneum lipid phase transitions by cosmetic additives – differential scanning calorimetry, optical microscopy and water evaporation studies. *J Soc Cosmet Chem* 1993; **44**: 89–100.

10. Rawlings A, Harding C, Watkinson A et al, The effect of glycerol and humidity on desosome degradation in stratum corneum. *Arch Dermatol Res* 1995; **287**: 457–64.

11. Stiller MJ, Bartolone J, Stern R et al, Topical 8% glycolic acid and 8% L-lactic acid creams for the treatment of photodamaged skin. *Arch Dermatol* 1996; **132**: 631–6.

12. Imokawa G, Asasaki S, Kawamata A et al, Water retaining function in the stratum corneum and its recovery properties by synthetic pseudo-ceramides. *J Soc Cosmet Chem* 1989; **40**: 273–85.

13. Imokawa G, Abe A, Jin K et al, Decreased level of ceramides in stratum corneum of atopic dermatitis: An etiologic factor in atopic dry skin. *J Invest Dermatol* 1991; **96**: 523–6.

14. DiNardo A, Sugino K, Wertz P et al, Sodium lauryl sulfate (SLS) induced irritatant contact dermatitis: a correlation study between ceramides and in vivo parameters of irritation. *Contact Dermatitis* 1991; **35**: 86–91.

15. Elias PM, Holleran WM, Mennon GK et al, Normal mechanisms and pathophysiology of epidermal permeability barrier homeostatis. *Curr Opin Dermatol* 1993; 231–7.

16. Sah A, Mukherjee S, Wickett RR, Effects of product structure and formulation on delivery of AHA to skin. *J Soc Cosmet Chem* 1997; **48**: 55–6.

17. Prall JK, Theiler RF, Bowser PA, Walsh M, The effectiveness of cosmetic products in alleviating a range of dryness conditions as determined by clinical and instrumental techniques. *Int J Cosmet Sci* 1986; **8**: 159–74.

18. Boisits EK, Nole GE, Cheney MC, The refined regression method. *J Cutan Aging Cosmet Dermatol* 1989; **1**: 155–63.

19. Grove GL, Skin surface hydration changes during a mini regression test as measured in vivo by electrical conductivity. *Curr Ther Res* 1992; **52**: 556–61.

20. Grove GL, Jackson R, Czernielewski MD, Tuley M, Poster presentation at the 53rd Annual Meeting of the American Academy of Dermatology, 1995.

21. Appa Y, Hemingway L, Orth DS et al, Poster presentation at the 53rd Annual Meeting of the American Academy of Dermatology, 1995.

22. Highley DR, Savoyka VO, O'Neil JJ, Ward JB, A stereomicroscopic method for the determination of moisturizing efficacy in humans. *J Soc Cosmet Chem* 1976; **27**: 351–63.

23. Hannuksela A, Kinnunen T, Moisturizers prevent irritant dermatitis. *Acta Derm Venereol (Stockh)* 1992; **72**: 42–4.

24. Potts RO, Stratum corneum hydration: experimental techniques and interpretation of results. *J Soc Cosmet Chem* 1986; **37**: 9–33.

25. Kajs TM, Gartstein V, Review of the instrumental assessment of skin: effects of cleansing products. *J Soc Cosmet Chem* 1991; **42**: 249–71.

26. Frosch PJ, Kligman AM (eds), *Non-Invasive Methods for the Quantification of Skin Functions.* New York: Springer-Verlag, 1993.

27. Serup J, Jemec GBE (eds), *Handbook of Non-Invasive Methods and the Skin.* Boca Raton, FL: CRC Press, 1995.

28. Berardesca E, Elsner P, Wilhelm K-P, Maibach HI (eds), *Bioengineering of the Skin: Methods and Instrumentation.* Boca Raton, FL: CRC Press, 1995.

29. Barel AO, Clarys P, Measurement of epidermal capacitance. In: *Handbook of Non-Invasive Methods and the Skin* (Serup J, Jemec GBE, eds). Boca Raton, FL: CRC Press, 1995:165–70.

30. Tagami H, Measurement of electrical conductance and impedance. In: *Handbook of Non-Invasive Methods and the Skin* (Serup J, Jemec GBE, eds). Boca Raton, FL: CRC Press, 1995:159–64.

31. Distante F, Berardesca E, Transepidermal water loss. In: *Bioengineering and the Skin: Methods and Instrumentation* (Berardesca E, Elsner P, Wilhelm K-P, Maibach HI, eds). Boca Raton, FL: CRC Press, 1995:5–12.

32. Morrison BM, Scala DD, Comparison of instrumental methods of skin hydration. *J Toxicol Cut Ocular Toxicol* 1996; **15**: 305–14.

33. Loden M, Lindberg M, The influence of a single application of different moisturizers on the skin capacitance. *Acta Derm Venereol (Stockh)* 1991; **71**: 79–82.

34. Agache PG, Twistometry measurement of skin elasticity. In: *Handbook of Non-Invasive Methods and the Skin* (Serup J, Jemec GBE, eds). Boca Raton, FL: CRC Press, 1995:319–28.

35. Barel AO, Courage W, Clarys P, Suction methods for measurement of skin mechanical properties: the cutometer. In: *Handbook of Non-Invasive Methods and the Skin* (Serup J, Jemec GBE, eds). Boca Raton, FL: CRC Press, 1995:335–40.

36. Elsner P, Skin elasticity. In: *Bioengineering and the Skin: Methods and Instrumentation* (Berardesca E, Elsner P, Wilhelm K-P, Maibach HI, eds). Boca Raton, FL: CRC Press, 1995:53–64.

37. Omata S, Terunuma Y, New tactile sensor like the human hand and its applications. *Sensors and Actuators* 1992; **35:** 9–15.

38. Schatz H, Altmeyer PJ, Kligman AM, Dry skin and scaling evaluated by D-Squames and image analysis. In: *Handbook of Non-Invasive Methods and the Skin* (Serup J, Jemec GBE, eds). Boca Raton, FL: CRC Press, 1995:153–7.

39. Meilgaard M, Civielle GV, Carr BT, *Sensory Evaluation Techniques*. Boca Raton, FL: CRC Press, 1987.

40. Smithies RH, Moisturization claims challenged through the NAD. *J Toxicol Cut Ocular Toxicol* 1992; **11:** 205–11.

41. Adams RM, Maibach HI, A five year study of cosmetic reactions. *J Am Acad Dermatol* 1985; **13:** 1062–9.

42. Frosch PJ, Kligman AM, A method of apprising the stinging capacity of topically applied substances. *J Soc Cosmet Chem* 1977; **28:** 197–210.

43. Basketter DA, Griffiths HA, A study of the relationship between susceptibility to skin stinging and skin irritation. *Contact Dermatitis* 1993; **29:** 185–9.

44. Phillips L, Steinberg M, Maibach HI, Akers WA, A comparison of rabbit and human skin response to certain irritants. *Toxicol Appl Pharmacol* 1972; **21:** 369–82.

45. Berger RS, Bowman JP, A reappraisal of the 21-day cumulative irritation test in man. *J Toxicol Cut Ocular Toxicol* 1982; **1:** 109–15.

46. Nilsson E, Mikaelsson B, Andersson S, Atopy, occupation and domestic work as risk factors for hand eczema in hospital workers. *Contact Dermatitis* 1985; **13:** 216–23.

47. Freeman S, Maibach HI, Study of irritant contact dermatitis produced by repeated patch testing with sodium lauryl sulfate and assessed by visual methods, transepidermal water loss and laser doppler velocimetry. *J Am Acad Dermatol* 1988; **19:** 496–501.

48. Kligman AM, The invisible dermatoses. *Arch Dermatol* 1991; **127:** 1375–82.

49. Lee CH, Maibach HI, Study of cumulative contact irritant contact dermatitis in man utilizing open application on subclinically irritated skin. *Contact Dermatitis* 1994; **30:** 271–5.

50. Frosch PJ, Kligman AM, The chamber scarification test for irritancy. *Contact Dermatitis* 1976; **2:** 314–24.

51. Christensen M, Kligman AM, An improved procedure for conducting lactic acid stinging tests on facial skin. *J Soc Cosmet Chem* 1996; **47:** 1–11.

52. de Groot AC, Nater JP, van der Hende R et al, Adverse effects of cosmetics and toiletries: a retrospective study in a general population. *Int J Cosmet Sci* 1988; **9:** 255–9.

53. Jackson EM, Paraben paradoxes. *Am J Contact Dermatitis* 1993; **4:** 69–70.

54. Marzulli FN, Maibach HI, Contact allergy predictive testing in humans. In: *Dermatolotoxicology*, 4th edn (Marzulli FN, Maibach HI, eds). New York: Hemisphere, 1991:415–39.

55. Kligman AM, Epstein W, Updating the maximization test for identifying contact allergens. *Contact Dermatitis* 1975; **1:** 231–9.

56. Morris WE, Kwan SC, Use of the rabbit ear model in evaluating the comedogenic potential of cosmetic material. *J Soc Cosmet Chem* 1983; **34:** 215–25.

57. Mills OH, Kligman AM, Human model for assessing comedogenic substances. *Arch Dermatol* 1982; **118:** 903–5.

58. Strauss JS, Jackson EM, American Academy of Dermatology Invitational Symposium on Comedogenicity. *J Am Acad Dermatol* 1989; **20:** 272–7.

59. von Krogh C, Maibach HI, The contact urticaria syndrome. *Semin Dermatol* 1982; **1:** 59–66.

60. Nethercott JR, Holness DL, Adams RM et al, Patch testing with a routine screening tray in North America: 1985 to 1989. I. Frequency of response. *Am J Contact Dermatitis* 1991; **2:** 122–9.

61. Storrs F, Rosenthal LE, Adams RM, et al, Results of patch tests in North America 1983–1985. *J Am Acad Dermatol* 1989; **20:** 1038–44.

62. Simion FA, Babulak SW, Morrison BM et al, Experimental method for soap induced dryness in the absence of erythema. Poster presentation at the 49th Annual Meeting of the American Academy of Dermatology, 1991.

63. Hannuksela M, Sensitivity of various skin sites in the repeated open application test. *Am J Contact Dermatitis* 1991; **2:** 102–4.

25

Infrared irradiation: Skin effects and protection

Kenneth D Marenus, Daniel H Maes

INTRODUCTION

The solar electromagnetic spectrum is a continuum of wavelengths ranging from ultraviolet (UV, 280 nm) to infrared (IR, >700 nm). Exposure of the skin to energy of these wavelengths can cause both specific and some generalized responses. It is the purpose of this chapter to review these responses and then to discuss what can be done, in practical terms, to prevent them.

Figure 25.1 illustrates the electromagnetic spectrum. It is important to note that even though there are arbitrary definitions, such as the one dividing UV-A from UV-B, this spectrum is composed of a range of energies of specific wavelengths. It is always seductive to view these phenomena in terms of experiential associations (i.e. visible light or heat), but in fact, for the purposes of biochemical and clinical studies, it is far better to remain within the conceptual framework of a continuum of energies of defined wavelength.

Much is known about the effects of UV-B and UV-A on skin. Less is known about the impact of IR and even still less about visible light. Since approximately 40% of the energy impinging on the Earth's surface is in wavelengths greater than 700 nm,[1] it is important that the effects of this energy be given careful consideration.

Studies of the effects of IR and the effect of IR + UV have been conducted. The results of these studies clearly lead to two general conclusions. First, the type of damage inflicted by IR alone is very similar to that imposed by UV-B. This would include everything from dermal elastosis to skin cancer. Second, IR can add to UV-B-induced damage in much the same way that UV-A adds to UV-B damage.

In terms of IR alone, it has long been recognized that chronic exposure to elevated temperatures can result in an increased number of cancerous lesions. The classic example of thermal skin cancer is described in an epidemiological study by Cross[2] in elderly Irish

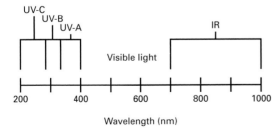

Figure 25.1 The electromagnetic spectrum.

women who worked at home and spent long hours in front of peat fires. Another IR syndrome, erythema ab igne, described by Findlayson et al,[3] demonstrates that the effects of IR can be distinct from those of other wavelengths, but result in similar morphological changes.

The first definitive work demonstrating the epidermal and dermal effects of chronic IR was that of Kligman.[4] After exposing guinea pigs to a defined regimen of IR or IR + UV-B for a period of 45 weeks, it was clear that the general dermal damage from IR alone resembled that of UV. An IR elastosis, of distinct morphology somewhat different from UV-induced elastosis, was observed.

According to Kligman, like UV, the IR caused an early increase in elastic fiber deposition, which was cumulative with time. In addition to the normal thickening of the fibers, dense accretions of fine feathery fibers were also seen. The study also points out that there was a general increase in acid mucopolysaccharides as well as epidermal hyperplasia in response to IR, much like that observed after chronic UV exposure.

In another study by Juhlin et al,[5] panelists were exposed to a moderate degree of heat (38°C) from an IR lamp for a period of one hour. When raised blisters were made and the exudate examined, there was a significant increase in free arachidonic acid as well as assorted prostaglandins (PGE2, PGD2, PGF2a and 6-oxo-PGF1a). These results further suggest that the mechanism of IR damage is similar to that of UV. Finally, work by Sauder[6] has indicated that interleukin-1 (IL-1) can be produced as a result of thermal injury.

In the Estée Lauder laboratories, extensive effort has been made to understand the effect of IR at the cellular as well as the clinical levels. Numerous in vitro experiments with human dermal fibroblasts and human keratinocytes have been conducted. The results of these studies serve to reinforce the concept that the mechanisms involved in IR damage to skin are much the same as those of UV.

Table 25.1 Release of arachidonic acid at 24 hours in keratinocytes and fibroblasts in response to IR

Condition	Fibroblasts	Keratinocytes
Control (37°C)	2%	13%
Heat (45°C/60 min)	198%	55%
IR with heat (45°C/60 min)	210%	66%
IR without heat (37°C/60 min)	183%	34%

Specifically, in studying the effects of IR on these two cell populations, it is clear that fibroblasts are more sensitive than keratinocytes to equivalent doses of IR. One set of studies examined the effects of heat (45°C), IR exposure combined with heat (45°C), IR exposure without increased heat (37°C) and a control. Cells were prelabeled with [³H]arachidonic acid, and the release of this marker was taken as an indication of membrane perturbation, as demonstrated previously with UV exposure by DeLeo et al.[7] The results are illustrated in Table 25.1. They indicate that

- keratinocytes are somewhat resistant to IR and heat perturbation;
- the response of the fibroblasts appeared to be independent of the stimulus; that is, the response was independent of the type of stimulus.

The relative resistance of the keratinocytes to perturbation by IR also suggests a protective role of these cells for fibroblasts in skin. Recent work has shown that within the keratinocyte there is a system of 'heat shock' or stress proteins. Upon exposure to IR, these proteins (e.g. HSP 72) are synthesized and are then available to play a role in downregulating the cell's response to the heat stimulus.[8] In fact, pretreating keratinocytes with heat can result in a reduction in the number of UV-B-induced apopototic (sunburn) cells.[9] Investigations into the functional aspects of this unique heat-induced cellular protective system promise to provide interesting discoveries in the near future.

A second series of experiments was conducted using the same in vitro system to evaluate the role of UV in combination with IR. In these experiments, the cells were exposed to low doses of UV and IR separately, and the same low doses of UV and IR together.

The amount of arachidonic acid was followed over a 24-hour time period as well as the amount of lactic dehydrogenase release, an indication of cytoplasmic disruption, at 24 hours. Figures 25.2 and 25.3 illustrate the results. It is clear in both cases that the low doses of UV-B and IR separately were not adequate to provoke a response, while the combination of IR and UV-B at the same low dose did stimulate release of arachidonic acid as well as lactic dehydrogenase. These results confirm in vitro what had been observed by Kligman and others histologically – namely that there is an additive response to the combination of UV and IR. In practical terms, this means that sunscreen products that only protect from UV are only doing part of the job.

CLINICAL RESULTS

Similar studies were conducted in a clinical panel. In these studies, markers of IR effect were determined. The results indicated that erythema as well as capillary blood flow were responsive to both UV and IR as stimuli. In these experiments, after giving panelists low doses of either UV or IR, limited increases in both blood flow and erythema were observed. When these same low doses of IR and UV were administered simultaneously, it was apparent that the effects of each type of irradiation were additive. Figures 25.4 and 25.5 illustrate the results obtained from a panel of 20 panelists. Again, the importance of the additive contribution of these wavelengths to skin damage is apparent.

IR PROTECTION

It is clear from both the clinical as well as the in vitro studies that IR can contribute significantly as a form of actinic skin damage. It can contribute as an additive effect with UV, and it can contribute on its own. Not only is it clear that IR can create damage, but the

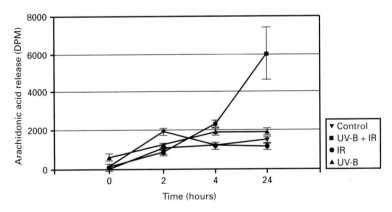

Figure 25.2 The release of arachidonic acid from keratinocytes irradiated with either UV-B or IR was insignificant at the lower doses and at all time points. The combined low dose of UV-B and IR, however, caused a significant increase in the release of arachidonic acid at 24 hours.

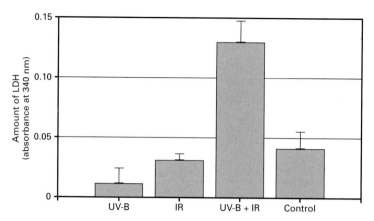

Figure 25.3 At 24 hours, release of lactate dehydrogenase (LDH) in keratinocytes treated with low-dose UV-B or IR was not significantly higher than controls. UV-B and IR administered simultaneously caused a significant release of this enzyme.

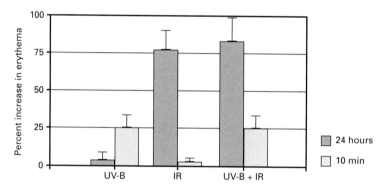

Figure 25.4 Immediately after irradiation, UV-B has no effect on skin redness. After 24 hours, an erythema was visible but did not meet the criteria defining a MED (minimal erythemal dose). Immediately after irradiation, sites treated with IR alone and IR + UV-B both developed significant erythema. The site treated with IR + UV-B had a higher degree of erythema than the site treated with IR alone. Equivalent erythema developed at 24 hours on the sites treated with UV-B and IR + UV-B.

mechanism by which it occurs is also clear. Like UV, when even a low dose of IR interacts with the skin, it evidently triggers the series of events known as the 'inflammatory cascade'. It is this series of reactions, beginning with activation of phospholipase A2 and ending with the production of variety of bioactive intermediates such as the prostaglandins and leukotrienes, that is common to many types of skin stimuli. It is important to understand the mechanism of IR action on the skin, because only in this way is it possible to design products that can prevent it.

There are two basic approaches to protection of the skin from IR: either by the use of physical blocks externally or the use of bioactive blocks internally.

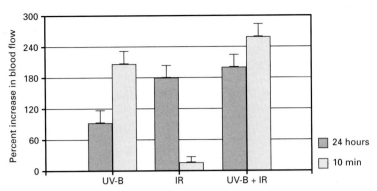

Figure 25.5 UV-B caused an immediate increase in blood flow, which increased further after 24 hours. IR also caused a greater increase immediately, but this had mostly disappeared within 24 hours. The combination of UV-B + IR resulted in a significant increase in blood flow, which was sustained for 24 hours.

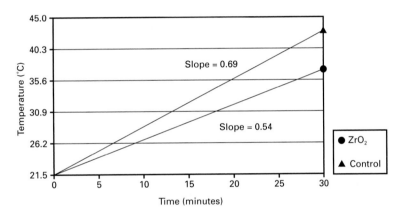

Figure 25.6 Water-heating rates in covered dishes with and without ZrO_2 paste. The lower heating rate in the dish with ZrO_2 indicates the ability of scattering elements to reduce thermal heating.

Sunscreens with physical blocks

A first approach is to simply block as much IR as possible from hitting the skin. This may be accomplished with significant amounts of physical blockers such as titanium or zirconium oxides. Figure 25.6 illustrates the reduction in heating rates that can occur owing to the presence of a thin film of ZrO_2. It is clear that even a small amount of this type of block can do a lot to reduce the amount of IR entering the skin.

Clinical studies have been conducted to evaluate the ability of sunscreen products based on ultrafine TiO_2 to provide protection from IR as well as UV-B and UV-A. In these experiments, panelists were exposed to an IR bulb at three sites with a total dose of $37\,J/cm^2$ at 800 nm. Both erythemal development as well as increases in capillary blood flow were monitored as markers of IR-induced activity in the skin.

On each of the panelists, one site served as an untreated control and the other two were

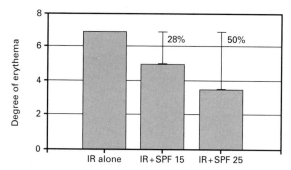

Figure 25.7 Demonstration of the ability of a TiO₂-based sunscreen to provide IR protection in a dose–response manner. Here, erythema in response to IR is reduced significantly.

treated with TiO₂-based sunscreens of SPF 15 and SPF 25 respectively. Figures 25.7 and 25.8 demonstrate the results of the study. It is clear from these figures that both erythema and capillary blood flow were significantly reduced on the TiO₂ sunscreen-treated sites. In addition there was a dose–response relationship between the amount of TiO₂ in the sunscreens and the degree of IR protection.

Antioxidants

As mentioned above, the mechanism of IR-induced damage involves the generation of inflammatory mediators such as PGE2 and IL-1α. There are many reports in the literature demonstrating the ability of antioxidants to prevent inflammation. In the Estée Lauder laboratories we have worked extensively to evaluate the ability of antioxidants to reduce UV-B-induced skin damage at many levels.[10] Since antioxidants such as vitamin E, vitamin C and BHT are effective at reducing UV damage and since this damage in part is mediated by the inflammatory cascade, it is not unreasonable to suppose that antioxidants would also be effective against IR-induced skin changes.

In another clinical study, volunteers were treated with a mixture of antioxidants, including vitamin E, vitamin C, BHT and nordihydroiguariaretic acid (NDGA). It is important to note that spectrophotometric analysis of this mixture in the vehicle indicated no direct UV or IR absorption by the material. Another site was treated with the vehicle only at the same dose of 2 mg/cm² and a third site served as an untreated control. The markers of IR damage, as before, were erythemal development and increases in capillary blood flow.

The results of the study are illustrated in Figures 25.9 and 25.10. It is clear from these results that the antioxidants were highly effective in preventing an IR-induced inflammatory response in the skin.

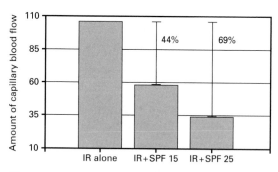

Figure 25.8 A TiO₂-based sunscreen provides IR protection in terms of preventing increases in capillary blood flow – an indication of inflammation.

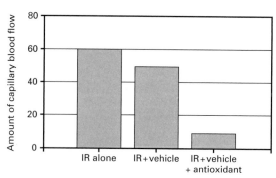

Figure 25.9 Effectiveness of a blend of common antioxidants in providing IR protection as demonstrated by prevention of an increase in capillary blood flow.

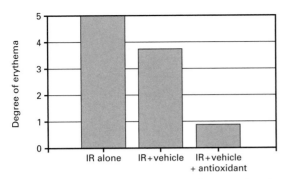

Figure 25.10 Antioxidants provide IR protection in terms of prevention of erythema.

SUMMARY

It is clear from many studies that the potential for skin damage from IR is significant. The type of damage that can occur ranges from elastosis to skin cancer. More research must be done in order to elucidate where the mechanisms of this damage may depart from those involved in UV. In addition, IR effects in terms of lipid perturbation in the stratum corneum may yield some insight into the barrier damage that often accompanies solar exposure.

Even though some are aware of this damage, few manufacturers of skin care products have made this a consideration when designing products. One particular class of products where IR protection is essential is in sunscreens. It is necessary to understand how to provide adequate and full-spectrum solar protection in these products so that the consumer is fully protected in the sun. This will be achieved to a greater extent, first, when the cosmetic industry learns how to best use the ingredients it currently has and, second, when even better solar protection materials are discovered.

ACKNOWLEDGEMENTS

The authors gratefully acknowledge the efforts of all those who have contributed to this work (in alphabetical order): Susan Jadlos, Tom Mammone, Neelam Muizzuddin and Scott Rothstein.

REFERENCES

1. Koller LR, *Ultraviolet Radiation*. New York: Wiley, 1965:105.
2. Cross F, On a turf (peat) fire cancer. Malignant change superimposed on erythema ab-igne. *Proc R Soc Med* 1967; **60:** 1307–8.
3. Findlayson GR, Sams WM Jr, Smith JG, Erythema ab-igne, a histopathologic study. *J Invest Dermatol* 1966; **46:** 104–7.
4. Kligman LH, Intensification of ultraviolet-induced dermal damage by infrared radiation. *Arch Dermatol Res* 1982; **272:** 229–38.
5. Juhlin L, Civier A, Shroot S, Hensby C, Effect of infrared irradiation on the recoverable levels of free arachidonic acid and prostaglandins in human forearm skin. *J Invest Dermatol* 1983; **81:** 297–300.
6. Sauder DN, Biologic properties of epidermal cell thymocyte-activating factor (ETAF). *J Invest Dermatol* 1985; **85:** 176s–82s.
7. DeLeo VA, Horlick H, Hanson D et al, Ultraviolet radiation induces changes in membrane metabolism of human keratinocytes in culture. *J Invest Dermatol* 1984; **83:** 323–6.
8. Murmatsu T, Hada H, Kobayashi N et al, Induction of 72 kD heat shock protein in organ-cultured normal human skin. *J Invest Dermatol* 1992; **98:** 786–90.
9. Maytin E, Wimberly J, Kane K, Heat shock modulates UV-B induced cell death in human epidermal keratinocytes: evidence for a hyperthermia-inducible protective response. *J Invest Dermatol* 1994; **103:** 547–53.
10. Pelle E, Marenus K, Maes D, Antioxidant protection against ultraviolet light induced skin damage. *In: Oxidative Stress in Dermatology* (Fuchs J, Packer L, eds). New York: Marcel Dekker, 1993:127–40.

26

Efficacy of sunscreens

Nicholas J Lowe

INTRODUCTION

The incidence of sunlight-induced skin aging and skin cancers has been increasing in many parts of the world. In particular, the incidence of melanoma skin cancer has shown a well-documented increase in several continents over the last several years.[1]

Many authorities are recommending primary prevention programs to reduce cutaneous photodamage and skin carcinogenesis. An integral component of these programs is the use of protective clothing[2] and effective sunscreens.[3,4]

Most modern sunscreens have highly efficient absorption or reflecting capabilities throughout ultraviolet B (UVB), partly ultraviolet A (UVA) and, in some instances, infrared wavelengths. Over the last several years, more efficient sunscreening ingredients have been developed for improved skin protection.[5–8]

More recently, direct evidence has been derived, from a large population study in Australia, of the effectiveness of sunscreens in their ability to reduce the incidence of solar keratoses.[4]

This chapter will review the protectiveness of sunscreens and assays that predict their levels of protection.

HISTORY OF SUNSCREENS

In 1928, the world's first commercial sunscreen – an emulsion of benzyl salicylate and benzyl cinnamate – was developed in the United States. In the 1930s, a phenyl salicylate appeared on the Australian market. In 1935, lotions of quinine oleate and quinine bisulfate were available in the United States. In 1943, *p*-aminobenzoic acid (PABA) was patented, introducing this popular agent and subsequently its derivatives. The US military used red petrolatum, a physical blocking agent, as a sunblock during World War II. A variety of other UV-filtering agents, including glycerol–PABA, 2-ethylhexyl salicylate, digalloyl trioleate, homomenthyl salicylate and dipropylene glycol salicylate, were subsequently developed.[5] Most of the early agents were directed toward UVB, the portion of the solar spectrum responsible for the most obvious effect, the familiar sunburn.

Parsol 1789 (avobenzone or 4-t-butyl-4'-methoxydibenzoylmethane), an agent broadly effective against the UVA spectrum, is now marketed in combination with UVB-blocking agents. These formulations provide broad-spectrum chemical sun protection to the US consumer.[6,7]

Micronized reflecting powders have more

recently been made available from a variety of manufacturers. Unlike traditional physical blockers, micronized reflecting powders are less visible, yet provide broad-spectrum protection against UV radiation.

Antioxidants such as tocopheryl acetate and vitamin C products are also being incorporated with sunscreens as putative free-radical scavengers.

EVALUATION OF SUNSCREENING AGENTS

Evaluation of sunscreen protection factor

The US Food and Drug Administration (FDA) approved technique to assess the efficacy of a sunscreen against sunburn is determination of the sunscreen protection factor (SPF).[8] The SPF is defined as the ratio of the time of UV exposure necessary to produce minimally detectable erythema in sunscreen-protected skin to that time for unprotected skin.

A typical testing protocol is as follows. Skin in a non-exposed area, such as the buttocks or lower back, is covered with lightproof adhesive foil; $1 \, cm^2$ areas of foil are removed sequentially so that each area receives a defined dose of UVB. The following day, the patient returns to be examined, and the areas are assessed for erythema. The amount of exposure necessary to generate uniform but barely detectable erythema is determined.

The following day, sunscreen is applied uniformly with a pipette at $2 \, mg/cm^2$ or $2 \, \mu l/cm^2$. The sunscreen is allowed to dry for 15 minutes, and then the subject is irradiated for incrementally increasing times, based on the estimated SPF, which is usually determined spectrophotometrically. The volunteer is asked to return again 24 hours later, at which time the skin is re-examined. The SPF is then calculated from the ratio of the protected MED to the unprotected MED.[8]

There is some controversy about whether SPF thus defined accurately reflects the action spectra for induction of skin cancer in humans. Also, application of $2 \, mg/cm^3$ correlates with using at least 29.6 ml (1 oz) over the body's surface. Since studies have revealed that most individuals apply about 22.2 ml (0.75 oz, $1.5 \, mg/cm^2$ or $1.5 \, \mu l/cm^2$), the usage SPF may be significantly less than the listed in vivo SPF.[9]

It is also important to recognize that the SPF is a measure of UVB plus UVA protection, provided that a suitably filtered xenon arc solar simulator is used. For SPF assays we use a 1000 W xenon-arc solar simulator (Oriel) and a 2 mm thick Schott WG 320 nm filter plus a UG 11 filter.

Evaluation of protection against UVA

Currently, there is no consensus regarding an ideal in vivo assay to assess protection against UVA. The UVB spectrum readily causes erythema, and can be used for the SPF assay;[8] UVA can cause erythema, but only after a much larger dose. However, the action spectra for other UVA-induced phenomena (e.g. photosensitivity dermatitis, photoaging, and development of melanoma and non-melanoma skin cancer) are not specifically defined. A variety of different assays have been described for evaluation protection against UVA.[10]

Phototoxic protection factor

The phototoxic protection factor (PPF) was developed to try to decrease the UVA dose necessary to achieve a detectable difference in erythema.[6] This involves sensitizing the subject's skin with 8-methoxypsoralen (8-MOP) either topically or orally, and then comparing the MED, as for UVB sunscreen testing. This is a reliable assay, with clearly defined visual erythema, but can result in long-term pigmentation of skin sites.[6] This has a minimal risk for the volunteers, because each skin site is irradiated only once.

UVA erythema protection factor

The UVA erythema protection factor (APF) is defined analogously to SPF, and assesses the time to induce erythema in UVA-exposed skin. The reliability of such testing is of some question because of the inadequacy of current filters and the long deviation of irradiance with many solar simulators. However, Cole and Van Fossen[11] have described a high-intensity UVA source that they contend is a more effective method to assess UVA protection based on either erythema or tanning in an unsensitized individual.

We have also evaluated this assay using a 1000 W xenon-arc solar simulator (Oriel) filtered with 2 mm thick WG 345 nm plus UG 11 filters. We find the assay to be reproducible, and it can also be used for evaluating water-resistant sun protection against UVA.

Pigment-darkening protection factor

Immediate pigment darkening (IPD), a UVA and visible spectrum-mediated transient oxidation of pre-existing melanin, has also been used to evaluate UVA sunscreen efficacy.[12] This method has been criticized because it must be performed on individuals with darker skin, since pale-skinned individuals – who are the most in need of protection – do not demonstrate easily measurable IPD.[13]

The delayed pigment-darkening response evaluated 2 hours after UVA radiation may be more reproducible.[14] We have also investigated this assay. It requires more UVA energy than for IPD, but it is more reproducible, and is practical with a greater variety of skin phototypes than the ID assay.

In vitro transmission protection factor

The transmission protection factor is defined as the ratio of the photocurrent measured by a spectroradiometer through Transpore TM tape (3M Company, St Paul MN) to the photocurrent measured through sunscreen-coated tape at a given wavelength. According to Diffey and Robson,[15] this in vitro method provides close agreement with in vivo recorded SPF data. Other techniques include spectrophotometrically comparing sunscreen applied to either a quartz crystal or excised epidermis.

SUBSTANTIVITY

Substantivity is the characteristic of a sunscreen that reflects how effectively the advertised degree of protection is maintained under adverse conditions, including repeated water exposure of sweating. According to the US FDA, a sunscreen is declared water-resistant if it can maintain its original SPF after two 20 minute immersions. A sunscreen is very water-resistant if it retains its protective integrity after four 20 minute immersions.[8] Substantivity is of enormous importance, because sunscreens are used outdoors in settings where abundant sweating and repeated immersion in water is common.

ACTIVE SUNSCREEN INGREDIENTS (Table 26.1)

Protectants against UVB

p-Aminobenzoic Acid

p-Aminobenzoic acid (PABA) has been available since 1943, and was popular in the 1950s and 1960s. Nowadays, PABA is used infrequently as a sunscreen for a variety of reasons. Its absorption peak at 296 nm is relatively far from the UVB-induced erythema peak at 307 nm. It is poorly soluble in water, and must be used as a 5–15% solution in alcohol. After application, PABA penetrates the stratum corneum effectively, where it is trapped and remains bonded by hydrogen bonding to epidermal proteins. This greatly enhances its substantivity, but also increases the risk of contact or photocontact dermatitis. Sensitivity of this sort is seen in up to 4% of the population.[16] It can cause a stinging sensation when applied and stains both cotton and synthetic fabrics. After photo-oxidation, this can leave a permanent yellow discoloration. PABA is no longer commonly used in sunscreens.

Table 26.1 FDA-approved sunscreen ingredients in the United States (1997)

Chemical	Approved (%)
UVA absorbers	
Oxybenzone	2–6
Sulisobenzone	5–10
Dioxybenzone	3
Methyl anthranilate	3.5–5
Avobenzone	2–3
UVB absorbers	
Aminobenzoic acid (PABA)	1–5
p-Amyldimethyl PABA (padimate A)	1–3
2-Ethoxyethyl-p-methoxcinnamate	8–10
Digalloyl trioleate	2–5
Ethyl 4-bis(hydroxypropyl)aminobenzoate	1–5
2-Ethylhexyl 2-cyano-3,3-diphenylacrylate	7–10
2-Ethylhexyl p-methoxycinnamate	2–7.5
2-Ethylhexyl salicylate	3–5
Glyceryl p-aminobenzoate (glyceryl PABA)	2–3
Homomenthyl salicylate	4–25
Lawsone with dihydroxyacetone	0.25% with 3%
Octyldimethyl PABA (padimate O)	1.4–8
2-Phenylbenzimidazole-5-sulfonic acid	1.4
Triethanolamine salicylate	5–12
Physical blockers ⎫	
Red petrolatum ⎬	30–100
Titanium dioxide ⎭	

PABA derivatives

PABA esters are created by the addition of hydrocarbon groups to the PABA molecule. Many of these molecules are improvements over PABA, in that they are water-soluble and do not penetrate the stratum corneum. In the past, the most widely used of the PABA derivatives was padimate O, or octyldimethyl PABA, although it is now employed in few current sunscreens.

Salicylates

The salicylates are *ortho*-distributed aromatic compounds with a peak absorption of about 300 nm. Two compounds of this type, octyl salicylate and homomenthyl salicylate (homosalate), are currently approved in the United States. Although not very effective as sunscreens, they have the benefit of being exceptionally stable, essentially nonsensitizing and water-insoluble, leading to high substantivity. They are also useful as solubilizers of other poorly soluble sunscreen ingredients, such as the benzophenones.

Cinnamates

2-Ethylhexyl-*p*-methoxycinnamate (Parasol MCX; absorption maximum 310–311 nm), 2-ethoxyethyl-*p*-methoxycinnamate and octyl methoxycinnamate are available in the United States. These are effective in blocking UVB, but have poor substantivity and are generally found in combination with other agents. Cinoxate, the cinnamate most often seen with other cinnamates, is found in balsam of Tolu, coca leaves and cinnamon oil.

Protectants against UVA

Benzophenones

Benzophenones are aromatic ketones that absorb predominantly in the UVA portion of the spectrum, between 320 and 350 nm. For example, oxybenzone has an absorption maximum of 326 nm in polar solvents, compared with 352 nm in nonpolar solvents. Benzophenone-3 (sulisobenzone) and dioxybenzone are also approved for the US market. Oxybenzone is frequently implicated as the etiologic agent in photocontact allergy, although reactions have also been reported with dioxybenzone.[16,17]

Dibenzoylmethanes

Dibenzoylmethanes are substituted diketones that undergo keto–enol tautomerism on absorption of UV radiation. The keto forms have a UV absorption maximum of 260 nm, whereas the enol forms absorb above 345 nm. Parasol 1978 (avobenzone or 4-t-butyl-4'-methoxydibenzoylmethane), with an absorption maximum at 355 nm, is the only agent of this class available in the United States.

Although these compounds are capable of a high degree of UV absorption,[8] they are unstable and can undergo photoisomerization to compounds that are not protective. Parsol 1789 suffers a loss of protective power through photodegradation.[18] Even Parsol 1789 does not provide significant protection against UVA radiation close to 400 nm.[6]

Photoinstability of sunscreens

Concerns have recently been expressed about the stability of certain sunscreen ingredients when exposed to sunlight. Some examples of photo-unstable sunscreen filters include combinations of Parsol 1789 and octyl-methoxycinnamate. The formulation and the choice of other active ingredients are of key importance in stabilizing some filters, for example Parsol 1789 stabilized with Mexoryl.

PHYSICAL BLOCKERS

Physical blocking agents, such as zinc oxide, titanium dioxide, iron oxide, kaolin, ichthammol, red veterinary petrolatum, talc $(MgSiO_x)$, and calamine are composed of particles of a size that scatter, reflect or absorb solar radiation in the UV, visible and even infrared ranges. Twenty percent zinc oxide, 20% titanium dioxide as well as 1% iron oxide have been spectrophotometrically demonstrated to reduce transmittance in the UVA and visible ranges to a maximum of approximately 20%. The combination of the zinc and iron oxides is synergistic, effectively reducing transmittance in the UVA and visible ranges to as low as 1.5%.

Older physical blockers had the disadvantage that they were comedogenic, had to be applied in a relatively thick layer, and melted in the sun, staining clothing. They were opaque and therefore visible, making them cosmetically undesirable for many individuals.

Recently developed micronized preparations now available in the United States provide an excellent option within this class of sunscreens. Micronized physical blockers are suspensions of finely ground material, such as titanium dioxide, that reflect at wavelengths shorter than the visible spectrum. Because they do not reflect in the visible spectrum, they are invisible and thus more cosmetically acceptable. Micronized titanium dioxide is chemically stable and does not cause any photoallergic or contact dermatitis.

Micronized sunscreens are more effective at the shorter UV wavelengths. A major difficulty in formulating micronized sunscreens is preventing agglomeration of the particles. If this occurs, the portion of the spectrum reflected will shift into the visible range and the product will have characteristics of traditional opaque physical blockers.

SYSTEMIC PHOTOPROTECTION

Over the years, a variety of systemic agents have been investigated as oral agents for sunscreening purposes. The appeal is threefold. First, oral agents are convenient. Second, they provide coverage for the entire body. Finally, oral agents are likely to eliminate the concern over substantivity so critical for topically applied products. Included in the list of these products are PABA, antihistamines, aspirin, indomethacin, retinol, ascorbic acid and α-tocopherols (i.e. vitamins A, C and E), corticosteroids, psoralens, β-carotene, and antimalarials. The last three are used in some individuals afflicted with certain photosensitivity dermatoses.

SUNSCREEN: CLINICAL USAGE AND EFFICACY

Sun protection for normal skin

It is well established that prolonged exposure to UVB leads to deleterious effects on human skin, including photoaging and non-melanoma skin cancers (NMSC). We recommend that patients use sunscreens, depending on their skin phototype as described in Table 26.2.

Additionally, all individuals should be encouraged to stay indoors or seek shade during the peak hours of solar radiation flux from 10 a.m. to 2 p.m. A hat or a sun visor is a useful addition. Patients with pale complexions should be reassured that 'fair' skin is attractive. Those who insist on darker skin should use a self-tanning lotion containing dihydroxyacetone (DHA). Tanning salons should be avoided, since intense UVA exposure provides limited protection, and induces photoaging and photoallergic responses.

Persons who spend a significant amount of time outdoors, particularly in areas of high solar flux, should be cautious about the immediate and long-term risks from UV exposure, and should be advised about how to properly protect themselves. Such individuals include naturalists, skiers, hikers, bicyclists, fishermen, mountain climbers and gardeners, as well as members of certain professions (e.g. farmers and farm workers, lifeguards and postal delivery persons).

Finally, this information should be disseminated to children at an early age. Childhood is typically the time of life when maximal sun exposure occurs. Childhood sunburns are implicated in increasing risk for malignant melanoma and NMSC, and thus should be avoided assiduously. It has been calculated biostatistically that if children consistently used an SPF 15 sunscreen through to the age of 18, the occurrence of NMSC could be reduced by 78%.

Table 26.2 Skin types and suggested sunscreen protection factors				
			Suggested SPF	
Type	Characteristic	Examples	Routine day	Outdoor activity
I	Always burns easily, never tans	Celtic or Irish extraction; often blue eyes, red hair, freckles	15	25–30 (waterproof)
II	Burns easily, tans slightly	'Fair-skinned' individuals; often have blond hair	12–15	25–30 (waterproof)
III	Sometimes burns, then tans gradually and moderately	Most Caucasians	8–10	15 (waterproof)
IV	Burns minimally, always tans well	Hispanics and Asians	6–8	15 (waterproof)
V	Burns rarely, tans deeply	Middle Easterners, Indians	6–8	15 (waterproof)
VI	Almost never burns, deeply pigmented	Blacks	6–8	15 (waterproof)

Sunscreen protection against actinic keratoses

In previous animal studies, sunscreens possessing an SPF of 15 or greater were found to be capable of reducing the incidence of cutaneous preneoplasia and neoplasia.[4]

In a recent investigation of a large population of Australians, the daily use of a sunscreen that contained a combination of 8% 2-ethylhexyl-*p*-methoxycinnamate and 2% avobenzone (which had an SPF of 17) resulted in a significant reduction in the number of new actinic keratoses appearing in the sunscreen-protected population, compared with the placebo-cream control population.[4] This study was conducted in 588 individuals over one Australian summer. It confirmed the importance of daily sunscreen protection and the ability of human skin to undergo apparent repair during sunscreen protection. The reversal of epidermal dysplasia suggests that the daily use of effective sunscreens should be an important part of any community program for reduction of UV-induced skin carcinogenesis and aging.

Drug photosensitive skin reactions

There is a special need for photoprotective measures, including sunscreens and sun-protective clothing. Because the action spectra for many photosensitive reactions or photosensitive disease lie within the UVA, sunscreens are needed that efficiently protect individuals from these UV wavelengths. Table 26.3 lists drugs that can precipitate a photosensitive skin reaction.

Phototoxicity reactions

Phototoxicity can occur in any individual exposed to photosensitive agents and radiant energy of sufficient intensity. The action spectra usually involves UVA, and it is wise to use a broad-spectrum sunscreen as well as removing the offending phototoxic agent.

Table 26.3 Agents that may cause photosensitivity

Anticancer drugs
  Dacarbazine (DTIC-Dome)
  Fluorouracil (Fluoroplex; and others)
  Methotrexate (Mexate; and others)
  Procarbazine (Matulane)
  Vinblastine (Velban)
Antidepressants
  Amitriptyline (Elavil; and others)
  Amoxapine (Asendin)
  Desipramine (Norpramin: Pertofran)
  Doxepin (Adapin; Sinequan)
  Imipramine (Tofranil; and others)
  Isocarboxazid (Marplan)
  Maprotiline (Ludiomil)
  Nortriptyline (Aventyl; Pamelor)
  Protriptyline (Vivactil)
  Trimipramine (Surmontil)
Antihistamines
  Cyproheptadine (Periactin)
  Diphenhydramine (Benadryl; and others)
Antimicrobials
  Antifungals (Fentichlor, Multifungin, Jadit)
  Demeclocycline (Declomycin; and others)
  Doxycycline (Vibramycin; and others)
  Griseofulvin (Fulvicin-U/F; and others)
  Methacycline (Rondomycin)
  Minocycline (Minocin)
  Nalidixic acid (Negram)
  Oxytetracycline (Terramycin; and others)
  Sulfacytine (Renoquid)
  Sulfadoxine-pyrimethamine (Fansidar)
  Sulfaguanidine
  Sulfamethazine (Neotrizine; and others)
  Sulfanilamide
  Sulfapyridine
  Sulfasalazine
  Sulfathiazole
  Sulfisoxazole (Gantrisin; and others)
  Tetracycline (Achromycin; and others)
Antiparasitic drugs
  Bithionol (Bitrin)
  Chloroquine (Aralen)
  Hydroxychloroquine
  Pyrvinium pamoate (Povan)
  Quinine
  Oxybenzone
  PABA esters
  p-Aminobenzoic acid
Others
  Amiodarone (Cordarone)
  Bergamot oil, oils of citron, lavender, lime, sandalwood, cedar (used in many perfumes and cosmetics; also topical exposure to citrus rind oils)

Contd

Table 26.3 Continued
Benzocaine
Captopril (Capoten)
Carbamazepine (Tegretol)
Chlordiazepoxide (Librium)
Coal tar and derivatives (containing acridine, anthracene, naphthalene, phenanthrene phenols, thiophene)
Contraceptives, oral (Norethynodrel)
Cyclamates (calcium cylcamate, sodium cyclohexylsulfamate)
Antipsychotic drugs
Chlorpromazine (Thorazine; and others)
Chlorprothixine (Taractan)
Fluphenazine (Pernitil; Prolixin)
Haloperidol (Haldol)
Perphenazine (Trilafon)
Sulfamethizole (Thiosulfil; and others)
Sulfamethoxazole (Gantanol; and others)
Sulfamethoxazole–trimethoprim (Bactrim; Septra; and others)
Thiothixene (Navane)
Trifluoperazine (Stelazine; and others)
Triflupromazine (Vesprin)
Trimeprazine (Temaril)
Diuretics
Acetazolamide (Diamox)
Amiloride (Midamor)
Bendroflumethiazide (Naturetin; and others)
Benzthiazide (Exna; and others)
Chlorothiazide (Diuril; and others)
Cyclothiazide (Anhydron)
Furosemide (Lasix)
Hydrochlorothiazide (HydroDIURIL; and others)
Hydroflumethiazide (Diucardin; and others)
Methyclothiazide (Aquatensen; Enduron)
Metolazone (Diulo; Zaroxolyn)
Polythiazide (Renese)
Quinethazone (Hydromox)
Thrichlormethiazide (Methahydrin; and others)
Hypoglycemics
Acetohexamide (Dymelor)
Chlorpropamide (Diabinese; Insulase)
Glipizide (Glucotrol)
Glyburide (DiaBeta; Micronase)
Tolazamide (Tolanase)
Tolbutamide (Orinase; and others)
Nonsteroidal anti-inflammatory drugs
Benoxaprofen (Oraflex)
Ketoprofen (Orudis)
Piperacetazine (Quide)
Prochlorperazine (Compazine; and others)
Promethazine (Phenergan; and others)
Thioridazine (Melleril)

Table 26.3 Continued
Naproxen (Naprosyn)
Phenylbutazone (Butazolidin; and others)
Piroxicam (Feldene)
Sulindac (Clinoril)
Sunscreens
6-Acetoxy-2,4-dimethyl-*m*-dioxane (preservative in sunscreens)
Benzophenones
Cinnamates
Diethylstilbestrol
Disopyramide (Norpace)
Dyes (acridine, acriflavine, anthraquinone, eosin, erythrocine, fluorescein, methylene blue, methyl violet, orange red, rose bengal, toluidine blue, trypaflavin, trypan blue)
Furocoumarins; psoralens (trioxsalen, methoxsalen, psoralen)
Gold salts (Myochrysine; Solganal)
Hexachlorophene (pHisoHex; and others)
Isotretinoin (Accutane)
6-Methylcoumarin (used in perfumes, shaving lotions, and sunscreens)
Mestranol
Musk ambrette (used in perfumes)
Quinidine sulfate and gluconate
Saccharine
Tattoo dye (red or yellow cadmium sulfide)

Many plants produce photoactive substances, such as furocoumarins (particularly psoralens), that can induce phototoxic reactions (Table 26.4). This particular category of phototoxic reactions is termed *phytophotodermatitis*. It has been noted in vegetable pickers and other food handlers, as well as naturalists. Flower leis given to visitors in Hawaii have also been implicated.

Phytophotodermatitis is commonly exploited by dermatologists as part of a therapeutic regimen to control psoriasis and to repigment the skin of persons with vitiligo. Patients are administered psoralens either topically or orally, and are then exposed to controlled doses of UVA as photochemotherapy.

Psoralens in combination with UVA

Table 26.4 Common plants and lichens causing photodermatitis

Common name	Botanical name	Family
Lime	*Citrus aurantifolia*	Rutaceae
Citron	*Citrus medica (C. acida)*	Rutaceae
Bitter orange	*Citrus aurantium*	Rutaceae
Lemon	*Citrus limon*	Rutaceae
Bergamot	*Citrus bergamia*	Rutaceae
Gas plant; burning bush	*Dictamnus albus (D. fraxinella)*	Rutaceae
Common rue	*Ruta graveolens*	Rutaceae
Persian lime (Tahitian)	*Citrus aurantifolio, "Persian"*	Rutaceae
	Phebalium argenteum	
Cow parsley, wild chervil	*Anthriscus sylvestris*	Umbelliferae
Celery	*Apium graveolens*	Umbelliferae
Giant hogweed	*Heracleum mantegazzianum*	Umbelliferae
Parsnip (garden variety)	*Pastinaca sative (P. urens)*	Umbelliferae
Cow parsley	*Heracleum sphondylium*	Umbelliferae
Parsnip (wild parsnip)	*Heracleum giganteum*	Umbelliferae
Fennel	*Foeniculum vulgare*	Umbelliferae
Dill	*Anethum graveolens*	Umbelliferae
	Peucedanum ostruthium	Umbelliferae
Wild carrot, garden carrot	*Daucus carota*	Umbelliferae
Masterwort	*Peucedaum ostruthium*	Umbelliferae
	Ammin majus	Umbelliferae
Angelica	*Angelica archangelica*	Umbelliferae
Figs	*Ficus carcia*	Umbelliferae
Milfoil, yarrow	*Achillea millefolium*	Composiate
Stinking mayweed	*Anthemis cotula*	Composiate
Buttercup	*Ranunculus* spp.	Ranunculaceae
Mustard	*Brassica* spp.	Cruciferae
Bind weed	*Convolvulus arvensis*	Convolvulaceae
Agrimony	*Agrimonia eupatoria*	Rosaceae
Goose foot	*Chenopodium* spp.	Cheopodiaceae
Scurfy pea, bavchi	*Psoralea corylifolia*	Leguminosae
St John's wort	*Hypericum perforatum*	Hypericaceae
	Hypericum crispum	Hypericaceae
	Schinopsis quebrachocolorado	
Red quebracho	*Schinopsia lorentzii*	Anacardiaceae
Lichens	*Parmelia* spp.	Lichen (symbiotic
	Hypogymnia spp.	association between
	Pseudovernia spp.	fungi and algae)
	Cladonia spp.	commonly grouped
	Platismatia spp.	with fungi
	Physcia spp.	
	Umbilicaria spp.	
	Cetrania spp.	

increase the risk of development of NMSC. Therefore it is important to protect patients with UVB- and UVA-protecting sunscreens following PUVA phototherapy sessions.

Photoallergy reaction

Photoallergy involves interaction of the immune system and solar radiation. Photoallergic reactions are rare, and are usually triggered by UVA exposure. Individuals with these disorders have previously been exposed to the responsible agent, and, after re-exposure to it and UV radiation, develop the dermatitis. Because UVA is most often responsible, it is important to use an effective UVA sunscreen product.[6]

Photosensitivity skin disorders

Photodermatoses include several disorders. Since afflicted persons are extremely sensitive to the sun, it is essential to provide them with efficacious sunscreens and sun-protective clothing.

Polymorphous light eruption (290–365 nm)

Polymorphous light eruption (PMLE) is a common, idiopathic skin eruption that occurs in susceptible individuals on exposure to solar irradiation that is more intense than usual. It affects 10–14% of the white population, most of them female, with onset usually in the first three decades of life. Typically, PMLE manifests as some combination of pruritic papules, mascules, vesicles, plaques or confluent erythema 1–2 days (2 hours to 5 days) after sun exposure on areas of unprotected skin. It is seen most commonly at the beginning of summer or during a visit to a geographic clime with a higher solar flux. The reaction resolves over 7–10 days if additional sun exposure is avoided. As the name suggests, the reaction is polymorphic, although, in a given individual, it is usually a single morphology that remains constant.

Investigators have variously implicated UVA, UVB, UVC, visible radiation, X-rays, and even α-particles in the action spectrum. Often, PMLE flares can be prevented by using newer broad-spectrum sunscreens.

It must be kept in mind that sunscreens that provide modest UVA protection (e.g. benzophenones) are poorly effective for those who suffer with PMLE. More UVA protective sunscreens containing agents such as Parsol 1789 are often effective. Many patients benefit from prophylactic PUVA photochemotherapy, whereas others respond to oral agents, including antimalarials or β-carotene.

For some, it may be necessary to avoid the sun entirely and to wear effective sun-protective clothing.

Porphyrias (400–410 nm)

Porphyrias are caused by an inherited or acquired abnormality in the heme metabolic pathway. Substrates for the effected enzyme accumulate, leading to the clinical manifestations. There are a wide variety of porphyrias because of the complexity of heme biosynthesis.

Photosensitivity begins in childhood on sun-exposed areas, with the acute development of vesicles, bulae, and hyperpigmentation or hypopigmentation. The skin is also more sensitive to trauma than is normal. Chronically, the skin scars atrophically, with mutilating deformities of exposed areas, including cicatrizing alopecia.[20] The action spectrum is in the visible range from 400 to 410 nm (Soret band), and thus these unfortunate individuals must be protected by a physical blocking agent or by adequate clothing. Some sufferers do respond to oral β-carotene.

Solar urticaria (290–515 nm)

Solar urticaria is a rare, rapidly developing reaction to sun or UV exposure. Minutes after exposure, sensitive individuals develop pruritus, followed by the urticaria and erythema. The reaction quickly runs its course, rarely lasting longer than 24 hours.

Persons with this syndrome encompass different subsets. Some produce a serum factor that, after inoculation into a normal subject, transiently permits induction of solar urticaria in the recipient. This group appears to generate an immunoglobulin of the IgE class, which causes the reaction. These subjects can rightfully be classified among those with photoallergies. Others cannot transfer the reaction passively, and the mechanism for the development of solar urticaria is unknown.

Antihistamines are effective at high doses in a few patients. Maintenance solar exposure and PUVA therapy have also been used successfully in some. Patients should be phototested to determine the wavelengths that promote their reaction, and then provided with a protective sunscreen. Alternatively, or additionally, they may be instructed to avoid the sun whenever possible.

Chronic actinic dermatitis (290 nm–visible)

Chronic actinic dermatitis encompasses the gamut of disease previously described as chronic photosensitivity dermatosis, and manifests initially as erythematous macules and plaques in sun-exposed areas, including the face, exposed areas of scalp, rim of the ears, back of the neck, forearms and back of the hands. Over time, this leads to superimposed areas of edema and vesiculation during acute flares. Clinical evaluation in these patients should be conducted by phototesting across a broad portion of the UV and visible spectrum.

Histologically, the skin initially resembles a contact dermatitis, but can progress with actinic reticuloid to the pattern of a cutaneous T-cell lymphoma. The portion of the spectrum causing the reaction varies from one person to another. Therefore phototesting and careful selection of sunscreens or avoidance of the sun are mandated in the management of these patients. Treatment options include oral azathioprine, PUVA, with or without prednisone, etretinate, and cyclosporin.[21]

Persistent light reaction (290–400 nm)

Most patients who develop a chemical photosensitivity dermatitis note that their reaction resolves within a week or two if the offending agent is eliminated. A subset of individuals continue to overreact to the sun in spite of careful avoidance of the putative photosensitizer.

This condition is called persistent light reaction, and sometimes resolves in months, although it may persist indefinitely. For some persons, the reaction is so severe that it results in a generalized exfoliate dermatitis. Histologically, the tissue shows a dense perivascular round cell infiltrate.

In some cases, the mechanism of this reaction is ongoing exposure to some chemical that is not correctly identified and eliminated.

In other instances, the offending agent has bonded to dermal proteins in such a way that it cannot be eliminated. Often the reaction is idiopathic. The action spectrum may be in the UVB, and UVA is common. Phototesting to determine appropriate protective sunscreens and avoidance of the sun are usually effective in minimizing flares.

Lupus erythematosus (290–330 nm)

Cutaneous lupus erythematosus (LE) occurs in two broad forms: discoid LE and subacute cutaneous LE. The lesions of discoid LE are typically found on the head and neck, and are well-defined, variably sized scaly patches that heal leaving atrophy, scarring and pigmentary changes. Subacute cutaneous LE manifests as papulosquamous or polycyclic lesions around the neck, the outer aspects of the arms, and the trunk. These lesions are more mild than discoid LE, and heal without scarring or atrophy. Although UVB appears to be more prominent in LE, UVA also plays a role in some individuals.[22]

Interestingly, exacerbations of noncutaneous lupus (e.g. nephritis) are sometimes seen after sun exposure. Therefore it is necessary to provide these patients with broad-spectrum sunblock and encourage them to avoid the sun. Oral antimalarials, such as chloroquine, have been used with limited success. Recently, an open-label trial of a broad-spectrum sunscreen containing padimate O and avobenzone reduced the clinical severity of cutaneous LE over a 4-week period.[22]

Xeroderma pigmentosum (290–340 nm)

The autosomal recessive disorder xerodermic pigmentosum (XP) stems from a genetic defect in the ability to repair DNA. Patients are subject to premature development of skin neoplasms, including malignant melanoma as well as basal cell and squamous cell carcinoma.

Patients should aim for careful protection against the sun and vigilant detection of skin cancer. Eye protection should also be emphasized.

Albinism

Oculocutaneous albinism is an autosomal recessive defect in the formation of melanosomes. Although melanocytes are present, these individuals are either hypomelanotic or amelanotic in the skin and hair. Patients living in areas of high solar flux uniformly develop premalignant (i.e. actinic keratoses) or malignant (i.e. nonmelanoma skin cancer) skin lesions by early adulthood if they are not careful to apply sunscreen and avoid unnecessary sun exposure. Melanoma is rare, although the reason for this is unclear.

CONCLUSIONS

A relation between UVB exposure and the development of basal cell and squamous cell carcinoma has been documented. It appears likely that high-dose exposure to UV radiation increases the risk of development of malignant melanoma. Prolonged exposure to either UVA or UVB increases the rate of skin aging.

Development continues of new, highly effective sunscreens of both the traditional chemical kind and newer micronized physical blockers. Meanwhile, physicians may benefit their patients most by discouraging sun exposure and encouraging prudent and regular use of sunscreens.

ACKNOWLEDGEMENT

Part of this chapter has been adapted, with permission, from Friedlander J, Lowe NJ, In: *Sunscreens, Development, Evaluation and Regulatory Aspects* (Lowe NJ, Shaath N, Pathak M, eds). New York: Marcel Dekker, 1997.

REFERENCES

1. Scotto J, Fears TR, Fraumeni JF, *Incidence of Non-Melanoma Skin Cancer in the United States*. Washington, DC: US Department of Health and Human Services Publication, 1983:82–2433.

2. Sayre RM, Lowe NJ, Scientific poster presentation at the American Academy of Dermatology Meeting, December 1992.

3. Stern RS, Sunscreen use and non-melanoma skin cancer. In: *Sunscreens, Development, Evaluation and Regulatory Aspects* (Lowe NJ, Shaath N, eds). New York: Marcel Dekker, 1990:85–92.

4. Thompson SC, Jolley D, Marks R, Reduction of solar keratoses by regular sunscreen use. *N Engl J Med* 1993; **329:** 1147–51.

5. Shaath NA, Evolution of modern sunscreen chemicals. In: *Sunscreens, Development, Evaluation and Regulatory Aspects*, 2nd edn (Lowe NJ, Pathak M, Shaath N, eds). New York: Marcel Dekker, 1997:3–35.

6. Lowe NJ, Dromgoole SH, Sefton J et al, Indoor and outdoor efficacy testing of a broad spectrum sunscreen against ultraviolet. A radiation in psoralen-sensitized subjects. *J Am Acad Dermatol* 1987; **17:** 224–30.

7. Lowe NJ, USA photoprotection. In: *Sunscreens, Development, Evaluation and Regulatory Aspects* (Lowe NJ, Shaath N, eds). New York: Marcel Dekker, 1990:459–68.

8. Griffin ME, Bourget TD, Lowe NJ, Sunprotection factor determination in the United States. In: *Sunscreens, Development, Evaluation and Regulatory Aspects*, 2nd edn (Lowe NJ, Shaath N, Pathak M, eds). New York: Marcel Dekker, 1997:499–512.

9. Gotlieb A, Borget T, Lowe NJ, Sunscreens: effects of amounts of application of sun protection factors. In: *Sunscreens, Development, Evaluation and Regulatory Aspects*, 2nd edn (Lowe NJ, Shaath N, Pathak M, eds). New York: Marcel Dekker, 1997:583–600.

10. Lowe NJ, Ultraviolet A claims and testing procedures for OTC sunscreen. In: *Sunscreens, Development, Evaluation and Regulatory Aspects*, 2nd edn (Lowe NJ, Shaath N, Pathak M, eds). New York: Marcel Dekker, 1997:527–36.

11. Cole C, VanFossen R, Measurement of sunscreen USA protection; an unsensitized human model. *J Am Acad Dermatol* 1992; **26:** 178–84.

12. Kaidbey KH, Barnes A, Determination of USA protection factors by means of immediate pigment darkening in normal skin. *J Am Acad Dermatol* 1991; **25:** 262–6.

13. Agin PP, Stanfield JW, Letter. *J Am Acad Dermatol* 1992; **27:** 136–7.

14. Chardon A, Moyal D, Houseau C, Persistent pig-

ment darkening response. In: *Sunscreens, Development, Evaluation and Regulatory Aspects,* 2nd edn (Lowe NJ, Shaath N, Pathak M, eds). New York: Marcel Dekker, 1997:559–82.

15. Diffey BL, Robson JJ, A new substrate to measure sunscreen protection factors throughout the ultraviolet spectrum. *Soc Cosmet Chem* 1989; **40:** 127–33.

16. Dromgoole SH, Maibach HI, Contact sensitization and photocontact sensitization of sunscreening agents. In: *Sunscreens, Development, Evaluation and Regulatory Aspects* (Lowe NJ, Shaath N, eds). New York: Marcel Dekker, 1990:313–40.

17. Dromgoole SH, Maibach HI, Sunscreening agent intolerance: contact and photocontact sensitization and contact urticaria. *J Am Acad Dermatol* 1990; **22:** 1068–78.

18. Diffey BI, Stokes RP, Forestier S et al, Suncare product photostability. *Eur J Dermatol* 1997; **7:** 226–8.

19. Mosher DB, Fitzpatrick TB, Ortonne JP et al, Disorders of pigmentation. In: *Dermatology in General Medicine,* 3rd edn (Fitzpatrick TB et al,

eds). New York: McGraw-Hill, 1987.

20. Bickers DB, Pathak MA, The porphyrias. In: *Dermatology in General Medicine,* 3rd edn (Fitzpatrick TB et al, eds). New York: McGraw-Hill, 1987:1660–715.

21. Roelandsts RJ, Chronic actinic dermatitis. *J Am Acad Dermatol* 1993; **28:** 290–94.

22. Callen JP, Roth DE, McGrath MA, Dromgoole SH, Safety and efficacy of a broad spectrum sunscreen in patients with dixcoid or subacute cutaneous lupus erythematosus. *Cutis* 1991; **47:** 130–6.

Additional references

Sunscreen drug products for over the counter human use. Amendment to the tentative final monograph. *Fed Register* 61.180.48645–53341, 1996.

Marketing status of products containing avobenzene sunscreen drug products for over the counter human use. Amendment to the tentative final monograph. *Fed Register* 62.83.23350–23356, 1997.

27

The vulva

Peter Elsner, Howard I Maibach

ANATOMY AND PHYSIOLOGY OF THE VULVA AS RELATED TO COSMETOLOGY

Anatomy of the human vulva and of vulvar skin

The female external genital organs consist of the mons pubis, the labia majora, the labia minora, the clitoris and the glandular structures (Figure 27.1). The size and shape of

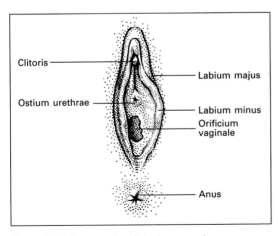

Figure 27.1 Topography of the human vulva.

these structures, their pigmentation and the distribution of hair show considerable variations, depending on hormonal status, pelvic architecture, race and age.[1]

Vulvar skin is not a biologically uniform entity. On the contrary, there are considerable anatomical and physiological differences between the skin covering the mons pubis, labia majora and labia minora, clitoris and perineum (Table 27.1). Even within the individual structures, there are differences between lateral and medial and anterior and posterior locations. Furthermore, vulvar skin is more influenced than other skin sites by occlusion (skin-to-skin and skin-to-garment), sweating, vaginal and urethral secretions, and mechanical trauma during sexual activity.

Age-dependent changes in vulvar skin are significant even though this skin is not subject to photoaging.[2] Rete ridges are missing until puberty. In the postpubertal woman, they gradually develop and increase in depth until menopause, when involution begins. The stratum corneum of labium majus skin increases in thickness with age, followed by post-menopausal atrophy.[3] Vulvar dermis shows elastotic degeneration similar to actinic damage in elderly women. While a stratum corneum is found at the lateral side of the labia minora in 100%, this is only true in two-

Table 27.1 Site-dependent anatomical characteristics of human vulvar skin

Anatomical structure	Type of epithelium	Sweat glands	Sebaceous glands	Terminal hair
Mons veneris	Cornified	+	+	+
Labia majora (lateral)	Cornified	+	+	+
Labia majora (medial)	Cornified	+	+	±
Labia minora (lateral)	Cornified	+	+	−
Labia minora (medial)	Cornified or mucous membrane	±	+	−
Perineum	Cornified	+	+	±

thirds for the medial side.[3] In specimens from healthy women below 20 years of age, a dermal inflammatory infiltrate is not observed, but it is a regular finding in menstruating women, with a maximum around the fourth or fifth decade, followed by gradual involution with age.[2] Plasma cells in limited numbers are regularly found in genital skin.

In vulvar swabs, parakeratotic cells are regularly observed – most frequently in the third and only very rarely in the eighth decade.[4,5] The frequency of parakeratotic cells seems to depend on the hormonal situation,[6] and it is decreased under topical testosterone therapy.[7]

PHYSIOLOGY OF VULVAR SKIN

Surface pH of vulvar skin

Vulvar skin surface pH is more than one unit higher than forearm pH (5.99 ± 0.45 compared with 5.02 ± 0.50).[8] Thus vulvar skin is like other intertriginous areas, which show pH values significantly higher than on non-occluded skin.[9] Occlusion seems to enhance stratum corneum ion permeability, thus neutralizing the normally acid skin surface. The higher skin surface pH of vulvar skin is an important cause of the high density of microbial colonization.

Barrier function of vulvar skin

Early work on transepidermal water loss (TEWL) as an indicator of barrier function of vulvar skin revealed the mean TEWL to be 1.45×10^3 µg water/cm^2/h, while that of the forearm was 7.7×10^2 µg water/cm^2/h ($p < 0.0001$).[10] Thus, the vulva appears far more permeable to water than the forearm. To eliminate possible eccrine sweat contamination, subjects received subcutaneous injections of atropine in both forearm and vulva test sites. The average mean forearm TEWL was 8.7×10^2 µg/cm^2/h and the vulvar TEWL was 1.4×10^3 µg/cm^2/h.[10]

Since TEWL may be influenced by anatomical or garment-related occlusion, TEWL of labia majora skin was studied over an extended period (Figures 27.2 and 27.3).[11] It was indeed found that vulvar TEWL decreased following de-occlusion. However, the stabilized final value was still significantly higher at the vulva than at the forearm. It should be noted that periodic bursts of markedly increased water loss were noted at vulvar test sites, but none in forearm sites (see Figure 27.2). It is unclear whether this increased emotional sweating in the vulva is simply a function of increased number of eccrine sweat glands in the vulva or an intrinsic property of vulvar tissue. Further studies

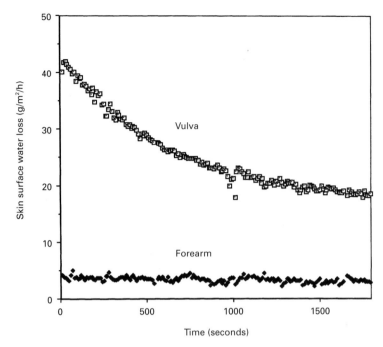

Figure 27.2 Long-term registration of transepidermal water loss (TEWL) of human vulvar skin.

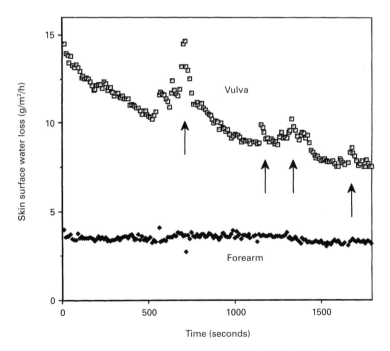

Figure 27.3 Long-term registration of TEWL of human vulvar skin. The spikes in the TEWL (arrows) represent sweating episodes.

using a topical drying chamber applied to vulvar skin over several days confirmed the increased intrinsic vulvar TEWL.[8] On the basis of these findings, the barrier function of vulvar skin seems to be imperfect compared with other body sites such as the forearm.

This was confirmed by dermatopharmacological data that showed a higher percutaneous penetration of hydrocortisone through vulvar skin compared with forearm skin.[12] The magnitude of the difference in percutaneous penetration between vulvar and forearm skin, however, is only 3–4-fold, compared with a more than 40-fold higher penetration in scrotal skin.

Irritant reactivity of vulvar skin

Impaired barrier function means less protection from the harmful effects of irritants and thus a higher proclivity to irritant dermatitis. Several studies have sought to determine whether vulvar skin is more or less susceptible to irritation from chemical agents in comparison with the ventral forearm.

Britz and Maibach[13] used two irritants, benzalkonium chloride (17%) and maleic acid (20%), for their ability to induce erythema without gross destruction of skin. These chemicals were applied at the labia majora and ventral forearm unoccluded. Vulvar skin was significantly more reactive than the forearm to these compounds. In addition, subjective complaints of burning and stinging were frequently noted with chemical application to the vulva, but not the forearm. In a number of studies, Elsner et al[14–16] investigated the effect of sodium lauryl sulfate (SLS), an anionic surfactant widely used in skin cleansing products, on vulvar compared with forearm skin. They patch-tested 20 healthy women, 10 before and 10 after menopause, with SLS for 24 hours. In forearm skin, irritant dermatitis developed in the majority of subjects. In vulvar skin, only 50% of the women developed irritant dermatitis. Postmenopausal women reacted less frequently and more slowly to SLS than premenopausal women in the forearm, whereas no age-related differences were observed in the vulva. The authors concluded that vulvar skin is not more reactive to SLS than forearm skin (Figure 27.4), and that age-related differences in irritant reaction are apparent in the forearm, but not in the vulva.[14] The reported studies indicate that vulvar irritant reactivity may not be higher than that of the forearm for all irritants, and that data from irritation tests in the arm should not simply be extrapolated to vulvar skin.

If irritant dermatitis does develop in vulvar skin, it tends to heal more quickly than forearm skin upon removal of the irritant. This is the case not only for chemically induced trauma but also for mechanical trauma.[17]

Microbiology of vulvar skin

Skin moisture and pH, which are increased on vulvar compared with forearm skin, are important factors for microbial growth. Another factor is microbial adherence to keratinocytes. Bibel et al[18] found a high adherence of *Staphylococcus aureus* to the larger, rougher cells of the labium majus, matched only by the adherence to fully keratinized nasal epithelial cells. *S. aureus* adherence both to labium minus and to vaginal epithelia was low, as was the adherence to forearm keratinized cells. Compared with the adherence of *S. aureus* to labium majus cells, other microorganisms (*Streptococcus pyogenes*, *Escherichia coli*, *Pseudomonas aeruginosa*, *Acinetobacter calcoaceticus* and *Candida albicans*) showed far lower adherence scores. Whereas *C. albicans* failed to attach to nasal cells and clung poorly to forearm and labium minus cells, there was a significant adherence of the organism to labium majus cells.

Aly et al[19] investigated the flora of 18 healthy female volunteers with a mean age of 39 years. Samples from mid-labium majus skin and forearm were collected by the detergent scrub method. Microbial counts were higher on the vulva ($2.8 \times 10^6/cm^2$) than on the

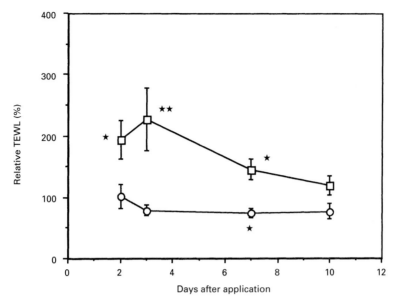

Figure 27.4 Influence of sodium lauryl sulfate (SLS) irritation on forearm (□) and vulvar (○) TEWL as an indicator of barrier damage: relative TEWL after 5% SLS-induced irritation (premenopausal women, $n = 10$).[16] Whereas a significant TEWL increase occurs in the forearm, this is not the case in the vulva, where a TEWL reduction was observed on days 7 and 10 with 5% SLS. Significant differences between treated and control sites evaluated by the paired *t*-test are indicated by stars: ★, $p<0.05$; ★★, $p<0.01$.

forearm ($6.4 \times 10^2/cm^2$). The prevalence data (Figure 27.5) show a higher prevalence of *S. aureus*, α-hemolytic streptococci, lipophilic and non-lipophilic diphtheroids, lactobacilli, Gram-negative rods and yeasts on vulvar compared with forearm skin, whereas the micrococci were less prevalent in the vulva.

The quantitative results from the same study[19] are shown in Table 27.2. Lipophilic diphtheroids, coagulase-negative staphylococci, micrococci, non-lipophilic diphtheroids and lactobacilli composed the dominant flora of the vulva.

We investigated the bacterial population dynamics of labium majus skin during the menstrual cycle.[20] In 20 women, samples were taken on days 2 and 4 of their menstruation and on day 21 of the menstrual cycle. The results confirm the previous work both as far as the approximate density of the aerobic

flora and the prevalence and densities of the various organisms are concerned. There was a small, though insignificant, reduction of total organisms during the menstruation from 2.0×10^6 on day 2 to 8.9×10^5 on day 4. This is more obvious for β-hemolytic strepto-

Table 27.2 Bacterial counts (organisms/cm²) on vulvar (mid-labium majus) and forearm skin ($n = 18$) (data are taken, with permission, from Aly et al[19])

Organism	Vulva	Forearm
Staphylococcus aureus	4.1×10^4	14
Coagulase-negative staphylococci	5.7×10^5	180
Micrococci	5.1×10^5	290
Streptococci	370	5
Lipophilic diphtheroids	7.9×10^5	110
Non-lipophilic diphtheroids	4.6×10^5	11
Lactobacillus spp.	4.6×10^5	10
Baccillus spp.	0	12
Gram-negative rods	1800	1
Yeasts	82	8

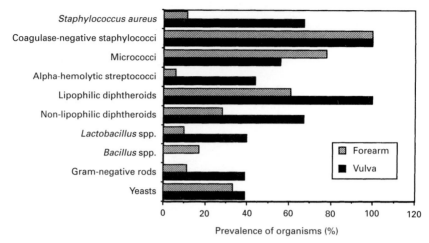

Figure 27.5 Prevalence of microorganisms in human forearm and vulva skin (*n* = 18) (based on data from Aly et al[19]).

cocci and both Gram-negative and Gram-positive rods. Lower numbers of micrococci and non-lipophilic diphtheroids were found on day 21 than during menstruation, whereas the opposite was true for α-hemolytic streptococci and non-pathogenic *Neisseria*. The numbers of *S. aureus* and coagulase-negative staphylococci showed little changes over the menstrual cycle. The numbers of lactobacilli and *Gardnerella vaginalis* were also relatively constant during the investigation period.

The microbial colonization of human skin is an important variable influencing body odors.[21] While sterile apocrine sweat is odorless, odors are developed by bacterial degradation of sweat. With the high and relatively stable density of bacteria on vulvar skin, the microbial generation of odors is a physiological, though cosmetically important, feature of this area. A fishy odor, especially after alkalinization by sexual intercourse and during menstruation, is an important symptom of bacterial vaginosis (BV), a frequent condition additionally characterized by a thin, homogenous vaginal discharge, vaginal pH > 4.5 and the presence of 'clue cells' (i.e. vaginal epithelia densely covered by bacteria) in a wet mount.[22] The fishy odor is attributed to

amines produced by the vaginal flora, which is marked by a lack of lactobacilli and an overgrowth of *G. vaginalis* and anaerobes in BV patients.

COSMETOLOGY OF VULVAR SKIN

The range of external products that are either specifically made for application on vulvar skin or that may regularly come into contact with the genital region is very extensive, ranging from fabrics (garments and towels) and paper products (menstrual pads) to chemicals (detergents and deodorants) and medicaments (Table 27.3). While human vulvar skin is an example of very specialized skin, many products designed for or regularly used on vulvar skin are not tested systematically for safety on this type of skin. This is especially evident for menstrual protection aids, which are regulated as medical devices in the USA, but not in Europe. Only recently has the safety of these products on vulvar skin been studied systematically.[23,24]

The dermatologist is mainly concerned about three conditions as possible side-effects of external products on vulvar skin: contact

Table 27.3 External products coming into contact with vulvar skin

Fabrics:
    Garments
    Towels

Cleansing agents
Deodorants and antiperspirants

Menstrual protection aids:
    Menstrual pads
    Tampons

Contraceptives:
    Condoms
    Barrier creams
    Douches

Medicaments for the treatment of vulvar and vaginal conditions

urticaria, and irritant and allergic contact dermatitis.

Contact urticaria

The contact urticaria syndrome (CUS) has been defined as a spectrum of externally induced immediate-type reactions of the skin and the mucous membranes, ranging from the simple wheal to anaphylactic shock.[25] Depending on the mechanism involved, contact urticaria may be immunologically or nonimmunologically induced. Whereas the latter remains limited to the application site of an agent to the skin, immunologically mediated contact urticaria may spread or may even result in generalized anaphylaxis presenting as rhinitis, conjunctivitis, asthma, gastrointestinal edema or even shock.

Schimkat et al[26] showed that human semen and latex are the two most commonly cited causes of contact urticaria in the vulvovaginal region. Most patients seem to have a personal or family history of atopy. The contact urticarial reactions both to semen and latex tend to be severe and sometimes life-threatening, and an immunological cause can be demonstrated by skin and/or in vitro tests in most cases. With the increasing use of latex gloves and condoms related to the HIV epidemic, the frequency of immediate-type contact allergy to latex has increased considerably in recent years.[27] Combinations of type I and type IV (protein contact dermatitis) allergic reactions to semen have been reported.[28]

Further case reports on contact urticaria of the female genital regions mention chlorhexidine, nifuroxime, cow milk constituents, copper and silk as additional causes.[26]

Diagnosis of contact urticaria

Since the symptoms of contact urticaria tend to be transient, the diagnosis is made on the basis of the typical history, skin tests (prick, scratch and intracutaneous tests), in vitro tests (RAST) and possibly controlled allergen exposure to the shock organ (provocation test). While latex is commercially available for in vivo and in vitro tests, this is not the case for allergens in human semen. In the latter cases, tests with the patient's partner's semen have to be performed, taking into account the possible infectious risk from body fluids.[26]

Contact dermatitis

Irritant contact dermatitis

Exposure of vulvar skin to strong irritants is a rare event, since the genital region is well protected from the environment. Occasionally, patients with neurological diseases such as quadriplegia resulting in hypo- or anesthesia of the lower part of the body may not notice contamination of their clothes and skin with strong irritants such as household cleaners, thus leading to acute irritant dermatitis. Another scenario may be the use of potassium permanganate for baths. When patients sit on incompletely dissolved potassium permanganate crystals, they may develop acute toxic reactions. In the older American gynecologic literature, toxic vulvovaginitis was described following the use of potassium permanganate as an abortifacient.[29,30] Potassium permanganate tablets were introduced into the vagina in the belief that abortion might be induced. As a consequence, sharply demarcated ulcers of the vagina and of the vulva with painless bleeding occurred, possibly leading to clinical shock.

Far more frequent than acute vulvar irritant dermatitis is chronic irritant dermatitis, where many subliminal insults may lead to cumulative skin damage if the time between them is too short for complete restoration of the barrier. Clinical symptoms will develop only when the damage exceeds a certain 'manifestation limit', which is individually determined. Persons with 'sensitive skin' are characterized by a decreased manifestation limit and/or a decreased restoration time, leading to earlier development of clinical irritant dermatitis. The etiological factors in cumulative vulvar irritant dermatitis are manifold, and are both endogenous and exogenous (Figure 27.6). Obesity will lead to increased occlusion, resulting in increased skin moisture, which in turn enhances the penetration of hydrophilic irritants into the skin. Friction is increased by

Table 27.4 Possible irritants on vulvar skin
Deodorants/hygiene sprays
Dermatological topical preparations
Garments and vulvar pads
Shower gels
Soaps
Spermicides
Vaginal douches

humidity, thus adding a mechanical irritating factor.[31] Another endogenous risk factor may be incontinence, resulting again in increased skin wetness, but at the same time providing urine and ammonia as irritants.

Exogenous factors are the multiple (low-grade) irritants that may come into contact with vulvar skin. The most frequent vulvar irritants are listed in Table 27.4. As far as cosmetics are concerned, the products that cause problems most frequently seem to be skin-care products, followed by personal cleanliness products, and deodorants and antiperspirants.[32] These data, however, are based on general consumer complaints about adverse reactions to cosmetics, and are not specific for vulvar disease. A number of years ago, several papers appeared on the vulvar side-effect of deodorants and female hygiene sprays.[33–35] Most of the reactions seem to have been irritant in nature, although patch testing was not performed in these studies. Fisher performed patch tests on 30 women who had developed vulvar dermatitis after the application of female hygiene sprays, and observed positive reactions in only four patients. Fisher[37] stresses that the propellants in the hygiene sprays (generally fluorinated hydrocarbons) are the most common cause of irritant dermatitis when the spray is applied too closely to the vulvar area.

Modern vaginal contraceptives consist principally of nonoxynol 9 and benzalkonium chloride, and are considered generally safe.[38]

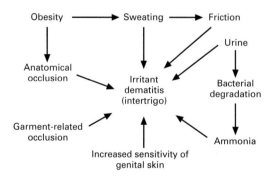

Figure 27.6 Multifactorial pathogenesis of vulvar irritant dermatitis.

However, they may occasionally cause irritant reactions such as pruritus, burning, erythema and edema, but serious dermatitis seems to be rare.[39]

Allergic contact dermatitis

Little is known about the spectrum of allergens causing vulvar allergic contact dermatitis, although sensitizations do not seem to be rare in vulva clinic patients.

Marren et al[40] patch-tested 135 patients with vulval symptoms using a standard tray, a medicaments tray, and a facial and preservative tray. Of these patients, 66 (49%) had positive results, and 30 of the test-positives (46%) had multiple positive tests. The most frequent sensitizations were found to be to medicaments (37 patients, 27%), with relevance of test results in most cases. Positive reactions to fragrances or to balsam of Peru were observed in 20 patients (14%). Steroid sensitivity was detected in 2.2% of patients. The authors considered most of the reactions as being due to secondary (iatrogenic) sensitization following the treatment of an underlying vulvar disorder. The reactions to fragrances, however, may well have been primary vulvar sensitizations causing vulvar dermatitis. The considerable incidence of sensitizations to topical corticosteroids is in line with recent reports on glucocorticosteroid sensitivity indicating sensitization rates of up to 5%. As topical corticosteroids are often prescribed in vulvar diseases, corticosteroid allergy should always be suspected when lesions do not improve or worsen under therapy. A group of medicaments not specifically mentioned by Marren et al are topical antiherpetic medications. These may cause both irritant and allergic dermatitis. Zovirax cream, the medication most frequently used nowadays to treat herpes, contains the anionic detergent sodium lauryl sulfate, a well known irritant, to enhance penetration of acyclovir into the skin. Dermatitis due to Zovirax cream has been described,[41] and is usually irritant in nature.

In a report from France,[42] perfumes, chlorhexidine, hexamidine, benzylalkonium chloride and latex are mentioned as the most frequent causes of allergic contact dermatitis in vulvar skin.

In the study by Fisher[36] on patients with vulvar dermatitis subsequent to the use of female hygiene sprays, he observed relevant sensitizations to benzethonium chloride, chlorhexidine, isopropyl myristate and perfume.

In our experience, vulvar menstrual pads have rarely caused allergic contact dermatitis. In 1985, Schmoll and Sterry[43] reported a case of contact dermatitis to copper(II) acetylacetonate that had been added to a brand of vulvar pads for its disinfectant properties. The fact that no more cases have been described may be because copper is a weak sensitizer. In a recent report from Canada,[44] sanitary napkins containing absorbent gel material were implicated as the cause of vulvar itching, burning and eruptions in a case series of 28 women. However, since this gynecological study was uncontrolled and lacked allergological workup, and since reactions could be reproduced by a provocation test in only 25% of the women, the causal relationship between napkin use and vulvar symptoms remains unclear.

To assess the possible importance of allergens in vulvar dermatitis, the frequency of sensitizations in large patch-test populations should be kept in mind. Sensitizations may be acquired at other skin sites, but dermatitis may manifest at the vulva if there is contact with the allergen. Poison oak and poison ivy may be cited as a typical example. More than half of the adult US population is considered to be sensitized to these plants through outdoor activities. The allergen may be transmitted to the vulva by contaminated hands, leading to allergic contact dermatitis.[39]

Diagnosing vulvar irritant and allergic dermatitis

While acute irritant dermatitis develops minutes to hours after exposure to the irritant, acute allergic contact dermatitis as a delayed reaction requires usually 24–48 hours after allergen contact before symptoms appear. The irritant reaction reaches its peak quickly, and then starts to heal ('decrescendo phenomenon'). The allergic reaction, in contrast, is more retarded ('crescendo phenomenon'). As for subjective signs, burning tends to be more associated with irritant dermatitis and pruritus with allergic dermatitis – but no safe distinction can be made.

In contrast to other sites of the human body, the morphology of irritant and allergic dermatitis at the vulva is very similar, so the diagnosis cannot be based on clinical grounds. Both forms of dermatitis show erythema, edema, vesicles that may coalesce, bullae and oozing. Necrosis and ulceration is only seen with primary irritants. Crusting, a typical secondary lesion of contact dermatitis at other sites, is usually absent in the vulvar region because of occlusion and increased skin moisture.

The clinical features of chronic irritant and allergic dermatitis include redness, lichenification, excoriations, scaling and hyperkeratoses. Gardner[39] stresses that many cases of chronic contact dermatitis tend to be misdiagnosed as hyperplastic vulvar dystrophy.

Since there is no specific diagnostic test for irritant dermatitis, the diagnosis is based on history, especially regarding contact to irritants, clinical examination and exclusion of other causes, notably contact allergy and infectious diseases.

The diagnosis of contact allergy can be made or excluded with patch testing. A skin biopsy may be useful to establish the diagnosis of contact dermatitis, but it is usually not helpful for differential diagnosis between irritant and allergic dermatitis.[45]

Complications of vulvar irritant and allergic dermatitis

The main complication of irritant dermatitis is allergic contact dermatitis. Possible mechanisms of the development of allergic dermatitis are the enhanced penetration of allergens into damaged skin and the presence of activated key elements of the immune system in the skin.

Female myelodysplastic patients sometimes develop hypertrophy of the labia minora, which is possible caused by long-term irritant dermatitis ('diaper dermatitis'). Intermittent catheterization may be difficult, and the risk of urethrovesical infections may increase. In these cases, labioplasty may be indicated.[46]

Both irritant and allergic contact dermatitis may be superinfected by pathogenic bacteria or fungi. The risk of superinfection is increased at the vulva, where the microbial density is high and *Staphylococcus aureus* is frequently present even in healthy skin.[19]

CONCLUSIONS

The vulvar skin is a form of specialized skin with unique morphological and functional properties. Vulvar dermatological diseases can show a different morphology, and occasionally manifest solely at this site. The vulva tends to be more permeable than other sites, and has a specific proclivity to irritant activity, unique microbial ecology and increased blood flow. Regarding unwanted effects of products applied to vulvar skin, both the spectrum of irritants and allergens and the clinical presentation of contact urticaria, irritant and allergic contact dermatitis may be different from other sites of the human body. One must be aware of these differences of this specialized skin, especially in cosmetic dermatology.

REFERENCES

1. Hoyme UB, Buehler K, Anatomy and physiology of the vulva, the vagina and the cervix. In: *Vulvovaginitis* (Elsner P, Martius J, eds). New York/Basel: Marcel Dekker, 1993:275–84.

2. Harper WF, McNicol EM, A histological study of normal vulvar skin from infancy to old age. *Br J Dermatol* 1977; **96**: 249–53.

3. Jones IS, A histological assessment of normal vulvar skin. *Clin Exp Dermatol* 1983; **8**: 513–21.

4. Nauth HF, Boon ME, Significance of the morphology of anucleated squames in the cytologic diagnosis of vulvar lesions. A new approach in diagnostic cytology. *Acta Cytol* 1983; **27**: 230–6.

5. Nauth HF, Böger A, New aspects of vulvar cytology. *Acta Cytol* 1982; **26**: 1–6.

6. Nauth HF, Haas M, Zytologische und histologische Untersuchungen zur Hormonabhängigkeit der Haut des äußeren weiblichen Genitales. *Geburtshifte Frauenheilkd* 1984; **44**: 451–9.

7. Nauth HF, Zur lokalen Testosterontherapie des Lichen sclerosus et atrophicus der Vulva. *Geburtshifte Frauenheilkd* 1982; **42**: 476–81.

8. Elsner P, Maibach HI, The effect of prolonged drying on transepidermal water loss, capacitance and pH of human vulvar and forearm skin. *Acta Dermatol Venereol (Stockh)* 1990; **70**: 105–9.

9. Ude P, Topographische hautphysiologische Meßwerte. *Z Hautkr* 1976; **51**(Suppl 2): 81–97.

10. Britz MB, Maibach HI, Human labia major skin: transepidermal water loss in vivo. *Acta Dermatol Venereol* 1979; **85**(Suppl): 23–5.

11. Elsner P, Wilhelm D, Maibach HI, Physiological skin surface water loss dynamics of human vulvar and forearm skin. *Acta Dermatol Venereol (Stockh)* 1990; **70**: 141–4.

12. Britz MB, Maibach HI, Human percutaneous penetration of hydrocortisone: the vulva. *Arch Dermatol Res* 1980; **267**: 313–16.

13. Britz MB, Maibach HI, Human cutaneous vulvar reactivity to irritants. *Contact Dermatitis* 1979; **5**: 375–7.

14. Elsner P, Wilhelm D, Maibach HI, The effect of low-concentration sodium lauryl sulfate on human vulvar and forearm skin: age-related differences. *J Reprod Med* 1990; **36**: 77–81.

15. Elsner P, Wilhelm D, Maibach HI. Multiple parameter assessment of vulvar irritant contact dermatitis. *Contact Dermatitis* 1990; **23**: 20–6.

16. Elsner P, Wilhelm D, Maibach HI, Study of sodium lauryl sulfate-induced irritant contact dermatitis in vulvar and forearm skin of pre- and postmenopausal women. *J Am Acad Dermatol* 1990; **23**: 648–52.

17. Wilhelm D, Elsner P, Maibach HI, Standardized trauma in human vulvar and forearm skin: effects on transepidermal water loss, capacitance and pH. *Acta Dermatol Venereol* 1990; **122**: 607–14.

18. Bibel DJ, Aly R, Lahti L et al, Microbial adherence to vulvar epithelial cells. *J Med Microbiol* 1987; **23**: 75–82.

19. Aly R, Britz MB, Maibach HI, Quantitative microbiology of human vulva. *Br J Dermatol* 1979; **101**: 445–8.

20. Elsner P, Maibach HI, Microbiology of human vulvar skin. *Semin Dermatol* 1990; **9**: 300–4.

21. Lukacs A, Korting HC, Antitranspirantien und Deodorantien – Wirkstoffe und Bewertung. *Dermatosen* 1989; **37**: 53–7.

22. Martius J, Bacterial vaginosis. In: *Vulvovaginitis* (Elsner P, Martius J, eds). New York/Basel: Marcel Dekker, 1993:345–64.

23. Hanke-Baier P, Johannigmann J, Levin RJ, Wagner G, Evaluation of vaginal and perineal area during the use of external sanitary protection throughout the menstrual cycle. *Acta Obstet Gynecol Scand* 1994; **73**:486–91.

24. Wilhelm D, Elsner P, Pine HL, Maibach HI, Evaluation of vulvar irritancy potential of a menstrual pad containing sodium bicarbonate in short-term application. *J Reprod Med* 1991; **36**: 556–60.

25. Maibach HI, Jones HL, Contact urticaria syndrome: contact urticaria to diethyltoluamide (immediate type hypersensitivity). *Arch Dermatol* 1975; **111**: 726–30.

26. Schimkat HG, Contact urticaria. In: *Vulvovaginitis* (Elsner P, Martius J, eds). New York/Basel: Marcel Dekker, 1993:83–110.

27. Fabro L, Mühletaler K, Wüthrich B, Anaphylaktische Reaktion of Latex, ein Soforttypallergen von zunehmender Bedeutung. *Hautarzt* 1989; **40**: 208–11.

28. Kint B, Degreef H, Dooms Goossens A, Combined allergy to human seminal plasma and latex: case report and review of the literature. *Contact Dermatitis* 1994; **30**: 7–11.

29. Shull JC, Vaginal bleeding from potassium permanganate burns. *Am J Obstet Gynecol* 1941; **41**: 161.

30. Vandergriff W, Diddle AW, Intravaginal use of potassium permanganate as an abortifacient: the error in diagnosis. *Obstet Gynecol* 1966; **28**: 155.

31. Elsner P, Wilhelm D, Maibach HI, Frictional properties of human forearm and vulvar skin:

Influence of age and correlation with transepidermal water loss and capacitance. *Dermatologica* 1990; **181:** 88–91.

32. Groot ACD, Beverdam EG, Ayong CT et al, The role of contact allergy in the spectrum of adverse effects caused by cosmetics and toiletries. *Contact Dermatitis* 1988; **19:** 195–201.

33. Kaye BM, Hazards of feminine hygiene sprays for women. *J Am Med Assoc* 1970; **121:** 2121.

34. Davis BA, Irritancy from feminine hygiene sprays. *Obstet Gynecol* 1970; **36:** 812.

35. Gowdy JM, Feminine deodorant sprays. *N Engl J Med* 1972; **287:** 203.

36. Fisher AA, Allergic reaction to feminine hygiene sprays. *Arch Dermatol* 1973; **108:** 801.

37. Fisher AA, *Contact Dermatitis.* Philadelphia: Lea & Febiger, 1986.

38. Zufferey MM, Risques vrais et faux de la contraception locale: spermicides, diaphragme. *J Gynecol Obstet Biol Reprod* 1985; **14:** 359–63.

39. Gardner HL, Contact vulvovaginitis: primary irritant and allergic reactions. In: *Benign Diseases of the Vulva and the Vagina,* 2nd edn (Gardner HL, Kaufman RH, eds). Boston: GK Hall, 1980:431–2.

40. Marren P, Wojnarowska F, Powell S, Allergic contact dermatitis and vulvar dermatoses. *Br J Dermatol* 1992; **126:** 52–6.

41. Robinson GE, Weber J, Griffiths C et al, Cutaneous adverse reactions to acyclovir: case reports. *Genitourin Med* 1985; **61:** 62–3.

42. LeSellin J, Drouet M, Bonneau JC, Sabbah A, Enquete allergologique dans les dermatoses de contact genitales. *Allerg Immunol Paris* 1991; **23:** 127–8.

43. Schmoll M, Sterry W, Kontakturtikaria und Kontaktdermatitis auf Cu(II)-Azetylazetonat in Slipeinlagen. *Akt Dermatol* 1985; **11:** 178.

44. Eason EL, Feldman P, Contact dermatitis associated with the use of Always sanitary napkins. *Can Med Assoc J* 1996; **154:** 1173–6.

45. Lever WF, Schaumburg-Lever G, *Histopathology of the Skin.* Philadelphia: Lippincott, 1983.

46. Kato K, Kondo A, Gotoh M et al, Hypertrophy of labia minora in myelodysplastic women. Labioplasty to ease clean intermittent catheterization. *Urology* 1988; **31:** 294–9.

PART SIX

COSMETIC TREATMENT OF SPECIAL CONDITIONS

28

Sensitive skin: What is it?

Smita Amin, Patricia Engasser, Howard I Maibach

INTRODUCTION

'Sensitive skin' is a neologism for consumers' and patients' feelings about their intolerance to skin care and cosmetic products applied to skin. Far from being a rarity, consumer studies in all races and continents identify a complex entity involving from one-quarter to one-half of the adult population. The dermatologic and cosmetic science literature abounds with confusion; the signs and symptoms are best understood when one approaches the syndrome as being multifactorial – composed of exogenous and endogenous features (Table 28.1). The latter might be considered phenotypic and the former genotypic. Status cosmeticus and the cosmetic intolerance syndrome represent uncommon and extreme forms of this disorder.

Occasionally, patients complain bitterly of facial burning and discomfort: their skin may show overt inflammation or they may have only subjective symptoms. This group challenges the practitioner's diagnostic acumen and ability to be empathetic when the severity of the patient's symptoms does not match the objective signs.

Fisher[1] coined the term *status cosmeticus* for the condition in which the patient no longer tolerates the use of cosmetics. Indeed, some patients experience subjective or objective irritations from cosmetics but they also become intolerant to many topical agents. Some patients have irritant dermatitis syndrome, occult allergic contact dermatitis, allergic photocontact dermatitis, or contact urticarial reactions, or combinations thereof, and the causal agents can be documented by careful clinical review and patch testing.

Other patients have seborrheic-rosacea diathesis that flares when soap and water are abandoned and cleansing and emollients are overused. This condition may be accompanied by facial erythema or scaling. Some of these patients require anti-inflammatory therapies, as do some atopic patients who develop this state.

Prolonged cosmetic elimination programs aid some women, who are able to gradually return to the use of other cosmetics – but only after 6–12 months or more. Subsequent additions of skin care to their regimens should be made one at a time, no more frequently than every two weeks. The final program should remain limited in the number and frequency of cosmetics used.

Another group of patients experience continuous facial burning without objective signs. Cotterill[2] describes these patients as having *dermatologic non-disease*. Many of these patients

Table 28.1 Causes of sensitive skin	
Exogenous	
Subjective irritation (burn, sting and itch)	Common, but difficult for patients to understand
Objective irritation	Common, but often difficult morphology to observe on the face
Allergic contact dermatitis; photoallergic contact dermatitis	Less common; often defined retrospectively by closed and open patch testing and photopatch testing
Contact urticaria	Open testing for rapid onset wheal-and-flare reaction
Endogenous	
Seborrheic diathesis; psoriasis	Common disorders, although a small percentage of patients have an atypical morphology
Rosacea and perioral dermatitis	Common, but morphology may be atypical
Atopic dermatitis	May be only residual from atopic dermatitis
Status eczematous[a] (status cosmeticus)	Some patients may have no other definable endogenous or exogenous factors
Dysmorphophobia[a]	Rare diagnosis that is made by exclusion

[a] These patients are the most difficult to treat successfully.

have a disturbed body image or dysmorphobia, and complain of physical defects without objective evidence. Frequently, these patients are depressed and require psychiatric help, but reject the skilled care they require. We stress that *cosmetic intolerance syndrome (CIS)* is not a single entity, but rather a symptom complex of multiple exogenous and endogenous factors. *Sensitive skin* covers the same range of pathophysiology, but generally is less severe. The term was coined to categorize consumers who are intolerant to cosmetic usage. Sensory irritation is the most common presentation. The consumer defines by their perception what is and is not sensitive skin; the dermatologist identifies the mechanism(s). Thus the consumer demarcates the 'phenotype' (i.e. appearance of symptoms), and the dermatologist the 'genotype' (i.e. mechanism(s)).

Careful delineation of endogenous and exogenous factors permit a rational approach to the syndrome.

EXOGENOUS FACTORS

Subjective irritation (burn, sting and itch not due to contact urticaria)

We define *subjective irritation* as chemically induced burning, stinging, itching, or other skin discomfort without visible signs of inflammation. This is a beguilingly simple definition. The complicated aspect resides in our ability to observe subtle inflammatory changes in specialized skin sites, such as the face and scalp, that have a proclivity to hide such alterations. The time course of subjective irritation aids identification: onset is typically rapid – within minutes; only occasional patients note symptoms hours later (Table 28.2). Propylene glycol and butylene glycol are common offending subjective irritants in cosmetics and skin care products.

Insights concerning its mechanism may be garnered by the fact that local anesthetics

Table 28.2 Causes of irritant dermatitis

Irritation	Onset	Characteristics	Prognosis
Acute primary irritant dermatitis	Acute: often single exposure	Vesicles/bullae, erythema/edema	Good
Irritant reaction	Acute: often multiple exposure	Erythema, vesicopapules, papules	Good
Delayed acute irritant dermatitis	Delayed: 12–24 h or longer	Vesicles/papules, erythema	Good
Cumulative irritant contact dermatitis	Slowly developing (weeks to years)	Erythema/papules, vesicopapules, scaling, lichenification	Variable
Traumatic irritant dermatitis	Slowly developing after preceding trauma	Erythema/papules, vesicopapules/scaling	Variable
Pustular and acneiform dermatitis	Acute to moderately slowly developing (weeks to months)	Papules/pustules, whitehead and blackhead comedones	Variable
Nonerythematous irritation	Acute to slowly developing	No visible changes	Variable
Friction	Slowly developing		Variable

block the response (unpublished data) and that, as a group, stingers react more vigorously to vasodilators than controls do.[3]

Note that subclinical contact urticaria must also be ruled out, since this mimics sensory irritation. Appropriate testing with higher concentrations of the ingredients of the formulation should identify contact urticaria.

Subjective irritation is not merely a mild form of objective irritation. Chemicals, such as alcohol, are capable of causing subjective irritation but are not commonly responsible for objective irritation. Sodium lauryl sulfate is a strong objective irritant, but does not routinely cause stinging. Until more basic information becomes available, subjective irritation will include other mechanisms that we presently lack insight to remove. The thermal sensory analyzer (TSA) may be a tool to help define the pathophysiology of subjective irritation. Recent studies with menthol, corticosteroids and acetylsalicylic acid (aspirin) have provided insight into their action of cutaneous sensation.[4–6] Similar studies with sensory irritants and their inhibitors may be productive.

At present, subjective irritation, with all its mechanistic imprecision, remains the most common cause of sensitive skin and CIS. Cosmetic and skin care manufacturers – even those with rudimentary toxicologic testing interest and epidemiologic feedback on their products – observe that 1–10% of all facial cosmetic users note and often complain of this discomfort. Some chemicals responsible for inducing subjective irritation and the toxicologic techniques for identifying the components and products have been reviewed by Frosch and Kligman.[7]

Before finalizing the diagnosis of subjective irritation in a patient who complains of immediate discomfort on application of cosmetics and skin care without readily detectable signs of inflammation, the patient should be

Table 28.3 Management of sensitive skin
1. Examine every cosmetic and skin care product
2. Patch and photopatch test to rule out occult allergic and photoallergic dermatitis; test for contact urticaria
3. Treat endogenous inflammatory disease
4. Limit skin care to:
(a) water washing without soap or detergent
(b) lip cosmetics – ad libidum
(c) eye cosmetics – ad libidum – if the eyelids are asymptomatic
(d) face powder – ad libidum
(e) glycerin and rose water as a moisturizer – only if needed
(f) 6–12 months of avoidance of other skin care products and cosmetics
5. Watch for and treat (if necessary) depression and other neuropsychiatric aspects

patch-tested to rule out subtle subclinical manifestations of allergic contact dermatitis. Management involves temporarily limiting skin care agents until the skin can tolerate simple formulations (Table 28.3). We prefer frankness in managing patients with CIS, because they may need to stay on this program up to a year or longer. We do not prohibit all skin care, but provide a positive suggestion list. Convincing patients to use this positive approach requires patience and tact.

Objective irritation

Objective irritation is defined as nonimmunologically mediated skin inflammation. In this condition, nonvisible or occult dermatopathology is the problem. It can be extremely difficult and often impossible with current technology to accurately identify low-grade inflammatory changes on the face. A high index of suspicion must be combined with careful physical examination enhanced by slight magnification. Ruling out contact allergy with patch testing is a scientific *sine qua non* of this diagnosis. Photomediated irritation or phototoxicity should also be considered in patients with this condition. Subclinical damage to skin may last for weeks after a single exposure.[8–11] This long-lasting

abnormality is difficult for the patient and the physician to understand.

Management is more difficult than might be appreciated. Almost any chemical can be an irritant, depending on the concentration, method of exposure, and other chemicals in the final formulation. Some chemicals evoke an inflammatory response only after repeated exposures at the same site to produce a cumulative irritation. Environmental and constitutional factors modify patients' responses.[12] We believe that our approach to skin care in these patients is rational (Table 28.3). Learning which skin care items have a low or high irritancy potential for a given patient requires some knowledge of formulation chemistry combined with judicious clinical trials to limited test areas.[13] As one generic example, triethanolamine stearate-emulsified formulations are significant causes for skin irritations in this group of patients.

Recent insights into the biologic complexity of irritant dermatitis syndrome may be found in references 14–16.

Allergic and photoallergic contact dermatitis

These mechanisms are generally the easiest to diagnose and simplest to manage in sensitive skin and the cosmetic intolerance syndrome.

Details of the patch testing of individual cosmetics and their ingredients are beyond the scope of this chapter, but the methodology is reviewed elsewhere.[17] Such testing should include all the patient's cosmetics and skin care items. Testing only with a routine series will miss the all-important uncommon allergen – a disservice to the affected patient.[18]

It is uncommon to patch-test patients more than once. Consequently, the first procedure should be complete, testing both screening series and all the patient's cosmetics and skin care products. In addition, the workup should include repeat testing of multiple positive patch tests to check reproducibility and to rule out the 'excited skin syndrome'.[19] Judicious use of provocative-use testing for cosmetic products helps to separate mild irritant reactions from allergic contact dermatitis. The provocative-use test (PUT) or the repeat open application test (ROAT) consists of twice-daily application for 14 days to the upper back or antecubital fossa.

Physicians not prepared to perform photopatch testing should refer patients to suitably equipped specialized units.

Management of patients with cosmetic allergic or photallergic contact dermatitis is aided by cosmetic ingredient labeling. Some dermatologically oriented cosmetic manufacturers provide special, allergen-free formulations for a given patient. Although fragrance allergy technically may still be troublesome to identify, fragrance-free formulations provide a convenient way around a general lack of technical expertise in this area.

Contact urticaria syndrome (CUS)

Diagnosis involves a high index of suspicion and appropriate open testing for 'immediate'-onset lesions.[20] The diagnosis is often missed because the transient erythema or urtication is masked by the face. However, when a small amount of material is applied to a limited area, careful observation with minimal magnification will reveal lesions – usually within 20 minutes.

Nonimmunologic contact urticaria (NICU)

Prototypic agents of nonimmunologic contact urticaria (NICU) are preservatives, such as benzoic acid and sorbic acid, and fragrances, such as cinnamic aldehyde. Management consists of identification and avoidance. Skin may react far more dramatically after bathing with surfactants.

Immunologic contact urticaria (ICU)

Contact urticaria resulting from an immunologic mechanism can be demonstrated by appropriate open immediate testing and passive transfer (to monkey) as well as radioallergosorbent (RAST) tests. Immunologic contact urticaria (ICU) to cosmetic ingredients with appropriate passive transfer or RAST tests have been performed infrequently to verify the mechanism. Parabens have been documented by passive transfer to cause ICU.[21] Immunologic contact urticaria may be more common in patients with atopy, but nonatopic or psoriatic persons are not exempt.

Natural product cosmetics contain food, plant, or dairy constituents, and are not rare inducers or eliciters of ICU and NICU.[22] We believe that future observers will identify numerous cases of this type.

Additional details on the contact urticaria syndrome can be found in reference 23.

ENDOGENOUS DERMATOSES

Effective dermatologic diagnosis depends on a clear understanding of morphology. All dermatologists comfortably diagnose classic manifestations of seborrheic dermatitis, rosacea, atopic dermatitis and psoriasis (or seborrhiasis) on the face. However, as expected in any biologic distribution, some patients have atypical morphologies, lesions masked by topical therapies (usually corticosteroids), or exacerbations from other topical preparations. These present a difficult challenge for those physicians who emphasize classic morphologies excessively in their diagnostic approaches.

Contrary to common expectation, the face and scalp (and the genitalia, palms, and soles) hide pathophysiology. Rampant inflammation can be seen, but minor-to-moderate inflammation is often masked. Perhaps the fact that the face has a greater blood supply than most other body parts (as measured by laser–Doppler velocimetry[24]) may partially account for the difficulty in observing all but the most marked inflammatory changes. This occult aspect of many facial dermatitides complicates the definition of the atypical endogenous eczema.

Complete physical examination and detailed personal and family history will sometimes direct the clinician to the 'correct' diagnosis. Often months to years are required for other stigmas to surface and make a disease process become obvious.

When all else fails – and certainly after complete patch testing – and after detailed counseling regarding cosmetic substitution, therapeutic measures may be indicated. We have often been forced to use the more potent topical corticoids on the face for a short period to break a cycle of the cosmetic intolerance syndrome. Isotretinoin has proven valuable in treating rosacea variants not responsive to oral antibiotics, such as tetracycline. Topical tar or sulfur can also be a helpful adjunct when managing seborrheic dermatitis and its variations.

STATUS COSMETICUS – COSMETIC INTOLERANCE SYNDROME

After patients have been thoroughly screened for endogenous and exogenous causes of cosmetic intolerance, the remaining group is not easily categorized. Excluding those patients with a disturbance of body image, we attempt to counsel patients when the mechanism of cosmetic intolerance remains entirely uncertain.

Initially, status cosmeticus patients often have mild difficulties with cosmetic use that intensifies as the number of products used multiplies in an effort to find a regimen of facial skin care that does not cause erythema, stinging, burning or discomfort. As the number of discarded cosmetics soars, the patient's and physician's frustration spirals, and the intensity of symptoms seems to increase – perhaps by some feedback mechanism. Additionally, any damage to the stratum corneum allows greater penetration of the topically applied chemicals. A partial solution seems to be prolonged strict adherence to a simple skin care program (Table 28.3). Even

after many months, when symptoms subside, patients must be counseled firmly to add cosmetics only one at a time and ultimately maintain a simple regime.

Cosmetic intolerance syndrome (CIS) represents the extreme example of status cosmeticus.[25]

DERMATOLOGIC NON-DISEASE

Cotterill[26] described a group of patients with dermatologic non-disease. These patients have significant symptomatology but no objective evidence of disease.

In his original group of 28 patients, 8 had facial symptoms, and 4 of these complained of intense burning, redness and discomfort. Cotterill states that these patients often suffer from a disturbed body image or dysmorphophobia, and commonly are depressed. Because several of his female patients with complaints of facial burning were suicidal, this serious disorder must be recognized by all clinicians who see patients with these complaints. Such patients who elect to seek dermatologic care have decided that their problems reside in their skin, and it is often difficult to convince them to seek the psychiatric care they require.

The method outlined here for properly evaluating these patients to detect causes of facial inflammation can help build rapport. Cotterill[26] noted that when these patients complain of redness and scarring of the face, they may refuse to use cosmetics for camouflage, and their symptoms are then used as a reason to withdraw from social contact. Unfortunately, their response to topical medications and systemic antidepressants is often very unsatisfactory.

SUMMARY

Sensitive skin and cosmetic intolerance represents a heterogeneous syndrome, perplexing to both patient and physician. This chapter has provided a systematic attempt at defining removable and treatable causes, ultimately leading to therapeutic interventions. Much remains to be done to define the pathophysiology of the all too common sensitive skin syndrome.

REFERENCES

1. Fisher A, Cosmetic actions and reactions: therapeutic, irritant, and allergic. *Cutis* 1980; **26:** 22–9.

2. Cotterill JA, Dermatological non-disease: a common and potentially fatal disturbance of cutaneous body image. *Br J Dermatol* 1981; **104:** 611–19.

3. Lammintausta K, Maibach H, Wilson D, Mechanisms of subjective (sensory) irritation. Propensity to non-immunologic contact urticaria and objective irritation in stingers. *Derm Beruf Umwelt* 1988; **36:** 45–9.

4. Yosipovitch G, Szolar C, Hui X, Maibach HI, Effect of topically applied menthol on thermal, pain and itch sensation and biophysical properties of the skin. *Arch Dermatol Res* 1996; **288:** 245–8.

5. Yosipovitch G, Szolar C, Hui X, Maibach HI, High-potency topical corticosteroid rapidly decreases histamine-induced itch but not thermal sensation and pain in human beings. *J Am Acad Dermatol* 1996; **35:** 118–20.

6. Yosipovitch G, Ademola J, Lui P et al, Topically applied aspirin rapidly decreases histamine-induced itch. *Acta Dermatol Venereol (Stockh)* 1997; **77:** 46–8.

7. Frosch P, Kligman A, A method for appraising the stinging capacity of topically applied substances. *J Soc Cosmet Chem* 1977; **28:** 197–209.

8. Maibach HI, Lammintausta K, Berardesca E, Freeman S, Tendency to irritation: sensitive skin. *J Am Acad Dermatol* 1989; **21:** 833–5.

9. Effendy I, Kwangsukstith C, Lee J, Maibach HI, Functional changes in human stratum corneum induced by topical glycolic acid: comparison with all-*trans* retinoic acid. *Acta Dermatol Venereol (Stockh)* 1995; **75:** 455–8.

10. Effendy I, Weltfriend S, Patil S Maibach HI, Differential irritant skin responses to topical retinoic acid and sodium lauryl sulphate: alone and in crossover design. *Br J Dermatol* 1996; **134:** 424–30.

11. Ale S, Laugier J, Maibach HI, Differential irritant skin responses to tandem application of topical retinoic acid and sodium lauryl sulphate: II. Effect of time between first and second exposure. *Br J Dermatol* 1997; **137:** 226–33.

12. Mathias CG, Maibach HI, Dermatoxicology monographs I. Cutaneous irritation: factors influencing the response to irritants. *Clin Toxicol* 1978; **13:** 333–46.

13. Hannuksela M, Allergic and toxic reactions caused by cream bases in dermatological patients. *Int J Cosmet Sci* 1979; **1:** 257–63.

14. Elsner P, Maibach HI, *Irritant Dermatitis: New Clinical and Experimental Aspects* Basel: Karger, 1995.

15. van der Valk PGM, Maibach HI, *Irritant Contact Dermatitis Syndrome.* Boca Raton, FL: CRC Press, 1995.

16. Marzulli F, Maibach HI, *Dermatoxicology,* 5th edn, Washington, DC: Taylor & Francis, 1996.

17. Engasser P, Maibach HI, Cutaneous reactions to cosmetics. In: *Contact Dermatitis* (Fisher A, ed.). Philadelphia: Lea & Febiger, 1986:368–93.

18. Adams RM, Maibach HI, A five-year study of cosmetic reactions. *J Am Acad Dermatol* 1985; **13:** 1062–9.

19. Maibach HI, The E.E.S. – excited skin syndrome (alias the angry back). In: *New Trends in Allergy* (Ring J, Burg J, eds). Berlin: Springer-Verlag, 1981.

20. von Krogh G, Maibach HI, The contact urticaria syndrome – 1982. *Semin Dermatol* 1982; **1:** 59–66.

21. Henry JC, Tschen EH, Becker LE, Contact urticaria to parabens. *Arch Dermatol* 1979; **115:** 1231–2.

22. West I, Maibach HI, Contact urticaria syndrome from multiple cosmetic components. *Contact Dermatitis* 1995; **32:** 121.

23. Amin S, Lahti A, Maibach HI (eds), *Contact Urticaria Syndrome.* CRC Press: Boca Raton, FL, 1997.

24. Tur E, Tur M, Maibach HI, Guy RH, Basal perfusion of the cutaneous microcirculation: measurements as a function of anatomic position. *J Invest Dermatol* 1983; **81:** 442–6.

25. Maibach HI, The cosmetic intolerance syndrome. *Ear, Nose Throat J* 1987; **66:** 49–53.

26. Cotterill JA, Clinical features of patients with dermatologic non-disease. *Semin Dermatol* 1983; **2:** 203–5.

29

Role of lipids in irritant dermatitis

Anna Di Nardo, Philip W Wertz, Howard I Maibach

INTRODUCTION

Stratum corneum integrity is of prime importance in preventing irritation, and the biochemical composition of the epidermis is important in the distribution and penetration of skin irritants. The stratum corneum has a predominantly lipid intercellular composition derived from complex biochemical modifications that allow the transformation from basal cells, with no intercellular lipid contents, to corneocytes, with a lipid rich composition. The corneal intercellular space occupies 20% of the stratum corneum volume.[1]

As keratinocytes differentiate, they produce increasing numbers of lamellar granules formed of lipid bilayers. Just before cornification, these granules move to the periphery of the cells and extrude their contents into the intercellular space. Each lipid bilayer connects with the next; some, enriched in covalently bound sphingolipids, connect with the corneocyte envelope.[2,3] The structure that results from this arrangement is the so-called 'brick-and-mortar' model – the name indicating that the stratum corneum forms a continuous combination of keratin-rich corneocytes with a lipid-rich matrix.[4]

The lipid composition of the different layers changes dramatically on moving to the surface. The basal cell lipid composition is mainly composed of phospholipids. During differention, other lipid classes are added: the transformation takes place under corneocyte, enzymatic control, post nuclear loss. A progressive depletion of phospholipids is coupled with increases in sterols and sphingolipids. Cholesterol sulfate occurs in significant quantities, with peak levels immediately beneath the stratum corneum in the stratum granulosum.[5]

Ceramides, important structures in the constitution of skin barrier function, can be separated into seven classes on the basis of polarity. The least-polar and least-abundant (7.5%) ceramide 1 is derived from acylglucosylceramide by removal of the sugar, and has the same long structure as its precursor. Ceramide 1 stabilizes different contiguous bilayers; the hydrogen bonds created by the ceramide hydroxyl groups help in this. The lateral chains of ceramides allow interconnections, and the absence of double bonds in *cis* positions enhances this. Moreover, the presence of the bonds between ω-hydroxy acids and cell membranes allows cohesion between corneocytes.[6]

With cholesterol, cholesterol sulfate and free fatty acids, ceramides form a non-phospholipid bilayer structure that is highly resistant to diffusion and oxidation. It is generally accepted that this structure acts as a barrier to transcutaneous water loss, the diffusion of toxic substances, as well as enhancing water-holding capacity.

The 'domain mosaic' model of the skin barrier depicts the bulk of the lipids as being segregated into crystalline/gel domains bordered by 'grain boundaries' where lipids are in a liquid-crystalline state. The bulk of the barrier, which is mainly in the crystalline/gel state, allows water to be lost from the organism, while, in the liquid state, grain boundaries allow some water to permeate the barrier towards the corneocytes, providing moisturized keratin.[7]

IRRITANT STUDIES

Several experimental models for studying biochemical changes in irritant contact dermatitis have been developed. Inflammatory response to irritants can be shown by testing in vitro chemotaxis, phagocytosis, enzyme release and complement activation. For example, dithranol-induced skin irritation provokes the release of lactate dehydrogenate, while high concentrations of sodium hydroxide, acetic acid and hydrochloric acid increase the uptake of lysine and isoleucine, and the release of acid phosphatase, neutral protease and lactate dehydrogenase. Some irritants, such as croton oil, release the prostaglandins PGE_2 and PGF_2 and prostacyclin.

Information on the complex relationship between chemicals and the skin aids the understanding of the pathogenetic mechanisms of irritation. This is a complex phenomenon resulting from the solvent properties of the vehicle, transport phenomena, biological response and clearance. Factors that are predictive of the degree of irritation include transport properties, partition coefficient, clearance, melting point, molecular weight and pK_a.[8]

To study the defence mechanism of the skin against irritation, we have focused atten-

tion on what happens during minimal irritation and how the skin acts to neutralize the insult. Irritant contact dermatitis models are easily studied in the mouse because of the possibility of obtaining skin samples. Humans are studied using non-invasive techniques, investigating the skin physiological parameters and the surface lipid component of the skin barrier both before and after a chemical insult.

We consider some organic solvents and, as a surfactant, sodium dodecyl sulfate (SDS).

ORGANIC SOLVENT IRRITATION

Organic solvents are commonly used in the extraction of lipids or in degreasing in industry. Such solvents range from the water-miscible methanol, ethanol and acetone to the water-immiscible aliphatic hydrocarbon hexane and various chlorohydrocarbons such as chloroform and carbon tetrachloride. Mixtures of these solvents efficiently extract skin lipids. Acetone alone is less effective in increasing water permeation, especially when mixed with diethyl ether. Schueplein and Ross[9] graded the effectiveness of delipidizing solvents on water permeation as follows: ethanol < acetone < diethyl ether < chloroform–methanol mixture. The fact that the chloroform–methanol mixture is more active in lipid extraction, and, at the same time, also more efficient in enhancing TEWL, was also shown by Abrams et al.[10]

Acetone

The application of acetone is performed by gently scrubbing the mouse flank for 10 minutes with a rayon ball, removing 0.7–1.4 mg of lipids per 7 cm^2. Water loss increases from a base control value of 5–10 ppm/cm^2 per hour to a value of 235–665 ppm/cm^2 per hour. Barrier recovery reaches 60% after 6 hours,[11] and normalizes in 24–33 hours.[12]

Permeation experiments show that lanthanum (which generally shows minimal flux) gains access to the stratum granulosum.

Barrier perturbation with acetone is followed by rapid secretion of lamellar body contents from the uppermost granular cell layer, leaving the cytosol largely devoid of lamellar bodies. At this time, the basic unit structure of the lamellar body bilayers appears disorganized and spaced with large lacunae, reflecting solvent extraction. New lamellar bodies appear in the granular layer in 30–120 minutes and well-organized intercellular lipids in 60–360 minutes. They normalize in 24 hours.[13]

Histochemistry performed with Oil red O (a marker for neutral lipids) and Nile Red (a fluorescent probe, which is yellow-gold for non-polar and reddish-brown for polar lipids) demonstrates that immediately after acetone treatment, the stratum corneum is depleted of lipids; this is followed by a slow recovery of stainable non-polar lipids, which decreases slowly in 48 hours and normalizes in 96 hours.[14] The recovery of the staining in the stratum corneum parallels the time course of barrier repairs as measured by TEWL.[11,14]

Lipid recovery can be followed in the epidermis using incorporation of tritiated water for 3 hours, and expressed in grams. After acetone application to mice, there is increased incorporation of tritiated water in cholesterol, non-saponifiable lipid (NSL) and fatty acid that is significant after 7 hours but not at 12 hours, reverting to normal in over 24 hours.[12,14]

Acetone treatment is also followed by an increase in HCG CoA reductase activity, which reverts to normal as barrier recovery occurs. Since barrier function recovers in a short time, reductase activity is also short-lived.[15] Immediately after the application of the irritant, the enzyme moves from the inactive state to the active state, even with minimal irritation. With greater irritation, the concentration of the enzyme increases mainly in the lower epidermis.[16]

Modifications of sphingolipids and their rate-limiting enzymes occur – but in a delayed manner. Sphingolipid synthesis occurs 5–7 hours after barrier impairment by acetone, and the time course of serine palmitoyl transferase activity parallels the increase in sphingosine synthesis and normalizes in 24 hours.[17]

It is also possible to study the affinity of solvents towards the different lipid classes and to quantify the amount of each kind of lipid removed from the skin in comparison with the whole stratum corneum extracts.[18] Acetone has a higher affinity for sterol esters, than for triglycerides, free sterols and sphingolipids. The amount of lipid extraction correlates with barrier function: increased lipid extraction leads to greater barrier impairment.

In vivo irritation by organic solvents

A few studies have been performed on human volunteers to evaluate the influence of skin lipids on the development of skin irritation. We employed xylene and toluene to induce irritation after one acute 24-hour application, to study the clinical parameters in humans utilizing non-invasive methods:[19] colorimetry to quantify the colour and TEWL to quantify the barrier impairment. Serial samples of stratum corneum lipids were assayed. Stratum corneum sheets were obtained from the volar forearm with cyanoacrylate glass resin; lipid analysis and quantification were performed using thin-layer chromatography and video-densitometry. The controls were performed at 24, 48, 72 and 96 hours from irritant application. The lipid values before and after application were correlated with irritation values obtained by instrumental evaluations. TEWL showed a significant increase at 24 hours and a rapid normalization at the following controls. Colorimetry produced a maximum increase at 24 hours, followed by a gradual decrease, which was still present at 72 hours. On correlating the absolute value and the percentage composition of the different classes of lipids with the irritation parameters

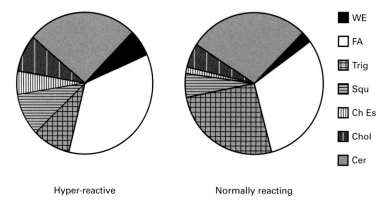

Figure 29.1 Lipid composition of hyper-reactive versus normally reacting subjects: WE, wax esters; FA, fatty acids; Trig, triglycerides; Squ, squalene; Ch Es, cholesterol esters; Chol, cholesterol; Cer, ceramides. (Modified from DiNardo et al.[19])

for each volunteer at 24 hours, a negative correlation was obtained between the quantities of ceramides and the visual score for both solvents.

Based on clinical observations, two populations were selected: less-reactive and hyper-reactive. Statistical differences were found in the total weight of lipids, in ceramides and in triglycerides (Figure 29.1). Considering the different classes of ceramides, we observed a significant reduction in both the percentage and the weight of ceramides 3, 4, 5 and 6II (Figure 29.2).

These data suggest that, in vivo, the proclivity to irritation by organic solvents depends on the lipid composition of the stratum corneum, especially on ceramides. The mechanism by which solvents penetrate the stratum

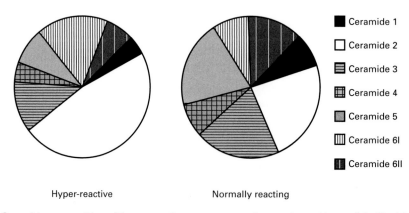

Figure 29.2 Ceramide composition of hyper-reactive versus normally reacting subjects. (Modified from DiNardo et al.[19])

corneum is unknown: solvents may induce transient conformational changes in lipid bilayer structures. Ceramides play an important role in the organization of these intercellular bilayers, so the significant decrease in the total weight of ceramides in subjects showing the greatest tendency to irritation seems to be important.

We also analysed the behaviour of surface lipids after solvent application. Changes in the percentage composition of surface lipids (an increase in polar and a decrease in nonpolar lipids) were observed after solvent application. Occlusion, which itself can be considered a type of irritant, presented a similar tendency – however, it did so at an early time period after the occlusion and to a lesser extent.

SODIUM DODECYL SULFATE IRRITATION

Grubauer et al[12] studied the application of sodium dodecyl sulfate (SDS) 10% in distilled water on mice flanks, performed by a 10-minute scrubbing with a rayon ball, followed by a saline wash. TEWL increased from a baseline value of 5–10 to a value of 184. The increase was lower than that after treatment with acetone.[12] Histochemistry performed using Oil red O (a marker for neutral lipids) shows that a single application removed all stainable material, with recovery at 24 hours.[14]

Epidermal lipid recovery was followed using incorporation of tritiated water for 3 hours, and expressed in grams. After SDS application on mice flank, there was a high incorporation of tritiated water in cholesterol, NSL and fatty acids in the first 4 hours, to about 30% of the control value.[12] When only non-saponifiable lipids and cholesterol are considered over a 96-hour time period, the incorporation remains high at 96 hours, despite TEWL normalization,[14] and produces a sustained increase in the activity of HMG CoA reductase consistent with a slower repair

of the barrier and a prolonged increase in cholesterol synthesis.[15]

In vivo irritation by SDS

Changes in surface lipids have been investigated with the application of SDS 5% on human volunteers. SDS was applied with occlusion for 4 hours, and changes in sphingolipids and free amino acids were examined 1 week later. The amount of amino acids was lower than that in the control skin, but the total amount of sphingolipids did not differ from the control. The composition of sphingolipids changed significantly.[20] Fulmer and Kramer[21] reported that in surfactant-treated stratum corneum, surfactant-induced perturbation of keratinization led to abnormal ceramide biosynthesis and that the proportion of ceramide species was significantly altered, although the total amount of ceramides did not change.

In skin with scaling induced with SDS, the quantity of sphingolipids does not differ from that in controls.[22] Denda et al[23] studied variations in the lipid chain arrangements in surfactant-induced scaly skin and their relation with TEWL using attenuated total-reflectance infrared spectroscopy. They found a clear relationship between TEWL and the lipid chains when TEWL is in the range of 0–9 g/cm^2 per hour, but not after the application of SDS. They proposed that the degree of order of the intercellular lipid structure in healthy skin is related to the TEWL; however, neither the decline in barrier function nor the decreased water content in SDS-induced scaly skin is directly due to intercellular lipid structural abnormalities but rather to an abnormal stratum corneum morphology and abnormalities of amino acids and/or proteins in cornified cells.

We studied the influence of ceramide composition on SDS-induced irritant contact dermatitis and the modification of stratum corneum physiology after detergent application[24] by applying SDS patches on the forearms of volunteers, utilizing TEWL and colorimetry (the *a** value for redness) to evaluate physiological parameters: skin barrier function and skin colour. We experimentally induced acute irritant contact dermatitis in order to correlate clinical irritation and barrier disruption with ceramide baseline composition and to study the modification induced on skin surface ceramides after SDS application. Stratum corneum lipids were separated and analysed by TLC and densitometry.

With 3% SDS, the baseline ceramide composition showed a correlation between the colorimetric *a** value and ceramide 6I and a correlation between TEWL and ceramide 1. Analysis of ceramide behaviour after SDS application revealed an increase at 24 hours, which was proportional to the concentration applied.

We found a correlation between ceramide and skin barrier impairment at 24 hours for the SDS 3% irritation, confirming that ceramide 1 may have a protective effect on skin barrier impairment as measured by TEWL.

UVA AND UVB IRRITATION

Exposure of human skin to UV radiation leads to changes in the physiology and biochemistry of the skin. In animals, increasing doses of UV led to a concomitant increase in TEWL.[25] Wefers et al[26] irradiated the lumbar region of volunteers with 9 times the minimal erythema dose – on one site with UVA and on another with UVB. The skin lipid modifications were evaluated using lipid extraction and thin-layer chromatography. They noticed a dramatic change in the barrier composition, which, for UVB, was also accompanied by an increase in skin thickness. There was a significant increase in tryglycerides, free fatty acids and squalene (mostly of sebaceous origin according to the sample area) and in total quantity and composition of ceramides. The ceramides were mainly ceramides 2, 3 and 5, and two classes not usually present in normal skin.[26] An interesting result was the absolute enhancement of the ceramide fraction and the appearance of two new bands in the non-polar ceramide region following irradiation.

The influence of UVA and UVB upon skin reactivity has been investigated using three different test systems: the alkali-resistance test, the dimethyl sulfoxide test and the SDS test. In all tests, UVA- and UVB-irradiated areas were found to be more resistant to primary irritants than non-irradiated skin. According to this work, the beneficial effects of UV can be explained by the enhanced level of ceramides and, as a consequence of this, by an improved barrier function.[27]

CONCLUSIONS

We speculate that the levels of skin lipids, and especially of ceramides, may play a preventive role in irritation in normal human skin. The analysis of baseline skin lipid composition may be a predictive test to identify heightened sensitivity to irritants in the occupational setting, with practical implications for workers in at-risk occupational sectors. Detailed information should clarify what can and cannot be accomplished with the addition of ceramides to skin care products.

REFERENCES

1. Elias PM, Leventhal M, Intercellular volume changes and cell surface expansion during corneification. *Clin Res* 1979; **27:** 525a.

2. Landmann L, The epidermal permeability barrier. *Anat Embryol* 1988; **178:** 1–13.

3. Wertz PW, Madison KC, Downing DT, Covantly bound lipids of human stratum corneum. *J Invest Dermatol* 1989; **92:** 109–11.

4. Elias PM, Grayson S, Lampe MA et al, The intercorneocyte space. In: *Stratum Corneum* (Marks R, Plewig G, eds). Berlin: Springer-Verlag, 1983:53–67.

5. Lampe MA, William ML, Elias PM, Human epidermal lipids: characterization and modulations during differention. *J Lipid Res* 1983; **24:** 131–40.

6. Wertz PW, Epidermal lipids. *Semin Dermatol* 1992; **2:** 106–13.

7. Forslind B, A domain mosaic model of the skin barrier. *Acta Dermatol Venereol (Stockh)* 1994; **74:** 1–6.

8. Berner B, Wilson DR, Guy R et al, The relationship of primary skin irritation and pK_a in man. In: *Exogenous Dermatoses: Environmental Dermatitis* (Mennè T, Maibach HI, eds). Boca Raton, FL: CRC Press, 1991:37–49.

9. Scheuplein RJ, Ross L, Effects of surfactant and solvents on the permeability of epidermis. *J Soc Cosmet Chem* 1970; **21:** 853–9.

10. Abrams K, Arvell JD, Shriner D et al, Effect of organic solvents on in vitro human skin water barrier function. *J Invest Dermatol* 1993; **101:** 609–13.

11. Grubauer G, Elias PM, Feingold KR, Transepidermal water loss: a signal for recovery of barrier structure and function. *J Lipid Res* 1989; **30:** 323–33.

12. Grubauer G, Feingold KR, Elias PM, Relationship of epidermal lipogenesis to cutaneous barrier function. *J Lipid Res* 1987; **28:** 746–52.

13. Menon GK, Feingold KR, Elias PM, Lamellar body secretory response to barrier disruption. *J Invest Dermatol* 1992; **98:** 279–89.

14. Menon GK, Feingold KR, Moser AH et al, De novo sterologenesis in the skin. II. Regulation by cutaneous barrier requirements. *J Lipid Res* 1985; **26:** 418–27.

15. Proksch E, Elias PM, Feingold KR, Regulation of 3-hydroxy-3-methylglutaryl-coenzyme A reductase activity in murine epidermis: modulation of enzyme content and activation state by barrier requirement. *J Clin Invest* 1990; **85:** 874–82.

16. Proksch E, Elias PM, Feingold KR, Localization and regulation of epidermal 3-hydroxy-3-methyl-glutaryl-coenzyme A reductase activity by barrier requirements. *Biochim Biophys Acta* 1991; **1083:** 71–9.

17. Holleran WM, Feingold KR, Mao-Qiang M et al, Regulation of epidermal sphingolipid synthesis by permeability barrier function. *J Lipid Res* 1991; **32:** 1151–8.

18. Grubauer G, Feingold KR, Harris MR, Elias PM, Lipid content and lipid type as determinants of the epidermal permeability barrier. *J Lipid Res* 1989; **30:** 89–96.

19. Di Nardo A, Sugino K, Ademola J et al, Role of ceramides in proclivity to toluene and xylene induced skin irritation in man. *Dermatosen* 1996; **44:** 119–25.

20. Denda M, Hori J, Yoshida S, Nanba R et al, Stratum corneum sphingolipids and free amino acids in experimentally-induced scaly skin. *Arch Dermatol Res* 1992; **284:** 363–7.

21. Fulmer AW, Kramer GJ, Stratum corneum lipid abnormalities in surfactant induced dry skin. *J Invest Dermatol* 1986; **86:** 377–80.

22. Horii I, Yamamoto A, Stratum corneum sphingolipids and free amino acids in experimentally induced scaly skin. *Arch Dermatol Res* 1992; **284:** 363–7.

23. Denda M, Koyama J, Namba R, Horii I, Stratum corneum lipid morphology and transepidermal water loss in normal skin and surfactant induced scaly skin. *Arch Dermatol Res* 1994; **286:** 41–6.

24. Di Nardo A, Sugino K, Ademola J et al, Sodium lauryl sulfate (SLS) induced irritant contact dermatitis: a correlation study between ceramides and in vivo parameters of irritation. *Contact Dermatitis* 1996; **35:** 86–91.

25. Lamaud E, Schalla W, Influence of UV-irradiation on penetration of hydrocortisone in hairless rat skin. *Br J Dermatol* 1984; **27**(Suppl): 152–7.

26. Wefers H, Melnik BC, Flür M et al, Influence of UV irradiation on the composition of human stratum corneum lipids. *J Invest Dermatol* 1991; **96:** 959–62.

27. Lehemann P, Hölzle E, Melnik B, Plewig G, Human skin response to irritants: the effect of UVA and UVB on the skin barrier. In: *The Environmental Threat to the Skin* (Marks R, Plewig G, eds). London: Martin Dunitz, 1992:203–9.

30

Ichthyosis

Rudolf Happle

INTRODUCTION

The term 'ichthyosis' is applied to a group of inherited disorders of keratinization characterized by scaling and more or less diffusely involving the entire surface of the body. The Greek word *ichthyosis* means 'fish-like disease', and poetically compares a human genetic disorder to the scales of a fish.

The mild forms of ichthyosis are of importance for cosmetic dermatology because they can serve as a model of dry skin. On the other hand, the more severe types of ichthyosis may constitute a considerable cosmetic handicap and psycho-social burden.

It is not the purpose of this chapter to give an overview of all the many different types of ichthyosis. Rather, some prototypic examples of these disorders will be considered. Firstly, two very mild forms – autosomal dominant ichthyosis vulgaris and X-linked recessive ichthyosis – are described because they occur very frequently and represent a major cause of the problem of 'dry skin'. Secondly, the story of the Lambert family from England will be reported. The skin disorder present in this family was so severe that during several generations the affected male members earned their living by presenting themselves on penny shows at fairs. The story of this family

stands at the beginning of the written history on the ichthyoses.

A PROTOTYPE OF DRY SKIN: AUTOSOMAL DOMINANT ICHTHYOSIS VULGARIS

Autosomal dominant ichthyosis vulgaris (ADI) constitutes a relatively mild medical problem.[1] Most individuals affected with this disease will never consult a dermatologist, and they would be surprised to hear that the state of their skin bears a long-winded scientific name. They simply feel that their skin is 'a bit dry', and they try to alleviate this dryness by application of smoothening ointments or creams.

Clinical features of ADI

At birth and during the first weeks of life, the skin of affected children is of normal appearance. During the following months, however, a mild diffuse scaling develops. An experienced specialist can establish the diagnosis by firmly rubbing his thumbs over the baby's soles. In most patients, however, the first signs of ADI are not recognized before the second year of life. In older children and adults, a

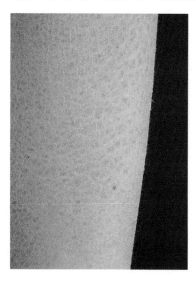

Figure 30.1 Autosomal dominant ichthyosis vulgaris.

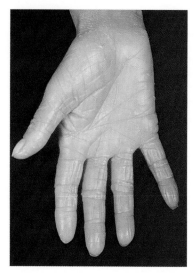

Figure 30.2 Accentuated palmar creases as a characteristic feature of autosomal dominant ichthyosis vulgaris.

fine translucent scaling involves the entire integument, but is particularly pronounced on the back, the extensor surface of the arms (Figure 30.1) and the shins. The large flexural folds are usually free from scaling. A very characteristic sign of ADI is the presence of accentuated palmar creases (Figure 30.2). Moreover, affected children and adolescents may show follicular hyperkeratoses mainly involving the extensor surface of the upper arms and the thighs.

A major problem caused by ADI in adult patients is hyperkeratosis of the heels, resulting in painful cracking and fissures. Similar fissures may develop during winter time at the paronychial area of the fingers.

Relationship between ADI and atopic eczema

Individuals affected with ADI are especially prone to develop atopic eczema.[2] Remarkably, this risk is absent in other types of ichthyosis. The accentuated palmar creases present in many patients affected with atopic eczema are usually a sign of ADI. When we consider the fact that atopic eczema constitutes a major conundrum in clinical dermatology, the impact of ADI on skin problems becomes evident. It should be noted, however, that not every individual affected with ADI will develop atopic eczema and that, conversely, many children may develop atopic eczema without having ADI.

Formal genetics of ADI

The trait shows a classical Mendelian pattern of inheritance. Affected individuals transmit the disorder to 50% of their offspring. The sex ratio of the disease is equal. When the issue of genetic counseling is considered, one should bear in mind that the psychosocial burden of this disease is very mild. The disease occurs so frequently because there is virtually no handicap of reproduction. The mildness of the disorder may be illustrated by the following story. A dermatologist specializing in the field of inherited skin diseases became himself the father of a nice little girl and proudly took over the task of changing the baby's diapers. On this occasion, his thumbs examined the soles of the child and signaled to his brain that ADI may be present. So he called his wife who was working in the kitchen: 'My dear, I feel that our daughter may have ichthyosis.' To his surprise, the wife who was also a physician called back from the kitchen: 'Oh, you finally got it! She has ichthyosis because she is my daughter!' Indeed, the dermatologist had up to then overlooked the presence of this cutaneous trait in his own wife.

Laboratory findings of ADI

Microscopic examination of ADI shows a thickening of the horny layer, which otherwise looks normal – a phenomenon called orthohyperkeratosis. As a characteristic feature, the granular layer that is situated beneath the horny layer is markedly reduced and may in some areas even be absent. On electron-microscopic examination, the keratohyalin granules that form a structure inherent to the granular layer are scarce and of abnormal appearance, looking spongy or crumbly.[3]

A major protein component of keratohyalin is called filaggrin. This protein is particularly rich in basic amino acids. It has been shown that filaggrin and its precursor profilaggrin are markedly reduced or even absent in biopsies obtained from ADI patients. It seems reasonable to assume that this filaggrin defect may play a major role in the pathogenesis of ADI.

Treatment of ADI

Topical treatment of ADI consists of the application of ointments or creams containing substances that deal with keratolysis and hydration of the horny layer. A backbone of treatment is the application of urea-containing creams. Alternatively, sodium chloride in a concentration of 5–10% may be applied.

Some patients prefer a prescription of 5% lactic acid incorporated in an aqueous cream. The topical application of retinoids is usually not necessary, and oral retinoids are never advisable because the benefit would not outweigh the undesirable effects of such therapy.

Some patients benefit from bathing in water containing sodium chloride in a concentration similar to that found in sea water. In my experience, however, it is preferable to apply the sodium chloride after the bath, incorporated in a cream.

A DISORDER SPARING THE FAIR SEX: X-LINKED RECESSIVE ICHTHYOSIS

The features of X-linked recessive ichthyosis (XRI) are a little more severe than those of ADI, but still rather mild. When compared with ADI, the significance of XRI for cosmetic dermatology is limited because this disorder affects only male individuals, who are, as a rule, less concerned about cosmetic problems.

Clinical features of XRI

In contrast to ADI, XRI may already be noted at birth. On rare occasions, the newborn may be encased in a translucent, collodion-like membrane, a phenomenon called 'collodion baby'.[4] During the neonatal period, this collodion-like membrane cracks and is shed. (It should be noted, however, that in most cases the collodion baby is a phenomenon heralding one of the other types of ichthyosis.) Later on, the boys show rather large, thick, brownish scales forming an imbricated pattern and being particularly pronounced on the trunk and the extensor surface of the limbs (Figure 30.3). In contrast to ADI, the palmar creases are normal.

Extracutaneous features associated with XRI

The birth of boys affected with XRI may be complicated by weakness of labour, and a cae-

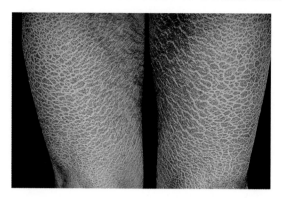

Figure 30.3 X-linked recessive ichthyosis characterized by brownish scales.

sarian section is often performed. This can be explained by the fact that XRI is caused by a steroid sulfatase deficiency.[5] Because this enzyme is lacking in the placenta belonging to the affected male child, the childbearing woman has abnormally low levels of oestriol, resulting in weakness of labour. In fact, a disease called placental sulfatase deficiency is well known to obstetricians, who may not be aware of the fact that this disorder exclusively occurs when boys are born, and that these boys will later develop XRI. An additional associated feature is cryptorchidism, which may be unilateral or bilateral.[6]

Formal genetics of XRI

The underlying X-linked gene is transmitted by clinically unaffected women to half of their sons, who will be clinically affected, and to half of their daughters, who will be clinically unaffected. Affected men cannot transmit this trait to their sons because these do not inherit their X chromosome. On the other hand, an affected man will transmit the gene to all of his daughters, who become clinically unaf-

fected carriers. This mode of inheritance results in a characteristic pedigree showing skipping of one generation.

Laboratory findings of XRI

Light- and electron-microscopic examination does not reveal any abnormal features of the skin. However, biochemical analysis of various tissues, including hair roots or blood cells, shows absence of steroid sulfatase. Female carriers show reduced levels of steroid sulfatase approximately corresponding to that observed in normal males.[7] The gene locus of steroid sulfatase has been mapped on the short arm of the X-chromosome at Xp22.3.[8]

The 'brick and mortar' model

The stratum corneum is composed of two components, and has been compared with a brick wall.[9] The 'bricks' are the corneocytes, and the 'mortar' is made up of lipids. For a normal barrier function of the stratum corneum, a regular composition of the 'mortar' is of utmost importance. Cholesterol metabolism plays a pivotal role in a normally functioning horny layer. Apparently, excess amounts of cholesterol sulfate present within the stratum corneum give rise to the increased scaling as observed in XRI.

Treatment of XRI

The treatment of XRI is similar to that described for ADI.

A SEVERE TYPE OF ICHTHYOSIS EXHIBITED AT PENNY SHOWS: THE STORY OF THE LAMBERT FAMILY

Some congenital types of ichthyosis are so severe that they attract public attention. A historical example is the family of Edward Lambert, who was born in 1727. He suffered from an extreme ichthyosis involving the entire skin, with the exception of the face, the palms, the soles and the penis. His skin was covered with brown hystrix-like hyperkeratoses. At the age of 14 years, he was presented to the Royal Society of London.[10]

Because the disease of the Lambert family no longer exists, it is difficult to categorize this trait according to a modern classification of the ichthyoses. Traupe[1] has suggested that Edward Lambert and his kinsmen suffered from ichthyosis hystrix of the Curth–Macklin type.

In spite of the handicap of his severe genetic disease, Edward Lambert was able to find a wife and to give life to six affected children. For several decades to come, Edward Lambert and other male members of his family (Figure 30.4) presented themselves in penny shows at fairs.[11] They travelled throughout the United Kingdom as well as the European continent, and were presented as 'porcupine men'.

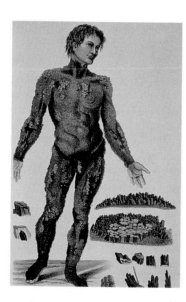

Figure 30.4 A member of the Lambert family as published in 1802 by Tilesius.[11]

A handbill from the year 1820, announcing the appearance on stage of a certain Francis Lambert, has been preserved:[12] see Box. Two statements made in this handbill were incorrect. The great grandfather and founder of this family was not found 'savage in the woods of North America', but was born to English parents from Suffolk. Secondly, the peculiar skin disease was not transmitted only in the male line. The disease affected the women of this family in the same way. It is not known why the family decided to conceal this fact. Did they intend to make the trait more interesting and to attract more attention? Or was it a case of male chivalry protecting the affected female relatives?

The true mode of transmission of this disorder was disguised by the Lambert family in such an effective way that even 150 years later, Edward Lambert's disease was taken as an example of Y-linked inheritance. However, in 1958 Penrose and Stern[12] published additional data on the Lambert family obtained by examination of the parish registers of the county of Suffolk. The revised pedigree data showed a regular autosomal dominant transmission of this trait.

For obvious reasons, the ichthyosis present in the Lambert family constituted a substantial handicap. The stigma of this ichthyosis was so spectacular that the affected male members of the family earned their living by exposing themselves at fairs. Notwithstanding this, the affected individuals were able to transmit the trait through at least five consecutive generations. On the other hand, the reproductive disadvantage caused by this disease was so severe that the trait vanished after some generations.

Today patients affected with a severe type of ichthyosis similar to that reported in the Lambert family are seen on rare occasions by dermatologists. Most of these patients suffer from epidermolytic hyperkeratosis of Broq.[1] The cause of this disorder is a point mutation involving the gene of either keratin 1 on chromosome 12q or keratin 10 on chromosome

---

New Species of Man.

Among the Wonders of Nature, which have from time to time tempted the Curiosity of the Public, perhaps no object more worthy of attention has been offered to their notice, than a Singular Variety of the Human Species, now exhibiting at the *Great Room*, 182, *Fleet Street*, near St. Dunstan's Church. This Young Man is 30 years of age, covered with Scales, with the exception of the face, soles of the feet, and palms of the hand, which are like those of any other man. These Scales, nearly half an inch long, are so hard and firm, that with a touch of the finger they make a sound like stones striking together; those on the stomach are short, round and distant; those on the arms, on the contrary, approach each other like the bristles of an hedge-hog. The great grandfather of the singular family to which this man belongs, was found savage in the woods of North America. The peculiarity descends only in the male line. *(For a description of this Species see the Works of Buffon.)*

Physicians and Natural Philosophers will find an extensive field opened to their enquiries, and every arrangement is made with regard to Dress to aid their Researches, without violating Decency.

ADMISSION One shilling each person. Doors open from 9 o'Clock in the Morning till 8 o'Clock in the Evening.

17q.[13] The patients tend to exude an offensive body odour. The story of the Lambert family illustrates the fact that such types of ichthyosis constitute a considerable psycho-social burden.

REFERENCES

1. Traupe H, *The Ichthyoses. A Guide to Clinical Diagnosis, Genetic Counseling, and Therapy.* Berlin: Springer-Verlag, 1989.
2. Hofbauer M, Schnyder UW, Zur Differential-diagnose von autosomal dominanter Ichthyosis vulgaris and X-chromosomaler Ichthyose. *Hautarzt* 1974; **25:** 319–25.
3. Anton-Lamprecht, Zur Ultrastruktur hereditärer Verhornungsstörungen. III. Autosomal-dominante Ichthyosis vulgaris. *Arch Dermatol Forsch* 1973; **248:** 149–72.
4. Larrègue M, Ottavy N, Bressieux JM, Lorette J, Bébé collodion: trente-deux nouvelles observations. *Ann Dermatol Venereol* 1986; **113:** 773–85.
5. Koppe JG, Marinkovic- Ilsen A, Rijken Y et al, X-linked ichthyosis: a sulphatase deficiency. *Arch Dis Child* 1978; **53:** 803–6.
6. Traupe H, Happle R, Clinical spectrum of steroid sulfatase deficiency: X-linked recessive ichthyosis, birth complications and cryptorchidism. *Eur J Pediatr* 1983; **140:** 19–21.
7. Müller CR, Migl B, Ropers HH, Happle R, Heterozygote detection in steroid sulphatase deficiency. *Lancet* 1980; **i:** 546–7.
8. Ross JB, Allderdice PW, Shapiro LJ et al, Familial

X-linked ichthyosis, steroid sulfatase deficiency, mental retardation, and nullisomy for Xp223-pter. *Arch Dermatol* 1985; **121:** 1524–8.

9. Elias PM, Epidermal lipids, barrier function, and desquamation. *J Invest Dermatol* 1983; **80:** 44S–9S.

10. Cockayne EA, *Inherited Abnormalities of the Skin and its Appendages.* London: Oxford University Press, 1933.

11. Tilesius WG, Ausführliche Beschreibung und Abbildung der beiden sogenannten Stachel-schweinmenschen aus der bekannten englischen Familie Lambert oder the porcupine man. Altenburg: im Literarischen Comtoir, and *JH Voigt's Mag f d neuesten Instanz d Naturk* 1802; **4:** 422–32.

12. Penrose LS, Stern C, Reconsideration of the Lambert pedigree (ichthyosis hystrix gravior). *Ann Hum Genet* 1958; **22:** 258–83.

13. Cheng J, Syder AJ, Yu QC et al, The genetic basis of epidermolytic hyperkeratosis: a disorder of dif-ferentiation-specific epidermal keratin genes. *Cell* 1992; **70:** 811–19.

31

Atopic dermatitis

Georg Rajka

INTRODUCTION

In the complex mechanism of atopic dermatitis (AD), in addition to genetic constitutional factors, a multiple immunoregulatory defect is of obvious importance, resulting in itching and inflammatory changes in the skin. However, it has been strongly emphasized that there are several changes in the clinically normal-appearing skin in AD that may be of primary and mostly non-immunological character or secondary to immunological and pathophysiological changes presented in the disease. Consequently, a definition of symptom-free skin seems to be necessary.[1]

The functional changes observed in symptom-free skin include a lowered itch threshold, which thus contributes to the basic trait of the disease – the itch – which links together immunological and non-immunological traits. First, however, alterations of skin structure and certain functions should be pointed out.

In symptom-free AD skin, the skin structure is altered and there are changes in barrier function and sensitivity to irritants as well as minimum blister time. These changes also occur in several other inflammatory conditions, but are particularly pronounced in AD; they include lowest corneocyte values and greatest epidermal thickness.[2,3]

From the clinical point of view, the reduced barrier function plays the major role here, since it may lead to higher colonization with *Staphylococcus aureus* and a lowered threshold to irritants. These are characteristic aspects of the disease, and explain many complaints of the AD patient. Furthermore, it has been shown that certain changes, such as epidermodermal hyperkeratosis, epidermal hyperplasia, intercellular oedema, alteration of venules, occasional fibrosis and focal demyelinization of cutaneous sensory nerves, occur in the symptom-free skin in AD; in addition, a slight dermal infiltrate consisting primarily of lymphocytes has been seen.[4,5]

Of great clinical significance are observations pointing to an altered water exchange in AD, indicating the barrier function located in the stratum corneum. Water exchange in a broad sense includes sweat secretion and transepidermal water loss (TEWL). A large amount of experimental work has been devoted to sweat secretion and/or TEWL in symptom-free skin in AD. These were performed with different techniques, and so it is difficult to judge their value, but some basic conclusions can be drawn:

- Sweat secretion seems to be normal (in contrast to some earlier claims regarding higher acetylcholine-induced sweating,[6] which were later not confirmed), but it is impaired by periosteal oedema or parakeratotic plugging, giving rise to pseudoanhidrotic conditions.[7] Furthermore, sweat loss is reduced in dry skin in AD.[8]

- According to several experiments,[9–12] TEWL is increased in symptom-free AD.
- Different estimates of the water content in the stratum corneum in AD have been obtained: both higher and lower values (particularly in dry skin) have been observed.[11,13–16]

The dominant clinical feature is that thermal or emotional sweating leads to itching in the majority of AD patients.

Sebum excretion is altered in AD, contributing to the generally very dry skin of AD patients (who also frequently have associated xerosis). As with water exchange, different techniques of investigation have been used – ranging from paper absorption to photometry. However, the major conclusions here are generally the same: sebaceous secretion is lower than normal,[17–19] with a lower number of sebaceous glands per unit skin area.[20]

SKIN DRYNESS

The clinical diagnosis is primarily based on visual observation; however, the pathophysiology of dry skin is complex (Table 31.1). There are, in fact, objections to the assumption that dry skin really is dry, that is, it has lower water content. For example, in the aged with dry skin, the stratum corneum has a higher rather than a lower water content and TEWL is reduced.[21] Piérard[22] is probably correct in saying that the term 'dry skin' is a misnomer, and the condition should be understood as the sum of changes in lipids and (unrelated) hydration, and also involves the degree of roughness of the stratum corneum. It may be studied by densitometry, computer image analysis or cohesometry.

In addition to those mentioned above, there are a number of changes in vascular phenomena (together with increased pilomotor reaction) that occur in AD. Table 31.2 lists the major changes found in symptom-free skin in AD.

MANAGEMENT

Therapy of AD is aimed at counteracting the itching, the inflammatory and immunological changes, and the complications of the disease, as well as reducing skin dryness. In the following some measures against dryness are mentioned.

Moisturizers/emollients

Products aimed at counteracting dry skin and improving softness and lubrication are called

---

Table 31.1 Possible causes and mechanisms of dry skin in AD

Major causes
Lowered humidity
Lowered ambient temperature
Epidermal cell damage (due to lipid solvents, friction etc.)

Major mechanisms
- *Disturbances of water content*
  Increased TEWL
  Increased hydration of stratum corneum/low electrical impedance
  Reduced hydration of stratum corneum/deficiency of water-binding substances?

- *Disturbances of epidermal functions*
  Disturbances of keratinization/epidermal hyperplasia
  Increased cohesion between corneocytes

- *Disturbances of sebaceous gland functions*
  Reduction in number of sebaceous glands
  Reduction of cell proliferation in sebaceous glands
  Reduction of sebaceous lipid secretion

Possibilities of combination
Interaction: for example, between water/lipids
Association with follicular keratosis/ichthyosis
Association with inflammatory changes

Consequences/correlations to dry skin
Impaired barrier function
Increased colonization of *Staphylococcus aureus*

Table 31.2 Alterations in symptom-free AD skin
• Increased itchiness (lower itch threshold) • Increased epidermal thickness • Impaired barrier function • Lowered resistance to contact irritants • Increased staphylococcal colonization • Increased TEWL • Coexistence with dry skin • Slight dermal lymphocyte infiltrate, alteration in venules • IgE on antigen-presenting cells[a] • White dermographism[b] • Nicotinate white reaction[b] • Delayed blanch[b] • Acral vasoconstriction • Absence of flare after histamine or allergen injection • Increased pilomotor reaction

[a] Found by one group.
[b] Not unanimously stated.

moisturizers, emollients or lubricants. They are similar, although often interpreted differently by dermatologists, cosmetologists and consumers. Moisturizers are considered to add water to the skin and counteract skin roughness, whereas emollients (lubricants) hydrate the skin by occlusion and thereby conserve the water content of the stratum corneum. Lipid ingredients of cream bases either prevent any loss of skin lipids or replace them.

The usual emollients include mineral oils, petrolatum, fatty alcohols and esters, and lanolin and its derivatives. Classically, they are divided into oil-in-water (o/w) and water-in-oil (w/o) emulsions: the former are used mostly during the day, while the latter are used in the form of night (cold) creams. In order to increase stability and improve consistency, non-ionic emulsifiers such as glyceryl monostearate are added to w/o emollients, whereas anionic o/w emulsions (containing, for example, triethanolamine stearate) are used on their own.[23] Lotions are used instead of creams on the face and as body lotions for reasons of cosmetic acceptability.

Urea 10–20% in a cream base is considered to be an effective substitution therapy for dry skin,[24] and has a fairly significant antipruritic effect.[25] 12% Ammonium lactate has also been recommended.[26] Borage oil (with high content of α-linolenic acid) was found effective on barrier function (in infantile seborrhoeic dermatitis[27]) and canola oil and its fractions had a favourable effect on irrition or barrier repair.[28] In double-blind evaluation cream E45 was superior to the control (R Graham Brown, personal communication). Since the ceramide fraction of stratum corneum may increase a deranged water-holding property,[29] ceramide-containing products are the focus of some interest – including the interest of the public.

There are several in vivo techniques for measuring skin hydration in human or animal skin and thus testing the efficacy of emulsions. Because of methodological problems, however, it is difficult to determine which tests are most appropriate for this purpose. Furthermore, the water content of the stratum corneum in AD is, as mentioned above, still a matter of controversy, even though the prevailing view is that it has a low value. Thus at present there are no generally accepted tests of the effect of emollients on the dry skin of AD patients. Therefore an empirical approach is still dominant, among both dermatologists and especially consumers, in the selection of a given emollient. The choice among countless products is strongly influenced by the local or national drug or cosmetic industry and its advertising campaign, by geographical and climatic factors (for example the need for greasier products in cold areas), by pricing, and by the subjective opinions of patients regarding the moisturizing capacity and tolerance of products.

From the dermatological point of view, it is assumed that w/o products are more helpful, but o/w creams may sometimes be better tolerated. This can be observed, for example, when patients select preparations with greater fat content (creams) instead of lotions as hand emollients. In the author's opinion, it is of value to create a certain degree of occlusion after emollient application by wearing cotton gloves for longer periods during the afternoon and evening or (provided they do not cause sweat retention and thus itching) during the night. In this case the possibility of an increase in *Staphylococcus aureus* skin levels should be considered,[30] and therefore alternation with antibacterial creams may be useful. This is advisable as a therapeutic measure, in view of the known high staphylococcal colonization values.[31-33]

Many products also contain antioxidants to prevent rancidity. Preservatives such as parabens, Bronopol, Germall II and 115, triclosan, Grotan HD2 and particularly Kathon CG included in emollients may sometimes cause sensitization, and added fragrances may present a still greater sensitizing potential. Because of their possible sensitizing and irritant properties, scents like cinnamic alcohol, cinnamaldehyde, eugenol and geraniol should be avoided.

The question of how often an emollient should be applied, for example to the hands, is not easy to answer. A reasonable balance is recommended between too few applications, and thus little effect, and frequent renewals, hindering sweat evaporation, particularly in inflamed skin areas.

It should be mentioned here that it is necessary to distinguish between inflammatory phases possibly combined with dry skin on the one hand and simple chapping on the other. In the first case more hydrated products (or a urea–hydrocortisone combination) are required, whereas the presence of chapping indicates the use of greasier preparations. In more expressed xerosis or for hyperlinear thickened palms (and frequently for plantar areas) keratolytics should be considered.

Bathing/bath oils

Dispersible bath oils containing mineral oils with emulsifiers (which are responsible for the dispersion) are useful as bath additives for AD patients. They may contain perfumes. Other bath oil types, like floating or beads, are less often used in dermatology. Long hot baths are not indicated for AD patients because of the induction of sweating, and short showers with not so hot water are preferable.

Soaps

Opinions concerning the usefulness of soaps, particularly for children with AD, are strongly divided, since (excessive) exposure to water and skin lipid solvents may aggravate the particularly dry skin of AD patients. Soaps are useful in reducing the staphylococcal colonization of AD skin, but are, in general, considered to be irritating to dry atopic skin;[34,35] this can also be shown by patch and chamber testing,[36,37] which, however, differs from the way in which soaps are used.

In a recent study 130 AD patients were allowed to use common toilet soap, and, immediately after bathing, topical medication (steroid creams and, for patients with dry skin, petrolatum) was applied. The study was conducted over two consecutive years, but after just one week 91% of patients showed a considerable improvement in skin lesions; no deterioration was observed, and thus the topical medications were found to be more effective than they were before the use of soap.[38]

It is possible that, in this interesting study, the potentially irritative effect of soaps was counteracted by topical steroids. In any case, it shows that short-term use of soaps can, in general, not be considered as contraindicated in the management of AD patients. Several clinicians recommend soap substitutes (soapless cleansers), or neutral, acid and soft/mild soaps, or water with colloidal additives, such as soda, corn starch or oatmeal. It is uncertain whether or not detergents are more appropriate for AD skin than soaps; they are non-alkaline but remove skin lipids more efficiently than soaps. Arachis oil or paraffin oil may be used to clean off pastes, for example, from the skin.

REFERENCES

1. Rajka G, *Essential Aspects of Atopic Dermatitis.* Berlin: Springer, 1989.

2. Al-Jaberi H, Marks R, Studies of the clinically uninvolved skin in patients with dermatitis. *Br J Dermatol* 1984; **111:** 437.

3. Frosch PJ, Kligman AM, Rapid blister formation in human skin with ammonium hydroxide. *Br J Dermatol* 1977; **96:** 461.

4. Mihm MC, Soter NA, Dvorak HF et al, The structure of normal skin and the morphology of atopic eczema. *J Invest Dermatol* 1976; **67:** 305.

5. Soter NA, Mihm MC Jr, Morphology of atopic eczema. *Acta Derm Venereol (Stockh)* 1980; **92**(Suppl): 11.

6. Warndorff J, The response of sweat glands to beta-adrenergic stimulation. *Br J Dermatol* 1972; **86:** 282.

7. Gordon BI, Maibach HI, On the mechanism of the inactive human sweat gland. *Arch Dermatol* 1968; **97:** 66.

8. Parkinnen MU, Kiistala R, Kiistala U, Baseline water loss and cholinergic sweat stimulation in atopic dermatitis: a gravimetric measurement of local skin water loss. *Arch Dermatol Res* 1991; **283:** 382.

9. Rajka G, Transepidermal water loss on the hands in atopic dermatitis. *Arch Dermatol Res* 1974; **251:** 111.

10. Abe T, Ohikido M, Yamamoto K, Studies on skin surface barrier functions: skin surface lipids and transepidermal water loss in atopic skin during childhood. *Jap J Dermatol* 1978; **5:** 223.

11. Finlay AY, Nicholls S, King CS et al, The 'dry' non-eczematous skin associated with atopic eczema. *Br J Dermatol* 1980; **102:** 249.

12. Werner Y, Lindberg M, Transepidermal water loss in dry and clinically normal skin in patients with atopic dermatitis. *Acta Derm Venereol (Stockh)* 1985; **65:** 102.

13. Gloor M, Strack R, Geissler H et al, Quantity and composition of skin surface lipids and alkaline-resistance in subjects with contact allergy and healthy controls. *Arch Dermatol Forsch* 1972; **245:** 184.

14. Werner Y, Lindberg M, Forslind B, The water-binding capacity of stratum corneum in dry non-eczematous skin of atopic dermatitis. *Acta Derm Venereol (Stockh)* 1982; **62:** 334.

15. Werner Y, The water content of the stratum corneum in patients with atopic dermatitis. Measurement with the corneometer CM 420. *Acta Derm Venereol (Stockh)* 1986; **66:** 281.

16. Kölmel K, Nicolaus A, Giese K, Photoacoustic determination of the water uptake by the upper horny layer of non-eczematous skin in atopic dermatitis. *Bioeng Skin* 1985; **1:** 125.

17. Mustakallio KK, Kiistala U, Piha J et al, Epidermal Lipids in Besnier's prurigo (atopic eczema). *Ann Med Exp Biol Fenn* 1967; **45:** 323.

18. Wheatley VR, Secretion of the skin in eczema. *J Pediatr* 1965; **66:** 220.

19. Rajka G, Surface lipid estimation on the back of the hands in atopic dermatitis. *Arch Dermatol Res* 1974; **251:** 43.

20. Wirth H, Gloor M, Stoika D, Sebaceous glands in uninvolved skin of patients suffering from atopic dermatitis. *Arch Dermatol Res* 1981; **270:** 167.

21. Kligman AM, Perspectives and problems of cutaneous gerontology. *J Invest Dermatol* 1979; **73:** 39.

22. Piérard GE, What does 'dry skin' mean? *Int J Dermatol* 1987; **26:** 167.

23. Idson B, Moisturizers, emollients, and bath oils. In: *Principles of Cosmetics for the Dermatologist* (Frost R, Horwitz SN, eds). St Louis: Mosby, 1982:37.

24. Swanbeck G, New treatment of ichthyosis and other hyperkeratotic conditions. *Acta Derm Venereol (Stockh)* 1968; **48:** 123.

25. Swanbeck G, Rajka G, Antipruritic effect of urea solutions. *Acta Derm Venereol (Stockh)* 1970; **50:** 225.

26. Vilaplana J, Coll J, Trullas C et al, Clinical and non-invasive evaluation of 12% ammonium lactate emulsion for the treatment of dry skin in atopic and non-atopic subjects. *Acta Derm Venereol (Stockh)* 1992; **72:** 28.

27. Tollesson A, Frithz A, Borage oil, an effective new treatment for infantile seborrhoeic dermatitis. *Br J Dermatol* 1993; **129:** 95.

28. Lodén M, Andersson A, Effect of topically applied lipids on surfactant-irritated skin. *Br J Dermatol* 1996; **134:** 215.

29. Imokawa G, Akasaki S, Hattori M et al, Selective recovery of deranged water-holding property by stratum corneum lipids. *J Invest Dermatol* 1986; **87:** 758.

30. Rajka G, Aly R, Bayles C et al, The effect of short-term occlusion on the cutaneous flora in atopic

dermatitis and psoriasis. *Acta Derm Venereol (Stockh)* 1981; **61:** 160.

31. Leyden JJ, Marples RR, Kligman AM, Staphylococcus aureus in the lesions of atopic dermatitis. *Br J Dermatol* 1974; **90:** 525.

32. Kligman AM, Leyden JJ, McGinley KJ, Bacteriology. *J Invest Dermatol* 1976; **67:** 160.

33. Aly R, Maibach HI, Shinefield HR, Bacterial flora of atopic dermatitis. *Arch Dermatol* 1977; **113:** 780.

34. Hellerström S, Rajka G, Clinical aspects of atopic dermatitis. *Acta Derm Venereol (Stockh)* 1967; **47:** 75.

35. Sulzberger MB, Atopic dermatitis. In: *Current Dermatologic Management* (Maddin S, ed). St Louis: Mosby, 1975:106.

36. Rostenberg A, Sulzberger MB, Some results of patch tests. A compilation and discussion of cutaneous reactions to about five hundred different substances as elicited by over ten thousand tests in approximately one thousand patients. *Arch Dermatol Syph* 1937; **35:** 433.

37. Frosch PJ, Kligman AM, The soap chamber test: a new method assessing the irritancy of soaps. *J Am Acad Dermatol* 1979; **1:** 35.

38. Uehara M, Takada K, Use of soap in the management of atopic dermatitis. *Clin Exp Dermatol* 1985; **10:** 419.

32

Telangiectases

Albert-Adrien Ramelet

INTRODUCTION

Telangiectases frequently occur on the face or legs. This benign condition may represent a major cosmetic concern for patients and a difficult therapeutic challenge for their physician.

On the face, most telangiectases appear in adulthood as a manifestation of an inflammatory disease, rosacea. True angiomas are less frequent. Telangiectases of the legs are mainly dependent on venous insufficiency.

TELANGIECTASES OF THE FACE

Telangiectases are permanently dilated, fine superficial blood vessels, and can be divided into primary and secondary types. Telangiectases may be so close together that they appear as homogenous redness, which fades on vitropression.

The major causes of telangiectases are listed in Table 32.1. Diagnosis does not usually represent a major problem for an experienced dermatologist.

Couperose and rosacea

In adulthood, couperose (telangiectatic flare), an early stage of rosacea, is the most frequent cause of facial telangiectases. Rosacea appears mainly during the third or fourth decade, with a slightly higher prevalence in Caucasian women.[1–3]

Rosacea is a symmetrical inflammatory disease of the convexities of the face and neck,

Table 32.1 Classification of telangiectases
Primary
Naevus flammeus
Sturge–Weber syndrome
von Hippel–Lindau syndrome
Klippel–Trenaunay–Weber syndrome
Bloom's syndrome
Osler–Weber–Rendu disease
Ataxia telangiectasia
Essential telangiectasia
Naevus araneus (spider naevus)
Angioma serpiginosum
Secondary
Couperose (rosacea)
Heliodermatitis
Chronic radiodermatitis
Xeroderma pigmentosum
Steroid dermatitis
Trauma
AIDS
Scleroderma
Lupus erythematosus
Dermatomyositis
Leg telangiectases

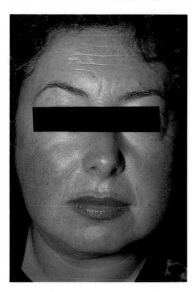

Figure 32.1 Erythrosis and couperose.

which develops in four stages. Transitional erythema (*flushing*) first occurs after non-specific stimuli such as stress, sun or cold exposures, hot foods or beverages, and alcohol intake. Progressively redness becomes persistent (*erythrosis*), and telangiectases (*couperose*) appear, mainly on the cheeks (Figure 32.1). Later stages include papular and pustular eruptions (formerly called '*acne rosacea*'), lupoid granulomas, chronic facial oedema, or hypertrophic changes such as *rhinophyma* and *gnathophyma*. The complaint may be complicated by migraine (in post-menopausal women)[4] and ophthalmic attacks.

The aetiology of rosacea is unknown. The appearance and evolution are probably governed by a vascular disorder, related to a microcirculatory disturbance of the facial angular veins, which are directly involved in the brain-cooling system. *Demodex* infestation might play an additional role in granulomatous rosacea.[2]

Basic treatment of rosacea

Protection

Protection against ultraviolet light (sun protection factor higher than 10) and extreme temperatures, and avoidance of topical steroids are imperative.

Prevention of flushing

This is also important, with avoidance of alcohol and of hot or spicy food or beverages. Ice sucking may contribute to the control of flushing.

Drug treatment

Topical application of *metronidazole* and systemic administration of *antibiotics* for several weeks (tetracycline hydrochloride, 250 mg bid; metronidazole, 250 mg bid) or, in refractory cases, of *isotretinoin* (0.2–1.0 mg/kg for 4–6 months; pregnancy is to be totally avoided during and one month after this teratogenic therapy), control the inflammatory component of the disease, but are only mildly effective on telangiectases.

Older treatments such as vitamin B_2 are obsolete. Alpha-sympathomimetic drugs could be valuable in the future.

Besides basic treatment of rosacea, *destruction of telangiectases* both relieves the patient and contributes to the control of the disease.

Treatment modalities for couperose

Any dermatosurgical treatment may lead to scarring (though this is generally minimal), and the patient must be warned about this. Several sessions are usually necessary to obtain an appreciable result.

Electrosurgery

This is the treatment of choice for small and medium-sized telangiectases of the face, using a biterminal monopolar device or a programmed diathermocoagulation (Timed). Ectatic capillaries can be eliminated with multiple microcoagulations of low energy and short duration at a distance of 1–2 mm from each other. One should begin to destroy the most prominent telangiectases going from the outer zones towards the centre of the face. The treatment may have to be repeated several times until fading of the couperose occurs.

Lasers

Laser-beam treatments (mainly with KTP, argon and pulsed dye lasers) give better results than electrosurgery, but are more expensive.

Fine-needle sclerotherapy

Larger vessels fade after fine-needle sclerotherapy (30.5 G needle; diluted Scleremo, Aethoxysclerol 0.25–0.5%, as discussed below).

Other treatments

These include *chemoscarification* (fine oblique scarification with half a razor blade, followed by application of 33% trichloroacetic acid), *cryotherapy* (particularly for erythrosis) and *crenotherapy* (showers of fine high-pressure water jets – 'douches filiformes').

Topical treatment

Creams containing flavonoids or digoxin have a minor effect, but are a valuable help, as female patients want to adapt their cosmetic habits to the disease.

Camouflage make-up

This may be required. Covermark totally disguises erythrosis, but its application is cumbersome. Some new cosmetic day-creams include green pigments that can hide the red congestive aspect of erythrosis.

Naevus flammeus (hemangioma planum, port wine stain)

Naevus flammeus is congenital or early-developing. One or several circumscribed plaques of red or purplish colour fade under diascopy. Naevus flammeus may be associated with severe malformations, including Sturge–Weber, von Hippel–Lindau and Klippel–Trenaunay–Weber syndromes, among others.

Medical camouflage make-up such as Covermark and green colour creams is a valuable help. Laser therapy (argon, KTP or pulsed dye laser) is the treatment of choice, although it may lead to scarring.

Progressive disseminated essential telangiectasia

This rare disease occurs at any age, and is of unknown aetiology. Superficial venectases spread progressively over the face and extremities (Figure 32.2).

Other telangiectases

The major causes of telangiectases are listed in Table 32.1. Many of them can be treated with sclerotherapy, fine-needle diathermy or laser beams. In some cases, dermabrasion or cryotherapy can be considered.

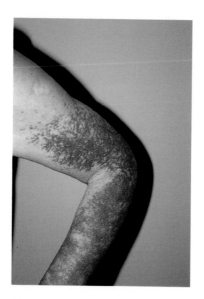

Figure 32.2 Progressive disseminated essential telangiectasia.

VENOUS TELANGIECTASES OF THE LEGS

Venous telangiectases, also known as sunburst veins, venous stars, shooting stars, spider veins and cutaneous arborizing venules, may be cosmetically very unattractive. Mostly asymptomatic, they are frequently associated with reticular and truncal varicose veins,[5] or may reveal deep vein insufficiency.[6] They start in young and middle-aged patients, their prevalence increasing with age. They may arise as a result of local trauma, pregnancy, inadequate dressing (tight garments) and prolonged standing at work.[5] Patients, mainly women, often seek medical advice and therapy for venous telangiectases of the legs because of their unsightliness.

Anatomy and physiopathology

Venous telangiectases are small (0.1–1 mm) dilated veins of the dermis localized 175–280 μm under the stratum granulosum.[7] Histological abnormalities of their vessel walls are very similar to those of varicose veins. The dilatation of the venules is consecutive to the extension to distal vessels of the venous hyperpressure and reflux in the superficial or deep venous system.[5]

A 'feeding' venule is visible in most cases of sunburst veins, especially at the latero-exterior or posterior side of the legs and thighs. A long blue reticular vein divides into several distal branches, which bear the telangiectases at their extremities (Figure 32.3).

Definitive treatment of spider veins depends wholly on the eradication of their drainage 'feeding' vein. Therefore a precise knowledge of venous anatomy is mandatory. The venous drainage of the legs[5] is shown in Figure 32.4.

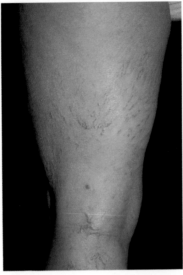

(a)

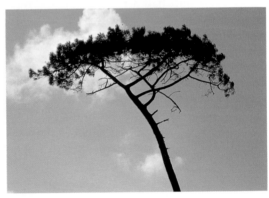

(b)

Figure 32.3 (a) Telangiectases of the leg and their 'feeding' veins. (b) Maritime pine, a natural example of telangiectatic venous drainage and 'nourishing vein'. (Courtesy of Alain Dessarps, Lausanne.)

'Ankle flare' (corona phlebectatica paraplantaris)

This is a special aspect of leg telangiectases. A crown of dilated venules surrounds the ankle, generally denoting chronic venous insufficiency (CVI).

Flare of new telangiectases ('matting')

This is one of the most feared complications of any treatment of all types of varicosities. 'Matting' occurs after sclerotherapy of vari-

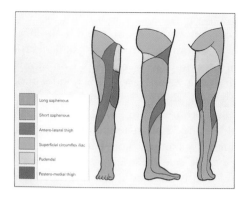

Figure 32.4 Venous drainage of the leg (With kind permission of P Griton, Paris, and of Editions Masson, Paris.) 1, long saphenous; 2, short saphenous; 3, antero-lateral thigh; 4, superficial circumflex iliac; 5, pudendal; 6, postero-medial thigh.

cose veins as well as after their surgical or microsurgical removal. The reason why the unpredictable angiomatous plaques or telangiectases present is unknown: it could be persistence of a perforator, localized venous hypertension, arteriovenous microshunt, or the presence of neoangiogenic activation factors. Whatever the reason, treatment (sclerotherapy or laser beam) is generally difficult, while prevention is somewhat uncertain. As oestrogens might play a role in the aetiology, some people recommend a halt to any oestrogen intake during treatment of leg telangiectases.

Patients with leg telangiectases may ignore the fact that they are often suffering from more severe venous disorders such as long or short saphenous veins, or deep vein incompetence. Meticulous examination of patients is therefore essential.

Diagnosis

The extent and connections of superficial varicosities to the saphenous and deep veins must be determined in a precise manner. *No treatment should be undertaken without a previous thorough examination of the patient.* This allows the choice of an adequate and successful treatment and prediction of its long-term results or risks of recurrences.[5]

Inspection
The whole of both lower limbs from the groins to the toes must be inspected: first standing, then lying (reticular 'feeding' veins are often more visible in the supine position).

Palpation and percussion
These detect dilated saphenous veins. In particular, the short saphenous vein is often more easily felt than seen. Palpation also reveals fascial defects (e.g. perforator incompetence). The cough impulse test and Schwartz test (percussion test) determine reflux and truncal insufficiency.

Directional Doppler ultrasound
This detects sapheno-femoral and sapheno-popliteal reflux, and deep veins or perforator insufficiency.

Duplex ultrasound scanner
This shows exactly the topography of the saphenous and deep veins, the presence of a reflux and the competence of valvules. It has progressively replaced phlebography.

Plethysmography
This analyses microcirculatory disturbances, detects saphenous incompetence and predicts the success of saphenous and perforator surgical operation previous to telangiectatic treatment.

Treatment modalities

The treatment of venous telangiectases is often disappointing, and relapses are frequent. The patient is to be reassured, since the condition is a benign impairment of the superficial venous system.

Camouflage make-up

Covermark can conceal telangiectases.

Most *self-tanning agents* are derived from dihydroxyacetone and react with the horny layers of the skin. They do not have a sun-protective effect, but can provide a tanned complexion, which diminishes the unattractive aspect of telangiectases.

Venoactive drugs[5]

These only have an effect on venous symptoms. They are ineffective in preventing or attenuating leg telangiectases.

Sclerotherapy[5,8]

This is the basic treatment of venous telangiectases. One should never forget to destroy the 'feeding' venule of the spider veins. Very fine needles (30.5 G) allow intravenous injection of a sclerosing solution, which damages the vessel wall (Figure 32.5). The affected venule can be resorbed, but it can also repermeabilize – particularly if the venous hyperpressure has not been corrected.

The sclerosing agent should not be too strong or concentrated, to avoid complications such as venular thrombosis, skin necrosis, brown staining and 'matting'. Commonly used sclerosing agents are 0.5% polidocanol (*Aethoxysclerol*), diluted chromated glycerol (*Scleremo*), a combination of 25% dextrose, 10% saline and 2-phenylethanol (*Sclerodex*). The value of a compression bandage following fine-needle sclerotherapy is debatable. As the vessel wall is affected a few minutes after injection, compression is not mandatory in sclerotherapy of telangiectases.

Muller's phlebectomy

This allows removal of the 'feeding' vein of telangiectases, ensuring a lasting result.[5,8,9] The 'feeding' reticular veins are carefully drawn with an indelible marking pen and anaesthetized after skin disinfection.

The venule is grasped with a special phlebectomy hook (Figure 32.6) through tiny cutaneous incisions (1 mm) or needle puncture

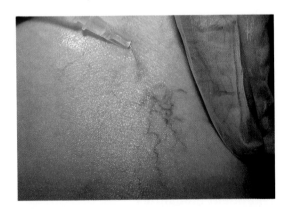

Figure 32.5 Fine-needle sclerotherapy (the needle is bent to ensure better catheterization of the venule).

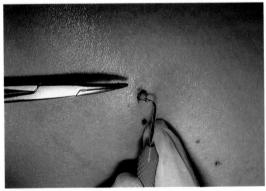

Figure 32.6 Muller's phlebectomy: eradication of a reticular varicose vein with Ramelet's phlebectomy hook (Salzmann AG, Unterstrasse 52, CH-9001 St-Gallen, Switzerland; Venosan North America Inc, 1617 N Fayettoville Street, PO Box 4068, Asheboro, NC 27204–4068, USA).

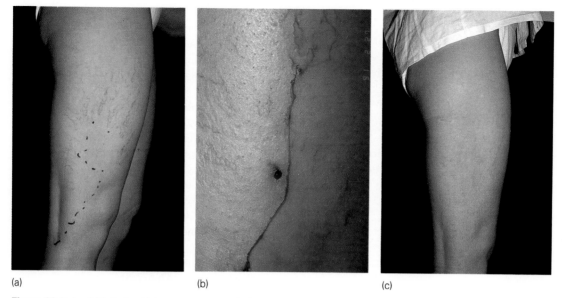

(a) (b) (c)

Figure 32.7 (a–c) Muller's phlebectomy: removal of the 'feeding' vein of telangiectases; latest result.

and extracted from one incision to the other.[8–10] Complementary fine-needle sclerotherapy of telangiectasias can be performed immediately before or after the eradication of their 'feeding' venules. Larger spider veins may also be destroyed with gentle subcutaneous 'curetage' with the sharp edge of the hook.

An elastic bandage secures compression for three weeks, preventing postoperative haemorrhage and complications. The scars are usually totally invisible after a few months (Figures 32.7a–c). Complications are exceptional.[11]

Electrocautery
This is disappointing and provokes hypopigmented, atrophic, visible scars. It should be avoided in this indication.

Laser photocoagulation and Photoderm
Although these expensive treatments are highly fashionable, their value is debatable. Laser therapy with a pulsed dye laser is indicated only as a complementary treatment after suppression of venous reflux, and should be limited to venules with a diameter smaller than 0.4 mm.[7] The value of KPT/YAG (532 nm) and Photoderm has still to be defined.

Prevention of venous telangiectases of the leg

This is quite difficult. Sunbathing is to be avoided, while local heating of the skin can cause dilatation of the superficial venules and venous stasis. Tight-fitting clothes are inappropriate.

General prevention of venous disorders, by cold showers, exercise, wearing elastic support stockings, etc., is also beneficial

CONCLUSIONS

The approach to the treatment of couperose and of leg telangiectases varies, although both conditions respond to relatively similar treatment modalities. A good knowledge of diathermy, sclerotherapy, laser beam surgery and microsurgery allows a trained practitioner to effectively relieve patients. As such treatments do not correct the aetiology of these benign malformations, the patient has to be informed about the almost unavoidable relapses of the condition.

REFERENCES

1. Grosshans E, La rosacée. *Presse Méd* 1988; **17:** 2393–8.
2. Ramelet A-A, Rosacea: disease or reaction pattern? *Dermatologica* 1986; **173:** 53–6.
3. Wilkin J, Rosacea, pathophysiology and treatment. *Arch Dermatol* 1995; **130:** 359–62.
4. Ramelet A-A, Rosacea, a reaction pattern associated with ocular lesions and migraine? *Arch Dermatol* 1994; **130:** 1448.
5. Ramelet A-A, Monti M, *Phlébologie*, 3éme édn. Paris: Masson, 1994.
6. Winters I, Marshall M, Risikofaktor Alter für die Leitvenen bei Venen-gesunden und bei Patienten mit Besenreiservaricosis. *Phlebol* 1993; **22:** 228–9.
7. Wiek K, Vanscheidt W, Ishkanian S et al, Selektive Photothermolyse von Besenreiservarizen und Teleangiektasien der unteren Extremität. *Hautarzt* 1996; **47:** 258–63.
8. Weiss RA, Weiss MA (eds), *Guide to Diagnosis and Treatment of Varicose and Telangiectatic Veins.* New York: McGraw-Hill, 1998, in press.
9. Ramelet A-A, Le traitement des télangiectasies: indications de la phlébectomie selon Muller. *Phlébologie* 1994; **47:** 377–81.
10. Ramelet A-A, Muller phlebectomy, a new phlebectomy hook. *J Dermatol Surg Oncol* 1991; **17:** 814–16.
11. Ramelet A-A, Complications of ambulatory phlebectomy. *Dermatol Surg* 1997; **23:** 947–54.

33

Hirsutism

Rodney Dawber

A general discussion of hirsutism is given by Dawber and Van Neste.[1]

ANDROGENS AND HIRSUTISM

There have been several attempts to correlate hair growth in women with plasma androgen levels, but these reports have yielded conflicting results. Reingold and Rosenfield[2] noted a considerable variability between hair growth scores and free testosterone, but no significant relationship. Others have calculated a complex formula for multiple plasma androgen levels:

testosterone/sex hormone binding globulin
+ androstenedione/100
+ dehydroepiandrosterone sulphate/100

This correlates with hair growth only in women with idiopathic hirsuties. In another study, a relationship was found between hair growth and salivary testosterone levels.

These relationships are clearly unsatisfactory, because they cannot explain the differential response to androgens by hair follicles at different sites on the body. The development of hair follicle and dermal papilla models in vitro may help answer these questions.

The physiological mechanisms for androgenic activity may be considered in three stages:

1. production of androgens by the adrenals and ovaries;
2. their transport in the blood on carrier proteins – principally sex hormone binding globulin (SHBG);
3. their intracellular modification and binding to the androgen receptor.

The first sign of androgen production in women occurs 2–3 years before the menarche, and is due to adrenal secretion. The signal for this development is unknown; there may be increased activity of C_{17-29} lyase, which directs glucocorticoid precursors towards the androgen pathway, or there may be a reduced forward metabolism of dehydroisoandrosterone (DHA) as a result of reduced activity of Δ^5-3β-hydroxysteroid dehydrogenase; this process represents a maturation of the adrenal zona reticularis. The major androgens secreted by the adrenal are androstenedione, DHA and DHA sulphate (DHAS). Their control during postpubertal life is unknown, but it is thought that androstenedione and DHA may be controlled by ACTH, since their serum levels mirror those of cortisol.

Ovarian androgen production begins

under the influence of the pubertal secretion of luteinizing hormone (LH), and takes place in the theca cells. The predominant androgen secreted by the ovaries is androstenedione during the reproductive years and testosterone after the menopause. Androgen secretion continues throughout the menstrual cycle, but peaks at the middle of an ovulatory cycle. Androstenedione secretion is greater from the ovary containing the dominant follicle.

In normal women, the majority of testosterone production (50–70%) is derived from peripheral conversion of androstenedione in skin and other extraplanchnic sites. The remaining proportion is secreted directly by the adrenals and ovaries. The relative proportion estimated from each gland varies between studies: 5–20% from the ovary and 0–30% from the adrenal. DHA is a source of less than 10% of circulating androstenedione and 1% of circulating testosterone.

Androgen transport proteins

In non-pregnant women, the majority of circulating androgens are bound to a high affinity β-globulin, SHBG. A further 20–25% is transported loosely bound to ablumin, and about 1% circulates freely. The free steroid is believed to be active, and the binding protein is therefore of paramount importance. The affinity of the androgens for SHBG is proportional to their biological activity.

The function of SHBG is unknown. It is probable that its main role is to buffer acute changes in unbound androgen levels and to protect androgens from degradation. Burke and Anderson have suggested that it also acts as a biological amplifier. High oestrogen levels increase SHBG and therefore reduce available androgen; high androgen levels reduce SHBG and increase available free androgen.

Androgen pathophysiology in hirsuties[3]

Hirsutism is a response of the hair follicles to androgenic stimulation, and increased hair growth is therefore often seen in endocrine disorders characterized by hyperandrogenism. These disorders may be due to abnormalities of either the ovaries or adrenal glands. It is likely that the majority of hirsute women have underlying polycystic ovary syndrome (PCO). A small proportion of hirsute women have no detectable hormonal abnormality, and are usually classified as 'idiopathic' hirsuties (see Figure 18.2 in Chapter 18, 'Facial and body hair'). This subgroup is gradually becoming smaller as diagnostic techniques become more refined, and the condition here is probably due to more subtle forms of ovarian or adrenal hypersecretion alterations in serum androgen binding proteins or in the cutaneous metabolism of androgens.

Although many hirsute women are obese, the role of adipose tissue is undefined, but it is clinically recognized, though undocumented, that weight loss by obese hirsute women with menstrual irregularities may result in regulation of menses and a reduction in body hair growth.

Polycystic ovary syndrome

The perception of polycystic ovary syndrome (PCO; Figure 33.1) has changed dramatically since it was first described in 1935 by Stein

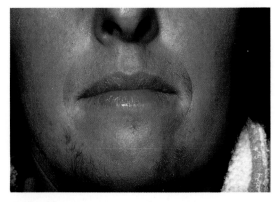

Figure 33.1 Hirsutism in a subject with polycystic ovary syndrome.

and Leventhal, who defined a syndrome consisting of obesity, amenorrhoea, hirsutism and infertility associated with enlarged plycystic ovaries. This disorder has been a controversial diagnosis, since it is defined by the appearance of organs that are difficult to visualize. This has led to the use of multiple diagnostic formulations based on clinical and biochemical abnormalities. A more fundamental issue has been raised by modern imaging techniques, which have revealed the presence of polycystic ovaries in apparently normal women. Ideas concerning the pathogenesis of PCO have been as controversial as the diagnosis, and different authorities embrace the belief that it is primarily due to an ovarian abnormality, inappropriate gonodotrophin secretion, a disorder of the adrenal glands, or increased peripheral aromatase activity resulting in hyperoestrogenaemia. Whether the increased androgen is of adrenal or ovarian origin remains controversial.

The pattern of clinical features of patients with PCO will depend to an extent on the diagnostic definition of the disorder and upon the presenting symptom, be it dermatological, endocrine or gynaecological. Using ultrasound visualization of polycystic ovaries as the diagnostic criterion, the following clinical features were found in a series of 556 patients: hirsuties (61%), acne (24%), alopecia (8%), acanthosis nigricans (2%), obesity (35%), menorrhagia (1%), obligomenorrhoea (45%), amenorrhoea (26%) and infertility (>29%). However, those patients who present to a dermatologist will almost invariable have acne and/or hirsuties.

Laboratory investigations in PCO usually reveal an elevated level of luteinizing hormone, often with an increased ratio of luteinizing hormone to follicle-stimulating hormone, and testosterone, androstenedione and oestradiol levels are often raised. The demonstration by ultrasound examination of multiple peripheral ovarian cysts around a dense central core will depend on the expertise of the operator.

Ovarian tumours

Hirsuties is a nearly universal feature in virilizing ovarian tumours; however, functioning tumours that cause virilization represent approximately 1% of ovarian tumours. Amenorrhoea or oligomenorrhoea develop in all premenopausal patients, and alopecia, cliteromegaly, deepening of the voice and a male habitus develop in about half of the patients. The majority of patients with virilizing ovarian tumours have raised plasma testosterone levels.

Hirsuties in pregnancy

Hirsuties has only rarely been reported to develop during pregnancy; it may be due to the development of PCO or a virilizing tumour. PCO has been reported to present with virilization during the first or third trimester, and may regress post-partum. Androgens freely cross the placenta, and virilization of a female fetus may occur. The range of tumours occurring during pregnancy has been reviewed by Novak and co-workers.[4]

Congenital adrenal hyperplasia

Cholesterol is metabolized in the adrenal cortex, via a complex pathway, into aldosterone, cortisol, androgens and oestrogens. A defect in a pathway results in a reduction of the product of the pathway involved, with a redistribution of the precursors to other pathways, which results in over-production of other hormones. Complete absence of a particular enzyme may be incompatible with life, and severe reduction in enzyme activity is usually apparent at birth or early childhood due to dehydration with a salt-losing state and/or virilization.

Partial reduction in enzyme activity may present after childhood, and, during the past decade, a small proportion of women presenting with postpubertal hirsuties have been demonstrated to have subtle forms of 'late-onset' congenital adrenal hyperplasia (CAH). The diagnosis cannot be made clinically, and dynamic endocrine investigations are required to differentiate between PCO and idiopathic hirsuties. Women with late-onset CAH may have normal menstrual cycles; however, approximately 80% will have polycystic ovaries.

21-Hydroxylase deficiency

This is the commonest defect association with late-onset CAH. As many as 3–6% of women presenting with hirsuties may be affected with this form. It is an allelic variant of the classic childhood salt-wasting type; the classic form is associated with HLA-Bw47 and the late-onset form with HLA-B14. Of women with this abnormality, 75% will present with hirsutism, with or without menstrual irregularities. 3β- and 11β-hydroxylase deficiencies are less common forms of CAH, and are consequently less frequently found in hirsute women.

Acquired adrenocortical disease

Adrenal carcinomas usually present with abdominal swelling or pain; however, 10% of both adenomas and carcinomas may present with isolated virilization. The combination of virilization and Cushing's syndrome strongly suggests the presence of a carcinoma. The testosterone level is usually markedly raised in the latter.

Patients with Cushing's syndrome are said to have both hypertrichosis, a generalized diffuse growth of fine hair due to hypercortisolaemia, and androgen-induced coarse hair in the usual male pattern.

Gonadal dysgenesis

One group described six patients with 46, XY gonadal dysgenesis. All had unambiguously female genitalia but male skeletal characteristics: wide span, broad shoulders and chest; two were hirsute, two had temporal recession and three had deep voices. Other workers reported a further 30 patients with gonadal dysgenesis, of whom three (with Y chromosome material) presented with slowly progressive hirsuties and secondary amenorrhoea.

Hyperprolactinaemia

The exact relationship between prolactin and hirsuties in the amenorrhoea–galactorrhoea syndrome has been reported as 22–60%. This may be due to a direct effect of prolactin or adrenal androgen production or to PCO, with which it is frequently associated; prolactin has also been reported to attenuate cutaneous 5α-reductase activity both in vivo and in vitro.

Idiopathic hirsuties

Idiopathic hirsuties is the diagnostic category given to those hirsute women in whom no underlying endocrine disorder can be detected. There are a number of subtle dynamic alterations in the androgen metabolism of hirsute women compared with non-hirsute women; daily testosterone production is increased by 3.5–5-fold; the majority of androgen is secreted as testosterone (hirsute 75% versus normal <40%) rather than as androstenedione; increased androgens in hirsute women are associated with lower levels of SHBG, which binds less testosterone and increases its free level. More free testosterone is therefore available for peripheral metabolism and clearance; these two factors disguise the increased rates of testosterone production. Free testosterone is a more sensitive measure of testosterone status, and is approximately three-fold greater in hirsute than in non-hirsute women.

Normal values for total testosterone are found in 25–60% of hirsute women and in 80% of those with regular menstrual cycles. This may be due to the effect of SHBG or to the wide fluctuations in plasma testosterone seen in hirsute women. Consequently, multiple measurements are often required to detect the increased levels. However, some women will not demonstrate elevations of testosterone despite exhaustive investigation. Paradoxically, in these women, the growth of hair by their skin is the only, and most sensitive, androgen bioassay.

Cutaneous virilism

Alterations in the cutaneous sensitivity to androgens is the reason cited for the existence of hirsuties in the presence of normal serum androgens and the lack of hirsuties in women with raised androgens. However, there has been no systematic study of hyperandrogenized non-hirsute women to determine whether or not they have other cutaneous features of androgen excess. The skin is a complex structure containing many different tissues, and it is now recognized that all the structures within the skin are modified by androgens. The eccrine and sebaceous glands are more active and the skin is thicker and contains more collagen in men than in women. Inflammation of the apocrine glands in hidradenitis suppurativa is associated with hyperandrogenism, as is occlusion of the follicular duct in both vellus and terminal hairs. It is therefore possible that the skin of non-hirsute hyperandrogenized women does respond to androgens, but not by the development of terminal hairs.

Shuster proposed a primary role for the skin. He suggested that in some individuals, the genetically determined level of cutaneous enzymes is sufficient to produce a negative feedback on the ovaries and adrenals and so enhance androgen production; he offered no evidence to support this hypothesis. However, some studies have provided data for a primary increase in cutaneous androgen metabolism, noting that the only androgen abnormality in women who have a very short history of hirsuties (less than one year) is an increase in the cutaneous androgen products: dihydrotestosterone (DHT) and 3α-androstanediol. The metabolic activity of skin in hirsuties is increased both in direct incubation assays of skin and by measurements in vivo of, for example, 3α-androstanediol glucuronide. Whole skin homogenates from genital and pubic skin of hirsute women have been demonstrated to express increased conversion of testosterone to DHT. However, isolated hair follicles from hirsute women do not appear to have different enzyme activities from controls. As the pilosebaceous units contain considerable androgen metabolizing ability, the increased conversions of testosterone by whole skin homogenates may merely reflect the increased mass of pilosebaceous tissue in hirsute women.

3α-Androstanediol glucuronide has been proposed to be a specific marker of cutaneous androgen metabolism; early studies suggested that it was raised only in hirsute women with polycystic ovaries but not in controls or non-hirsute women with polycystic ovaries; there has been little confirmatory work, and a recent study has cast doubt on its infallibility.

Hirsute women have a number of metabolic and systemic abnormalities that suggest that hirsuties is not only a cosmetic disability but may have a more serious prognosis. Hirsute women have body shapes that tend towards the male form, and, with this, they have altered lipid profiles that would suggest an increased risk of cardiovascular disease. A relationship between diabetes and hyperandrogenism in women, or 'diabetes of bearded women', has been recognized for many years. However, it has now been established that the disordered carbohydrate metabolism is due to insulin resistance (IR). Furthermore, acanthosis nigricans (AN) acts as a cutaneous marker for the IR. The combination of AN and IR occurs in 5% of women with hyperandrogenism (HA) and in 7% of women presenting with hirsuties. Women with HAIR–AN have marked features of virilism – namely muscular physique, acne, alopecia and hidradenitis suppurativa.

Insulin may play an important role in the pathogenesis of hyperandrogenism. Studies in vitro have demonstrated that insulin exerts a stimulatory effect on ovarian androgen production and that it inhibits the synthesis of sex-hormone-binding globulin by the liver. Its mode of action may be through the receptors for insulin-like growth factors, which are present both in the ovaries and in the skin. Stimulation of these may result in AN. It is, however, unknown whether the hyperinsulinaemia and insulin resistance are primary or secondary.

DIAGNOSTIC APPROACH TO THE HIRSUTE WOMAN

Most hirsute women have probably been aware of excess hair since puberty; some will give a shorter history, but it will be of the order of years. Some women are so good at cosmetic procedures that they do not appear hirsute at all. It is important to obtain facts from the history regarding patterns of hirsuties and alopecia or other features of cutaneous virilism and evidence for PCO – for example, irregular menses or infertility. A family history of childhood dehydration or precocious puberty in a brother might be a feature of congenital adrenal hyperplasia. A drug history may point to an ingested source of androgens, for example glucocorticoid or anabolic steroids. The progestogenic components of many contraceptive preparations are relatively androgenic, and this is often cited as a cause of hirsuties although it has not been a relevant factor in our experience.

The cutaneous examination will include the pattern and severity of hair growth and the associated presence of acne, androgenetic alopecia and acanthosis nigricans. Features suggestive of systemic virilization will include a deepening of the voice, increased muscle bulk and loss of the smooth skin contours, hypertension, striae distensae and cliteromegaly. This last feature, cliteromegaly, is probably the most important physical sign pointing towards systemic virilization. The implication of systemic virilization, especially where there is a short history (e.g. less than one year) is that there is a tumour causing it, which is quite different from 'cutaneous virilism'.

The extent to which it is necessary for hirsute women to be investigated is debatable. The main reason for the depth of investigation of hirsute women is the inability to differentiate between idiopathic hirsuties, PCO and CAH on clinical grounds, and it is out of this quagmire that the standard of over-investigation has arisen. The therapeutic tools available at present are too clumsy to warrant such diagnostic definition.

THERAPY

Most women will be satisfied with the assurance that they are not 'turning into men', and may not require any medical help or may only need advice about local destructive measures; however, many women will already have tried these methods.

Cosmetic measures

The easiest measure is to bleach the hair with hydrogen peroxide. This produces a yellow hue due to the native colour of keratin, and may be as unacceptable as the original colour. Hair plucking is widely performed, but the act of plucking not only removes the hair shaft but also stimulates the root into the anagen phase, and there is only a brief delay whilst the shaft grows through the epidermis. Shaving avoids this problem by removing all the hairs, but is followed by growth only of the hairs that were previously in anagen.

Waxing is performed by the application onto the skin of a sheet of soft wax, which, as soon as it has hardened with the hair shafts embedded, is abruptly peeled off the skin, removing all the shafts. This is a painful method, and is often complicated by folliculitis. Certain natural sugars, long used in parts of the Middle East, are becoming popular in place of waxes, since they appear to depilate as effectively, but with less trauma.

Electrolysis is the only permanent method for removal of hair. A fine electrical wire is introduced down the hair shaft to the papilla, which is destroyed by an electrical current. Laser destruction is being widely investigated, but the efficacy of this method requires further studies.

Systemic anti-androgen therapy

Since hirsuties is a condition mediated by androgens, attempts have been made to ameliorate the growth of hair using drugs with anti-androgenic properties. The complete spectrum of therapeutic agents evaluated in the treatment of hirsuties is described below. It is, however, common practice to use cyproterone acetate and spironolactone as first-line therapy for those women whose hirsuties is so severe as to warrant systemic therapy.

It is important that hirsute women be carefully selected prior to initiating therapy, for the following reasons. First, the effect on hair growth takes several months to become apparent, and only partial improvements may be expected. Secondly, anti-androgens feminize male fetuses, and it is essential that the women do not become pregnant. Thirdly, these drugs only have a suppressive, and not curative, effect, which wears off a few months after cessation of therapy, and therapy may need to be taken indefinitely if a favourable improvement occurs. Finally, the long-term safety of these drugs is unknown, and tumours in laboratory animals have been reported with several of the following agents.

Cyproterone acetate

Cyproterone acetate (CPA)[5,6] is both an anti-androgen and an inhibitor of gonadotrophin secretion. It reduces androgen production, increases the metabolic clearance of testosterone and binds to the androgen receptor; in addition, long-term therapy is associated with a reduction in the activity of cutaneous 5α-reductase. Cyproterone acetate is a potent progestogen, but does not reliably inhibit ovulation. It is usually administered with cyclical oestrogens in order to maintain regular menstruation and to prevent conception in view of the risk of feminizing a male fetus.

Several dose regimens have been advocated. Low-dose therapy (Dianette, Schering AG) is an oral contraceptive containing 35 µg ethinyloestradiol and 2 mg CPA, taken daily for 21 days in every 28. However, all of the dose-ranging and efficacy studies have been performed using a preparation containing 50 µg ethinyloestradiol; this may be relevant, since only the higher dose of oestrogen increases SHBG. Current dosage recommendations for CPA usually advise that 50 or 100 mg CPA should be administered for 10 days/cycle. However, there have now been many dose-ranging studies that suggest that there is no dose effect. Objective studies comparing Dianette with and without extra CPA found no difference, either in the reduction of the overall hirsuties grades or in the reduction in hair shaft diameters.

Side-effects of CPA include weight gain, fatigue, loss of libido, mastodynia, nausea, headaches and depression. All of these are more frequent with a higher dose. Contraindications to its use are the same as for the contraceptive pill, and include cigarette smoking, age, obesity and hypertension.

Spironolactone

Spironolactone has several antiandrogenic pharmacological properties. It reduces the bioavailability of testosterone by interfering with its production, and increases its metabolic clearance. It binds to the androgen receptor, and like cyproterone acetate, long-term therapy is associated with a reduction in cutaneous 5α-reductase activity. It was an act of serendipity that demonstrated its therapeutic advantage in hirsuties. A 19-year old hirsute woman with polycystic ovary syndrome was treated with spironolactone (200 mg daily) for concurrent hypertension, and she noted after three months that she needed to shave less frequently. This report was soon followed by studies demonstrating that spironolactone reduced testosterone production and subjectively reduced hair growth in hirsute women.

Different dose schedules of spironolactone have been studied, varying between 50 and 200 mg taken either daily or cyclically (daily for three weeks in every four). Within this dose range, the one chosen will depend on the severity of the hirsuties.

There have been no formal clinical trials comparing the two treatments, but comparative reports claim that both agents are equally effective. It is not known whether the two agents have an additive effect.

Corticosteroids

These are first-line therapy for congenital adrenal hyperplasia, and were the first endocrine therapy to be employed in the treatment of hirsuties with the rationale of suppressing the production of adrenal androgens. Corticosteroids are effective in reducing plasma androgen levels, but there are contradictory reports regarding their therapeutic effect on hair growth.

Medroxyprogesterone acetate

Medroxyprogesterone acetate (MPA) is a synthetic progestogen that was introduced as an anovulatory agent because of its ability to block gonadotrophin secretion. It reduces androgen levels by reducing the production of testosterone and increasing its metabolic clearance.

A comparison of topical (0.2% ointment) with systemic therapy either by intramuscular injection of MPA (150 mg every 6 weeks) or subcutaneous injection (100 mg every 6 weeks) gave a beneficial response in most patients. MPA given alone may result in menorrhagia.

Desogestrel

This is the progestogen used in the Marvelon contraceptive pill (Organon Ltd), which contains 30 µg ethinyloestradiol and 150 mg desogestrel. All the studies undertaken have reported subjective and/or objective reductions in hair growth of 20–25% after 6–9 months therapy, with a high degree of patient satisfaction.

Ketoconazole

This is a potent inhibitor of adrenal and ovarian steroid synthesis. There have been only isolated reports of its use in hirsuties, but these have demonstrated a marked reduction in hair growth after 6 months. However, this treatment cannot be recommended in view of the risks of hepatic toxicity during long-term therapy.

Flutamide

This acts as a pure anti-androgen, and works by binding to androgen receptors. However, it has no antigonadotrophic effect, and the result of binding to central androgen receptors is that it prevents the negative feedback effect of testosterone, and consequently androgen levels rise. There has been a single study in hirsuties in which flutamide (250 mg twice daily) was administered with an oral contraceptive for seven months: 12 out of 13 patients demonstrated a subjective improvement in hair growth and acne.

Gonadotrophin-releasing hormone agonists

Gonadotrophin-releasing hormone (Gn-RH) agonists inhibit LH production, and this results in profound suppression of androgen production. These agents are presently under investigation, but preliminary studies suggest that they effectively reduce hair growth and acne in women with PCO.

Cimetidine

This is a weak anti-androgen as mediated by androgen receptor binding studies. A study of patients with idiopathic hirsuties demonstrated a marked reduction in hair growth using hair weight, whereas no such effect was seen in controls given only a placebo.

Bromocriptine

This is a dopamine agonist, and long-term therapy with bromocriptine regulates menstrual cycle length, but 12 months therapy produced no measurable effect on linear hair growth in women with polycystic ovaries.

REFERENCES

1. Dawber RPR, Van Neste D, *Hair and Scalp Disorders*. London: Martin Dunitz, 1995:154–68.

2. Reingold SB, Rosenfield RL, The relationship of mild hirsutism or acne in women to androgens. *Arch Dermatol* 1987; **123:** 209–14.

3. Hauner H, Ditschuneit SB, Pal SB et al, Fat distribution, endocrine and metabolic profile in obese women with and without hirsuties. *Metabolism* 1988; **37:** 281–6.

4. Novak DJ, Lauchlin SC, McCawley JC et al, Virilization during pregnancy; case report and review of the literature. *Am J Med* 1970; **49:** 281–5.

5. Barth JH, Cherry CA, Wojnarowska F et al, Cyproterone acetate for severe hirsutism; results of a double-blind dose-ranging study. *J Clin Endocrin Metab* 1991; **35:** 5–10.

6. Crosignani PG, Rubin B, Strategies for the treatment of hirsutism. *Hormone Res* 1989; **4:** 651–9.

34

Pigmentation: Dyschromia

Sumar Kumit Bose, Jean-Paul Ortonne

INTRODUCTION

Any visible pigmentary change, whether hyper-, hypo- or depigmentation, is a cause for concern, leading to a visit to a dermatologist. Normal skin colour results from an admixture of several coloured pigments: haemoglobin carotenoids and melanins, of which the latter are most important.[1] The skin colour depends upon the types of melanin in an individual; these include eumelanins (brown-black), pheomelanins (yellow-red) and mixed melanins. They vary in their chemical and physical properties, and are produced by highly specialized dendritic cells of the basal layer of the epidermis called melanocytes. Melanin pigmentation is a multistep complex process involving both melanocytes and keratinocytes in the epidermal-melanin unit. Any pigmentary modulation from normal genetically programmed pigmentary control by exogenous (light, chemicals, local infection) or endogenous (hormones, drugs) factors leads to pigmentary abnormality. Various treatments include depigmenting agents, azelaic acid, retinoids, PUVA, bleaching agents, camouflage (cover-up), tattooing, skin grafts, transplantation of melanocytes, cautery and reconstructive surgery. It is important to judge the cosmetic deformity and type of skin before any procedure is undertaken, since post-inflammatory hyper- or depigmentation is common.

DISORDERS OF PIGMENTATION[2]

Classification

Pigmentary disturbances include epidermal hypopigmentation (leucoderma), epidermal hyperpigmentation (melanoderma) and grey, slate or blue discoloration (ceruloderma). Not all of these are related to the melanin pigmentary system – some may be only partially related or may not be related at all. Leucoderma can be either melanocytopenic (hypopigmentation with reduction or absence of melanocytes) or melanopenic (hypopigmentation with a normal number of melanocytes but an absence of, or reduction in, melanins), whereas in melanoderma (melanotic disease) there is an increase in the melanin pigment, and in ceruloderma (melanocytic disease) there is an increase in the number of melanocytes. Some of these hyperpigmentary disorders for which patients seek medical advice include freckles, melasma, actinic and senile lentigines, café-au-lait spots, post-inflammatory hypermelanosis, Becker's naevus, facial melanosis, lichen planus actinicus and iatrogenic melanosis. Among the hypopigmentations, the most common are vitiligo, idiopathic guttate hypomelanosis, post-inflammatory hypomelanosis, pityriasis alba, hypomelanotic tinea versicolor, iatrogenic depigmentation and contact hypomelanosis. Some of these disorders are common in day-to-day dermatological practice, and require careful evaluation, since they usually produce psychological, social and personality concerns. These cosmetic disfigurements may have disastrous effects in persons in certain professions that involve dealing with the public, such as receptionists, actors and secretaries. Drastic measures or over-treatment usually exaggerate these conditions. Case-to-case study helps.

Wood's lamp is perhaps the minimum requirement to differentiate both melanin hypo- and hypermelanotic pigmentary disorders. Epidermal hypermelanosis is accentuated, whereas the dermal type disappears or becomes less obvious. The contrast between normal and hypopigmented skin is greater under Wood's lamp examination, especially in light-skinned individuals.

Skin biopsy is of the utmost importance for classification and therapeutic management. Theoretically there are two situations:

- There are too many melanocytes or there is too much melanin in the skin. In this situation treatment is directed against melanocyte destruction – usually by bleaching and depigmenting agents.
- There is not enough melanin or there are too few melanocytes in the epidermis and/or hair follicles. Such cases require treatment leading to stimulation of melanin and/or melanocytes in the melanocytopenic macules. Photochemotherapy is the only effective treatment presently available for repigmentation of hypomelanotic areas. Other cosmetic methods include dyes and covering agents (camouflage, tatooing, etc.).

Leucoderma (Table 34.1)

Vitiligo (melanocytopenic)[3,4]

Vitiligo is an acquired hypomelanotic disorder characterized by well-circumscribed progressive cutaneous macules with hypo- or hyperpigmented border (Figure 34.1). It is frequently associated with circulating autoantibodies. The average incidence of vitiligo is between 1% and 2% but higher incidence is seen in certain populations (range

---

Table 34.1 Disorders of pigmentation with cosmetic importance

Leucoderma
- Vitiligo[3,4]
- Idiopathic guttate hypomelanosis (IGH)[9]
- Post-inflammatory depigmentation,[4] post-burn depigmentation,[4] psoriasis,[4] leprosy,[4] chronic lupus erythematosus[4]
- Pityriasis alba[13,14]
- Pityriasis versicolor[15]
- Chemical and drug-induced:
  hydroquinone and its derivatives,[2] corticosteroids,[28] mercury,[2] rubber slippers (mercaptobenzothiazole and/or thiuram mixture),[4,21] sandalwood oil,[34,36] butylphenol[4]

Melanoderma
- Becker's naevus[16]
- Freckles or ephelides[17]
- Solar lentigo[17]
- PUVA lentigines[3,4]
- Berloque pigmentation[4]
- Melasma[4]
- Post-inflammatory hypermelanosis:[3]
  trauma,[4] acne excoree,[4] lichen planus,[4] lupus erythematosus,[4] post-dermabrasion,[31] fixed drug eruption[4]

Cerulodermas
- Naevus of Ota[3,4]
- Riehl's melanosis:[4]
  occupational melanosis or melanoderma toxica[3,4]
- Macular amyloidosis[18]
- Drug-induced hyperpigmentation:
  minocycline,[4,19] phenothiazines,[4,32] silver,[4] clofazimine,[4,20] carotenoderma[4]
- Tattooing[11,38]
- Erythema ab igne[27]
- Dermal melasma[3,4]
- Oral contraceptives[3,4]
- Post-inflammatory:
  acne excoree,[4] perfume contact hypermelanosis,[4] fixed drug eruptions,[4] henna[4]

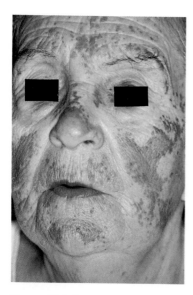

Figure 34.1 Extensive facial involvement in a patient with vitiligo. Only a few areas with normal pigmentation remain. This patient can benefit from permanent chemical depigmentation of normal skin on the face.

0.14–8.8%). Fifty percent of cases of vitiligo appear before 20 years of age. Family history is present in 30–40% of cases. Inheritance is thought to be autosomal dominant, with variable expression. Increased incidence of HLA-DR4 in blacks, B-13 in Moroccan Jews and BW 35 in Yemeni Jews has been reported. Vitiligo has been reported to follow emotional crisis, physical injury and sunburn. Areas of friction and trauma are characteristically involved, like knees, elbows, ankles, backs of hands, and feet. Other areas are cheeks, chin, eyes, nose, mouth, anal area, anterior tibial area, flexor of wrists, axilla and lower back. The distribution is symmetrical, but dermatomal arrangement may be seen. Wood's lamp determines the exact extent of depigmentation. Achromotrichia occurs in 9–45% of vitiligo patients. Associated abnormalities include mild iritis to ocular abnormalities in

10–40% of cases. Vitiligo has been associated with various autoimmune diseases, namely Grave's disease, hyperthyroidism, thyroiditis, myxoedema or thyroid carcinoma, diabetes mellitus, pernicious anaemia, multiglandular insufficiency, halo naevi and alopecia areata. Premature greying of hair occurs in 37% of cases. Dopa and haematoxylin–eosin staining shows absence of melanocytes but occasional lymphocytes at the active margins. Electron microscopy shows keratinocyte vacuolization, with extracellular granular material deposits adjacent to melanocytes in basal keratinocytes. Melanocytes from depigmented and pigmented areas of vitiligo show structural aberrations, with abnormal cytoplasmic filaments, mitochondria and cell membranes. Morohashi and co-workers have described changes of autophagocytosis of melanosomes, whereas Boissy and colleagues have suggested melanosome compartmentalization and aberration of the rough endoplasmic reticulum.[5] Various hypotheses for the cause of vitiligo has been suggested, including immune, self-destructive, neural and composite mechanisms.[3] Recently, new hypotheses have been proposed, including inherent structural defects in melanocytes, the role of growth factors in the non-functioning of vitiligo melanocytes,[6] the effective role of melatonin[7] and finally vitiligo being a disorder of T lymphocytes.[8] The actual mechanism of inhibition or destruction of melanocytes in vitiligo may in fact be much more complex than these suggested mechanisms. A patch of depigmentation due to vitiligo on exposed areas can give rise to cosmetic and social concerns, especially in racially pigmented skin. Photochemotherapy, cover-up and high sun protection factor (SPF) sunscreens to minimize the risk of sunburn on the achromic areas should be used.

Idiopathic guttate hypomelanosis (melanopenic)[9]

Idiopathic guttate hypomelanosis (IGH) is an asymptomatic and benign dermatosis charac-

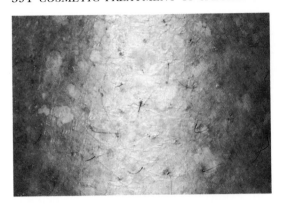

Figure 34.2 Idiopathic guttate hypomelanosis.

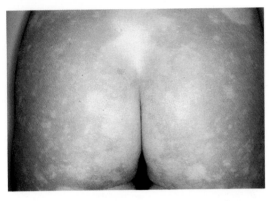

Figure 34.3 Macules in post-inflammatory hypomelanosis are characterized by ill-defined borders.

terized by numerous, usually small, hypopigmented and achromic spots on the extremities (Figure 34.2). The distribution on forearm and legs and the fear of vitiligo provoke aesthetic concerns. The aetiology of IGH remains obscure. Both hereditary and non-hereditary factors may play a role. Sunlight may induce the lesions of IGH, but there is no conclusive evidence for this. Aging, genetics and gradual spontaneous loss of melanocytes have been proposed as causes of IGH. The number of melanocytes is decreased, but, unlike in vitiligo, they are always present. Intralesional triamcinolone with or without small grafts improves the appearance of individual lesions.

Post-inflammatory depigmentation or hypomelanosis (melanopenic)[4]

Post-inflammatory hypomelanosis occurs in a variety of conditions with a reduced number of functional melanocytes, such as indeterminate leprosy of cheeks, chronic lupus erythematosus, and sarcoidosis (Figure 34.3).

Hypomelanosis, as in resolving psoriasis of face and extremities, is related to an increased mitotic rate of keratinocytes and diminished transfer of melanosomes.

Post-burn or post-traumatic depigmentation (melanocytopenic)[10]

Certain racially pigmented skins are highly prone to post-inflammatory depigmentation, especially following burns. This depigmentation is common in second- and third-degree burns, and causes permanent achromia, in particular on the hands, with absence of dopa-positive melanocytes and no hair follicles. This causes a serious cosmetic liability in dark-skinned people. Various methods of treatment include tattooing,[11] use of split-skin grafts of 0.1–0.2 mm thickness, homologous thin Thiersch skin grafts, and recently epidermal grafts containing melanocytes.[12]

Pityriasis alba (melanopenic)[13]

This is a non-specific dermatitis of unknown origin, characterized by erythematous scaly patches of the face, which is followed by depigmentation. Leucoderma may persist on the face for a year or more. Electron microscopy shows a reduced number of melanocytes and decreases in the number and size of melanosomes. Association with atopy is frequently seen. Treatment is unsatisfactory. In extensive pityriasis alba, PUVA therapy has been reported to be successful.[14]

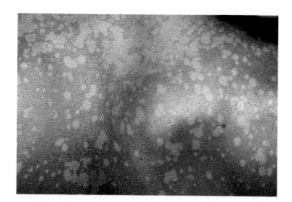

Figure 34.4 Achromic tinea versicolor. (Courtesy of Dr Strobel.)

Pityriasis versicolor (melanopenic)[15]

This is a chronic, mild, usually asymptomatic infection of the stratum corneum. The lesions are characterized by a branny or furfurous consistency; they are discrete or concrescent, and appear as discoloured or depigmented areas of the skin (Figure 34.4). Although chest, abdomen, upper limbs and back are usually affected, frequent consultations are sought for lesions on the neck and face. The disease is caused by a lipophilic yeast *Malassezia furfur*, which is a common endogenous saprophyte of normal skin. It is not known why certain individuals are susceptible to the disease. Genetic predisposition, poor nutrition, and accumulation of extracellular glycogen have been suggested. C9 to C11 dicarboxylic lipid fractions produced during metabolism of oleic acids inhibit the dopa tyrosinase reaction, causing depigmentation. Diagnosis is by Wood's lamp showing yellow fluorescence, and skin scraping with potassium hydroxide demonstrating branched mycelium with grouped small yeast cells. Most patients respond to local therapy with imida-zoles (miconazole, isoconazole, ketoconazole, etc.). Rarely, systemic therapy with oral ketoconazole is required. Resistant achromic patches require retinoid cream locally.

Melanoderma (Table 34.1)

Becker's naevus (melanotic)[16]

Becker's melanosis is a fairly common condition, affecting 0.5% of young men. Initially noticed as brown pigmentation during adolescence, it becomes conspicuous after exposure to the sun. It is most characteristically situated on the shoulders, anterior chest and scapular area (Figure 34.5). However, the face and neck may rarely be affected. After a couple of years, thick dark hairs develop. Females may develop associated unilateral hypoplasia of the breast, spina bifida and limb asymmetry. Histologically, basal and suprabasal keratinocytes are heavily pigmented; melanocytes have been reported to be normal or increased. Ultrastructure shows increased melanocyte activity and an increased number of melanosomal complexes in keratinocytes, consistent with enhanced melanin synthesis. Giant melanosomes have been reported in both melanocytes and keratinocytes. Camouflaging is recommended.

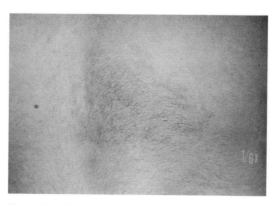

Figure 34.5 Typical Becker's naevus.

Freckles or ephelides (melanotic)[17]

Freckles are poorly defined pale-brown macules seen on exposed areas. Histologically, the melanocytes are normal in number compared with adjacent normal skin, but there is increased production of melanin due to ultraviolet stimulation.

Freckles are usually noticed in summer in fair-haired and fair-skinned individuals. Photoprotection is advised.

Solar lentigo (melanocytotic)[17]

These are areas of macular brown pigmentation 1 cm or more in diameter, appearing after both acute and chronic exposure to the sun (Figure 34.6). There is a linear increase in melanocytes at the dermo-epidermal junction, but no atypia or incontinence of pigment is seen. This condition either appears after sunburn or is seen in chronically sun-exposed elderly. The face and the backs of hands are affected. Treatment includes high-SPF sunscreens, retinoids and cryotherapy.

PUVA lentigines (melanocytotic)[3]

PUVA lentigines occur in more than 2% of patients after 2–3 years of extensive PUVA therapy. They are pigmented macules (stellate

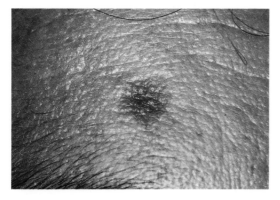

Figure 34.6 Actinic lentigo.

freckle-like), occurring in exposed areas frequently in the elderly of skin types I and II. The melanocytes are hypertrophic and may have cytological atypia.

Berloque pigmentation (melanotic)[4]

This results from intensification of melanogenesis by light as a result of 5-methoxypsoralen (bergapten) bergamot oil in perfumes (eau-de-cologne) by 320 nm light. Susceptibility depends upon absorption and duration of exposure to the sun after application of perfume. Lesions are deep-brown and follow the pattern of the application; they fade gradually over weeks to months. There is an increase in the number of functional melanocytes, which are more dendritic and dopa-positive. There is increased melanogenesis, and the distribution of melanosomes in the keratinocytes changes in Caucasoids from the aggregated to the non-aggregated form.

Melasma (melanotic)[3,4]

This is an acquired condition accompanied by irregularly shaped patches and plaques of light- to dark-brown pigmentation developing on the face, that is, on the cheeks, nose, forehead, upper lip, chin and sometimes neck (Figure 34.7). It is distressing and unsightly in racially pigmented skin. The aetiology remains obscure, but it is often attributed to solar exposure, genetics and hormones. Other causes implicated are oestrogens, progesterone, cosmetics and hydantoin. It usually develops during pregnancy or with the use of oral contraceptives. It also occurs in men. Wood's lamp distinguishes dermal, epidermal and compound (dermal + epidermal) forms of melasma. In epidermal melasma, the melanin deposits occur in the basal and suprabasal layers, but occasionally throughout the epidermis. In dermal melasma, melanin-laden macrophages are noticed around the superficial and mid-dermal vasculature. The ultrastructure shows increased melanocytes, melanogenesis, transfer of melanosomes, and size and percentage of melanosomes in ker-

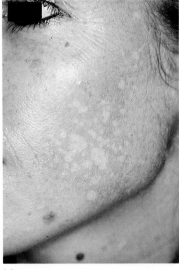

(a)

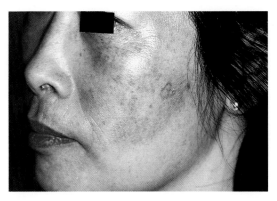

Figure 34.8 Post-inflammatory hypermelanosis of the face.

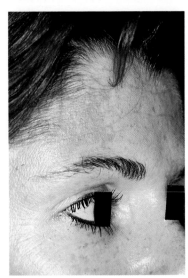

(b)

Figure 34.7 Melasma on the cheek (a) and forehead (b).

atinocytes. Treatment includes hydroquinone 2% locally, Kligman's formula, high-SPF sunscreens, Covermark or Dermablend.

Post-inflammatory hypermelanosis (melanotic)[4]

Any acute or chronic inflammatory process may give rise to hypermelanosis in predisposed individuals. This usually happens in disorders affecting the basal keratinocytes, such as lichen planus and lupus erythematosus. In racially pigmented skin, these two diseases produce disfiguring pigmentation of exposed areas such as the face and extremities (Figure 34.8). In fixed drug eruption, in addition to damage to basal cells, there is pigmentary incontinence, with melanophages in the upper dermis. Post-inflammatory hyperpigmentation follows trauma, acne excoree, and dermabrasion in dark-skinned individuals.

Ceruloderma (Table 34.1)

Naevus of Ota (melanocytotic)[3,17]

Naevus of fusucaeruleus ophthalmomaxillaris is an acquired, usually unilateral, blue or grey-brown macule occurring most characteristically in the eye and the surrounding skin innervated by the first and second branches of the trigeminal nerve (Figure 34.9). Although first described among Japanese in 1939, it has also been reported in other races. In milder forms, there is involvement of the upper and lower eyelids, and periorbital skin to the temple region; in others, in addition

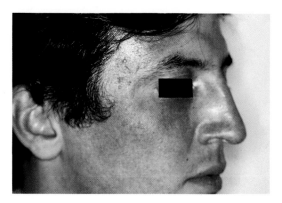

Figure 34.9 Typical naevus of Ota.

the zygomatic area of forehead, eyebrow and nose are involved. Frequently, female patients come for treatment with the colour of the lesions ranging from black, purple, blue-black, slate-blue, purplish brown and brown. Mottled or freckle-like pigmentation is also observed. Ocular melanosis is common. Histology reveals stellate, bipolar dermal melanocytes in the reticular dermis. Occasionally, epidermal melanocytes are increased in number. Electron microscopy shows the presence of stage IV melanosomes in the melanocytes, which are often surrounded by an extracellular sheath. CO_2 snow and argon lasers may reduce the colour intensity, and Covermark is successful as camouflage.

Riehl's melanosis (melanotic)[4]

This is a distinct pattern of non-pruritic pigmented dermatitis characterized by a brownish-grey pigmentation that develops rapidly over the face, forehead and temples. The pigmentation may extend to the chest, neck, scalp and hands. It is seen commonly in women, but occurs rarely in man and children. Histologically, it is characterized by liquefactive degeneration of basal cells accompanied by the formation of melanophages in the dermis. A moderate cellular infiltration of lymphoid cells and histiocytes is also usually present in the papillary dermis; these are perivascular or band-like. The aetiology of Riehl's melanosis is not yet clear. Nutrition, tar derivatives, ingredients in talcum powder, and perfumes have been blamed. Recent reports from Japan and elsewhere suggest that cosmetics or their ingredients may be responsible, since patch tests have been positive in all cases. In children, it is more likely that nutritional factors play a role, since there is no history of contact with cosmetics. Ultrastructurally, there is intracellular and intercellular oedema of keratinocytes, a multi-layered basal lamina and many dermal melanophages. Treatment is difficult. Improvement occurs slowly in cases of proven sensitivity to cosmetics after stopping their use.

Occupational melanosis or melanoderma toxica[3,4] is probably the same as Riehl's melanosis, with a similar aetiological background. Workers handling coal-tar products, such as pitch, asphalt, creosote and mineral oils, may develop diffuse melanosis of exposed skin, probably through the photodynamic action of anthracene, phenanthrene and other substances. A reticulate pigmentation develops slowly after prolonged exposure, and is associated with atrophy, telangiectasia, lichenoid papules and follicular keratosis. The diagnosis is established by history and photopatch testing. In addition to pigmentary incontinence, small amounts of amyloid are described. Keratosis and epitheliomas may subsequently form.

Lichen and macular amyloidosis (derived from epidermal cells) (melanotic)[18]

This is a common condition, exhibiting a familiar presentation in Asians, Chinese and Malaysians, but is rare among Europeans and North Americans. Lichen amyloidosis usually starts as intensely pruritic discretely small papules 1–3 mm in diameter. The colour is from yellowish-brown to grey. Lesions affect the extremities. Amyloid is seen by electron microscopy, closely associated with dermal papillae. Recent evidence shows amyloid to be derived from degradation products of keratin. Epidermal hyperplasia occurs.

Macular amyloidosis is less common, and is accompanied by greyish-brown macules. It gives a rippled appearance in some cases. Histology and amyloid deposits are similar to those of lichen amyloidosis, except for the absence of hyperkeratosis and papillomatosis.

Drug-induced hyperpigmentation (Table 34.1)

Minocycline (non-melanotic)[4]

Pigmentation with minocycline is seen in patients taking this drug for a long time. Pigmentation may involve inflamed tissue like acne scar or fish-tank granuloma, or may be diffuse, affecting sun-exposed areas. Histology shows brown-black granules, which stain positive for iron. Electron microscopy reveals electron-dense material in dermal macrophages. X-ray microanalysis confirms the presence of iron and calcium. Recently, minocycline has been detected along with iron and calcium in these granules.[19]

Chlorpromazine and related phenothiazines (non-melanotic)[4]

Chlorpromazine prescribed in high doses among certain patients results in bluish-grey pigmentation of sun-exposed areas of the skin. In addition, the affected individuals may develop cataracts, corneal opacities and pigmentation of the conjunctiva. Exposure to the sun causes this, and there is extensive melanin-like material throughout the reticulo-endothelial system and involving the parenchymal cells of internal organs. Electron microscopy shows an increase of melanin in the epidermis, and perivascular macrophages in the dermis contain electron-dense particles. Radiolabelled chlorpromazine is found in tissues containing melanin. D-Penicillamine

may diminish the pigmentation. Halting the use of chlorpromazine ultimately fades the colour.

Silver pigmentation (argyria) (non-melanotic)[4]

This occurs owing to deposition of silver in the skin from prolonged industrial exposure or a result of a medication with silver commonly called Asiatic pills. Pigmentation is a slate-grey colour, appearing after a few months to years. Increased pigmentation is most apparent in the sun-exposed areas, especially the forehead, nose and hands. The sclera, nails and mucous membranes are involved.

Electron microscopy shows numerous silver granules in the dermis in relation to the basal lamina of the eccrine sweat glands. These granules are readily visible with dark-field illumination. Pigmentation is permanent and difficult to treat.

Clofazimine[4]

This drug is used in the treatment of leprosy, and produces an initial pink to later brown coloration of the skin due to an accumulation of the drug. Later, with prolonged treatment, a violaceous brown colour develops in affected areas. Histochemical studies indicate a ceroid-like brown pigment in the foamy macrophages. The earlier reddish hue may be due to accumulation of the drug in the skin.[20] Halting the drug returns the colour to normal.

Carotenoderma[4]

Carotene, a lipochrome, contributes a yellow colour to normal skin. In the presence of excessive blood carotene levels, this yellow component is increased, and is most conspicuously accentuated where the horny layer is thick or subcutaneous fat is plentiful. Metabolic carotenaemia occurs in certain diseases like hyperlipaemia, diabetes, nephritis and hypothyroidism. Nowadays people with carotenaemia include food faddists and weight watchers taking oranges and carrots, and those taking carotenoids that contain canthaxanthin for photoprotection.

AETIOLOGICAL FACTORS IN DYSCHROMIAS (Table 34.2)

Occupationally induced dyschromia

Hyper- or hypomelanosis may have legal implications in relation to industrial workers. They are especially common in susceptible individuals. Vitiligo-like depigmentation of the extremities is seen in people working in

commercial rubber factories.[4,21] Patch tests show mercaptobenzothiazole and/or thiuram mixture-positive discoloration.[22] Factory workers handling phenol derivatives containing *p*-butylphenol often notice depigmentation of hands and feet or in the areas of contact.[23] A patch test is usually positive. Fibreglass workers and hydrofluoric acid workers have hyperpigmentation at the site of the entrance of the spicule of fibre or contact with the acid.[24,25] Similarly, gardeners,[26] perfumery workers,[4] pitch and tar handlers,[4] glass blowers and bakery workers[27] suffer from phytophotopigmentation,[26] berloque pigmentation,[4] melanoderma,[3,4] reticulated pigmented skin and erythema ab igne.[27]

Iatrogenic dyschromia

The commonest iatrogenic dyschromias include depigmentation due to injection of steroids[28] and excess use of hydroquinone or its derivatives.[2] Several cases have been reported following intralesional injection of steroids in lichen planus hypertrophicus, keloids, intra-articular injections and intrabulbar injections. Depigmentation persists for a long time, and may improve with local retinoid therapy.[29] Improper use of local psoralen lotions for vitiligo produces hyperpigmentation of neighbouring areas of contact.[30] Prolonged use of minocycline for acne may result in hyperpigmentation at the site of scars.[4] PUVA therapy may result in lentigo-like pigmentation on the exposed areas; sometimes pigmented macules are also seen.[3] Post-dermabrasion hyperpigmentation[31] is very common in individuals with phototypes IV and V, and produces disfiguring cosmetic results. Grey or slate-coloured pigmentation of the face is commonly seen with prolonged use of chlorpromazine,[4] and sometimes with imipramine.[32] Many surgical procedures may result in pigmentary changes: these include hyperpigmentation after sclerotherapy[33] and CO_2 laser therapy,[34] and depigmentation following cryotherapy.[2]

Table 34.2 Aetiological factors in dyschromias

Occupationally induced hyper- or hypopigmentation
- Rubber workers: vitiligo-like depigmentation (commercial rubber)[21]
- Factory workers handling phenols, catechols and guanonitrofuracin: depigmentation[4,23]
- Fibreglass workers: hyperpigmentation[24,25]
- Hydrofluoric acid burns: hyperpigmentation[24]
- Gardeners: phytophotodermatitis: hyperpigmentation 'Edger's rash'[26]
- Perfumery workers: hyperpigmentation of hands or/and face[4]
- Pitch or tar workers: hyperpigmentation of exposed areas[4]
- Glass and bakery workers: reticulate hyperpigmentation; erythema ab igne[27]

Iatrogenic hyperpigmentation and hypopigmentation
- Local or intralesional steroids: depigmentation[28]
- Hydroquinone: confetti-like depigmentation[2,4]
- Minocycline: hyperpigmentation[4,19]
- Psoralens, fluocoumarins: hyperpigmentation[4,30]
- PUVA lentigo, PUVA pigmented macules[36]
- Post-dermabrasion hyperpigmentation[31]
- Chloropromazine: slate-grey hyperpigmentation[4]
- Post-sclerotherapy hyperpigmentation[33]
- Cryotherapy depigmentation[2]
- CO_2 laser hyperpigmentation[34]

Social habits, cosmetics and dyschromia
- Bindi adhesive: depigmentation[23]
- Henna: hyperpigmentation[35]
- Sandalwood perfume, paste or oil: depigmentation[36]
- Asiatic pills (health pills) containing silver: slate-grey colour[37]
- Talcum powder: facial melanosis[4]
- Customary tattooing[38]

Social habits, customs and dyschromia

Social customs and habits may predispose certain individuals to cosmetic disfigurement. The best and commonest example is 'bindi' depigmentation seen on the foreheads of women in the Asian subcontinent owing to the habit of using flat round coloured plastic with adhesive on the centre of their forehead.[23] This is usually due to butylphenol in the adhesive. A patch test is usually positive. The use of henna for hand and facial decoration on certain festive occasions may cause photocontact dermatitis, resulting in residual hyperpigmentation in the areas exposed.[35] Sandalwood paste or oil in perfumes, when applied to the face and exposed areas during certain tribal marriages, may cause contact depigmentation or hypopigmentation.[36] Asiatic pills (health pills) commonly used in the past (and by a few people still) result in slate-grey coloration. This is due to silver deposition in the skin. Silver is converted by oxidation into silver oxide, which is slate-grey in colour.[37] The custom of using excess talcum powder on the face in racially pigmented skin causes facial melanosis.[4] Facial and decorative tattooing may cause photosensitization, infection and residual surrounding hyperpigmentation.[4,36,38]

MANAGEMENT OF HYPERPIGMENTATION (Table 34.3)

Depigmenting agents

Various chemical agents produce depigmentation of the human skin. A few of these, such as hydroquinone and its derivatives, are employed singly or in combination with other media in the management of hypermelanosis.

Hydroquinone[2]

Most cases of hypermelanosis have been treated with hydroquinone during the past two decades. Hydroquinone is commonly used in concentrations of 2–5%. Higher

Table 34.3 Management of dyschromias
Hypermelanosis
Depigmenting agents
• Hydroquinone and derivatives[2]
• N-Acetyl-4-S-cysteaminylphenol[4]
• Azelaic acid[2]
• Local steroids[2]
• Local retinoids[2]
• Bleaching agents[2]
• Miscellaneous:
photoprotection[4]
pulsed dye and Q-switched ruby lasers[53,54]
Physical and chemical treatment
• Trichloroacetic acid (TCA); glycolic acid[50,51]
• Dermabrasion[31]
• Plastic surgery[3,4]
• Argon laser[3]
Hypomelanosis
Medical
• Psoralen photochemotherapy[30]
• Khellin photochemotherapy[2]
• Phenylalanine[2]
• Camouflaging,[2,56,57] hair dye[2]
Surgical
• Grafting and transplantation of melanocytes[2]
• Tattooing[38]
• Plastic surgery[3,4]

concentrations up to 10–20% have been used singly or in combination, but they are more likely to produce adverse effects. Hydroquinone is commonly employed for the treatment of melasma, contact hypermelanosis due to perfumes in cosmetics, and post-inflammatory hypermelanosis. Melasma of epidermal type is found to be most responsive to hydroquinone. Treatment has to be continued for a long time before cosmetic benefits are obtained; these can be up to 70–90%. The preparation is given twice daily with a sunscreen of high SPF. It is possible to achieve normal colour with disappearance of hypermelanosis, but these may be reversible.

In certain individuals, hydroquinone may provoke sensitization and contact dermatitis, which is common with the higher concentrations (6, 8 and 10%). The safest has been found to be 2% hydroquinone, followed by

5%, but 10% produced constant irritation. The most frequently observed side-effects are irritation, sensitization, post-inflammatory hyperpigmentation (which gradually fades), ochronosis and confetti-like depigmentation. Others observed in Black patients are colloid degeneration and pigmented colloid milium.[39] Different formulas have been proposed by different authors for increasing the efficacy and reducing the side-effects. They are Eldopaque, Solaquin, Solaquin forte, and Chromatone with aloe vera.

The following formula was proposed by Kligman and Willis:[40]

- hydroquinone   5.00%
- tretinoin (retinoic acid)   0.10%
- dexamethasone 21-acetate   0.10%
- ethanol, 95%   47.40%
- propylene glycol   47.40%

The vehicle may be hydrophilic and the steroid may be less or more potent according to the response. The following guidelines have been proposed for the use of the above cream or solution:

- The preparation should be applied twice daily every day for several months.
- It is preferable to use a preparation not older than 30 days, or it may deteriorate.
- Concurrent use of medicines other than a photoprotective cream is not recommended.
- It should be kept in a cool dark place away from sunlight.
- Alteration of the colour of the preparation indicates decreasing potentiality.

Complete depigmentation of normal skin in adult Black men has been observed after a daily application of hydroquinone for 5–7 weeks. During the first week of treatment, erythema and desquamation usually precede depigmentation. In clinical use, 60–90% of patients with melasma, ephelides, post-inflammatory hyperpigmentation and (to a lesser extent) berloque pigmentation show improvement. This preparation has been successfully used for lightening the human skin, as with Kligman's formula.

Hydroquinone derivatives[2]

The monobenzyl ether of hydroquinone (MBEH or monobenzone) has also been used in the treatment of hypermelanosis in human subjects. This agent is well known to produce excessive depigmentation at sites distant from its application. Furthermore, in some patients the leucoderma continues for several months after application. Hence MBEH should be prohibited from use in hypermelanotic disorders like melasma, ephelides and post-inflammatory hyperpigmentation, and in cosmetic creams. MBEH produces vitiligo-like depigmentation, which may spread beyond its area of application. The only clinical use of MBEH recommended at present is to give normal pigmented areas in extensive vitiligo a uniform colour. This permanent chemical depigmentation of uninvolved skin in patients with vitiligo may be achieved with twice-daily applications of 20% MBEH in an ointment base. Permanent depigmentation takes place after several months to a year, and is complete and effective in every patient. The side-effects include a burning sensation, itching, erythematous eruption, dryness, contact dermatitis and oedema.

Although occasional areas of repigmentation may occur, the patient must understand that the depigmentation is permanent and irreversible.

The following guidelines for choice of patients for such treatment have been proposed:

- vitiligo patients having a desire for permanent depigmentation for uniformity of colour;
- patients over 40;
- patients with more than 50% of depigmented skin;
- willingness to accept the fact that repigmentation will no longer be possible.

Careful selection of patients must be made

before commencement of this kind of treatment. Correct use generally gives fairly good results, and most patients are pleased with these.

The monomethyl ether of hydroquinone (MMEH) is preferred in Europe and Africa because of its potent action and lower irritation potential compared with hydroquinone. It is used in 10% concentration. This compound can also produce confetti-like hypopigmentation indistinguishable from that of MBEH. Hence the same restrictions should be followed as for MBEH, and it should be stressed that these agents must only be used for this particular indication in humans.

The mechanisms of action of hydroquinone and its derivatives are not clear. The following have been suggested: selective destruction of melanocytes, inhibition of melanosome function and alteration of melanosome structure, inhibition of tyrosinase biosynthesis, inhibition of melanin formation, interference of transfer of melanosomes of keratinocytes, chemical effect on melanin or enhancement of melanin degradation, and conversion of hydroquinone and its derivatives to highly toxic radicals that cause melanocyte death.

Other depigmenting agents
N-Acetyl-4-S-cysteaminylphenol[41]

This is one of the most potent depigmenting agents, acting specifically only on functioning melanocytes with active synthesis of melanin. It is stable (even to boiling for more than 10 minutes), readily soluble in water and of low toxicity to experimental animals. The median lethal doses of 4-S-cysteaminylphenol and N-acetyl-4-S-cysteaminylphenol are 400 mg/kg and 1400 mg/kg of body weight respectively. The observed melanocytotoxicity of N-acetyl-4-S-cysteaminylphenol can be explained, at least in part, by a mechanism similar to that attributed to tyrosinase-activated cathechols and phenols. In one study out of 12, all but three melasma patients responded very well. The poor response in the three was related to dermal melanosis with dermal melanophages.

This agent does not cause permanent depigmentation of the skin, even after prolonged use. Its exact mechanism of action is not clear. N-Acetyl-4-S-cysteaminylphenol on exposure to tyrosinase forms a dark-brown pigment. This may be formed via oxidative cyclization of the side-chain to produce a benzothiazine-type structure.

It is possible that these pigments may function as filters of UV and visible light, as does melanin pigment in the skin. This new preparation is much safer than hydroquinone and its derivatives in the treatment of hypomelanosis.

Azelaic acid (AA)[2]

This is a naturally occurring medium-chain-length saturated nine-carbon dicarboxylic acid. It has an inhibitory effect on tyrosinase, the key enzyme in melanogenesis. It has been proposed that AA could be involved in the sequelae of hypochromia in pityriasis versicolor due to fungus *Malassizia furfur*, which is capable in culture of oxidizing oleic acid to AA. Hence AA was proposed as a depigmenting agent. Creams containing 10%, 20% and 35% of AA have been employed, but their detailed formulas are unknown.

AA is applied twice daily for several months, and has been shown to give satisfactory results in the management of melasma, post-inflammatory melanoderma and hypermelanosis caused by physical or photochemical agents. Several controlled trials on the effect of AA are in progress, and further data are needed to confirm the initial results. One of the hallmarks of AA treatment is its reported beneficial effect in the treatment of lentigo maligna melanoma and primary lesions of malignant melanoma. Many discrepancies are obtained in the therapeutic results of AA from different centres. These could be related to the use of different vehicles with different penetrating ability. Thus standardization of formulas and regimen is necessary for precise evaluation of this drug.

The mechanism of action is not clear. AA

does not have a selective effect on melanocytes. It may act by reversibly inhibiting essential oxidoreductive enzymes. Additional data are required before AA could be routinely used in the treatment of hypermelanosis.

Miscellaneous agents

Many drugs have been used to lighten skin colour and to give a red glow to the face. Hydrocortisone 0.1% cream has been freely available for this purpose. Mercurials are also used widely. Percutaneous absorption of mercurials can cause nephrotoxicity; hence they should be banned from use. Because of these side-effects, these various compounds have limited use as depigmenting agents. Furthermore, depigmentation is never total, and always regresses after discontinuation of therapy.[2]

Topical retinoids[42]

Topical retinoids have been widely used for multiple cutaneous disorders, including dyschromia. Topical tretinoin singly or in combination gave good results in actinic keratosis, lichen planus, melasma, freckles, post-inflammatory hyperpigmentation and pityriasis versicolor. Melasma has been treated successfully with a combination of 0.05% tretinoin cream, 0.1% betamethasone valerate and 2% hydroquinone. There was objective improvement in 65% of patients and subjective improvement in 95%. Beneficial results had previously been reported in a study involving a formula containing 0.1% tretinoin, 5% hydroquinone and 0.1% dexamethasone in ahydrophilic ointment or equal parts of an ethanol and propylene glycol solution. Twice-daily application induced lessening of pigmentation of melasma, ephelides and post-inflammatory hyperpigmentation within six weeks. The same regimen was effective in post-inflammatory hyperpigmentation secondary to surgery, which improved in 9 out of 12 patients treated with a combination of 4% hydroquinone, 0.05% retinoic acid and

0.25% triamcinolone acetonide. Tretinoin 0.5–0.1% cream has been very effective in treating pigmentary changes of photoaging.[43]

Topical 0.1% tretinoin significantly improves both clinical and microscopical manifestation of 'liver spots' associated with photodamage. Furthermore, these lesions do not return for at least six months after therapy is discontinued.[44] This topical treatment also lightens the hyperpigmentation of photoaging in Chinese and Japanese patients.[45] Furthermore, topical 0.1% tretinoin produces significant clinical improvement of melasma, mainly due to reduction in epidermal pigment, but this improvement is slow.[46] Finally, topical application of 0.1% tretinoin significantly lightens post-inflammatory hypermelanosis of the skin in Black patients to a clinically minimal but statistically significant degree. In the same study, it was noted that this topical treatment also lightens normal skin in Black patients.[47]

Bleaching agents[2]

Bleaching agents are commonly used for hair and skin lightening; they do this by oxidizing melanin pigments. If carried to extremes, this can lead to total solubilization and elimination. A variety of bleaching products are available in the form of solutions, emulsions, creams, shampoos, powders, pastes and oils. They contain hydrogen peroxide alone, with ammonia, or mixed with other oxidizing products such as peroxy salts or peroxides.

Physical and chemical treatments

These methods are used for removal of localized pigmented spots.

Liquid nitrogen cryotherapy

Melanocytes are particularly susceptible to freezing, and hence cryotherapy should be avoided in dark-skinned people because of the risk of permanent depigmentation. The freezing agent must be applied gently to avoid blistering and skin necrosis. Cryotherapy with liquid nitrogen is commonly used successfully to treat individual pigmented lesions. A randomized, controlled prospective trial comparing liquid-nitrogen cryotherapy and argon laser light delivered by a Dermascan shuttered delivery system and low-fluence CO_2 laser irradiation conclude that liquid nitrogen therapy was superior to the two lasers in the treatment of solar lentigines.[48] Although satisfactory results are common, cryotherapy for benign epidermal lesion is problematic because of hypopigmentation, hyperpigmentation atrophy, scarring and/or frequent recurrence.

Liquid nitrogen cryotherapy has also been used for the treatment of naevus of Ota, delayed naevus spilus and blue naevus. The cryotreatment was performed using a liquid nitrogen cryogenic instrument with a removable disc-shaped copper tip called CRYO-MINI.[49]

Chemabrasion and peeling

Chemabrasion or peeling using various chemicals is another therapeutic modality for removing freckles, solar lentigines and other localized patches of melanin hyperpigmentation. Glycolic acid peels are also useful for the treatment of dyspigmentation of photodamaged skin, of post-inflammatory hyperpigmentation in Black patients, and, to a lesser extent, of melasma among Asian women.[50,51] Both glycolic acid/kojic acid and glycolic acid/hydroquinone topical skin care products are effective in reducing melanin hyperpigmentation in melasma patients.[52] Chemabrasion using trichloroacetic acid (TCA) is another therapeutic modality for removing freckles, solar lentigines and other localized patches of pigmentation. The following procedure has been proposed.[2] A single application of a 25% solution of TCA is made on the test site. In the event of a burning sensation, the area is washed with soap and water and rubbed with a soap-impregnated cloth. If a 25% solution produces inadequate effects

or results, 50% or even 75% solutions are tested on subsequent areas. The concentration that produces desquamation and loss of the lesion without excessive injury is used as the treatment of choice. The solution is applied rapidly on the lesion by the physician, using a cotton-tipped swab, and washed off if irritation occurs. This procedure is effective in removing spotty hyperpigmentation. However, it should be used with extreme caution, since concentrated TCA may cause instantaneous necrosis of the epidermis and post-inflammatory hyperpigmentation, frequently seen in skin types V and VI.

Lasers for benign cutaneous pigmented lesions[53,54]

Melanins absorb light across the visible portion of the electromagnetic spectrum, and thus melanin-containing pigmented lesions can be treated with a variety of lasers. These lasers can be divided into three categories:

- green light lasers (both pulsed and non-pulsed systems);
- red light lasers;
- near-infrared lasers.

All of these can be used to quickly remove lentigines and ephelides.

Green light lasers do not penetrate as deeply into the skin as the red and near-infrared systems, which because of their longer wavelengths are more likely to lighten deeper dermal pigmented processes.

The flashlamp-pumped pulsed tunable dye laser (510 nm) gives satisfactory fading of a wide range of pigmented epidermal lesions, including lentigines, ephelides, café-au-lait spots and Becker's naevi. Good results have also been reported with post-inflammatory hyperpigmentation. Q-switched ruby lasers have also been used successfully to treat a similar range of pigmented lesions, as well as deeper lesions such as naevus of Ota and infraorbital pigmented skin. The long wavelength of the Q-switched Nd:YAG and alexandrite lasers makes these systems uniquely effective for the treatment of dermal melanocytosis, including naevus of Ota and post-inflammatory hyperpigmentation. Non-pulsed green light lasers (i.e. krypton, copper and argon), although efficacious in treating superficial epidermal pigmented lesions, do not produce the uniformly improved results seen following treatment with the other lasers.

Results with melasma have always been very disappointing. Pigment-specific lasers have also been used to treat congenital naevi or naevus spilus. However, this issue is very controversial. The long-term risk of the persistence of naevocellular cells in the treated areas is unknown, and should impose a strong limitation of the use of this treatment strategy.

It should be noted that some patients not responding to treatment with one Q-switched laser may respond to another pigmented lesion laser. Although several pigment-specific lasers are presently available, new long-pulsed pigment-specific systems may prove to further enhance the clinical results obtained in resistant pigmented lesions.

MANAGEMENT OF HYPOPIGMENTATION (Table 34.3)

Psoralen photochemotherapy (PUVA)[2,30]

PUVA is the most successful currently available treatment for vitiligo. It involves the use of psoralens followed by exposure to long-wavelength ultraviolet A irradiation. Numerous psoralens occur naturally in plant species. Of these, only a few are used therapeutically, including methoxalen (8-methoxypsoralen), 4,5',8-trimethoxypsoralen and recently bergapten (5-methoxypsoralen) – almost exclusively for vitiligo. Different responses to topical and systemic photochemotherapy have been reported by different investigators (Tables 34.4 and 34.5). Some degree of repigmentation is seen in about 60–80% of treated patients. A satisfactory cosmetic result is usually obtained in less than 20% of cases. Commencement of repigmentation begins with either perifollicular pigmented spots or spreading of pigment cells from the pigmented borders. Evidence of repigmentation is usually first seen after 1–4 months of treatment, but complete repigmentation usually requires 100–300 treatments.

Khellin photochemotherapy[2,30]

Khellin is a furochrome extracted from the seeds of *Ammi visnaga*, and was initially prescribed as a spasmolytic, antiasthmatic and coronary dilator. It has structural similarities to 8-MOP and has been used for the treatment of vitiligo both locally and systemically in combination with natural sunlight or artificial UVA. In one double-blind study 5–7 out of 30 patients receiving 100 mg khellin tablets daily showed 90–100% and 50–60% repigmentation of the vitiliginous areas after four months of treatment. The repigmentation was stable up to one year after discontinuation of treatment. Side-effects were nil. In another study, the khellin photochemotherapy was as effective as psoralen photochemotherapy. Some patients (30%) suffered nausea, hypotension and loss of appetite, but treatment could be continued. Asymptomatic elevation of transaminases may occur in one-third of patients during two or four weeks of therapy. A recent study using 3% khellin cream incorporated in poly(ethylene glycol) used locally on vitiliginous patches followed by exposure to UVA (1–10 J/cm²) gave satisfactory results without side-effects. More trials of khellin photochemotherapy are required before it can be used routinely. It could be a valuable alternative to psoralen photochemotherapy.

Table 34.4 Response to systemic PUVA therapy[30]

Study[a]	Psoralen derivative	UV source	Total number of patients	Patients with induced repigmentation (%)	Non-responses (%)	Cosmetically acceptable repigmentation (%)	Total repigmentation (%)
Sadi et al	8-MOP	Sun + artificial	219	73	?	11	11
El Mofty	8-MOP	Sun	75	61	9	6	20
Elliot	8-MOP	Sun + artificial	27	81.5		67	26
Fitzpatrick et al	TMP	Sun	84	70	23	41	25
Bleehen	TMP	Sun + artificial	32	47	53	19	0
Parrish et al	TMP/ 8-MOP	Artificial	26	73	27	23	0
Theodoridis et al	TMP	Sun or artificial	118	83.2	6.8	67	?
Pathak et al	8-MOP + TMP (0.3 mg + 0.6 mg/kg)	Sun	55	—	—	38	—
	8-MOP (0.3 mg/kg)	Sun	47	—	—	31	—
Wennersten and Hägermark	TMP	Sun	42	20	?	0	0
	TMP	Artificial	35	40	?	26	1 patient
Lassus et al	8-MOP	Artificial	139[b]	100	0	59	50
				85	15	54	20

[a] For details see Ortonne.[30]
[b] Focal vitiligo (22 cases) and generalized vitiligo (117 cases).

Phenylalanine[2]

Phenylalanine in a dose of 50 mg/kg body weight has been used in combination with UVA for repigmentation in one-quarter of cases of vitiligo. Phenylalanine increases the photo-tolerance of vitiliginous skin and the tanning ability of uninvolved skin.

Hair dyes[2]

Hair colorants may be used for colouring diffuse grey hair or a white or grey lock. The colour dye penetrates both white and normal hair. It is advised to use a shade slightly lighter than the natural hair colour. However, permanent colour dyes containing *p*-phenylene diamine dihydrochloride may produce contact reactions and hyperpigmentation of forehead in racially dark skin.

Liquid nitrogen cryotherapy

Liquid nitrogen cryotherapy has been proposed for the treatment of idiopathic guttate hypomelanosis.[55] In this common skin disor-

Table 34.5 Response to topical PUVA therapy[30]

Study[a]	Psoralen derivative	UV source	Total number of patients	Patients with induced repigmentation (%)	Non-responses (%)	Acceptable repigmentation (%)	Total repigmentation (%)
Kanof	8-MOP	Sun + artificial	85	26	74	7	?
Kelly and Pinkus	8-MOP	Sun + artificial	20	85	15	30	25
Fulton et al	8-MOP	Artificial	15	93	7	60	20
Africk and Fulton	TMP	Sun	20	93	7	55	25
Halder et al	8-MOP	Artificial	43[b]	?	?	16	?
			33[c]	?	?	15	?
			34[d]	?	?	14	?
			73[e]	—	—	36	?

Response is defined as ⩾50% return of pigmentation of all of the involved areas.
[a] For details see Ortonne.[30]
[b] Children, segmental type + cases with >20% involvement.
[c] Children non-segmental type + cases with >20% involvement.
[d] Children, all types with <20% involvement.
[e] Adults, non-segmental types with <20% involvement.

der of unknown cause, significantly fewer dopa-positive melanocytes are present in the white macules. After gentle freezing with liquid nitrogen to destroy the melanocytes remaining in the white macules, complete repigmentation occurred in 6–8 weeks in 91% of the treated lesions. More recently, a similar repigmentation has been reported following superficial dermabrasion of the lesions.

Tattooing,[38] micropigmentation

Tattooing or body art has been practised from ancient times for both mystical and religious purposes.

Cosmetic tattooing is the art of improving the appearance of eyelids, correction of a pigmentary defect, a scar, augmentation of thin eyebrows, and so on. Different tattooing equipment is available for such treatment for use by aesthetic dermatologists: Cooper Vision (Natural Eyes), Penmark, Dioptics (Accents), Vision Concepts (Glamour Eyes), Cosmedyne, Alltek and Eyelite, for example.

Although the technique is fairly simple, proper selection of cases is mandatory.

Only minimum pigmentation should be done to give the desired results. The pigments, if added in excess, can be difficult or even impossible to remove. It is better to perform cosmetic tattooing after several consultations. Pigmentation is usually permanent. Colour perception is very important for performing tattoo improvement in the case of scars, stable vitiligo and post-burn leucoderma.[11] Preoperative photographs should always be obtained for medical documentation. The pigments can be premixed, or mixed and matched. The colours used are slightly darker than the shade desired in general, because the final colour is usually lighter than anticipated.

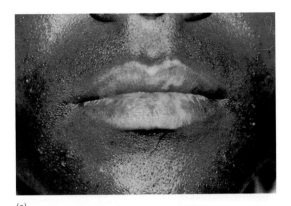

(a)

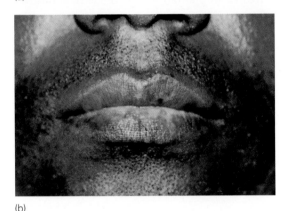

(b)

Figure 34.10 Vitiligo of the lips: (a) before and (b) after micropigmentation. (Courtesy of Dr C de Rivoyre.)

Micropigmentation tattooing is popularly used as a camouflage procedure. The technique is simpler than melanocyte transfer, and serves the purpose of hiding a white patch like stable vitiligo, leucoderma or post-traumatic depigmentation. The sites usually preferred for tattooing are lips (Figure 34.10a,b), eyebrows, hands and fingers. Inert pigments of matched skin colour are impregnated into the intradermal plane by the tattoo artist. In a recent study, no adverse side-effects such as allergy or fibrosis were noticed from

this procedure, and most patients were satisfied at the outcome. Other potential fields of micropigmentation surgery include

- permanent eyelining;
- eyelid pigmentation after cryosurgery;
- eyelash enhancement for sparse lashes;
- lid contour improvement after trauma or surgery;
- eyebrow enhancement or replacement;
- nipple replacement by tattooing.

Lip contour enhancement by lip lining is especially popular among young women. It is a simpler and permanent technique compared with collagen implants for the creation of French lips. Lip lining is done in a step-by-step manner to get the desired effect according to the individual choice.

The area of the skin to be tattooed is cleaned with benzalkonium chloride or alcohol. A small amount of local anaesthetic is injected into the site. A thin layer of antibiotic cream at the site is preferred before beginning the procedure. The instrument can be mains electric or battery operated, with a single needle or a three-needle set. The needles are dipped into the requisite pigments and brought to the site, usually held at a 45° or even 90° angle. The current is then turned on and the pigment is inserted. After this, the area is wiped. It is better to do less rather than more tattooing. Side-effects are rare, but can include bacterial infection, herpes simplex, warts, photosensitization (from cadmium in red pigments), Koebner's phenomenon and keloids.

Camouflaging[2,56,57]

Camouflaging is the art of using cosmetic products in order to hide cosmetic disfigurement due to hyper- and/or hypomelanosis. It is usually done on lesions in the exposed areas, such as the face and the dorsal regions of the hands. Hypomelanotic areas are covered by lotions containing dihydroxyacetone and certain aniline dyes (Vitadye, Dy-O-

Derm), but these have to be reapplied every few days. Corrective cosmetics such as Dermablend, Covermark and Continuous Coverage are available in various shades, allowing a perfect match to normal skin colour in most patients.

These preparations combine a water-resistant opaque base with a broad-spectrum sunscreen. They are helpful in hyperpigmented disorders in which sunlight plays an aggravating and perpetuating role. In hypomelanosis such as vitiligo, correct use can completely hide the depigmented macules. Skin-colouring creams or browning agents are not sunscreens, but contain dihydroxyacetone, which colours the stratum corneum brown owing to its oxidative properties. These brown pigments screen against UVA and visible light. This tanning preparation can be used effectively in vitiligo patients with skin types I and II.

The coloration is visible 3–4 hours following a single application, and lasts for 4–6 days. The colour fades slowly with desquamation of skin. The main disadvantage is that it does not give a uniform colour to the skin. β-Carotene and canthaxanthin (Phenoro, β-carotene 10 mg and canthaxanthin 15 mg per capsule) oral preparations have been used to treat cosmetic defects in vitiligo. By darkening vitiliginous skin, they reduce the contrast between involved and normally pigmented skin. Good cosmetic results are seen in vitiligo patients with skin types I and II.

In one study, 10–35% of patients gave very satisfactory responses, with the rest unsatisfactory. There is increased resistance to sun exposure in vitiligo. As canthaxanthin is reported to produce retinopathy, proper ophthalmic consultations are mandatory.

Eye shadows, mascaras and liners accentuate patients' eyes and draw attention to them to further distract from facial cosmetic defects such as those seen in vitiligo around the eyes and in naevus of Ota, while lipsticks can be used to cover vitiligo of lips.

Grafting and transplantation of melanocytes[2,58]

Surgical procedures for leukoderma related to vitiligo, post-burn depigmentation and idiopathic guttate hypomelanosis have been reported to be effective in resistant cases. These include grafting of suction-blistered epidermis within the white macules, thin Thiersch grafts or minigrafts, and transplantation of in vitro cultured epidermis bearing melanocytes (Figure 34.11). Another procedure is implantation of in vitro cultured

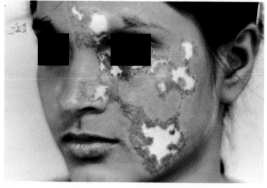

(a)

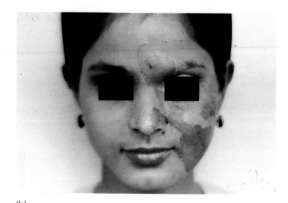

(b)

Figure 34.11 Thiersch grafts on stable vitiligo zosteriformis: (a) before and (b) 15 days after grafting. (Courtesy of Professor PN Behl.)

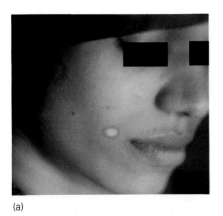

(a)

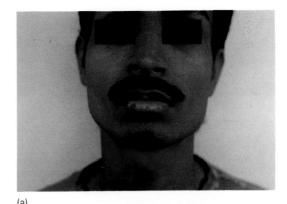

(a)

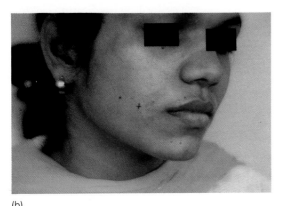

(b)

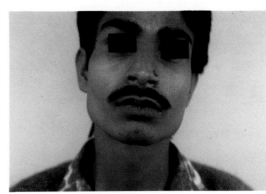

(b)

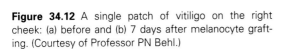

Figure 34.12 A single patch of vitiligo on the right cheek: (a) before and (b) 7 days after melanocyte grafting. (Courtesy of Professor PN Behl.)

Figure 34.13 Vitiligo mucosae treated with melanocyte grafting: (a) before and (b) 2 months after the operation. (Courtesy of Professor PN Behl.)

melanocytes. These are alternative methods for the treatment of vitiligo and post-burn leucoderma (Figures 12a,b; 13a,b).

THE RISK OF DYSPIGMENTATION AFTER COSMETIC SURGERY

Dermabrasion is not a good therapeutic strategy to treat hypermelanosis in dark-skinned individuals, because of the risk of dyspigmentation – either hyperpigmentation or hypopig-

mentation. However, a recent study[59] suggests that laser skin resurfacing can be used to treat rhytides and acne scars in skin phototypes III and IV. According to this paper, the proper pre- and postoperative management includes the use of tretinoin cream 0.05%, hydroquinone 5% and desomide 0.1% cream nightly for 2–4 weeks prior to the surgical procedure. The same topical treatment along with the use of a broad-spectrum sunscreen should also be applied postoperatively.

TATTOO REMOVAL[60,61]

Tattooing is a common practice among young people and military recruits, and in certain societies and jails. A change of profession or partner, or a previously hidden tattoo becoming visible, may lead an individual to turn to an aesthetic dermatologist. Various methods of tattoo removal have been practised, but all leave some scar marks. Among the various treatments available (excision, salabrasion, dermabrasion, lasers, cryosurgery, electrofulguration, grafting and tissue expansion), the use of lasers is at present the most acceptable.

Professional and newer tattoos are easier to remove than amateur and old ones. Site is also important, since deltoid, chest and art tattoos produce hypertrophic scars or keloids on removal. Below, we discuss only two of the most popular techniques practised today.

Laser treatment of tattoos[60,61]

This is the best treatment for tattoos. The concept of using lasers for tattoo removal is not new. Localized burning of tattooed areas using focused CO_2 and argon lasers involves destruction of tissue, and is associated with a high potential for scarring. An alternative and attractive technique employs the principle of selective absorption of incident laser energy (selective thermolysis) by the tattoo pigment, without destruction of the surrounding skin. In addition, the photoacoustic vibratory effect seen with newer lasers leads to the sonar-like selective explosion of tattoo inks.

The factors that determine the number of treatment sessions required for clearance include

- whether the tattoo is professional or amateur;
- the ink colour and density;
- the age of the tattoo;
- the patient's underlying complexion;
- the location of the tattoo.

Several currently available pulsed lasers can be used for tattoo removal. However, at pre-sent no single laser can optimally remove all tattoos. Several wavelengths remain necessary to optimally treat multicoloured tattoos. The Q-switched ruby laser (694 nm) is a red-light, 24–40 ns pulse-duration laser. This laser is best for removing black, green and blue inks, but relatively ineffective for red or yellow inks. Because light of this wavelength is absorbed well by melanins, transient hypopigmentation is very common following treatment. Transient hyperpigmentation is less common. Depigmentation is infrequent (1–5% of cases), but occurs more commonly on Black or Asian skin. Textural changes and scarring are rare.

The Q-switched Nd:YAG laser produces invisible laser energy at a 10 ns pulse duration. This laser is highly effective in treating black tattoos. It is fairly ineffective in treating green tattoo pigment. Complications from this laser are uncommon, but are similar to those seen with the Q-switched ruby laser. However, hypopigmentation is rarer following treatment with the Q-switched Nd:YAG laser. The frequency-doubled Q-switched Nd:YAG laser (532 nm) and the flashlamp-pumped dye laser (510 nm) effectively lighten red tattoo ink as well as orange and purple inks. However, they tend to be less effective in removing black ink, and are ineffective in removing green pigment. Post-laser pigmentation (hypo- and/or hyperpigmentation) can be a problem.

The Q-switched alexandrite laser (755 nm) works well for black and green tattoo pigments. Although not effective in lightening green ink, it does appear to have an effect on blue colour.

Dermabrasion with tannic acid (the French technique)[2]

This technique has been described by Penoff in a study of 85% patients with 207 tattoos observed over a period of 11 years. After the tattoo area has been anaesthetized, the area is very superficially dermabrated. As the tattoo becomes prominent and oozing occurs, tannic acid (Penoff's solution) is applied using a cotton swab. This is followed by a second dermabrasion to rub the tannic acid gently into the dermis. Tannic acid painting is then done using a hand-held tattoo needle. The site is washed with saline, followed by rubbing with a silver nitrate stick. A black dry eschar forms in 2–3 minutes and separates in 2–3 weeks. Residual pigment, if any, usually disappears over the ensuing 1–3 months.

REFERENCES

1. Quevedo WC Jr, Fitzpatrick TB, Szabo G et al, Biology of the melanin pigmentary system. In: *Dermatology in general Medicine*, 3rd edn (Fitzpatrick TB, Eisen AZ, Wolff K et al, eds). New York: McGraw-Hill, 1987:224–58.

2. Ortonne JP, Pigmentary changes. In: *Aesthetic Dermatology* (Parish LC, Lask GP, eds). New York: McGraw-Hill, 1991:74–83.

3. Mosher DB, Fitzpatrick TB, Ortonne JP, Hori Y, Disorders of melanocytes. In: *Dermatology in General Medicine*, 3rd edn (Fitzpatrick TB, Eisen AZ, Wolff K et al, eds). New York: McGraw-Hill, 1987; 810–54.

4. Bleehen SS, Ebling FJG, Champion RH, Disorders of skin colour. In: *Textbook of Dermatology*, 5th edn (Champion RH, Burton JL, Ebling FJG, eds). Oxford: Blackwell, 1992:593–618.

5. Boissy RE, Liu YY, Medrano EE et al, Structural aberration of the rough endoplasmic reticulum and melanosomes. Compartmentalization in long-term cultures of melanocytes from vitiligo patients. *J Invest Dermatol* 1991; **97**: 395–404.

6. Ramaiah A, Puri N, Mojamdar M, Etiology of vitiligo. A new hypothesis. *Acta Dermatol Venereol (Stockh)* 1989; **69**: 323–7.

7. Slominski A, Paus R, Bomirski A, Hypothesis: possible role for the melatonin receptor in vitiligo: discussion paper. *J R Soc Med* 1989; **82**: 539–41.

8. Goudie RB, Two views of the origin of vitiligo. *Lancet* 1991; **338**: 306–7.

9. Falabella R, Idiopathic guttate hypomelanosis. *Dermatol Clin* 1988; **2**: 241–7.

10. Taki T, Kozuka S, Izawa Y et al, Surgical treatment of skin depigmentation caused by burn injuries. *J Dermatol Surg Oncol* 1985; **12**: 1218–21.

11. Vadodaria SJ, Vadodaria BS, Tattooing for the management of white patches. *Ann Plast Surg* 1989; **23**: 81–3.

12. Kahn AM, Cohen MJ, Daplan L, Treatment for depigmentation resulting from burn injuries. *J Burn Care Rehabil* 1991; **12**: 468–73.

13. Burton JL, Eczema, lichenification, prurigo and erythroderma. In: *Textbook of Dermatology*, 5th edn (Champion RH, Burton JL, Ebling FJG, eds). Oxford: Blackwell, 1992:570–1.

14. Zaynoun S, Jaber LAA, Kurban AK, Oral methoxalen photochemotherapy of extensive pityriasis alba. *J Am Acad Dermatol* 1986; **15**: 61–5.

15. Rippon JW, *Medical Mycology, Superficial Infections*. Philadelphia: Saunders, 1988:154–9.

16. Atherton DJ, Naevi and other developmental defects. In: *Textbook of Dermatology*, 5th edn (Champion RH, Burton JL, Ebling FJG, eds). Oxford: Blackwell, 1992:462–3.

17. Mackie RM, Melanocytic naevi and malignant melanoma. In: *Textbook of Dermatology*, 5th edn (Champion RH, Burton JL, Ebling FJG, eds). Oxford: Blackwell, 1992:1526–39.

18. Calkins E, Amyloidosis of the skin. In: *Dermatology in General Medicine*, 3rd edn (Fitzpatrick TB, Eisen AZ, Wolff K et al, eds). New York: McGraw-Hill, 1987:1656–7.

19. Okada N, Nishida K, Sato S et al, Characterization of the pigmented granules in Minocycline induced cutaneous pigmentation. *J Invest Dermatol* 1991; **96**: 567 (abst).

20. Fitzpatrick JE, New histopathologic findings in drug eruptions. *Dermatol Clin* 1992; **10**: 19–36.

21. O'Malley MA, Mathias CG, Priddy M et al, Occupational vitiligo due to unsuspected presence of phenolic antioxidant by products in commercial bulk rubber. *J Occup Med* 1988; **30**: 512–16.

22. Zaitz ID, Proenca NG, Droste D et al, Dermatite de contato acromiante por sandalias de borracha. *Med Cutan Ibero Lat Am* 1987; **15**: 1–7.

23. Bajaj AK, Gupta SC, Chatterjee AK, Contact depigmentation from free paratertiary-butylphenol in bindi adhesive. *Contact Dermatitis* 1990; **22**: 99–102.

24. Adams RM, *Occupational Skin Diseases.* London: Grune & Stratton, 1983:159.

25. Koh D, Aw TC, Foulds IS, Fiberglass dermatitis from printed circuit boards. *Am J Ind Med* 1992; **21**: 193–8.

26. Ippen H, Phytophotodermatitis caused by plant trimming (edger's rash). *Derm Beruf Umwelt* 1990; **38**: 190–2.

27. Kligman LH, Kligman AM, Reflections on heat. Comments. *Br J Dermatol* 1984; **110**: 369–75.

28. Lemont H, Hetman J, Cutaneous foot depigmentation following an intra-articular steroid injection. *J Am Pediatr Med Assoc* 1991; **81**: 606–7.

29. De Lacharière O, Escoffier C, Gracia AM et al, Reversal effects of topical retinoic acid on the skin of kidney transplant recipients under systemic corticotherapy. *J Invest Dermatol* 1990; **95**: 516–22.

30. Ortonne JP, Psoralen therapy in vitiligo. *Clin Dermatol* 1989; **7**: 120–35.

31. Fulton JE Jr, The prevention and management of postdermabrasion complications. *J Dermatol Surg Oncol* 1991; **17**: 431–7.

32. Hashimoto K, Joselow SA, Tye MJ, Imipramine hyperpigmentation: a slate-gray discoloration caused by long-term imipramine administration. *J Am Acad Dermatol* 1991; **25**: 357–61.

33. Thibault P, Wlodarczyk J, Postsclerotherapy hyperpigmentation. The role of serum ferritin levels and the effectiveness of treatment with the copper vapor laser. *J Dermatol Surg Oncol* 1992; **18**: 47–52.

34. Spadoni D, Cain CL, Facial resurfacing. Using the carbon dioxide laser. *AORN J* 1989; **50**: 1007–13.

35. Natous AJ, Henna. *Cutis* 1986; **38**: 21.

36. Hayakawa R, Matsunaga K, Arima Y, Depigmented contact dermatitis due to incense. *Contact Dermatitis* 1987; **16**: 272–4.

37. Muller M, Wiedmann KH, Generalized argyria caused by targesin-containing drug used for stomach complaints. *Med Klin* 1991; **86**: 432–4.

38. Goldstein N, Micropigmentation surgery: cosmetic tattooing and removal. In: *Aesthetic Dermatology* (Paris LC, Lask GP, eds). New York: McGraw-Hill, 1991; 101–13.

39. Findlay GH, Morrison JGL, Sinson IW, Exogenous ochronosis and pigmented colloid milium from hydroquinone bleaching creams. *Br J Dermatol* 1975; **93**: 613–22.

40. Kligman AM, Willis I, A new formula for depigmenting human skin. *Arch Dermatol* 1975; **111**: 40–8.

41. Jimbow K, N-Acetyl-4-S-cysteaminylphenol as a new type of depigmenting agent for the melanoderma of patients with melasma. *Arch Dermatol* 1991; **127**: 1528–34.

42. Haas AA, Arndt KA, Selected therapeutic applications of topical tretinoin. *J Am Acad Dermatol* 1986; **15**: 870–7.

43. Olsen EA, Katz HI, Levine N et al, Tretinoin emollient cream: a new therapy for photodamaged skin. *J Am Acad Dermatol* 1992; **26**: 215–24.

44. Rafal ES, Griffiths CEM, Ditre CM et al, Topical tretinoin (retinoic acid) treatment for liver spots associated with photodamage. *N Engl J Med* 1992; **326**: 368–74.

45. Griffiths CEM, Goldfarb MT, Finkel LJ et al, Topical tretinoin (retinoic acid) treatment of hyperpigmented lesions associated with photoaging in Chinese and Japanese patients: a vehicle-controlled trial. *J Am Acad Dermatol* 1994; **30**: 76–84.

46. Griffiths CEM, Finkel LJ, Ditre CM et al, Topical tretinoin (retinoic acid) improves melasma. A vehicle-controlled, clinical trial. *Br J Dermatol* 1993; **129**: 415–21.

47. Bulengo-Ransby SM, Griffiths CEM, Kimbrough-Green CK et al, Topical tretinoin (retinoic acid) therapy for hyperpigmented lesions caused by inflammation of the skin in Black patients. *N Engl J Med* 1993; **328**: 1438–43.

48. Stern RS, Dover J, Levin JA, Arndt KA, Laser therapy versus cryotherapy of lentigines: a comparative trial. *J Am Acad Dermatol* 1994; **30**: 985–7.

49. Hosaka Y, Onizuka T, Ichinose M et al, Treatment of nevus Ota by liquid nitrogen cryotherapy. *Plast Reconstr Surg* 1995; **95**: 703–11.

50. Burns RL, Prevost-Blank PL, Lawry MA et al, Glycolic acid peels for postinflammatory hyperpigmentation in Black patients. *Dermatol Surg* 1997; **23**: 171–5.

51. Lim JTE, Tham SN, Glycolic acid peels in the treatment of melasma among Asian women. *Dermatol Surg* 1997; **23**: 177–9.

52. Garcia A, Fulton JE, The combination of glycolic acid and hydroquinone or kojic acid for the treatment of melasma and related conditions. *Dermatol Surg* 1996; **22**: 443–7.

53. Sheehan-Dare RA, Cotterill JA, Lasers in dermatology. *Br J Dermatol* 1993; **19:** 1–8.

54. Goldberg DJ, Laser treatment of pigmented lesions. *Dermatol Clin* 1997; **15:** 397–407.

55. Ploysangam T, Dee-Ananlap S, Suvanprakorn P, Treatment of idiopathic guttate hypomelanosis with liquid nitrogen: light and electron microscopic studies. *J Am Acad Dermatol* 1990; **23:** 681–4.

56. Sebire D, Marchand JP, Simoneau L et al, A propos des autobronzants. *Nouv Dermatol* 1989; **8:** 329–32.

57. Brauer EW, Coloring and corrective make-up preparations. *Clin Dermatol* 1988; **6:** 62–7.

58. Falabella R, Escobar C, Borrero I, Treatment of refractory and stable vitiligo by transplantation of in vitro cultured epidermal autografts bearing melanocytes. *J Am Acad Dermatol* 1992; **26:** 230–6.

59. Ho C, Nguyen Q, Lowe NJ et al, Laser resurfacing in pigmented skin. *Dermatol Surg* 1995; **21:** 1035–7.

60. Dover JS, Linsmeier Kilmer S, Anderson RR, What's new in cutaneous laser surgery. *J Dermatol Surg Oncol* 1993; **19:** 295–8.

61. Linsmeier Kilmer S, Laser treatment of tattoos. *Dermatol Clin* 1997; **15:** 409–17.

35

Camouflage cosmetics

Victoria L Rayner

INTRODUCTION

Make-up artistry can be categorized in the following three ways:

- enhancement
- theatrical
- camouflage.

Enhancement make-up accentuates facial features; theatrical make-up is used in stage productions, television, video and motion pictures; and camouflage make-up is used to conceal abnormalities on the face, neck and body. The goal of camouflage make-up is to normalize the appearance of a patient suffering from a disfigurement. Unlike traditional cosmetics, cover creams are used because of their unique properties. They are waterproof and opaque, and offer a wide variety of cosmetic shades from which to choose. Selecting the correct cover cream system and cosmetic shades to match the skin tone and texture of the patient's complexion insures a successful camouflage result. Enhancement make-up can also be incorporated to emphasize attractive features and to divert attention away from the problem area. Whatever it takes to achieve a satisfactory result should be considered an appropriate technique, as long as the make-up application is kept simple enough for the patient to perform independently and as long as the treatment complements the patient's lifestyle.

COSMETIC CAMOUFLAGE INDICATIONS

A patient can benefit from a camouflage make-up lesson if he or she has a congenital, traumatic or surgical lesion or abnormality. This would include hemangiomas, fine capillaries, birthmarks, dark circles, scars, pigmentary problems, tattoos, burn scars and indications of post-surgical acute trauma. Patients in the recovery phase from dermabrasions, laser abrasion, chemical peels, rhytidectomy, rhinoplasty and belphroplasty can all profit from the use of cosmetics to offset the temporary trauma resulting from these procedures. An application of opaque cover creams can temporarily conceal bruising and reduce the appearance of redness and swelling, improving the patient's appearance until the physical evidence of these procedures becomes inconspicuous. Many dermatologic conditions such as lupus, rosacea, and vitiligo can also be cosmetically improved upon (Figures 35.1–35.3).

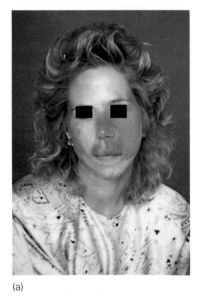

(a)

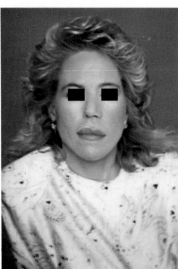

(b)

Figure 35.1 Portwine stain (a) before and (b) after application of camouflage make-up.

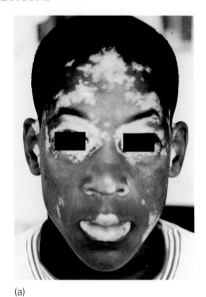

(a)

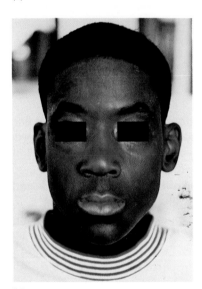

(b)

Figure 35.2 Vitiligo (a) before and (b) after application of camouflage make-up.

CLINICAL CONSIDERATIONS FROM THE REFERRAL SOURCE

The following information must be obtained before the camouflage treatment begins:

- the patient's medical history, revealing the disorder, its location, and the duration of the condition;
- any medication that may have been prescribed – topical or systemic (certain drugs

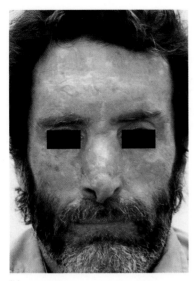

(a)

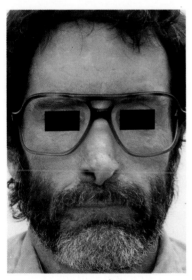

(b)

Figure 35.3 Basal cell carcinoma (a) before and (b) after application of camouflage make-up.

before anything is applied to their skin; for allergy-prone patients a special list of the ingredients used in treatment should be available for review;

- any skin care products the patient may have been instructed to use by the health care provider, such as cleansers, lotions, sunscreens, lubricating creams or α-hydroxy acids (AHAs).

CAMOUFLAGE THERAPIST'S CONSIDERATIONS

The camouflage therapist's considerations are as follows:

- the patient's perception of the problem;
- the patient's goals from the treatment;
- employment – the environmental conditions in which the patient will be viewed; the physical aspects of the patient's work environment (lighting, air quality, dry or humid atmosphere);
- the patient's social activities, hobbies and sports – the camouflage process must be compatible with the patient's lifestyle.

MATERIALS CHECK LIST

See Tables 35.1–35.4.

MAKE-UP KIT

The most efficient and practical container for camouflage materials is a large portable storage kit such as a fishing-tackle box with separate compartments. The sectional trays allow the materials to be transported without spillage or breakage. The kit should be large enough to accommodate all make-up tools, with additional space for extra items.

EQUIPMENT AND INSTRUMENTS

See Table 35.5.

temporarily alter the color of the patient's skin at the time of the application and can interfere with the correct color match);

- allergies or sensitivities – all patients should be questioned about any possible allergies

Table 35.1 Sterilization materials to sanitize instruments

Material	Available from
Ethanol (70%)	Drugstore
Quaternary ammonium compounds (QUATS)	Medical supply
Autoclave system	As above
Ultraviolet light	As above

Table 35.2 Skin care supplies

Material	Available from
Cleansers (oil/water, water/oil)	Department stores, pharmacies, distributors
Sunscreens, SPF 15 or higher (UVA and UVB protection)	As above
Astringent and toner	As above
Moisturizer (dry, normal, oil skin)	As above

Table 35.3 Cosmetics

Material	Available from
Powder blusher	Department stores, beauty supply, pharmacies
Cream rouge	As above
Lipsticks (pink, red, coral and terracotta)	As above
Lip-lining pencils (pink, red, sienna)	As above
Powder shadows: matte only (beige, brown, gray, dark green, navy blue)	As above
Eyebrow pencils (blonde, taupe, medium brown, dark brown, gray, black)	As above
Eyelash and brow dye (black, brown, light brown)	As above
Eyedrops	Pharmacies
Petrolatum	As above
Liquid mascara: waterproof (black and brown)	Department stores, beauty supply, pharmacies
Cake mascara (black and brown)	As above

Table 35.4 Disposable items

Material	Available from
Small plastic spatulas	Beauty product suppliers
Cotton swabs	Pharmacies
Cotton rolls	As above
Latex examination gloves	Medical supply

Table 35.5 Materials needed

Material	Available from
Medical examination table	Beauty supply, medical supply
Make-up station and wall-mounted mirror with lighting panels, using 17–40 W warm fluorescent bulbs on top and sides only	Lighting and fixture supply
Two portable free-standing goose-neck lamps with incandescent bulbs	As above
Hand-held mirror with one side magnifying	Pharmacy
Extension cord	Hardware store
High-backed director's chair	Furniture store
Trash receptacle	Hardware store

INTERVIEWING THE PATIENT

The purpose of interviewing the patient beforehand is to learn more about his or her goals for therapy. The patient's goals for treatment will fall into two categories: wants and needs. Each person has an idea of what beauty is and what will be cosmetically acceptable. This concept is generally based on the patient's ethnic, cultural and esthetic background.

It is the role of the camouflage therapist to help the patient recognize that sometimes not all desires can be met. If the camouflage therapist can get an idea of what it is that the patient wishes to achieve and what he or she will be amenable to, practical solutions can be devised. To prevent the patient from being disappointed with the final result, the camouflage therapist needs to be careful not to overstate what he or she can actually do.

FINANCIAL CONSIDERATIONS

The camouflage process should be tailored to meet the patient's individual budget. If the make-up is only required for short-term use, such as for postoperative care, obviously the financial factor will not need to be considered. However, over a period of months or even years, camouflage products can be quite costly if a variety of different tools must be used or several cover cream shades are required.

PHYSICAL CONSIDERATIONS

A careful examination must be made of the patient's skin and bone structure prior to the application of cosmetics. By first studying the patient's face, its contours and characteristic features, and by analyzing the skin surface, key factors that must be considered when selecting an appropriate cosmetic solution can be determined. A thorough evaluation of the actual disfigurement and the area surrounding it must be made. The size and location of the condition being treated, and the color, texture, moisture and oil content of the skin, are evaluated. Any evidence of physical irregularities or any suspicious abnormalities are documented and reported immediately to the patient's physician. While an irregularity may prove to be insignificant, it may be the symptom of a more serious condition or a complication after surgery, and may require immediate medical attention.

CLEANSING OF THE SKIN (Figure 35.4)

The first step is the preparation of the skin by cleansing, toning and moisturizing. Any residue left on the skin's surface can cause discoloration and ultimately affect coverage. The cleansing solution that is selected should correspond to the patient's skin type; for example, if the patient has oily or combination skin, a facial cleanser for oily skin is indicated. Cleansing should always be followed up with the use of an astringent to eliminate any remaining surface residue. An oil-free moisturizer that contains sunscreen should be applied prior to the camouflage application.

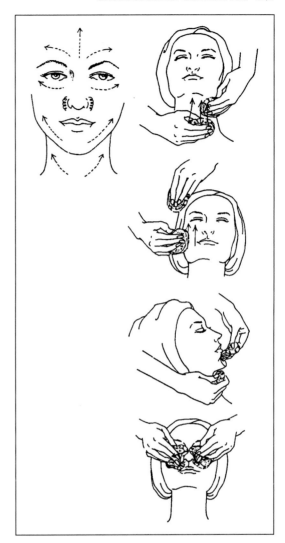

Figure 35.4 Procedure for cleansing the face.

CORRECTIVE COVER PRODUCTS WITH SETTING POWDERS (Figure 35.5)

Camouflage preparations have a thick, paste-like consistency and are more opaque than traditional make-up foundations. One or several of these cover creams are matched to the

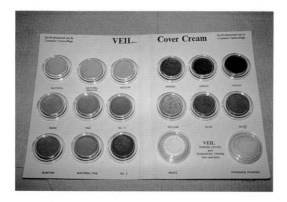

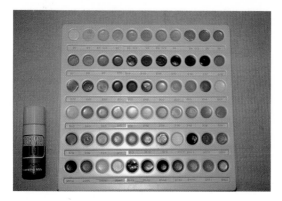

Figure 35.5 Two examples of cover cream palettes.

patient's skin and applied with a light tapping motion as opposed to the traditional rubbing method. A light translucent powder or a slightly tinted setting powder, sprinkled or lightly brushed over the top of the cover cream, stabilizes and waterproofs the application.

COLOR MATCHING AND APPLICATION OF COVER CREAMS

Cover cream products vary in cost, covering properties and color selection. The greater the variety of cover creams from which the camouflage therapist has to choose, the better is the chance of matching the right product to the patient's needs. The camouflage therapist should be equipped with at least three palettes from different cosmetic manufacturers in order to offer patients a full range of cover cream shades.

Cover creams will react differently once applied, depending on the pH of the patient's skin. Because of this, the color of the cover cream will differ noticeably from the original color as it appears in the container. Most manufacturers try to produce enough of a cover cream selection to match each patient's skin color, but unfortunately the appropriate cosmetic color usually falls somewhere in between two shades. Very rarely does an exact color match occur from using just one cover cream. The camouflage therapist should try to avoid selecting more than two shades when color blending. Working with three or more different cover creams would make the camouflage process too costly for the patient, and will require too much time to achieve the exact color match.

MATCHING COVER CREAMS TO THE SKIN (Figure 35.6)

To successfully match a cover cream to the patient's skin, the camouflage therapist must be able to identify the underlying colors that make up the patient's skin tone. Thin skin has a red undertone, which gives the appearance of ruddiness, whereas thick skin has more apparent traces of brown pigment in it.

Hemoglobin produces redness in the skin, keratin produces a yellowish cast and melanin brings forth a brown pigment. Patients from countries north of the equator will need cover creams in light shades such as ivory, natural, medium and peach; patients from countries south of the equator will wear darker shades such as suntan, tan, brown, chestnut, amber, copper and dark brown. Expertise in identifying undertones in the skin and being able to

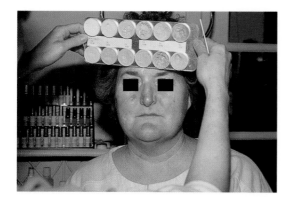

Figure 35.6 Identifying the underlying colors that make up the patient's skin tone to select the correct cover creams.

duplicate the varying degrees of color is mandatory when performing camouflage therapy.

THE PROCEDURE (Figure 35.7)

1. Patients are properly draped to protect their clothing during the procedure.
2. The cover cream palette is held by the therapist alongside the area of skin that is to be camouflaged. The therapist makes a quick scan of each cover cream shade to determine if it has the same amount of brown, yellow or red tones as the skin surrounding the lesioned area.
3. If the selected shade lacks some of the

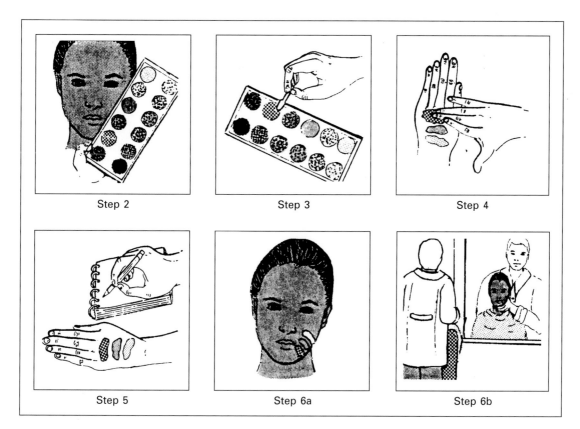

Step 2   Step 3   Step 4

Step 5   Step 6a   Step 6b

Figure 35.7 Procedure for matching cover creams to the skin.

yellow or pink undertones in a patient's skin, a second color is selected to fill the void, and is blended into the cover cream.

4. Once the correct shade or shades have been chosen, the therapist removes a small amount from the container using a spatula and places it on the back of the hand. The cream is rubbed onto the back of the hand in a circular motion until it is malleable and spreads easily.

5. Three different color combinations of no more than two blended colors each are selected and mixed. The formulas are recorded on a pad of paper.

6. A small sample of each of the three separate cover cream combinations is placed on the patient's skin. The therapist stands back and examines the application from a distance (if the irregularity is on the face, it is applied to the jaw area). By squinting, the therapist can ascertain if the cover cream meets the edges of the surrounding skin without detection. If the cover cream combination is the correct shade, it will blend in so well (not too light or too dark) that it will barely be noticeable. If the cover cream color combination is too dark, a little bit more of the lighter color of the two can be added until it matches the patient's skin tone. A pinhead amount of white cover cream can also be used to lighten it up. If it is too light, a little more of the darker shade of the two can be added until the color of the patient's skin tone is matched as closely as possible.

7. Once the correct color match has been selected, the area the patient wishes to conceal is covered, set and waterproofed. Setting the application involves waiting a few minutes after applying the cover creams for the powder to be absorbed. The setting time of the powder will depend on the patient's skin type (dry or oily). Patients who have more surface oil will require the powder to remain on their skin a little longer (approximately 8–10 minutes) to absorb some of their natural oils along with the oils in the cover creams. Patients with dry or aging skin will achieve a better result by having the cover creams on their skin longer (8–10 minutes) before setting the application with powder (the oil in the product helps to lubricate the surface of the skin), preventing the appearance of dryness. Patients with extremely dry (flaky and cracking) skin will not require setting powder to stabilize the cover creams. Using a setting powder will only accentuate fine lines and wrinkles and make the application appear more detectable.

8. After the cover creams have been set, the excess powder is removed with a powder brush or a cotton ball by using a gentle downward sweeping motion from the center outward.

9. If complete coverage is not achieved, re-application is necessary. The original camouflage steps are repeated, resetting the second application with powder. If the corrected result looks cakey and artificial, a moistened tissue is gently blotted over the area. Care must be taken not to rub over the cover creams, because friction can accidentally remove some of the make-up. After the cover creams have had time to settle on the skin (approximately one hour), the make-up application will appear more natural.

10. If a thick opaque is required, it may be necessary to duplicate the cover cream application slightly on the other (unaffected) side of the patient's face so as to achieve a completely natural result. This technique balances the two sides and prevents the camouflaged area from appearing 'made-up'.

11. Sometimes it is necessary to camouflage the entire facial area, which will automatically obliterate the natural color from the skin. To restore color tone and to give the skin a healthy appearance, the therapist applies a cream rouge of a powder

blusher. There are three types of blushers: powders, which are made from talc; water-based gels; and creams that are high in oil. Powder blushers are the most compatible with cover creams, because they absorb some of the oil in the make-up, which in turn helps set the make-up application. The powdered blush is applied to the cheeks with a brush or a disposable cotton ball in light, even strokes, extending the color into the hair line.

COSMETIC THERAPY FOR CHILDREN AND MEN

Sometimes camouflaging even minor irregularities on the faces of small children or on men can be difficult. For adolescent or male patients with hypopigmentation or vitiligo, a bronzing gel can be used to temporarily stain the skin, or a tinted powder can be applied to discreetly camouflage the lack of pigment. Although bronzing gel or tinted powder may not provide as much coverage as opaque make-up, it may be a better cosmetic solution because it may look more natural.

The duplication of natural imperfections on the skin

Concealing problem areas on men and children require a more complex set of make-up procedures to discreetly correct problem areas. These camouflage methods involve recognizing the subtle imperfections surrounding the treated area that constitute the natural appearance of the skin (freckles, veins and capillaries), and reproducing their appearance with make-up.

Skin imperfections are easily identified as the pink, yellow or brown undertones in the skin, such as capillaries, yellow undertones, patches of brown pigment, brown spots, freckles or uneven tanned areas. A more natural result is achieved by reproducing these common flaws over the cover cream application and on the areas surrounding the irregularity.

Imitating beard stubble, freckles and rosy cheeks

Imperfections can be re-created with the use of different types of sponges (stipple sponges, sea sponges, and synthetic sponges). Stipple sponges and sea sponges have larger pores than synthetic sponges. They can be used to dab on make-up rather than creating an overly made-up look.

Creating imperfections (Figure 35.8)

1. The camouflaged area is initially set with powder. After 8–10 minutes, the powder is lightly dusted off (powdering the area first prevents smudging).
2. To stipple-in color to imitate freckles, brown veins in the skin or an unshaven look such as a beard shadow, the camouflage therapist presses the stipple sponge into the cover cream solution. This must be done lightly to avoid completely filling in the holes in the sponge. A rose cover cream can be used for imitating broken capillaries, a brown and yellow mixture for freckles, and, depending on the beard color, brown, dark brown, gray or black for a beard shadow.
3. A preapplication test is performed by pressing the sponge down on the back of the hand to determine the amount of pressure that will be required to match the surrounding imperfections near or on the camouflaged site. If the pressure is correct, the therapist proceeds by pressing the sponge down onto the site.
4. Once the imperfection has been re-created, powder is re-applied to the area, but, instead of being brushed on, it is stippled on with the sponge.

Note that an eyebrow pencil can also be used to fill in freckles and beard stubble. If

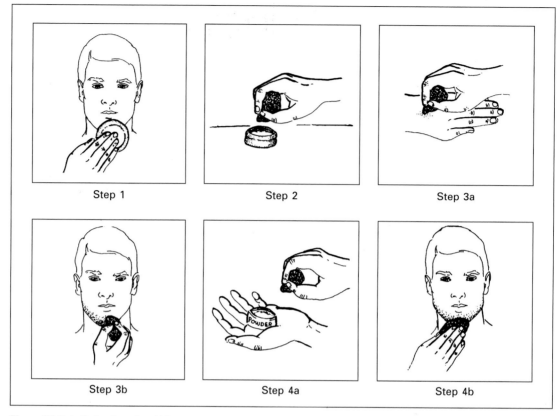

Figure 35.8 Imitating beard stubble.

the artificial freckles appear too thick, the pencil can be resharpened to create thinner marks. To prevent strokes from looking too bold and artificial, the pencil is held away from the tip. This reduces the pressure used during the application.

COLOR CORRECTORS

Most surgical or dermatologic surgery procedures result in temporary trauma to the skin, causing swelling and discoloration. Green color correctors will counterbalance redness or ruddiness, and mauve or lavender color correctors will offset sallow or yellow under-

tones in the skin. Color correctors are worn underneath make-up foundations or underneath cover creams. Neutralizing redness or concealing yellow undertones can be accomplished by selecting the appropriate color corrector, applying it over the discoloration, setting it with powder, and concealing it with a light application of cover cream or foundation.

Tattoos

To obliterate a red tattoo, a green color corrector is applied. To erase a blue tattoo, an orange color corrector is applied. The color corrector is applied to the area first, set with powder, concealed with a cover cream that matches the patient's skin, and reset with powder.

CONCEALING EYELID INCISION LINES

Acute trauma resulting from a blephroplasty produces a bright red discoloration on and around the incision area that is often difficult to conceal. If too heavy a make-up foundation is used, it will end up in the crease of the eyelids. To prevent this from occurring, a green or mauve color corrector can be applied instead of a heavy, opaque foundation. The corrector should be brushed directly over the incision line with a thin brush such as a lip or an artist's flat brush, set with powder, and the entire eye area covered with a light non-greasy foundation base that matches the patient's natural skin color.

COSMETIC THERAPY FOR PARTIAL BALDNESS

Cover creams can be applied directly to the scalp to eliminate the contrast between the patient's hair and scalp after a transplant or a scalp reduction. By selecting a cover cream that closely matches the patient's head, areas with low density of hair appear fuller. This procedure can also be very effective for patients who are recovering from alopecia areata.

CAMOUFLAGE AND THE MATURE PATIENT

Heavy applications of thick opaque cover creams will exaggerate lines and wrinkles on the face. Care should be taken to insure that cover creams are applied sparingly. Brightly colored eyeshadows and lipstick shades will make the mature female patient appear clownish. If colored eyeshadows and lipsticks are desired by the patient, muted, pale shades are best.

CONTOURING

Creating the illusion of light or dark is the basic principle behind highlighting and contouring. Light brings objects forward, making them appear as if they are closer, and dark makes objects recede, making them appear as if they are further away. Highlighters can be any cosmetic product (powder, cover stick, cream or foundation) that is two times lighter than the patient's natural skin tone. Shading can be created with the use of concealer creams, base foundations or powder cosmetics, as long as they are a shade-and-a-half to two shades darker than the patient's natural complexion. Highlighting and shading techniques can be used on patients who have traumatic scarring as a result of a car accident, bone cancer, burns, or any other condition that may have permanently altered the patient's bone structure and requires reconstruction through the application of cosmetics. If this is the case with the facial area, the make-up should create the illusion of perfect symmetry (both sides of the face being identical).

BRUSHES

A wide variety of brushes for contouring and shading is essential for corrective make-up and camouflage work. Synthetic and sable artist's flat brushes are recommended for the application of cover creams, whereas eyeshadow, contour and powder brushes are suggested for the application of shadows, powder blushers and setting powders.

PROSTHESES

Cosmetic prostheses are artificial devices that replace nails, eyelashes, eyebrows and other parts of the anatomy. A detailed description of how certain prosthetic devices can be used in the practice of camouflage therapy is given below, and the materials needed are listed in Table 35.6.

Table 35.6 Materials needed

Product	Available from
False eyelashes (individual and strip; upper and lower)	Theatrical make-up or hair replacement center
Artificial eyebrows (blonde, brown, black)	As above
Crepe hair (for eyebrows, mustaches and beards)	As above
Mustaches (blonde, brown, black)	As above

False eyelashes (Figure 35.9)

The eyes and the eyebrows are the most expressive part of the face. For many patients the loss of part or all of their eyelashes or eyebrows can be devastating. False eyelashes are considered a prosthesis in the practice of camouflage therapy. They are used to replace missing lashes or to conceal a scar along the

Select the appropriate type and color lashes.

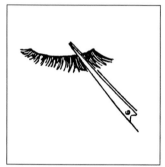

1. Trim to correct length.

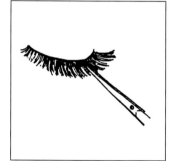

2. Feather the lashes by nipping into them with the points of the manicure scissors.

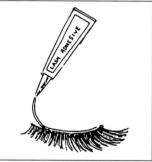

3. Apply a thin strip of adhesive to the lash.

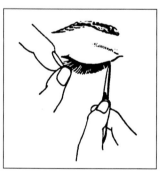

4. Apply the lash with the applicator or fingers.

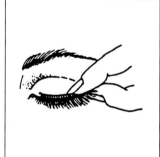

5. Press the lash into the lashline with fingers.

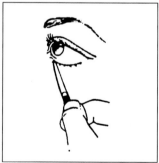

6. Use the same techniques to apply lower strip lashes.

Figure 35.9 Technique for applying strip lashes.

eyelid or the lower rim of the eye. There are different types of lashes, varying in size from full strip eyelashes to small clusters or individual lashes.

Re-creating eyebrows (Figure 35.10)

Crepe hair can be used to simulate natural eyebrows. In addition it can be used to make mustaches, beards and sideburns, and is an alternative to the pre-made hairpieces that can be purchased in a wig or theatrical make-up store. It is made from wool, and comes in braided strands in a variety of natural colors that can be blended together to create a more natural shade. To mix shades, several colors are combined, starting with the darkest color at the base and blending in the lighter ones

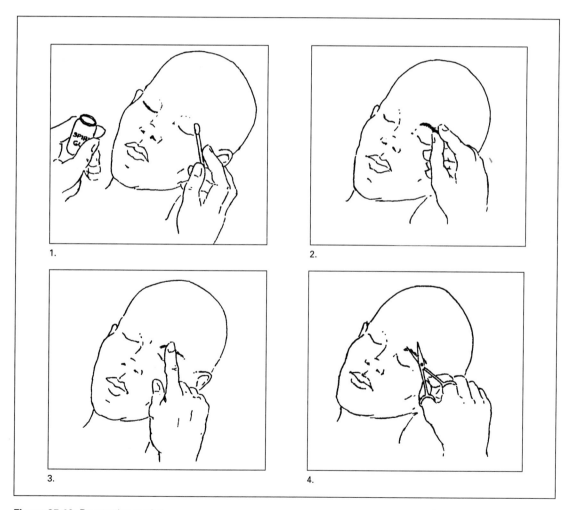

Figure 35.10 Re-creating eyebrows.

on the top. Crepe hair is attached to the skin with medical adhesive.

Ventilated eyebrows

Real or synthetic hair is individually knotted onto a thin lace net, cut, and shaped into a strip of hair that resembles an eyebrow. This type of artificial eyebrow is more practical for patients who will need to apply artificial eyebrows daily.

Reconstructing eyebrows (Figure 35.11)

Eyebrows should always be darkened slightly, and should only frame the eyes – not stand out. An eyebrow pencil is a wooden pencil filled with grease lead, although it is harder than an eyeliner pencil. For the best results, it is recommended that pencils be sharpened to a fine point before application. The following shades are recommended: blonde, taupe, medium brown, dark brown, gray and black, matching the natural hair and eyebrow color. The procedure is as follows:

- To completely reconstruct eyebrows, delicate, light strokes are applied with an eyebrow pencil that matches the patient's hair color to recreate the illusion of natural hairs.
- A gray eyebrow pencil can be used to buffer the harsh look that dark brown and black pencil marks can give. Gray pencil is applied first with light strokes, and followed up with gentle strokes of taupe, dark brown or black pencil, depending on which color is appropriate.
- Eyeshadows (matte, non-frost) can also be used to soften pencil lines or fill in very thin eyebrows by applying the eyeshadow to the brow with an angular brush in a color that matches the natural brow or the patient's hair color.
- Waterproof mascara is also used to fill in gaps in eyebrows or to imitate the appearance of eyebrows. To avoid an application that is too thick and obvious, mascara is

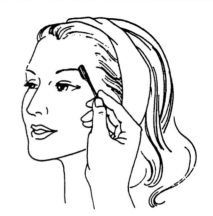

Before the application of eyebrow color, an eyebrow brush is used to brush away any make-up on the brows. The brows may be brushed upward and then across in the direction of the hair growth.

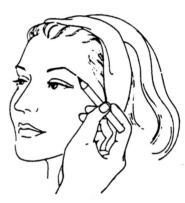

Brow color should be applied with light hair-like strokes. When brows are sparse, a finely pointed pencil is used to sketch in fine, hair-like strokes to resemble real brow hair. At first this takes practice in order to create the illusion of real brow hair

Figure 35.11 Reconstructing eyebrows with an eyebrow pencil.

applied by the following method: dip a disposable mascara wand into the applicator container; scrape the wand against the sides of the container to remove excess mascara; place the wand parallel to the brow bone, and lightly stroke the mascara onto the skin.

PATIENT INSTRUCTION

Only after the cosmetic application procedure has been completed and the patient is completely satisfied with the result does the instruction phase of the appointment begin.

Before attempting to repeat the procedure, the patient is asked to remove the application to insure that he or she will be able to properly perform the cleansing process. Because camouflage make-up is an oil-based formula, regular soap and water do not break down the oils in the cover creams. A thick cleansing emulsion (a water-in-oil emulsion) is the most efficient cleansing agent.

Cover cream removal method

1. The patient is asked to apply a liberal amount of cleansing cream directly over the cover cream, massaging it in a circular motion to loosen up the waxes and the oil in the product.
2. The patient is instructed to wipe off the make-up application with moistened cotton squares until the cover creams have been completely removed.
3. The cleansing cream will leave a filmy residue on the skin. This can be removed with a toner (without alcohol) for sensitive skin and an astringent (with alcohol) for oily skin.
4. Toning is followed up with a light moisturizer that contains a sunscreen.

Guiding the patient through the application process

After watching the camouflage therapist mix and apply the cover creams, the patient is ready to attempt the make-up process independently. A patient's previous experience with the application of cosmetics and prior knowledge of color determine the amount of appointment time that is needed for his or her instruction. The camouflage therapist evaluates the patient's color awareness by asking the patient questions regarding previous color studies or personal experimentation. Many patients have some prior knowledge of color theory, either through art courses or through hobbies such as landscaping, photography or interior design. To determine the patient's technical experience with cosmetics and how much of that experience can be incorporated into the camouflage lesson, the therapist inquires about the patient's current make-up routine.

RECOMMENDED READING

Allsworth J, *Skin Camouflage – A guide to Remedial Techniques.* Cheltenham, UK: Stanley Thornes, 1985.

Begoun P, *Blue Eyeshadow Should be Illegal.* Seattle: Beginning Press, 1988.

Boughton P, Hughes ME, *The Buyer's Guide to Cosmetics.* New York: Random House, 1981.

Brumberg E, *Save Your Money, Save Your Face.* New York: Facts On File, 1986.

Buchman H, *Stage Makeup.* New York: Watson-Guptill, 1971.

Corson R, *Stage Makeup.* Englewood Cliffs, NJ: Prentice-Hall, 1986.

Cosmetic, Toiletry and Fragrance Association, *Cosmetic Ingredient Dictionary,* 3rd edn. Washington, DC: CTFA, 1982.

Jellinek S, *Formulation and Function of Cosmetics.* New York: Wiley, 1980.

Place SC, *The Art and Science of Professional Makeup.* New York: Milady, 1989.

Rayner V, *Clinical Cosmetology: A Medical Approach to Esthetic Procedures.* Buffalo, NY: Milady, 1993.

Siedel L, Copeland I, *The Art of Corrective Cosmetics.* New York: Doubleday, 1984.

Traynor M, Seids D, *Mark Traynor's Beauty Book.* New York: Doubleday, 1980.

Trust D, *Overcoming Disfigurement – Part Three: The Cosmetic Component.* Wellingborough, UK: Thorsons, 1986.

Westmore M, *The Art of Theatrical Makeup for Stage and Screen.* New York: McGraw-Hill, 1987.

Winters R, *Consumer's Dictionary of Cosmetic Ingredients.* New York: Crown, 1976.

FURTHER DETAILS

For additional information on Camouflage Therapy as well as advanced certified training in this field please write to:

Center For Appearance & Esteem Training Institute
Victoria L Rayner
251 Post Street, Suite 420
San Francisco, CA 94108, USA
Tel: +1 415 398 6013
Fax: +1 415 398 7240

36

Acne

Robert Baran, Martine Chivot, Alan R Shalita

INTRODUCTION

Acne, whatever its severity, is a disease that requires medical care. Only such care is capable of making acne lesions go away. Nevertheless, advice with regard to skin hygiene and skin care can be of significant benefit to the acne patient. The goals of such cosmetic counselling in the acne patient are as follows:

- to clean the skin *gently* in order to prepare it for various treatments;
- to re-establish a more normal and comfortable skin surface often disturbed by acne treatments;
- to permit the application of make-up when necessary;
- to permit modest sun exposure.

SKIN CLEANING

The principle of skin cleaning for acne-prone skin is to gently remove surface debris and excess skin surface debris and excess skin surface lipids without irritating or drying the skin. We emphasize the gentle nature of such cleansing, since acne treatments are frequently accompanied by irritating side-effects. In addition, it has been clearly demonstrated that aggressive cleansing can often aggravate acne.[1]

As a broad categorization, acne-prone skin is seborrhoeic. Although there are obvious exceptions, individuals with acne, or a tendency towards acne, have higher levels of skin surface lipids than so-called normal controls. Indeed, sebum excretion tends to increase with the severity of the disease, so that patients with nodular acne and acne conglobata have, in general, the highest levels of sebum.[2] These results apply to both men and women. Thus one of the prime concerns of the individual with acne or acne-prone skin is the removal of the excess surface oil and the reduction of the resulting 'shine', either with or without make-up. An additional concern is to provide some measure of therapeutic benefit to the hygiene programme. Cosmetic science has now developed a wide array of ingredients and products that accomplish these goals in varying degrees.

Soaps

Soaps are the most commonly utilized personal hygiene products, and are adequate for cleansing the skin of sweat, skin surface lipid, surface bacteria and dust accumulated during the day. Soap is brought into intimate contact with the skin surface by mixing with water, and will generally emulsify whatever is on the skin surface. Further rinsing with water will remove all of this from the skin surface. Soaps are alkaline – mixed with water they liberate the free base from which they are formed and increase the skin surface pH, which is normally between five and six. The buffer capability of the skin allows the pH to return to normal in approximately half an hour. So-called 'natural' soaps such as the French Marseille soap are frequently used by patients, because they are thought to be ecologically safe and natural. However, they are not to be recommended, since they are generally strongly basic and promote excess drying of the skin. Super-fatted soaps alleviate this inconvenience. They are usually rich in lanolin and/or sweet almond oil, and usually contain a certain amount of glycerol. They may occasionally be used in acne patients with very thickened, treatment-resistant skin which is also very oily.

Dermatological bars or cakes

These products resemble soaps and are used in the same way, but strictly they are not soaps because they are chemically different. In general, these products contain surface-active ingredients, usually detergents, which have a variety of chemical modifications permitting easy and agreeable use. These compounds permit the addition of weak organic acids, which give them a pH close to that of normal skin. One can also add softeners and emollients to maximize their tolerability. Dermatological bars and cakes are therefore better tolerated than soaps. On the other hand, they do not lather so well, and are usually more expensive than soap because of their more sophisticated manufacturing process. Their use is certainly justified when soaps are not tolerated.

Finally, selected dermatological bars contain active anti-acne ingredients such as benzoyl peroxide, zinc sulphate and vitamin B_6.

Liquid 'soaps'

Chemically, these are strictly not soaps, but rather liquid forms of the bars discussed above.

Antiseptic foaming solutions
These are not recommended for daily use, and are not particularly useful in acne since they have never been demonstrated to have an effect on *Propionibacterium acnes* in vitro. In general, they have an acid pH.

Antibacterial 'washes'
Although a large number of cleansers for acne-prone skin incorporate antibacterial agents, most of them have activity against Gram-positive aerobic surface bacteria, and do not penetrate the follicle to achieve a predictable reduction in *P. acnes*. Thus, while these agents may prevent secondary infection in acne-prone skin, they have no real beneficial effect on acne lesions per se. In fact, overuse of those agents has been associated with Gram-negative folliculitis.

More recently, however, there has emerged a group of cleansers containing benzoyl peroxide as the active ingredient. Benzoyl peroxide is a potent oxidizing agent, which is bacteriacidal for *P. acnes* and appears to penetrate the follicle sufficiently to reduce the population of this organism. While cleansers containing benzoyl peroxide do not have the substantivity of topically applied benzoyl peroxide, they tend to be less irritating and less 'drying' than the topically applied creams, lotions and gels, and may be used in a cleansing regimen. Greater efficacy is achieved when the cleanser is left on for 4–5 minutes before rinsing.

Enhanced cleansing vehicles containing ingredients such as glycolic acid and zinc may improve the efficacy of benzoyl peroxide cleansers.

Cosmetic liquid soaps or gels
These are different from the above, and they can be used on a daily basis. They may have

some active ingredients, and generally have a pH close to that of normal skin.

'Emulsions'

These are milky liquid cleansers and cleansing creams, which also include make-up removal preparations. Emulsions have formed the basis of cosmetology. They are a mixture of two phases, one aqueous, the other lipid, which are brought together in stable, intimate contact by one or more emulsifying agents.

Cleansing milks are among the oldest of these products. The continuous phase is aqueous, and is designed to be rinsed off. The oil phase is less important, and represents only 20–30% of the final product. Cleansing milks can be utilized with or in the absence of make-up. They are applied with the fingers and massaged gently into the skin, and then rinsed either with water or a mild astringent lotion. Rinsing is essential, because this is what will finally remove everything from the skin surface. Some women still perform the cleansing ritual and then pat their skin dry with paper or a handkerchief in order to leave a thin film that will 'nourish the skin'. This would have the same effect as not rinsing soap off one's skin. Nevertheless, cleansing milks have excellent cosmetological properties, since they are gentle cleansers and do not disturb the normal pH of the skin.

Some make-up removers are provided in a compact format in which the aqueous phase of the emulsion is furnished with tap water at the time of use. They are used like soaps, but on mixing them in the hands with water, one obtains a light cream instead of a foam. They therefore offer the ease of use of a soap with the gentleness of milky cleanser. Foaming cleansing creams are a relatively new format, and offer the additional skin softening qualities of a cream.

Rinsing products

These can be tap water, waters from thermal baths in pressurized atomizers or astringent lotions.

Tap water is the most readily available of all rinsing products. Even when 'hard' tap water is well tolerated by oily skin and in those cases where it is somewhat drying to the skin, it can be supplemented by the application of an emollient cream. Certain women who have used a cleansing lotion or cream like to finish with a toner or astringent lotion. In the case of patients with oily skin these toners can be somewhat alcoholic (less than 20%), and may also contain other astringents such as tannins, witch hazel or a variety of so-called extracts like cucumber, sage and lemon. They may also contain camphor or allantoin, which are alleged to have anti-inflammatory as well as astringent properties. Many cleansers, toners and astringents now contain α-hydroxy acids, usually glycolic acid. These may provide additional exfoliative action in those patients requiring such treatment.

Finally, one should mention the problem of shaving in men, which can be problematic in patients with acne. In general, such patients should be advised not to shave too closely and not every day unless absolutely necessary. This is particularly important in patients with significant numbers of inflammatory lesions. There are a variety of shaving foams and creams with antiseptic ingredients, including benzoyl peroxide. While the latter may be useful in selected patients (particularly those with sycosis barbae), they are usually not necessary in ordinary acne patients who are undergoing medical treatment.

In conclusion, the cleansing of acne-prone skin can be achieved quite well with gentle use of one of the products mentioned above. Our preference is for a mild soap or dermatological bar, but the cleansing regimen can be adapted to the needs of the individual patient. All cleansers should be rinsed off.

ADJUNCTIVE TREATMENT PRODUCTS

A variety of products exist that may either be used for early treatment of very mild acne or that may be adjunctive to a medical therapeutic regimen. These include a variety of cleansing lotions containing salicylic acid as the active ingredient and that have a mild comedolytic and anti-inflammatory effect. Salicylic acid is a comedolytic agent available in a wide variety of cleansers and astringent lotions. Although relatively weak as a comedolytic compared with tretinoin and isotretinoin, it offers the advantage of providing mild anti-inflammatory activity, is widely distributed, and well tolerated in concentrations up to 2%.[3] Salicylic acid is a desquamating agent, and may cause mild peeling and an appearance of 'dry skin'. It is suitable for those individuals who desire mild exfoliation and/or those with modest numbers of comedones.

The anti-inflammatory activity of salicylic acid may explain its tolerability in relation to its exfoliating properties. Similarly, products containing elemental sulphur or its derivatives may exhibit mild anti-inflammatory properties. Most frequently, sulphur is incorporated into anti-acne creams and lotions rather than cleansers. In addition, it has some antibacterial and antifungal effects. This is noteworthy, because the yeast *Pityrosporum* has been implicated in seborrhoeic dermatitis and may play a secondary role in acne. In addition, there are creams and lotions containing carboxymethylcysteine, which appears to have a surface-active effect, decreasing the appearance of oiliness on the skin surface. There are a number of other products, distributed in various countries around the world, that contain ingredients whose mechanism of action is not fully understood or whose efficacy is not yet established.

There also exist a wide variety of facial masks, most of which contain ingredients that adsorb skin surface lipids. Some of these masks may also contain active ingredients such as sulphurated lime or benzoyl peroxide. At best, these are of temporary benefit, but in patients who desire such treatment they may serve to enhance compliance with the remainder of the therapeutic regimen.

Finally, in a number of countries products are available that physically abrade the skin. These may consist of microspheres of polyethylene or particles of aluminium oxide as well as abrasive sponges, brushes and so on. In the USA the use of this type of product has been discouraged for acne-prone skins, since they tend to rupture microcomedones and aggravate inflammatory acne.

MAKE-UP

When cosmetic acne was a more common phenomenon than it is today, much of it was due to the regular use of heavy, occlusive make-ups, whose comedogenic or acnegenic potential had not been studied.[4] More recently, the cosmetic industry has paid much closer attention to the acnegenic potential of their products, and a wide range of make-ups specifically designed for oily or acne-prone skin have been developed. These are usually labelled 'non-comedogenic' or 'non-acnegenic'. Women with acne-prone skin can therefore apply adequate coverage from a wide range of products offering maximum safety.[5]

In general, we recommend make-up designed for oily skin. These are usually oil-and-water emulsions, which may contain oil-absorbing substances such as kaolin, talc or micronized polyamide powders. Some make-ups are powder suspensions without any oil, but these tend to provide less adequate cover. There are also acne treatment creams that are tinted to provide cover while also giving a measure of benefit. Among other ingredients, these may contain sulphur and/or resorcin as well as bentonite. All make-up bases may be modified by a light application of face powder with a brush.

INCREASING TOLERANCE TO ACNE TREATMENT

The most common medically prescribed acne treatments (vitamin A acid and benzoyl peroxide) frequently have irritating side-effects. Not infrequently, patients will benefit from the application of an emollient cream or lotion, which will tend to diminish the irritation from these active ingredients. The physician who ignores the side-effects of these drugs and does not provide advice on how to minimize their side-effects will have considerably less success in achieving adequate patient compliance with the prescribed therapeutic regimen. There are now a large number of moisturizing creams and emollient lotions that have been adequately tested for comedogenicity and acnegenicity, so that the patient and the physician have a wide choice.

In addition, patients receiving oral isotretinoin for acne require advice concerning its side-effects:

- Cheilitis, or chapped lips, is the most common consequence of oral isotretinoin treatment. Again a wide range of lip pomades are available, some containing active ingredients such as sulpha and hydroxy acids, and others containing simple bland emollients. We generally allow patients to select their own preferences in this regard. For more severe cases application of an ointment containing hydrocortisone is usually beneficial.
- Dry eyes is another common side-effect of isotretinoin treatment. For these patients we recommend treatment with artificial tears or ophthalmological lubricants, of which there are now a large number. Patients who wear soft contact lenses usually have less of a problem than those wearing hard ones. Rarely, a bacterial conjunctivitis may ensue, for which treatment with antibacterial ophthalmological ointments is mandatory.
- Finally, generalized xerosis is not uncommon, and this is usually relieved by one of a number of emollient lotions or creams.

THE SUN AND THE ACNE PATIENT

The sun is a two-edged sword for most acne patients. While ultraviolet light may have a mild anti-inflammatory effect, and tanning tends to hide acne lesions, it is also comedogenic since exposure to it thickens the skin and promotes hyperkeratosis of both the skin surface and the follicle.[6] It is a well-known observation in clinical dermatological practice that acne patients tend to get worse shortly after returning from a summer vacation. Thus acne patients require careful counselling with regard to sun exposure. Specific advice depends on the individual case.

If the patient has been following a regular therapeutic programme throughout the winter and spring and enters their vacation with a totally pale skin, it is more than likely that they will attempt to get a good tan over the summer. Unfortunately this will result in the consequences described above. For this reason, we recommend a maintenance treatment programme over the summer including a non-comedogenic sun screen. Obviously one should also explain to the patient that the best protection for the back and shoulders is a light T-shirt, and one should always counsel against long exposure to intense sunlight.

If the patient is planning to continue a regular treatment programme throughout the summer, it is wise to limit the treatment applications to the evening while all the time continuing to explain the potential harmful effects of the sun (particularly if the patient is using vitamin A acid) and prescribing an adequate, non-comedogenic sun screen. It should be emphasized that all acne treatment can be continued during the summer if the appropriate precautions are taken. Patients who need to continue taking tetracycline antibiotics during the summer months should probably switch to minocycline, since this is the least phototoxic of all the tetracyclines.

For those patients who come for consultation just before going on vacation, it is most important to stress sun protection and avoidance of midday sun. Other constraints will be difficult to initiate in a patient who has not been seen before.

Bearing all of the above in mind, it is virtually impossible to totally interdict sun exposure – particularly during the summer vacation. One must therefore explain the problems associated with sun exposure and adapt recommendations according to the individual patients. For example, certain patients, particularly boys, will not like to use the creamier sunscreens. For these patients a gel may be more suitable, even if it provides less of a sun protection factor. One is better off with a product that will be used, even if it offers less protection than one that will not be used at all.

ACNE SURGERY

Another important step in acne hygiene is the removal of the unsightly lesions themselves.[7] Acne surgery is defined as the opening and evacuation of all acne lesions. In some countries this procedure is referred to as 'dermatological skin cleaning', but this is a less satisfactory terminology, since it may be confused with the skin cleaning performed in cosmetic or aesthetic salons.

Acne surgery most often involves the removal of open and/or closed comedones. Occasionally it may be necessary and/or desirable to open and drain inflammatory lesions as well. Ideally this procedure should be performed after the individual in question has used some form of comedolytic agent to soften and loosen the comedones. Alternatively, the lesions may be softened by the application of warm moist compresses and/or the application of a salicylic acid or sulphur–salicylic acid cream or lotion. The skin should first be cleansed with alcohol or another suitable antiseptic solution. Although it is common practice in many countries to

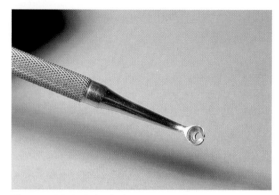

Figure 36.1 A keyhole extractor for the removal of comedones.

remove comedones by applying pressure with the fingertips or fingernails, this is no longer standard practice in the USA and many other countries. In particular, today's environment suggests that all procedures that may result in even pinpoint bleeding should be carried out by a physician wearing gloves. In this case it would be extremely difficult to remove comedones with the finger tips or nails. Rather, we prefer the use of a comedo extractor specifically designed for this purpose. Although one of us (Dr Shalita) prefers the use of a keyhole extractor (Figure 36.1), there are a variety of other comedo extractors available, and the choice depends upon individual preference. The advantage of the keyhole extractor is that it is easily cleaned by a simple gauze wipe when one is removing multiple comedones.

After cleansing the skin as described above, open comedones are easily removed by gentle but firm vertical pressure around the lesion. The comedo will then pop up into the orifice of the extractor. Patients who have been pretreated with topical tretinoin have comedones that are much more readily removable than patients who have not received such treatment. Similarly, if time permits, the application of a warm moist compress for 10–15

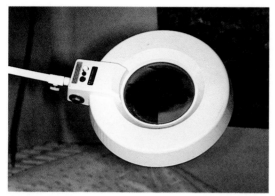

Figure 36.2 A magnifying lamp to aid comedone removal.

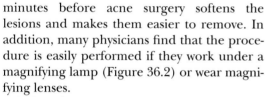

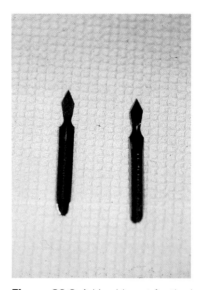

Figure 36.3 A blood lancet for the incision of comedones.

minutes before acne surgery softens the lesions and makes them easier to remove. In addition, many physicians find that the procedure is easily performed if they work under a magnifying lamp (Figure 36.2) or wear magnifying lenses.

Although occasionally the orifice of a closed comedone may be visible, it is frequently necessary to incise the lesion in order to simplify evacuation of the contents. Some small closed comedones may be removed without incision if one applies gentle pressure with the comedo extractor. However, if these lesions are not readily removable they should be incised. For this purpose a variety of instruments are available, such as the tip of a No. 11 scalpel blade, a Hagedorn needle, a blood lancet (Figure 36.3) or an ophthalmological foreign-body needle (Figure 36.4). Occasionally, closed comedones are not readily visible unless one stretches the skin. This is particularly true on the lateral aspects of the chin (Figure 36.5a,b).

We generally recommend that, following extraction of the lesions, the skin be cleansed again with alcohol or other antiseptic solution. Some dermatologists, however, apply a drop of 33% trichloracetic acid to the lesion,

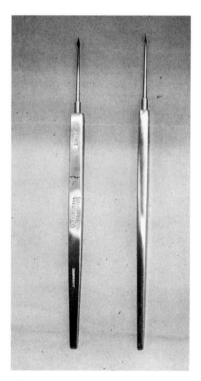

Figure 36.4 An ophthalmological foreign body needle for the incision of comedones.

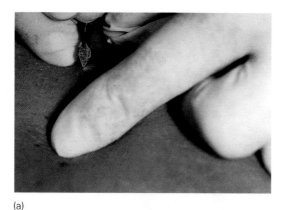

(a)

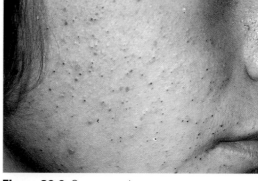

Figure 36.6 Open comedones.

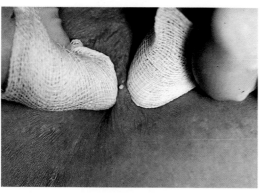

(b)

Figure 36.5 (a,b) Comedone removal on the lateral aspect of the chin. The skin occasionally needs to be stretched to reveal a closed comedone.

Although acne surgery does not have any effect on the overall course of the disease, it is of immediate cosmetic benefit to the patient. As such, it can significantly enhance patient compliance with the remainder of the therapeutic programme, since it demonstrates to the patient that rapid improvement is possible. Almost all forms of acne can benefit from some type of surgery – but, most notable among these, comedonal acne consisting of either open comedones (Figure 36.6), closed comedones (Figure 36.7) or a mixture of the two (Figure 36.8) will achieve significant and

followed by a wet compress to avoid blanching the skin.

Inflammatory lesions may also be incised and drained, but many of us prefer the use of intralesional corticosteroid injections to incision and drainage for this type of lesion. Small pustules, however, are easily removed with a comedo extractor, and this will achieve immediate cosmetic benefit. Similarly, the pressure from tense painful inflammatory lesions may be relieved by a tiny incision and gentle drainage of the contents, following which intralesional glucocorticoids may be injected.

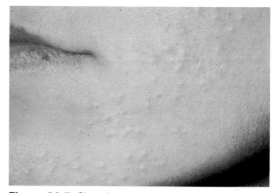

Figure 36.7 Closed comedones.

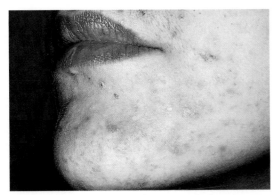

Figure 36.8 A mixture of open and closed comedones.

rapid improvement. Although acne surgery can be performed at any time during the course of treatment, it is preferable to wait until at least one month after treatment with a comedolytic agent such as tretinoin. Attempting acne surgery on the first visit is more painful, and may make the patient reluctant to pursue this form of treatment later. The patient should always be reminded that surgery is adjunctive to the medical treatment of their acne. Severe inflammatory acne is not infrequently accompanied by numerous comedonal lesions. Even in those patients who receive oral isotretinoin for their severe inflammatory acne, there may be a less pronounced effect on comedones. Some physicians prefer to treat such lesions by surgery early in the course of isotretinoin treatment while others prefer to wait until sometime after the course of isotretinoin has been completed and then to treat the remaining comedones by a combination of acne surgery and topical tretinoin. Acne surgery is also an ideal treatment for the lesions of Favre–Racouchot disease. Again a combination of topical tretinoin and surgery is the ideal treatment programme. Finally, it should be noted that, with routine antiseptic precautions, superinfection is almost never a problem following acne surgery – unless oral antibiotics are required for the acne condition itself, they are not required because of the surgery. Furthermore, the minuscule incisions performed as part of the procedure do not ordinarily leave scars, and the procedure is generally extremely well tolerated if practiced with intelligence and gentleness.

COSMETICS AND ACNE

The question of which cosmetics are best suited for individuals with acne or acne-prone skin has received considerable attention during the past 20 years – particularly since the subject of cosmetic acne was introduced.[4] Unfortunately, much confusion has resulted from misinformation, technical problems and exaggerated claims. Most important is the fact that cosmetics today are better formulated and better tested than they were in the past.

The concept of cosmetic acne derived from the observation that many women were presenting to dermatologists with acne after having used the heavy occlusive make-up and moisturizers popular in the 1940s and 1950s. Using the rabbit ear model, it was concluded that these agents in general, and selected cosmetic ingredients in particular, were comedogenic. It was also concluded that lipids, as a general class, were offensive compounds and that acne-prone individuals should use oil-free make-ups and avoid lipid-containing emollients.

It must be understood that the rabbit ear contains numerous sebaceous follicles, which readily become filled with horny material. Examination of these follicles by surface inspection, even with magnification, can lead to erroneous conclusions. For this reason the American Academy of Dermatology convened a panel of clinicians and investigators with particular interest and experience in the subject.[5] This group concluded that the problem of comedogenecity and acnegenecity of cosmetics had been overstated in the past, and that an accurate determination of these qualities in cosmetics and cosmetic ingredients was best made as a result of histological examination of the involved follicles. Furthermore, the comedogenecity and/or acnegenecity of individual ingredients may be modified by either the concentration in a given product and their mixture with other ingredients. What must one then conclude for the acne-prone consumer? Rather than recommending oil-free or water-based cosmetics and prohibiting all lipid-containing emollients, it is more prudent to advise the consumer to seek out those products tested for comedogenecity and acnegenecity and so labelled. Most major cosmetic manufacturers have the facilities to carry out such testing accurately, and the consumer may use them with a reasonable degree of confidence at the present time.

It should also be noted that therapeutic agents also exist that provide cosmetic cover while exerting a drying effect on acne or acne lesions. Thus most preparations containing sulphur and/or resorcin are incorporated into tinted bases, some of which also include the oil absorbent bentonite. Such products are designed to be applied to individual acne lesions, and appear to accelerate their resolution while providing cosmetic cover. Additionally, there are now benzoyl peroxide-containing lotions and creams, which are also provided in tinted bases to provide both effective medication and cosmetic cover at the same time.

In conclusion, the individual with acne or acne-prone skin can now achieve satisfactory cosmetic benefit from a broad range of cosmetic products without fear of provoking or aggravating acne and even while treating the underlying condition.

COSMETICS AND ACNE TREATMENT

Many acne treatments produce, as side-effects, dryness and peeling and occasionally erythema. It is therefore particularly important that acne hygiene and cosmetic cover be compatible with the therapeutic regimen pre-scribed. In addition, selective agents may result in photosensitivity, necessitating further precautions and sun screens.

Topical therapy

Topical therapy for acne consists primarily of comedolytic and antibacterial agents.[8] We have already discussed the use of salicylic acid and sulphur/resorcin preparations and will not repeat it here.

The most effective comedolytic agent available is topically applied tretinoin. Available in cream, gel and alcoholic lotion vehicles, tretinoin can be extremely irritating to the skin and is a photoirritant as well. Individual prescription of the proper concentration and dosage form can minimize these effects, but gentle cleansing with the least irritating or even emollient cleanser is essential. Patients using topical tretinoin will not infrequently require an emollient lotion or cream as well. This may be combined with a sunscreen for simple and maximum benefit. Although one would ideally select a non-acnegenic emollient and make-up for these individuals, in practice this is somewhat less important than with other acne therapy, since the comedolytic properties of tretinoin tend to overcome any comedogenic potential of cosmetics. Nevertheless, using non-acnegenic cosmetics is preferred.

Topical isotretinoin is also comedolytic, but less so than tretinoin. It also appears to be less irritating than the latter, but the same principles as for cosmetics apply. At the time of writing, the topical form of the drug had not been approved in the USA.

Adapalene and tazarotene are two new topical retinoids for acne treatment. Adapalene is a naphthoic acid derivative with retinoid activity. In clinical trials it has shown comparable efficacy to one form of tretinoin, with less irritancy. Animal models, however, show that it is less comedolytic than tretinoin. Tazarotene is a ligand-specific retinoid, which has been demonstrated to be effective in acne. We have no information on comparative trials against other retinoids.

Topical antibacterials

Topical antibacterials for acne include benzoyl peroxide and topical antibiotics, or a combination of these agents. As noted above, benzoyl peroxide, in creams, lotions and gels, may be quite irritating and occasionally a contact sensitizer. Topical antibiotics in hydroalcoholic vehicles may also be irritating, but less so than benzoyl peroxide. More recent gel, creamy lotion and ointment vehicles are even less irritating. A combination of benzoyl peroxide 5%/erythromycin 3% gel has recently been advocated.[9] Again, with these products, gentle cleansing is essential. Alkaline soaps are to be avoided, and neutral-pH cleansers are best for use with the antibiotics, which may be pH-labile. Non-acnegenic emollients and make-up should be used when necessary.

SYSTEMIC TREATMENT

Antibiotics

The most popular systemic antibiotic for acne treatment is tetracycline. The most important cosmetic consideration here is that tetracycline, doxycycline and demeclocycline are potentially phototoxic. Thus appropriate sun exposure precautions must be taken, and sunscreen use is recommended. Minocycline is much less likely to produce a photoreaction, if at all. Erythromycin is not phototoxic.

With the antibiotics, there are no specific cosmetic rules other than those applying to acne in general. Antibiotics decrease free fatty acids in skin lipids by decreasing *P. acnes.*

Hormonal treatment

Endocrine treatment has long been used for treatment of refractory acne in women, particularly when increased androgens are detectable. Oestrogens, antiandrogens and low-dose glucocorticoids in women can inhibit sebum production and provoke xerosis. Judicious use of non-acnegenic emollients may therefore be required. Titanium dioxide-containing sunblock make-up may be useful, since oestrogen can provoke melasma. It may need to be used with a bleaching agent such as hydroquinone for this problem.

Isotretinoin

Oral isotretinoin is indicated in severe refractory acne unresponsive to conventional treatment. Because of a profound effect on sebaceous glands, resulting in markedly decreased sebum production, isotretinoin produces xerosis, cheilitis, dry eyes, red chapped skin on the hands and increased skin fragility. Isotretinoin-treated patients are also more susceptible to sunburn. Thus such patients will require rich emollients, lipid-containing make-up, sunscreen and lip pomades to alleviate the normal side-effects of this treatment. The acnegenecity of these agents is probably less important here, because of the powerful anti-acne effect of the drug. Eye lubricants are frequently beneficial, but contact lenses may be difficult to use.

Acne prophylaxis

Although there is little evidence that anything, including active therapeutic intravention, actually prevents acne, it is certain that the disease can be modified by appropriate treatment. Similarly, it is logical to conclude that certain prophylactic measures should, at the very least, minimize or prevent aggravation of the disease.

Foremost among these prophylactic measures is the use of non-comedogenic and non-acnegenic cosmetics and the avoidance of agents known to promote acne, such as hair pomades. The latter are particularly popular in the black population, for whom non-acnegenic cosmetics have been slow to develop, and lead to a condition known as 'pomade acne'.[10] Certainly individuals with acne-prone skin are best served by careful selection from an increasingly large array of non-acnegenic cosmetics.

Secondly, there is a popular misconception that steaming the face improves acne and complexion. While it is true that brief exposure to moist heat will soften comedones prior to their physical removal, repeated and chronic exposure to moist heat actually aggravates acne, and may lead to a form of tropical acne.

Similarly, ultraviolet light has been thought to be beneficial in acne. In fact, short exposure to sunlight may hasten the resolution of inflammatory lesions, and suntan can mask the lesions. However, chronic exposure leads to thickening of the epidermis and follicle, with subsequent aggravation of acne.[6] In addition, ultraviolet exposure with certain acne treatments can lead to aggravated sunburn, as previously mentioned. Thus photoprotection is an important adjunct for individuals with acne or acne-prone skin.

In summary, acne and acne-prone skin require special attention with regard to cleansing, adjunctive treatment, cosmetics and photoprotection. The key concepts are gentle cleansing and the use of non-acnegenic cosmetics.

REFERENCES

1. Mills OH, Kligman AM, Acne detergicans. *Arch Dermatol* 1975; **111:** 65–8.
2. Pochi PE, Strauss JS, Sebum production, casual sebum levels, titratable acidity of sebum and urinary fractional 17-ketosteroid excretion in males with acne. *J Invest Dermatol* 1970; **102:** 267–75.
3. Shalita AR, Treatment of mild and moderate acne vulgaris with salicylic acid in an alcohol–detergent vehicle. *Cutis* 1981; **28:** 556–8.
4. Kligman AM, Mills OH, Acne cosmetica. *Arch Dermatol* 1972; **106:** 843–50.
5. American Academy of Dermatology Invitation Symposium on Comedogenicity (Special Report). *J Am Acad Dermatol* 1989; **20:** 272–7.
6. Mills OH, Kligman AM, Acne aestivalis. *Arch Dermatol* 1975; **111:** 891–2.
7. Shalita AR, Surgical methods for the treatment of acne vulgaris. *J Dermatol Surg* 1975; **1**(3): 46–8.
8. Leyden JJ, Shalita AR, Rational therapy for acne vulgaris: an update on topical treatment. *J Am Acad Dermatol* 1986; **15:** 907–15.
9. Chu A, Huber FJ, Todd Plott R, The comparative efficacy of benzoyl peroxide 5%/erythromycin 3% gel and erythromycin 4%/zinc 1.2% solution in the treatment of acne vulgaris. *Br J Dermatol* 1997; **136:** 235–8.
10. Plewig G, Fulton JE, Kligman AM, Pomade acne. *Arch Dermatol* 1970; **101:** 580.

37

Idiopathic hyperhidrosis

Daniel Lambert

INTRODUCTION

Idiopathic hyperhidrosis is defined as excessive sweating that is permanent and symmetrical, and localized in palms, soles and axillae. It is independent of thermoregulation phenomenona.

Idiopathic hyperhidrosis is increased by stress or emotion, and results from the stimulation of post-ganglionic-cholinergic fibres. It cannot be confined within the limits of a general illness like pathological hyperhidrosis, which accompanies fever, certain neurological disease (e.g. syringomyelia, Parkinson's disease and Riley–Day syndrome), endocrinopathy (e.g. diabetes mellitus, thyrotoxicosis and phaeochromocytoma) or trauma (e.g. medullary accidents and Frey's syndrome).

THERAPEUTIC POSSIBILITIES

General treatments, although theoretically feasible and attractive, pose practical problems of tolerance. For instance, anticholinergic compounds (e.g. atropine) are active, but the large doses required lead to unacceptable side-effects: dry mucous membranes, glaucoma, vesical retention and prostatic hypertrophy. Likewise, central inhibitors of the sympathetic nervous system (e.g. clonidine) appear to be effective by intravenous injection, but again only at toxic doses. The improvement induced by tranquillizers is insufficient. Thus tricyclic antidepressant drugs have been progressively abandoned. More recently, calcium-channel blockers (e.g. dilitiazem hydrochloride) at doses of 30–60 mg four times a day have given interesting results,[1] but our own experience has not allowed us to confirm these.

The failure of general therapies justifies the use of local treatments – medical, surgical or electrical.

LOCAL MEDICAL TREATMENT

For centuries unpleasant body odours have been hidden by intensive use of perfumes. However, the logical successors of perfumes – deodorant soaps and cosmetic deodorants – are not sufficiently strong or efficient over a long period of time. Antimicrobial fragrances have permitted the suppression of the microorganisms responsible for bromhidrosis (bad odour). Antiseptic benzalkonium chlorides and quaternary ammonium compounds, although very effective, are inactivated on the skin too rapidly. Hexachlorophene, a low-odour antimicrobial agent, was used in the development of the first soap bar, but has now been withdrawn for reasons of safety. Modern antiseptics (particularly triclosan and triclocarban derivatives) are efficient (but must be thoroughly rinsed off to avoid irritation). However, their effectiveness is limited, since the problem of permanent sweat production remains.

In practice, the products with the best performance are antiperspirant salts. Officinal tannin and formaldehyde in alcoholic solution act as anti-excretory antiperspirants, and are effective against axillary bacteria and work well as deodorants. Creams with formaldehyde base, with or without zinc oxide, are used on macerated palms and have identical results. Powders containing officinal tannin or trioxymethylene counteract plantar hyperhidrosis and control sweat production and body odours (for 12 hours).

Aqueous solutions of chromic acid or glutaraldehyde have been used, but their efficacy does not last, and a yellow coloration of the teguments, irritation and even allergic lesions are very frequent. They have therefore been supplanted by three groups of metallic salts: those of zinc, zirconium and aluminium. The first two groups have been withdrawn because of the formation of cutaneous granuloma. However, the well-tolerated aqueous forms of the aluminium salts are inefficacious.

The best results are obtained with hexahydrated aluminium chloride in 20–25% solution in absolute ethanol. The effect is optimal and lasts for several days. These very effective products used for axillary hyperhidrosis are less efficient on palmoplantar localization.[2] The mechanism of action is still enigmatic. The cause of anhidrosis could be a transient functional disturbance of the glands. It is possible that poral inflammation through chemical irritation causes the formation of an insoluble salt, whose deposition creates an operculum sufficient enough to stop sudoral gland activity.

LOCAL SURGICAL TREATMENT

There are no local surgical methods to control hyperhidrosis of palms and soles.

Surgery of the carpal duct gives transitory improvement, but does not appear to be a good solution in palmar hyperhidrosis at present.

The excision of axillary sudoral glands is still performed in cases of failure of local antitranspirants. An experienced surgeon may remove an appreciable percentage of the sudoral glandular group within the subcutaneous cellular tissue, keeping as much as possible of the recovering skin. This technique avoids complications due to total skin excision (unaesthetic antiphysiological retractions and paradoxical nauseous odour).

Resection of the cervical or thoracic sympathetic nerves has been used to control handicapping palmar and axillary hyperhidrosis. However, there are real risks of residual neuralgias, Claude Bernard–Horner syndrome, nerve inflammation or the appearance of compensation hyperhidrosis in un-involved areas. These sympathetic surgeries – all performed under general anaesthesia – are no longer considered appropriate.

Recently, endoscopic surgery of the sympathetic ganglia has been found to give the best results, without the side-effects of thoracotomy.

Severe hyperhidrosis of the palms, axillae and face has a strong, negative impact on the quality of life. Definitive cure can be obtained by upper thoracic sympathectomy. Performing sympathectomy was first reported by Hughes in 1942,[3] but strong side-effects were frequently registered.

In 1995 Drott et al[4] presented a new, efficient and safe method: endoscopic transthoracic sympathectomy. The patient is placed in a half-sitting position, under general anaesthesia. A small (7 mm) punch incision is made 2 cm caudal to the midportion of the clavicle or the anterior axillary line, and 2 l of carbon dioxide is insufflated into the pleural cavity through a Verres needle. A modified urologic transurethral electroscope (7 mm cannula) is then introduced through the same punch incision between the ribs.

In palmar hyperhidrosis the second and third thoracic sympathetic ganglia are destroyed by electrocautery. In axillary hyperhidrosis the fourth ganglion and in facial involvement the lower part of the first ganglion is destroyed.

The immediate postoperative result was excellent in 832 of 850 patients (98%). In complete transection of the nerve, no recurrences have occurred, more than 2 years postoperatively. Hemothorax is rare (in only 5 of 850 patients), pneumothorax occurred in four patients, and Horner's syndrome occurred in three cases with two permanent types.

Postoperative pain is observed for 3–4 days. Compensatory sweating, primarily of the trunk, occurred in 55% of the patients.

Endoscopic transthoracic sympathicotomy is easy, fast, inexpensive and efficient, with only rare and benign side-effects. It is the method of choice in the treatment of disabling hyperhidrosis of the palms, axillae and face.

ELECTRICAL TREATMENT

Galvanic currents have long been used in industry (electrolysis and electrotyping), and they have also been employed in medicine and kinesitherapy. Iontophoresis is a method allowing the introduction of salt ions in solution (electrolytes) into the tissues of an organism by a transcutaneous process. After a slow start, Shelley et al[5] confirmed the efficacy of the method, and Levit[6] and Shrivastava and Singh[7] improved it.

A generator delivers a constant current and automatically adjusts to any change in resistance in the external circuit during the procedure. The iontophoresis unit also incorporates a number of safety features for patients, such as limiting the maximum rate of change of current to 20 mA/s to prevent shock and requiring the current setting to be returned to zero before treatment can be commenced.

Currently three types of iontophoresis units are commercially available: line-operated units, simple battery-operated units and rechargeable power sources. The authorized voltage limit is 50 V.

Current is transmitted through wires and electrodes to two trays filled with tap water. Feet or hands needing treatment are plunged into these trays, where the current will flow, allowing Cl^- and Na^+ ions to migrate towards the opposite-sign electrode through the cutaneous tissue barrier.

The mechanism of action of tap-water iontophoresis remains unknown. The current densities are today much lower than those originally used, and are well below the threshold of damage to the acrosyringium.[8,9] As a consequence, mechanical obstruction is absent.

There are numerous techniques. The trays can be of various kinds and shapes, and electrodes can be attached to the tanks in various ways (but must not in any case be in contact with the skin, in order to avoid electrical burns). Metallic trays can be replaced by plastic trays or by sponges.

Examples of iontophoresis devices are given in Table 37.1 and shown in Figures 37.1–37.4.

Table 37.1 Examples of iontophoresis devices

Drionic	General Medical Company	Los Angeles (USA)	(Figure 37.1)
Anidro	Verbrugge Medical Service	Heusden (Belgium)	(Figure 37.2)
12M	12M	Caen (France)	(Figure 37.3)
Ionomatic	Dixwell	Lyon (France)	(Figure 37.4)

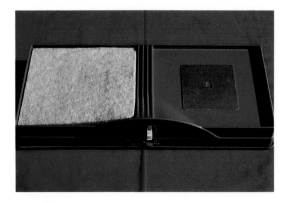

Figure 37.1 Drionic device.

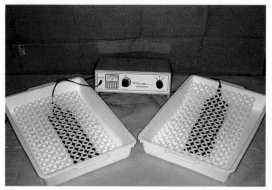

Figure 37.4 Ionomatic device.

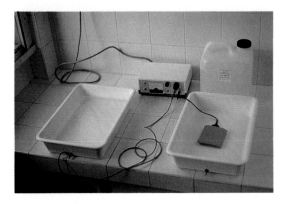

Figure 37.2 Anidro device.

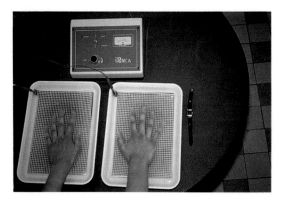

Figure 37.3 12M device.

Precautions for use

Besides the elementary precautions involved with the use of any electrical appliance (especially those connected to the mains network), several rules must be observed:

- all metal items (e.g. rings, bracelets, watches or any other jewellery) must be removed;
- skin must never directly touch the electrodes, to avoid the risk of burning;
- hands must not be removed abruptly from a tray when the current is on (this can lead to an unpleasant sensation like an electric shock) – this applies to devices connected to the mains and to rechargeable ones;
- any cutaneous lesions (wounds, fissures and cracks) must be protected with Vaseline – an unprotected lesion will show a smaller resistance when the current flows, and burns can appear even at low current intensity;

Contra-indications are as follows:[10]

- wearing a pacemaker (an absolute contra-indication for intensities greater than 10 mA);

- wearing a metallic intra-uterine device;
- wearing a metallic orthopaedic prothesis;
- patients with total arrhythmia;[11]
- pregnancy;[12]
- as the subject's active collaboration is necessary for the good follow-up of the treatment, young children or mentally handicapped patients cannot be treated;
- sensitivity of the hyperhidrosis area would disturb the optimal level of intensity, leading to greater risk of side-effects.

Method of treatment

Procedure

Hands or feet are placed flat on the bottoms of the trays. All metal items must have been removed prior to treatment to prevent iontophoretic burns. The trays are filled with tap water until the palms or soles are completely submerged, including the dorsum of the distal phalanges of fingers or toes.

In the case of a device with special electrodes (such as the Drionic) or one fitted with axillary electrodes, the felt pads must be water-saturated and in close contact with the skin.

Once the contact is made, the amperage is increased gradually with a potentiometer until the patient experiences slight discomfort: the average is 15 mA on palms and 20 mA on soles. Any abrupt intensity variation is painful. For this reason, hands or feet must not be removed before the intensity is gradually diminished. During the treatment, the amperage is maintained just below the threshold of discomfort. Adjustments can be made any time, if necessary. After 20 minutes, at the end of the treatment period, the current is slowly switched off. In case of an emergency, the patient can remove hands or feet from the water baths during treatment. The resulting electric shock is real but endurable.

Treatment should be carried out preferably once a day, at least three times a week. Sometimes the polarity is changed after 10 minutes, and the treatment then continues for another 10 minutes. New devices can automatically invert the polarity every two minutes – the results appear to be better and more rapid. Inversed polarity from one electrode to another has been used with identical results for both kinds of treatment. When sweating is sufficiently reduced, maintenance therapy is carried out on an individual schedule – usually once or twice a month. Ion mobility but also undesirable side-effects increase with current intensity. Shelley and Horvath[13] showed that miliaria appear at a 0.5 mA intensity. This was confirmed by Lowenthal.[14] The optimum intensity with maximum benefit result and with no undesirable effects depends on the following:

- the patient: 50 mA intensity has been used with pigs; however, adult humans do not easily tolerate intensities above 25 mA, while children and some sensitive patients cannot stand more than 10 mA;
- the location of the sweating: axillae are more sensitive than palms and soles; the optimum intensity is 15 mA for palms, 20 mA for soles and 10 mA for axillae.

Duration of therapeutic session[15,16]

This has varied between the various studies that have been performed (Table 37.2). The accepted duration in recent French studies[17–20] has been 20 minutes.

Table 37.2 Duration of therapeutic session

Authors	Duration (minutes)	Year
Levit[6]	20–30	1968
Shrivastava and Singh[7]	15–25	1977
Mitgaard[15]	10–20	1986
Hölzle[11]	20–30	1987
Vayssairat et al[16]	40	1983

Frequency of session and duration of attack treatment

An attack treatment is defined as the treatment necessary to achieve euhidrosis. It cannot be standardized, since it depends on the severity of the pathology and the patient's response to the iontophoresis. Our practice is for the treatment to comprise 2–6 sessions a week, with an average of 3 per week until euhidrosis. Usually the attack treatment lasts for four weeks.

A group of patients treated by Hölzle with two daily sessions presented a cutaneous inflammation, with the result that the intensity had to be reduced, diminishing the total efficacy of the treatment.

Results

Four examples of patients with good results after one month of therapy are shown in Figures 37.5–37.8.

Maintenance therapy

Necessity

Studies by Hölzle et al[21] showed that the euhidrosis obtained after three weeks of treatment lasts for only one week for feet and two weeks for hands; thus the treatment is not permanent. One or two months later, the sweating rate is the same as before the treatment. The more severe the hyperhidrosis, the shorter the delay. Among 36 patients followed by Bonerandi and Lota,[19] 30 (i.e. 86%) had recurrences after treatment lasting from a few days to several months (with an average of four weeks) after an attack treatment.

Among the 18 patients who received iontophoresis again, 16 improved completely. Thus iontophoresis only involves suspension of hyperhidrosis.

Frequency

The rhythm of the maintenance treatment is very variable, since it depends on each patient. In the opinion of the present author,

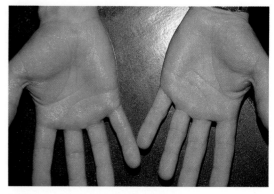

(a)

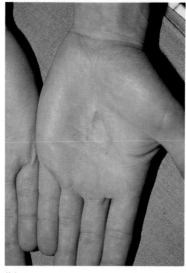

(b)

Figure 37.5 Patient 1 before (a) and after (b) iontophoresis.

it should be one session every one to two months.[10,18] The interval between two sessions should remain constant, because, as we shall see, there is no structural alteration in the sudoral glands.

Nevertheless, certain factors (such as stress, heat and humidity) may induce a patient to shorten the interval.

The average interval can be three,[16] four[22] or six[23] weeks.

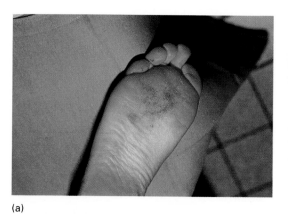

(a)

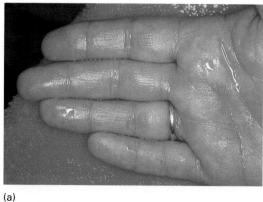

(a)

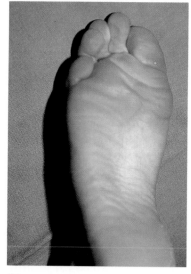

(b)

Figure 37.6 Patient 2 before (a) and after (b) iontophoresis.

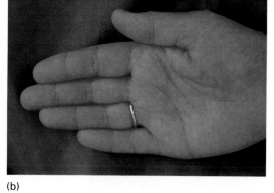

(b)

Figure 37.7 Patient 3 before (a) and after (b) iontophoresis.

Duration

In theory, the treatment should be carried on indefinitely,[22] although the pathology generally decreases with age. Few studies have been made over a long period, but it seems that the therapeutic effects remain as long as the treatment is continued. In the study by Hölze and Ruzicka[21] with a Hidrex device, the average duration of the treatment was 14 months without any relapse, with four patients having been followed for more than three years.

Place of treatment

This can be in hospital or a clinic, generally in a dermatological ward or at a dermatologist's surgery. This enables good follow-up of the patient, which is most important at the beginning of the treatment. However, the repeated attendances are very constraining, and in the long run are responsible for a new form of dependence – contrary to the aim of the treatment, which attempts to liberate the patient. It is also a constraint for the physician.

The cost of treatment is not a very serious consideration, since one session only lasts approximately 30 minutes (one period of 20

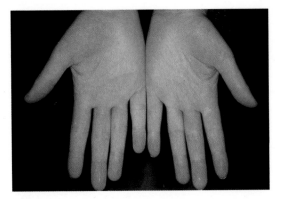

(a)

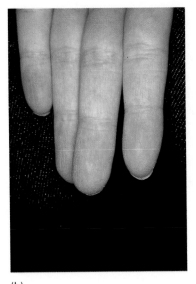

(b)

Figure 37.8 Patient 4 before (a) and after (b) iontophoresis.

minutes and 5–10 minutes to settle). For example, in France the Social Security quotation is K3 (two US dollars) for each session, and a series of treatment is 20 sessions.

Treatment by a chiropodist, a podologist or any other therapist is perfectly realizable. The necessary devices are perfectly adapted for home and office therapy. A hiring system is also possible.

It is advisable for a patient requiring long maintenance therapy to buy a device for home therapy, especially when several members of the same family are affected by the disease.

The purchase of such a device should only be decided after sufficient tests to confirm its efficacy and to be sure that the method is safe.

Simultaneous treatment of palms and soles

Patients often suffer from hyperhidrosis in both palms and soles. It would be convenient to treat all four extremities at the same time.

The Idromed 2 is the only device available that allows treatment of the two extremities at the same time, but two treatments may be carried out in sequence.

Note that one person at home can treat the left hand and foot for 20 minutes, and then the right hand and foot for the same time; this allows one hand to be kept free to regulate the intensity. However, treatment of the palms does not need the same intensity or the same number of sessions as treatment of the soles.

Side-effects

Once the major problem of electrical security is solved, tolerance is excellent.

Some difficulties have been observed. High amperage causes uncomfortable sensations, with burning and tingling on the submerged skin and pain in deeper tissue layers.

Apart from these immediate effects, skin irritation (Figure 37.9) and pruritis have occurred in some patients along the water surface. Transient erythema – a few small whitish vesicles sometimes associated with slight burning – have been observed. Xerosis and soreness last for no longer than a few hours. Deep burning has been reported, but is rare and has always been associated with defective devices and badly protected electrodes (Figure 37.10).

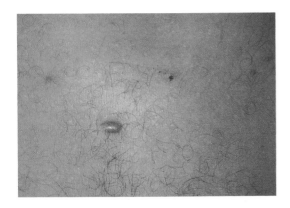

Figure 37.9 Irritated erythema.

No adverse effects of long-term maintenance therapy have been observed.

NEW POSSIBILITIES

Recently a new treatment was proposed by Boshara et al.[24] Subcutaneous axillary injections of botulinum toxin could be a worthwhile alternative in severe cases of axillary

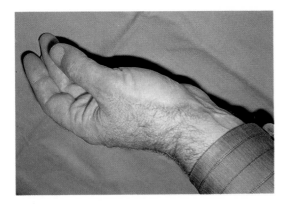

Figure 37.10 Scars after contact with electrode.

hyperhidrosis. The anhidrotic effect is expected to last for 6–8 months, with no significant side-effects. This modern treatment has not yet been compared with classical therapies of hyperhidrosis.

CONCLUSIONS

Following the introduction of the Drionic device in the United States in the 1980s, new generations of safe electrical devices have permitted the development of this technique worldwide.

All studies have shown identical results: over 85% success for a few weeks of attack treatment (average one month), with three sessions per week.

The duration of maintenance therapy varies widely, and depends fundamentally on patients' requirements and satisfaction.

On the whole, iontophoresis with tap water appears to be the most appropriate treatment presently available for both disabling and occasional palmoplantar hyperhidrosis.

REFERENCES

1. James WD, Schoomaker EB, Rodmann OG, Emotional eccrine sweating. *Arch Dermatol* 1987; **123:** 925–9.

2. Jensen O, Karlsmark T, Palmoplantar hyperhidrosis treatment with alcoholic solution of aluminium chloride hexahydrate. *Dermatologica* 1980; **161:** 133–5.

3. Hughes J, Endothoracic sympathectomy. *Proc R Soc Med* 1942; **35:** 585–6.

4. Drott C, Göthberg G, Claes G, Endoscopic transthoracic sympathectomy: an efficient and safe method for the treatment of hyperhidrosis. *J Am Acad Dermatol* 1995; **33:** 78–81.

5. Shelley WB, Howarth P, Weidmann F et al, Experimental miliaria in man. Production of salt retention anhidrosis and vesicles by means of iontophoresis. *J Invest Dermatol* 1948; **11:** 275–91.

6. Levit F, Simple device for the treatment of hyperhidrosis by iontophoresis. *Arch Dermatol* 1968; **98:** 505–7.

7. Shrivastava SN, Singh O, Tap water iontophoresis

in palmoplantar hyperhidrosis. *Br J Dermatol* 1977; **96:** 189–95.

8. Hölzle E, Alberti N, Long term efficacy and side effects of tap water iontophoresis of palmoplantar hyperhidrosis. The usefulness of home therapy. *Dermatologica* 1987; **175:** 126–35.

9. Reinauer S, Neusser A, Schauf G et al, Ionotophoresis with alternating current and direct current offset: a new approach for the treatment of hyperhidrosis. *Br J Dermatol* 1993; **129:** 166–9.

10. Lambert D, Ionophorèse: indications d'emploi. *Concours Méd* 1990; **112:** 2733–6.

11. Hölzle E, Tap water ionotophoresis for the treatment of palmoplantar hyperhidrosis. In: *Dermatology in five continents. Proceedings of the 17th World Congress of Dermatology, Berlin 1987* (Orfanos CE, Stadler R, Gollnick H, eds). Berlin: Springer-Verlag, 1988:464–9.

12. Lazareth I, Van ESP, Hyperhidrose palmoplantaire. *Quot Méd* 1990; Suppl 4650: 30–9.

13. Shelley WB, Horvath PN, Experimental miliaria in man: production of miliaria rubra (prickly heat). *J Invest Dermatol* 1950; **14:** 193–203.

14. Lowenthal LJA, Experimental miliaria: iontophoresis with salt solutions. *Arch Dermatol* 1962; **86:** 115.

15. Midtgaard K, A new device for the treatment of hyperhidrosis by iontophoresis. *Br J Dermatol* 1986; **114:** 485–8.

16. Vayssairat M, Cormier JM, Priollet P et al, L'ionisation doit-elle remplacer la sympathectomie dans le traitement de l'hyperhidrose palmoplantaire? *Presse Med* 1983; **12:** 301–2.

17. Desnos P, Henriet JP, Vigneron JL et al, Traitement de l'hyperhidrose par ionophorèse: principe, matériel, méthodologie, résultats. A propos de 93 cas. *Nouv Dermatol* 1988; **7:** 551–4.

18. Lambert D, Thulliez M, Dinet Y et al, Treatment of palmoplantar hyperhidrosis by iontophoresis. In: *Abstracts of 17th World Congress of Dermatology, Berlin, 1987*, Vol. 2 (Orfanos CE, Gollnick H, Stadler R, eds). Berlin: Department of Dermatology, University Medical Center, Steglitz, 1987:550.

19. Bonerandi JJ, Lota I, La ionophorèse. *Derm Prat* 1990; **48:** 2–3.

20. Yousry C, Jeanmougin M, L'éclectrothérapie en dermatologie: traitement de l'hyperhidrose palmoplantaire essentielle par galvanisation. *Dermatol Prat* 1990; **61:** 22–3.

21. Hözle E, Ruzicka T, Treatment of hyperhidrosis by a battery operated iontophoretic device. *Dermatologica* 1986; **172:** 41–7.

22. Levit F, Treatment of hyperhidrosis by tap water iontophoresis. *Cutis* 1980; **26:** 192–6.

23. Baran R, Drionic arrête la transpiration pendant 6 semaines. Un nouveau traitement contre l'hyperhidrose. *Nouv Dermatol* 1983; **2:** 36.

24. Boshara KO, Park DM, Jones JC, Schott HS, Botulinum toxin – a possible new treatment for axillary hyperhidrosis. *Clin Exp Dermatol* 1996; **21:** 276–8.

38

Aging and photoaging

William M Cunningham

INTRODUCTION

Cosmetic aspects of aging of the skin are of intense interest in most of our youth-oriented societies. The integument, as a most important presentation of the human to its counterparts, is essentially the visual calendar by which the years are measured. Although the young may temporarily wish to get older, the mature rarely wish to continue progress in that direction, and younger-looking skin becomes of major functional and psychological importance.

Organisms mature and manifest morphologic and functional changes, some of which have been attributed to intrinsic aging. Is there, in fact, inevitably programmed into the cells of the organism a chronological progression of change that occurs without outside influence and that could be truly classified as intrinsic? Does the mechanism of DNA replication itself or the generation of by-products of normal cellular metabolism such as free radicals and other reactive species lead to damaging events that 'age' the cell and eventually the entire organ and organism? These are difficult questions to definitively answer in the intact organism, particularly in the human, since there are ubiquitous, gross and minor extrinsic insults as well as internal disease processes that may partially or totally obscure intrinsic events.

Discoveries in molecular biology and clinical research have led to immortalized cell cultures and have allowed indefinite prolongation of organ survival after transplantation. The possible existence of longevity assurance genes (LAG) that putatively promote cell longevity and health has been theorized, and research efforts in this area have been organized in the LAG Interactive Network by the National Institute of Aging.[1] As with control over cell death by apoptosis, the continued life or rejuvenation of the cell is likely to be similarly under a strong and complex control. Exciting discoveries such as these in molecular genetics as well as progress in clinical research have led to a significant and accelerating interest in aging of the skin from both the scientific and commercial aspects.

Whereas the above comments no doubt apply to the skin as well as to other organs, the skin's lifelong, intense exposure to damaging extrinsic events, especially to ultraviolet solar radiation, may, in fact, largely overshadow intrinsic events and theoretical concerns. This chapter will thus only briefly describe the purported changes of intrinsic aging of the skin, and will principally focus on the various aspects of pathogenesis, gross and microscopic pathology, prevention, treatment and clinical study of photoaging of the skin.

INTRINSIC AGING OF THE SKIN

Aging of the skin, hair and nails is a continuum of change from embryo to senescence. We accept as normal and expect early maturational changes in these organs as the newborn becomes a child and loses its 'baby' skin and hair, and as the adolescent progresses to adulthood and manifests acne and temporal recession of the hairline. Those changes particularly associated with 'getting old', such as thinning and graying of the hair, are more grudgingly accepted, although still generally viewed as a normal part of the aging of the organism.

Past authors, on the basis of casual observations as well as scientific and clinical studies of variable quality, have concluded that intrinsic aging of the skin occurs, and have described various morphologic and physiologic changes. A comprehensive review of the subject in 1984 by Gilcrest[2] summarizes the changes attributed to aging in the gross morphology of the skin, including roughness, wrinkling, uneven pigmentation and various proliferative lesions. Microscopically, many changes have been described, the most obvious of which are variability of thickness and flattening of the epidermis with decreased rete ridge pattern and decrease in numbers of various cells, including melanocytes and Langerhans cells. Decreased dermal volume and cellularity, with fewer fibroblasts, mast cells and blood vessels, as well as capillary loop and nerve ending changes, have been observed.

A thorough scrutiny of the original literature upon which these conclusions are based is appropriate, in that although many conclusions have been drawn regarding intrinsic aging of the skin, a number of studies have not sufficiently excluded age-related environmental factors, especially ultraviolet radiation (UVR) exposure, and – importantly – age-associated disease states and hormonal changes. Although the skin is an important protector of the organism from outside insults, it is itself continuously assaulted from outside and within. Furthermore, its structure and function are intimately supported by the cardiovascular, endocrine, renal, hepatic and other organ systems. Exclusion of factors related to these systems is difficult even in seemingly 'normal' older individuals, and nearly impossible in hospital, nursing home and prison populations. The number of truly completely healthy, 40–80-year-old individuals with skin-supporting 'youthful' organ systems is limited for clinical studies of intrinsic aging of the skin.

Finally, although it had appeared intuitive to assume that intrinsic aging of all organs and cells is inevitable and irrevocable, the successful cloning of a sheep from somatic cells of an adult sheep occurred during the preparation of this chapter,[3] and clearly demonstrates that cell senescence and death may not always be irrevocably programmed for a specific time frame or unipolar direction. Is intrinsic aging of the skin inevitable? Perhaps no more so than the death of those sheep somatic cells – now a new and youthful organism.

These scientific and complicated musings force the current author to postpone further discussion of the increasingly complex topic of intrinsic aging of skin and to further elaborate on photoaging of the skin.

PHOTOAGING OF THE SKIN

Photoaging has been extensively studied experimentally and clinically in recent decades, and is, without doubt, a true entity – although, again, modified by other intrinsic events and extrinsic insults. Repeated observations at the molecular, cellular, animal and human experimental levels have substantiated the deleterious effects of solar radiation on the skin at each and all of these levels. Photoaging is presumably superimposed on any changes attributable to intrinsic aging, and appears, by the magnitude and profundity of its effects, to overshadow these changes in even minimally solar-exposed skin of most individuals. The spectrum of damage attributable to solar-induced damage encompasses cosmetic, functional and neoplastic changes, resulting in substantial medical and cosmetic problems in today's society.

It is abundantly clear that the development of malignant neoplasms of basal and squamous cell carcinomas and premalignant actinic keratoses of the skin is in large part related to UVR exposure. Although these are among the most important medical aspects of UVR damage, the topic is well discussed elsewhere, and this chapter will focus on the more cosmetic aspects of photoaging.

Pathogenesis

Photoaging may be defined as a gross, microscopic and functional condition of the skin produced in susceptible individuals by repetitive, chronic exposure to radiation of the electromagnetic spectrum, primarily ultraviolet radiation (UVR) from solar or artificial sources (Table 38.1). Until recently, it had been concluded to be solely a phenomenon of UVB exposure, but recent evidence from animal models and human experience has also strongly implicated at least UVA radiation.[4] In this regard, whereas it is well established that the acute effects of UVR, i.e. sunburn erythema, are most efficiently produced by UVB of wavelength 310 nm, there is less complete understanding of both carcinogenesis and photoaging, which are much longer-term consequences of UVR exposure and cannot be as easily reproduced experimentally in humans.

As understood at present, photoaging is produced by cumulative skin exposure to UVR, from various solar and artificial sources. For a number of reasons, including exposure and tissue penetration factors, solar-generated UVB (wavelengths 280–320 nm) is generally the most important spectrum in photoaging production. Increasingly, significant exposure to UVA (wavelengths 320–400 nm) is experienced from UV 'tanning booths' as well as from higher UVA doses experienced during longer total sun exposures allowed by UVB sunscreen use.

Certain wavelengths within these spectral regions have been demonstrated to be more damaging than others – particularly UVB of 310 nm, which most efficiently produces acute damage of sunburn, and shorter UVA wavelengths of 320–340 nm. UVB clearly damages the epidermis, and although it has limited penetration of the skin beyond the epidermis, probably has a cascade of effects well beyond this level due to consequences of DNA, membrane lipid and cellular protein perturbations of many cells, including keratinocyte and dendritic cells. As the epidermal cell is one of the body's richest sources of cytokines, release of these molecules resulting from UVR injury can have immediate, profound and far-reaching effects, as witnessed in the acute, painful and systemic condition of severe sunburn for example.

UVA penetrates well into the dermis, and, since 40–50% of the total exposure of UVA is transmitted, substantial damage from UVA

Table 38.1 Aspects of pathogenesis of photoaging

Cumulative UVR exposure
Generation of reactive oxygen species
DNA damage:
    thymidine-dimer production
    single-strand breaks
Perturbations of
    cell membranes (arachidonic acid release)
    enzymatic processes
    metabolic activities
Role of p53 tumor suppressor gene/protein?
Genetic predisposition:
    individual susceptibility
    melanization potential
    repair capabilities

alone is theoretically possible. UVC and other solar radiation may be highly damaging to cells, but ordinarily do not sufficiently penetrate the Earth's atmosphere and are not currently believed to substantially contribute to photoaging. This may change in the future as ozone-layer depletion allows more UVC and other damaging wavelengths to penetrate to the Earth's surface. Infrared radiation, on the other hand, is abundant and ubiquitous, and has been incriminated as adding to total UVR damage.[5] Definite proof of photoaging in human skin from visible light is presently lacking, although these wavelengths may be problematic in certain photosensitivities, especially of drug, metabolic disease or genetic causation.

It would be logical to assume that several spectral regions of radiation could be involved in the pathogenesis of photoaging, given the continuous nature of the electromagnetic spectrum with its various sources of exposure, wavelengths, flux, skin penetration depths, etc., and the wide variability in total skin exposure resulting from the variable geographic and indoor and outdoor exposure differences experienced by humans. The susceptibility of the individual to UVR damage is also probably highly variable, given the obvious profound differences in human genetic make-up, and thus in attendant variabilities in DNA and other cellular repair abilities, melanization potential and other unknown factors such as inflammatory cell responsiveness and general immunologic competence.

UVR exposure results in tissue damage at least partially through the mechanism of generation of reactive oxygen species, which in turn damage membrane lipids, cellular proteins and DNA.[6] DNA is a major chromophore for UV light and, after UVB exposure, formation of DNA photoproducts occurs, the most prevalent of which is a cyclobutylpyrimidine dimer (thymidine dimer). UVA exposure produces primarily single-strand breaks in DNA. Many of these DNA-damaging events are attributable to the formation of reactive oxygen species such as superoxide anion, hydrogen peroxide and hydroxyl radical. Although specific DNA-damaging effects are among the most important, other chromophores exist in skin, and UVR may disturb cellular activities both through DNA-related mechanisms and possibly, as in the case of release of arachidonic acid (AA) from cell membrane phospholipids, through mechanisms unrelated to DNA damage. Induction of enzymatic processes, alteration of metabolic activities and changes in gene expression result from UVR exposure, and have likely consequences in acute as well as chronic skin damage.[7] Synthesis and release of proteins, especially cytokines – which have a multiplicity of actions on various skin cells – is especially noteworthy. UVB radiation, as well as multiple other noxious stimuli, cause significant release from keratinocytes of cytokines, among which are interleukin (IL)-1, IL-6 and tumor necrosis factor (TNF)-α, all of which can increase synthesis of glycosaminoglycan (GAG) synthesis by fibroblasts and affect many other cellular functions. Additionally, demonstration of induction of proteases, gene expression regulation factors, growth factors, stress associated proteins and signal transduction proteins in mammalian cells in vitro leads to the inescapable conclusion that the pathogenesis of photoaging in human skin is of a highly complex nature and most likely involves multiple pathways. Furthermore, the relationship among the various processes of acute sunburn, carcinogenicity and photoaging is likely to be similarly complex, with sometimes unrelated as well as overlapping pathogenic mechanisms involved.

Although the most obvious clinical difference in skin is the natural spectrum of human skin color manifested in Fitzpatrick types I through VI, other genetically determined differences that affect all of the processes described above may be no less important in susceptibility to photoaging. It is likely that there are significant individual differences in basic response to UVR and in the multiple repair mechanisms operative after UVR damage to cells of the epidermis, dermis and immune system.

These inherent response factors, when combined with geographic and occupational extremes of UVR exposure, give rise to a virtual palette of photoaging. Whereas it is common to observe minimal photoaging in Black skin even in tropical environments – presumably due mostly to protection by melanin – many individuals do, in fact, demonstrate significant damage. The extensive photoaging inclusive of carcinogenicity observed in Whites of Celtic ancestry even in relatively northern latitudes with modest sun exposure is not always duplicated in Whites of Scandinavian origin, even with seemingly similar exposures. Even within individuals of similar and light skin color and similar exposure histories, there appear to be significant differences in propensity to develop neoplasia versus wrinkling or other cosmetic changes, and these differences cannot yet be explained.

On the other hand, the genetically determined and devastating disease xeroderma pigmentosum has, in its many subtypes, various known and defined DNA repair defects that result in dramatic skin changes of photoaging and cutaneous neoplasia after solar irradiation. This disease, as well as a number of other genetically determined skin diseases, are clearly at one pole of the spectrum of susceptibility to UVR damage. One would presume, in fact, as heterogeneous as humans are, that their genetically determined DNA repair ability might be a continuum of ability to repair the damage of various wavelengths, total exposures, etc. One might further expect that this factor, combined with susceptibility and repair capacity in other cellular and enzymatic systems and the individual's melanization capabilities, would determine not only the type of damage experienced but also the overall propensity to develop photoaging as well as the capability to reverse it.

The clinical manifestations of photoaging,

especially cutaneous carcinogenesis and photoaging after significant photochemotherapy with PUVA (psoralen plus UVA irradiation), have been well described, and are similar to those of solar causation.[8] This iatrogenic condition further affirms the damaging potential of UVA irradiation.

Clinical manifestations of photoaging

The clinical changes resulting from UVR exposure are highly variable in type and severity. Clinically, the spectrum of benign change in the skin encompasses fine and coarse wrinkles, irregular and mottled discrete and diffuse pigmentation changes, tactile and visual roughness and dryness, leathery texture, laxity, and sallowness[9] (Table 38.2). Telangiectasia, atrophy and purpura may be features in severe cases. Neoplastic lesions, ranging from benign to pre-malignant keratoses and malignant tumors, are a major result of UVR damage, although perhaps best classified separately from photoaging.[10] Dysplasia and malignancy may accompany even apparently mild cosmetic skin changes – no doubt indicating some unlinking of events

Table 38.2 Cutaneous manifestations of photoaging

Clinical changes
Roughness
Dryness
Laxity
Wrinkling – fine and coarse
Sallowness
Irregular, mottled hyper/hypopigmentation
Lentigines
Telangiectasias
Keratoses

Histologic changes
Uneven, thickened stratum corneum
Irregularly thinned epidermis
Rete ridge thinning
Dermal elastosis
Uneven, decreased/increased melanization

of DNA or other cellular or immunologic damage, which, as discussed above, results in structural, functional or malignant change or combinations thereof.

In this regard, the correlation between the obvious causation of UVR exposure and the end result of clinical epidermal and dermal change can be only partially made with certainty. It is clear that UVR can damage DNA and derange multiple systems of epidermal and dermal cells – probably by a number of different mechanisms. This damage, if not adequately repaired, likely results in some degree of keratinocyte and fibroblast malfunction. Epidermal dysplasia presumably results when damaged cells continue to replicate in the face of genetic damage that is insufficient to produce cell death but does continue to adversely affect cellular differentiation. Roughness, dryness and other epidermal changes may be manifestations of less profound keratinocyte malfunction, although this has not been established. Wrinkling, while clinically simple to define, has been more elusive from the histologic and pathogenic viewpoints. Presumably it is a result of fibroblast malfunction secondary to DNA and other cellular and protein damage, with consequent abnormal collagen, elastin and ground substance breakdown and re-synthesis, and thus abnormal dermal structure repair and remodeling. UVR may be highly damaging to cells of the immune system, with a presumptive relation to carcinogenicity, but there is, as yet, insufficient evidence for a direct role of the immune system in photoaging.[11]

The diagnosis of photoaging is based upon the presenting physical signs as well as the history of significant UVR exposure. Quantification of UVR exposure by history of past and present geographical location and estimated sun exposure from occupational and recreational exposure is imprecise, but to some extent unnecessary, given nearly universal exposure in many societies to excessive UVR from inadvertent and intentional sun exposure and the increasingly popular UVA tanning devices.

Photosensitivity secondary to medication, lupus erythematosis, porphyrias, etc. may require more careful history and laboratory investigation, and may result in further acceleration of photoaging. Genetic disease such as xeroderma pigmentosum may result in astonishing photoaging of both acute and chronic nature, including overwhelming and life-threatening malignancies.

Histologic changes of photoaging

The most characteristic histopathologic feature of photoaging has been designated 'solar elastosis'. This change in the papillary dermis results in an altered architecture partially due to replacement of the normal collagen of the papillary dermis with material that has staining characteristics similar to elastin and is, at least in part, altered elastic fibers. Other manifestations such as irregular stratum corneum, epidermal thinning, various degrees of keratinocyte dysplasia, and changes in dendritic cells and melanization have been reported with corresponding ultrastructural changes. Alterations of collagen structure, composition, function, synthesis and degradation have been variously observed by a number of methods, including immunohistochemistry and Northern and Western blot analyses, as have changes in the cutaneous microvasculature.[12-14] The relative roles of direct UVR damage, secondary reactive-species generation, collagenase production, and a host of cytokine-related effects and inflammatory events, in production of these changes are not completely clear at present, although some aspects of pathogenesis have been elucidated during attempts to explain retinoid reversal of these effects.[15]

Prevention of photoaging

It must be assumed that every absorbed photon of UVR, no matter what its source, wave-

Table 38.3 Prevention of photoaging
Meticulous sun avoidance
Protective clothing
Wide-brimmed hats
Correct use of sunscreens:
UVB filters
UVA filters
physical filters
Avoidance of 10 a.m.–4 p.m. exposure
Geographic change of domicile
Rescheduling of sports/occupation
Avoidance of UVA tanning

long sleeves and pants and materials of the tightest weave that do not allow transmission of light (potentially increased by incorporation of UV absorbers into the fabric). A line of clothing called SOLUMBRA has been specifically designed with a fabric weave that provides a simulated SPF above 30, is FDA-regulated as a device, and is available commercially from a US company. A hat is extremely important to reduce exposure to the vulnerable face, but gives inadequate protection unless it is truly wide-brimmed to more fully shade the face, ears and neck than the currently popular baseball cap. UV-blocking sunglasses protect the eyes and complement a hat, but should not give a false sense of security that permits even longer sun exposure.

Sunscreens of many types are now readily available, but, while widely utilized by the public, are usually inadequately applied in both amount and frequency.[17] They can clearly protect against acute events such as UVR-induced erythema, although conclusion of protection in carcinogenesis and photoaging in humans is more intuitive than scientifically established. To be most effective, they should be applied prior to each sun exposure and in sufficient quantity to achieve a uniformly thick layer over all exposed surfaces, which allows them to achieve their rated SPF. This regularity and meticulous application is not easy to achieve given the other rigors of daily life.

The use of sunscreens containing only UVB protectants appeared unassailable until more convincing evidence of the role of UVA as a contributor to photoaging became apparent. Liberal use of high-SPF UVB-blocking sunscreens is a conundrum. Whereas the protection from sunburn from UVB may be substantial, some skin-damaging effects occur at less than MED exposure, and thus are not eliminated.[18] Furthermore, the fact that UVB block allows a longer total time in the sun insidiously allows an exposure to higher total UVA when the limitation of perceived sunburn is removed. To some extent, the incor-

length or timing, potentially adds to cumulative photoaging of the skin. This caution must be explicitly given to patients who frequently demonstrate significant photoaging in spite of their vehement denial of a history of 'sunbathing'. At latitudes of Rome or New York, even 10 or 15 minutes of outdoor shopping in the summer sun at noon is more than sufficient to produce an MED in many individuals, and insidiously adds to the total and damaging UVR burden on the skin even in the absence of acute erythema.

Avoidance of UVR is possible but not easy, simple or complete (Table 38.3). In the most severe cases of sensitivity, such as in diseases like xeroderma pigmentosum, the person must be advised to remain indoors during all hours of sunlight. Others are wise to remain out of direct sunlight during peak irradiation times (variously between 11 a.m. to 2 p.m. or 10 a.m. to 4 p.m., depending on time of year and geographic location).[16] Seemingly adequate protective shelters such as shade from an umbrella may still allow reflected light from snow or beach and thus sufficient UVR to reach the skin to add to the total cumulative dose, even if they protect from acute sunburn. Clothing is variously protective, with simulated protection of up to SPF 15, although frequently much lower if of loose weave or if wet. The best protection is offered by adequate covering of body surfaces, such as with poration of UVA filters in sunscreens decreases this exposure, but does not eliminate infrared and visible-light exposure, which have both been theorized to contribute to the overall, total and damaging irradiation dose. Furthermore, the currently employed UVA filters are not as effective as those for UVB, and the establishment of universal standards for measurement of their blocking capability has not yet been achieved. Sunscreens that also incorporate a physical blocking ingredient such as micronized or nanosized zinc oxide or titanium dioxide can provide substantially more protection. These sunscreens have been improved over the previously available zinc oxide paste, but, in general, remain much less cosmetically acceptable because of their particularity and consistency.

Paradoxically, although a tan is partially photoprotective, with induction of an SPF increase between 2 and 4, achieving a tan requires initial damaging UV exposure, and maintaining a tan requires continued repetitive damaging UV exposures – therefore it is counterproductive. Additionally, the melanin achieved during tanning is only partially protective, and does not protect against all UVR effects and damage. Thickening of stratum corneum after UVB exposure may be more important than melanin in protecting from further UVR damage in that it absorbs or reflects up to 95% of incident UVB.[19] The fascinating discoveries that thymidine dimers, which are, in fact, products of UVR-induced DNA damage, induce both melanin formation and p53 protein led to the conclusion that their application may initiate not only a cosmetic tan but also some degree of photoprotection from carcinogenicity and photoaging.[20–22] Diacylglycerol application as self-tanning preparations offers cosmetic but minimal photoprotective benefits, although some melanogenesis is stimulated.[23]

Avoidance of tanning devices and prudent minimization of exposure to UVA during PUVA therapy are self-evident measures.

Table 38.4 Treatment of photoaging
Tretinoin
Isotretinoin
α-Hydroxy acids (AHA)
α-Keto acids
Chemical peels:
AHA
trichloroacetic acid and Jessners solution
Dermabrasion
Laser resurfacing
Botox
Collagen/gelatin matrix injections
Autologous fat transplantation
Theoretical:
topical/systemic hormones
anti-inflammatories/antioxidants
thymidine dimers/p53 protein
down/upregulation of elastin, collagen, collagenase by
cytokines, retinoids, growth factors, antisense
DNA/RNA technologies

Treatment of photoaging

Treatment of photoaging may involve treatment of all or some of its clinical manifestations of wrinkles, pigmentation, roughness, color and actinic keratoses (Table 38.4). Extensive discussion of the cosmetic surgical treatment for photoaging and of the treatment of malignant and pre-malignant change by 5-flurouracil, surgery, cryosurgery, elecrosurgery or laser surgery is beyond the scope of the present treatise. An underlying assumption of the following discussion is the frequent necessity for multiple or combined treatments to fully address the multiplicity of clinical defects.

Early clinical observations of the possible utility of tretinoin in photoaging were followed by the interesting observation that sunscreen application resulted in partial reversal of UV-induced photoaging in the hairless mouse and stimulated continued search for a pharmaceutical treatment for established photoaging.[24,25] Subsequent observations in this useful model demonstrated reversal of photoaging by topically applied all-*trans*-retinoic acid.[26] Confirmation of these results obtained in preliminary clinical trials[27,28] was followed by multiple, large, double-blind clinical trials, which have proven beyond doubt the efficacy of all-*trans*-retinoic acid[29] and 13-*cis*-retinoic acid[30] applied topically to photodamaged skin. Improvement in fine wrinkles, irregular pigmentation, roughness and laxity have been regularly substantiated – although all to a modest degree and usually after relatively prolonged use of at least 6 months.[31,32] Histologic changes after treatment include thickening of the total epidermis and its granular layer, transformation of the stratum corneum from its usual basket-weave pattern to a more compact morphology, and decreased melanin content of the epidermis. These treatments, aside from their short-term irritation, have not been shown to have longer-term side-effects, and are best recommended in conjunction with sun avoidance. A daily regimen of the mildest of cleansing and sufficient moisturization is used in conjunction with combination sunscreens containing UVA blocks and high-SPF UVB blocks. Tretinoin cream at a concentration of 0.05% is applied to the photoaged areas of the body each evening after skin cleansing routines are complete and the skin has been allowed to dry for several minutes. Tretinoin up to the 0.05% concentration each evening is frequently useful and sometimes mandatory, since irritation can be significant if the skin has not sufficiently hardened to the retinoid effects. A sample initial regimen of 3 times/week application of 0.01% or 0.025% tretinoin cream and subsequent upward steady progression allows tolerance to develop, and, since no immediate therapeutic effect is anticipated, does not significantly alter this essentially long-term therapy. Other retinoids, some selected on the basis of more selective retinoid receptor binding, will no doubt soon be demonstrated to have similar clinical effects, and will presumably become commercially available.

A host of other purported treatments has arisen in the knowledge that, in fact, photoaging is at least partially reversible, and that it is of major cosmetic and commercial importance. Many of these treatments appear promising, although most have not been as thoroughly subjected to the rigors of multiple, large, double-blind clinical trials as has tretinoin. Some treatments, however, may be much more effective for specific aspects of photoaging, be easier to utilize for extended periods of time, or demonstrate more complete or rapid reversal of important cosmetic parameters or concomitant treatment of actinic keratoses.

One of the most actively investigated treatments includes the daily use of low to moderate concentrations of various α-hydroxy acids (AHAs), which has been substantiated to effect some improvement in some of the clinical and histologic changes of photoaging, at least in the short term.[33–36] There has not yet been the same degree of substantiation of these agents as in the case of multiple large, double-blind clinical studies of tretinoin, and the data for longer-term gain have not yet been published.

Chemical peels utilizing phenol, high concentrations of AHA[37,38] or trichloroacetic acid[39] with Jessners solution, as well as skin resurfacing techniques utilizing laser resurfacing[40] and dermabrasion,[41,42] are all under active study for their immediate and long-term potential, have their rationale, and have shown some promise, especially when concomitant removal of actinic keratoses is desirable. These treatments mandate a higher level of skill and experience by the practitioner, and, if not correctly performed, can result in undesirable and lasting side-effects.

Short of the relatively major surgical procedures of lifts and blepheroplasties, a number of office surgical procedures can, for the right patients and with skilled practitioners, complement the more medical approaches to photoaging. Injection of various materials has been advocated for treatment of deeper wrinkles of the face, especially of the brow and nasolabial area. Botulinum toxin (Botox) paralyses the musculature under deep furrows of the brow, for example for several months, thus releasing tension on the skin and allowing the return of more normal surface skin contour.[43,44] Other materials, including collagen, gelatin matrix and autologous fat, have been successfully employed by injection under the wrinkle, with subsequent 'filling in' and lifting of the wrinkle to a plane more closely approximating the surrounding skin.[45]

Reports of the beneficial potential of anti-inflammatory agents[46] and antioxidants,[47] while fascinating from a theoretical point of view, require additional substantiation before their use can be recommended. Similarly, various topically administered hormones have been theorized to benefit aging skin, but convincing clinical results have not been generated in rigorous studies. Hypopigmenting agents such as the hydroquinones are usually of limited utility in treatment of the substantial and irregular pigmentary changes of photoaging.

As discussed above, the interesting observations of the effects of thymidine dimers on tanning and p53 protein will be exciting to follow. Antisense DNA and RNA, cytokines and multiple other technologies may similarly play a significant future role in the prevention and treatment of photoaging.

Clinical study of photoaging

A wide variety of clinical observations and instrumental techniques are currently available for detailed clinical study of photoaging and its therapeutic interventions[48] (Table 38.5). Although not all are completely validated, many are sufficiently precise and reproducible to ensure adequate documentation of the clinically important features of photoaging at baseline and during trials of various therapies.

The simplest observation of overall global response is frequently obvious to the investigator and subject, but may not be sufficient

Table 38.5 Photoaging study methodologies

Clinical evaluation:
    global response
    individual parameter changes
Photographs:
    baseline full face
    sequential
Grading systems:
    photonumeric scales
    clinical panel assessment
Investigator and self-assessment visual analog score (VAS)
Skin surface replicas, Silflo
Fluorescence, polarized-light photography

for adequate evaluation of comparative therapies. Use of a full-face baseline photograph is invaluable as a reference by which to judge progress at subsequent time points.[49]

A visual analog score (VAS), performed by either or both the investigator and subject, can be extremely useful, and surprisingly precise and reproducible in evaluation of both overall appearance and specific parameters of wrinkling, pigmentation and skin color.[50]

Very high-quality photography is the most useful and most utilized technique upon which are based serial clinical observations of wrinkles, pigmentation, color and overall appearance or global change. Investigator observations made over time can be supplemented and confirmed by third-party observations, comparing subjects' photos with previously developed photographic standards using photonumeric scales[51] or by clinical panel comparisons of baseline and subsequent time points performed by trained individuals in a blinded and randomized manner.[52] Both of these methods are sufficiently developed to allow one to expect that they are valid techniques.

A number of techniques have been developed to evaluate skin surface topography, especially utilizing skin surface replicas made of a dental impression material (Silflow).[53]

The reverse replicas thus obtained allow evaluation of skin contours by instrumentation (profilimeters) utilizing various image-analysis software programs, and may allow precise definition of therapeutic change.

Various photographic techniques using fluorescent, polarized and other light sources dramatically improve observations of certain parameters, especially of pigment distribution, intensity and concentration.[54,55]

The many and diverse clinical changes in photoaging allow the logical application of a multiplicity of other instrumental techniques, which subject will be explored in a future publication ('Photoaging' in *Cutaneous Biometrics*, Plenum Press, in press). Skin color, thickness, elasticity, hydration, transepidermal water loss, etc. can be qualified and quantified utilizing a number of available technologies.[56]

SUMMARY AND CONCLUSIONS

Rapid scientific progress in the past decade has more clearly elucidated aging, especially photoaging, of the skin. The availability of a reproducible and predictive animal model of photoaging, continued, rapid and profound progress in molecular genetics, and the availability of sensitive, valid clinical study methodologies will continue to foster the discovery of clinically relevant aspects of pathogenesis and treatments.

Meticulous avoidance of causative UVR, combined with a multiplicity of established medical and surgical treatments, can substantially benefit most patients with photoaging of the skin, reversing many of the troublesome cosmetic and functional aspects. We do not have the tools to completely reset the biological clock, but in this day of cloning of mammals and rapidly advancing medical and surgical technologies, can we hold out some hope for progression toward the, as yet, elusive fountain of youth?

REFERENCES

1. Hodes RJ, McCormick AM, Pruzan M, Longevity assurance genes: How do they influence aging and life span? *J Geriatr Dermatol* 1997; **5:** 26–32.
2. Gilchrest BA, *Skin and Aging Processes*. Boca Raton, FL: CRC Press, 1984.
3. Campbell KHS, McWhir J, Ritchie WA, Wilmut I, Sheep cloned by nuclear transfer from a cultured cell line. *Nature* 1996; **380:** 64–6.
4. Lowe NJ, Meyers DP, Wieder JM et al, Low doses of repetitive ultraviolet A induce morphologic changes in human skin. *J Invest Dermatol* 1995; **105:** 739–43.
5. Kligman LH, Intensification of ultraviolet-induced dermal damage by infrared radiation. *Arch Dermatol Res* 1982; **272:** 229–38.
6. Miyachi Y, Oxidative stress in cutaneous photoaging. In: *Frontiers of Photobiology* (Shima A, Ichahasi M, Fujiwara Y, eds). Amsterdam: Elsevier, 1993:443–6.
7. Kochevar IE, Molecular and cellular effects of UV radiation relevant to chronic photoaging. In: *Photoaging* (Gilcrest BA, ed). Cambridge, MA: Blackwell, 1995:51–67.
8. Stern RS, Thibodeau LA, Kleinerman RA et al, Risk of cutaneous carcinoma in patients treated with oral methoxalen photochemotherapy for psoriasis. *N Engl J Med* 1979; **300:** 809–13.
9. Drake LA, Dinehart SM, Farmer ER et al, Guidelines of care for photoaging/photodamage. *J Am Acad Dermatol* 1996; **35:** 462–4.
10. Rigel DS, Friedman RJ, Kopf AW et al, Lifetime risk for development of skin cancer in the U.S. population: current estimate is now 1 in 5. *J Am Acad Dermatol* 1996; **35:** 1012–3.
11. Streilein JW, UVB susceptibility: possible relationship to photoaging and photocarcinogenesis. In: *Photoaging* (Gilcrest BA, ed). Cambridge, MA: Blackwell, 1995:68–80.
12. Bernstein EF, Chen YQ, Kopp JB et al, Long-term sun exposure alters the collagen of the papillary dermis. *J Am Acad Dermatol* 1996; **34:** 209–18.
13. Kelly RI, Pearse R, Bull RH et al, The effects of aging on the cutaneous microvasculature. *J Am Acad Dermatol* 1995; **33:** 749–56.
14. Talwar HS, Griffiths CEM, Fisher GJ et al, Reduced type I and type III procollagens in photodamaged adult human skin. *J Invest Dermatol* 1995; **105:** 285–90.

15. Fisher GJ, Datta SC, Talwar HS et al, Molecular basis of sun-induced premature skin ageing and retinoid antagonism. *Nature* 1996; **379:** 335–9.

16. Goldsmith LA, Koh HK, Bewerse BA et al, Full proceedings from the National Conference to Develop a National Skin Cancer Agenda. *J Am Acad Dermatol* 1996; **35:** 748–56.

17. González E, González S, Drug photosensitivity, idiopathic photodermatoses, and sunscreens. *J Am Acad Dermatol* 1996; **35:** 871–5.

18. Lavker RM, Gerberick GF, Veres D et al, Cumulative effects from repeated exposures to suberythemal dose of UVB and UVA in human skin. *J Am Acad Dermatol* 1995; **32:** 53–62.

19. Harber LC, DeLeo VA, Prystowsky JH, Intrinsic and extrinsic photoprotection against UVB and UVA radiation. In: *Sunscreens, Development, Evaluation and Regulatory Aspects* (Lowe NJ, Shaath N, eds). New York: Marcel Decker, 1990:359–78.

20. Gilcrest BA, Zhai S, Eller ES et al, Treatment of human melanocytes and S91 melanoma cells with the DNA repair enzyme T4 endonuclease V enhances melanogenesis after ultraviolet irradiation. *J Invest Dermatol* 1993; **101:** 666–72.

21. Eller ES, Yaar M, Gilcrest BA, DNA damage and melanogenesis. *Nature* 1994; **372:** 413–14.

22. Tolbert DM, Kantor GJ, Definition of a DNA repair domain in the genomic region containing the human p53 gene. *Cancer Res* 1996; **56:** 3324–30.

23. Gordon PR, Gilcrest BA, Human melanogenesis is stimulated by diacylglycerol. *J Invest Dermatol* 1989; **93:** 700–2.

24. Cordero A, La vitamina A ácida en la piel senil. *Actua Ter Dermatol* 1983; **6:** 49–54.

25. Kligman LH, Akin FJ, Kligman AM, Sunscreens promote repair of ultraviolet radiation-induced dermal damage. *J Invest Dermatol* 1983; **81:** 98–102.

26. Kligman LH, Chen HD, Kligman AM, Topical retinoic acid enhances the repair of ultraviolet damaged connective tissue. *Connect Tissue Res* 1984; **12:** 139–50.

27. Kligman AM, Grove GL, Hirose R, Leyden JJ, Topical tretinoin for photoaged skin. *J Am Acad Dermatol* 1986; **15:** 836–59.

28. Weiss JS, Ellis CN, Headington JT et al, Topical tretinoin improves photoaged skin: a double-blind vehicle-controlled study. *J Am Med Assoc* 1988; **259:** 527–32.

29. Weinstein GD, Nigra TP, Pochi PE et al, Topical tretinoin for treatment of photodamaged skin. *Arch Dermatol* 1991; **127:** 659–65.

30. Cunningham WJ, Bryce GF, Armstrong RB et al, Topical isotretinoin and photodamage. In: *Retinoids: 10 Years On* (Saurat J-H, ed). Basel: Karger, 1990:182–90.

31. Bhawan J, Gonzalez-Serva A, Nehal K et al, Effects of tretinoin on photodamaged skin. *Arch Dermatol* 1991; **127:** 666–72.

32. Olsen EA, Katz HI, Levine N et al, Tretinoin emollient cream: A new therapy for photodamaged skin. *J Am Acad Dermatol* 1992; **26:** 215–24.

33. Ditre CM, Griffin TD, Murphy GF et al, Effect of α-hydroxy acids on photoaged skin: a pilot clinical, histological, and ultrastructural study. *J Am Acad Dermatol* 1996; **34:** 187–95.

34. Stiller MJ, Bartolone J, Stern R et al, Topical 8% glycolic acid and 8% L-lactic acid creams for the treatment of photodamaged skin. *Arch Dermatol* 1996; **132:** 631–6.

35. Griffin TD, Murphy GF, Sueki H et al, Increased factor XIIIa transglutaminase expression in dermal dendrocytes after treatment with α-hydroxy acids: potential physiological significance. *J Am Acad Dermatol* 1996; **34:** 196–203.

36. Perricone NV, DiNardo JC, Photoprotective and antiinflammatory effects of topical glycolic acid. *Dermatol Surg* 1996; **22:** 435–7.

37. Nelson BR, Fader DJ, Gillard M et al, Pilot histologic and ultrastructural study of the effects of medium-depth chemical facial peels on dermal collagen in patients with actinically damaged skin. *J Am Acad Dermatol* 1995; **32:** 472–8.

38. Piacquadio D, Dobry M, Hunt S et al, Short contact 70% glycolic acid peels as a treatment for photodamaged skin. *Dermatol Surg* 1996; **22:** 449–52.

39. Humphreys TR, Werth V, Dzubow L et al, Treatment of photodamaged skin with trichloroacetic acid and topical tretinoin. *J Am Acad Dermatol* 1996; **34:** 638–44.

40. Lowe NJ, Lask G, Griffin ME et al, Skin resurfacing with the Ultrapulse carbon dioxide laser. *Dermatol Surg* 1995; **21:** 1025–9.

41. Benedetto AV, Griffin TD, Benedetto EA et al, Dermabrasion: therapy and prophylaxis for the

photoaged face. *J Am Acad Dermatol* 1992; **27:** 439–47.

42. Nelson BR, Metz RD, Majmudar G et al, A comparison of wire brush and diamond fraise superficial dermabrasion for photoaged skin, *J Am Acad Dermatol* 1996; **34:** 235–43.

43. Carruthers A, Kiene K, Carruthers J, Botulinum A exotoxin use in clinical dermatology. *J Am Acad Dermatol* 1996; **34:** 788–97.

44. Matarasso SL, Carruthers A, Botulinum toxin: treatment for glabellar furrows. *J Geriatr Dermatol* 1997; **5:** 13–14.

45. Drake LA, Dinehart SM, Farmer ER et al, Guidelines of care for soft tissue augmentation: collagen implants. *J Am Acad Dermatol* 1996; **34:** 698–702.

46. Jurkiewicz BA, Bissett DL, Buettner GR, Effect of topically applied tocopherol on ultraviolet radiation-mediated free radical damage of skin. *J Invest Dermatol* 1995; **104:** 484–8.

47. Perricone NV, Aging: prevention and intervention, part 1: antioxidants. *J Geriatr Dermatol* 1997; **5:** 1–2.

48. Stern RS, Cooperman SA, The measure of youth. *Arch Dermatol* 1992; **128:** 390–3.

49. Griffiths CEM, Wang TS, Hamilton TA et al, A photonumeric scale for the assessment of cutaneous photoaging. *Arch Dermatol* 1992; **128:** 347–51.

50. Sendagorta E, Lesiewicz J, Armstrong RB, Topical isotretinoin for photodamaged skin. *J Am Acad Dermatol* 1992; **27** (No. 6, Part 2): S15–18.

51. Larnier C, Ortonne J-P, Venot A et al, Evaluation of cutaneous photoaging using a photographic scale. *Br J Dermatol* 1994; **130:** 167–73.

52. Armstrong RB, Lesiewicz J, Harvey G et al, Clinical panel assessment of photodamaged skin treated with isotretinoin using photographs. *Arch Dermatol* 1992; **128:** 352–6.

53. Grove GL, Grove MJ, Leyden JJ et al, Skin replica analysis of photodamaged skin after therapy with tretinoin emollient cream. *J Am Acad Dermatol* 1991; **25:** 231–7.

54. Muccini JA, Kollias N, Phillips SB et al, Polarized light photography in the evaluation of photoaging. *J Am Acad Dermatol* 1995; **33:** 765–9.

55. Kollias N, Gillies R, Cohen-Goihman C et al, Fluorescence photography in the evaluation of hyperpigmentation in photodamaged skin. *J Am Acad Dermatol* 1997; **36:** 226–30.

56. Serup J, Jemec GBE (eds), *Handbook of Non-Invasive Methods and the Skin.* Boca Raton, FL: CRC Press, 1995.

39

Modulation of inflammatory reactions in skin: A new approach to the treatment of premature aging

Daniel H Maes, Kenneth D Marenus

INTRODUCTION

The tremendous progress made over the past 10 years in biology, biochemistry, and dermatology has resulted in a new generation of skin care products. These modern products are able to provide significant and perceivable improvements in skin appearance and condition.

Today's cosmetic products provide the consumer with moisturization benefits due to specific lipids and water-binding agents. They also help improve the structure and appearance of the skin through the activity of agents designed to enhance specific skin functions.

Most technological developments thus far have taken place in what may be called 'repair technologies'. Specific ingredients, such as retinoids, are able to reduce damage induced by environmental exposure. In fact, many modern cosmetic products now contain specific agents that can increase dermal collagen and elastin synthesis, thereby reducing the appearance of lines and wrinkles and increasing firmness and elasticity.

The recent success of α-hydroxy acid or 'fruit acid technologies' is based primarily on the rapid visual and tactile benefits resulting from the keratolytic activity of these agents. This results from rapid elimination of dry skin cells on the uppermost layers of the stratum corneum, leaving behind a smoother feeling and more pleasant-looking skin surface.

To be a commercial success, today's product must quickly and safely create perceptible improvements in skin condition that are highly appraised by the consumer. Unfortunately, one-dimensional products often fail to provide essential benefits: that is, skin protection from a wide variety of environmental stresses. It is our opinion that the protection benefits imparted by a modern cosmetic product are as important as the repair benefits in providing the consumer with safe and effective skin care over the long term.

There is relatively little to be derived from repairing what has been damaged by years of over-exposure to sun and pollution, if at the same time protection from these same damaging factors is not provided.

There is now substantial evidence[1,2] that UV-B, UV-A and IR irradiation can generate significant damage to the skin and in fact the whole body at many levels. For example, UV-generated DNA damage and formation of apoptotic cells in the epidermis are well documented. In the dermis, environmental factors are responsible for the development of wrinkles and sagging skin. Even more threatening, immunosuppression linked with UV exposure has been proposed to play a role in generating both local carcinogenic activity and systemic immunosuppressive influences.

Similarly, long-term exposure to smoke has been shown[3] to induce a significant reduction of stratum corneum barrier function, resulting in an increase in skin dryness as well as premature formation of lines and wrinkles.

The need for protection is not well understood by the average consumer, since visible benefits are slow in accumulating from such activity. Still, it is important that modern cosmetic products combine both protection and repair activity in order to provide a complete range of treatment benefits for the consumer.

The last 10 years have seen remarkable advances in the understanding of biological processes that take place during and after exposure to the sun. The free-radical theory of aging is now widely accepted. Many antioxidants and free-radical scavengers have been tested and found to significantly reduce the extent of free-radical-based oxidation processes in the skin.[4,5] The combination of external protection provided by sunscreens, and internal protection provided by antioxidants is one obvious approach in daily-use skin care products aimed at reducing premature skin aging.

Although quite attractive, antioxidant technology alone has failed to provide strong enough protection from the damage caused by sun exposure. To date, antioxidants alone are capable of providing a protection equivalent to sun protection factor (SPF) 4. Only the combination of antioxidants with traditional sunscreens has been able to provide higher levels of UV protection (SPF 30 and above).[6]

For this reason, it became obvious that other processes were taking place in the skin during and after exposure to the sun, resulting in damage that was not controlled exclusively by free-radical reactions. It has been found[7–9] that these processes are related to a variety of inflammatory reactions that appear to develop in the skin in a more or less continuous manner.

In the first part of this chapter, we propose to review the factors that trigger inflammatory skin reactions, as well as to discuss the known mechanisms of these reactions. We then evaluate different methodologies currently available to assess the activity of the different pathways of the inflammatory reactions in vitro and in vivo.

The second part of this review will discuss the technologies and materials currently available to control inflammatory reactions. Further, we shall present an approach to providing wide-range skin protection from the variety of environmentally based stimuli through regular application of skin care products.

FACTORS TRIGGERING INFLAMMATORY REACTIONS

In everyday life, the skin is exposed to a multitude of challenges, including bacterial invasion and exposure to environmental contaminants such as cigarette smoke, car fumes, detergents and other irritants and sensitizers.

In order to defend the body from damage resulting from such exposure, the skin's immune system has developed a carefully balanced and elaborate defense mechanism, through which the rapid activation of leukocytes and concomitant development of various inflammatory reactions allows for the complete destruction of bacterial assailants.

It is obvious that the reaction of the immune system to bacterial aggression is necessary for the survival of the human species in an environment where the invasion of bacteria through cuts and wounds of the skin is practically a daily occurrence.

In such conditions, the various inflammatory reactions, which are an integral part of the skin's immune response, are to be considered necessary, since they play a key role in the elimination of the invading bacteria, but at the same time induce damage to the skin cells themselves.

The first line of defense of the skin against such continuous challenge is the stratum corneum. The structure and function of this unique skin region has been further clarified.[10,11] The key function of the stratum corneum is to act as a barrier preventing the penetration of the environmental agents into the epidermal and dermal spaces, where they may initiate reactions of the immune system.[12]

In the past, it was thought that only small molecules with molecular weights below 500 could penetrate the stratum corneum. It has now been documented[13] that fairly large molecules can find their way through this layer and therefore interact directly with the viable cells of the skin. In practice, barrier function is rarely optimal, and thus this is a relatively frequent occurrence.

In such situations, epidermal cells and even those of the deeper dermal layers are exposed to foreign and often immunogenic agents, which can trigger reactions ranging from simple irritation to full allergic induction.

Therefore one of the most important factors to consider when investigating the sources of specific skin reactions is the integrity of the stratum corneum. If this function is found to be weak, such as in the atopic patient, then it will be likely that the individual being examined will have a predisposition to suffer frequently from irritant contact dermatitis, which has potential to evolve into a full allergic reaction.

In addition to increased skin permeability caused by the disruption of the stratum corneum barrier, recent studies[14] have clearly demonstrated that increased mRNA levels of nerve growth factor (NGF) as well as tumor necrosis factor alpha (TFF-α) and interleukin-1 (IL-1) are observed in response to barrier abrogation.[15] As we shall discuss later, release of these growth factors and cytokines can activate epidermal proliferation, and trigger a series of inflammatory reactions with distinct consequences, especially related to premature aging.

Once a foreign molecule has penetrated into the living layers of the skin, it may trigger two distinct types of inflammatory reactions: acute and chronic.

The acute inflammatory reaction involves exclusively polymorphonuclear leukocytes (PMN), which rapidly migrate between endothelial cells and cross the basement membrane. PMN produce tissue damage through the release of substances including proteinases (collagenase, elastase) and free radicals.

Proinflammatory lipids, such as arachidonic acid, are associated with the acute inflammatory response. A significant increase of blood flow, and an augmentation of vascular permeability is generally caused by the activity of leukotriene B_4 (LTB_4) and prostaglandins.

Chronic inflammation, which involves mostly lymphocytes and macrophages, is activated by the myriad of antigens to which the skin may regularly be exposed. Once activated, T lymphocytes release many mediators of inflammation, such as arachidonic acid, through the activation of the phospholipase A_2. This results in the development of two independent metabolic pathways; cyclooxygenase and lipooxygenase, with the concomitant production of prostaglandins and leukotrienes.

When examining the interaction of the skin with its environment, a key point is that, whatever the mechanism, the end result will usually involve the release of free radicals and the activation of specific destructive enzymes such as collagenase and elastase.

The release of free radicals and the activation of proteases can result in a discrete amount of damage to the involved tissues, leading ultimately to the premature aging process.

It would be wrong to think that such events only take place when visible indications of inflammation develop. In fact, it has become more and more apparent that continual exposure to smoke, pollution and low doses of UV light results in the development of subclinical inflammatory processes that are not visible and can be detected only through histological examination. The importance of this type of reaction was initially presented by Dr A Kligman, who called this field 'Invisible Dermatology'. Invisible dermatology is the study of processes evolving at a subclinical level that, through their cumulative effects, can induce permanent changes in the structure and function of the skin.

Understanding the mechanisms of the skin's immune response as well as inflammatory reactions has become one of the most important issues in studying the processes involved in premature aging. It is essential to consider these events prior to developing any skin care products intended to control environmentally induced damage.

METHODOLOGIES TO INVESTIGATE MECHANISMS OF INFLAMMATORY REACTIONS

As we just have briefly reviewed, there are well-defined reactions that take place in the skin once it is exposed to UV or other environmental factors.

These reactions are:

- formation of lipid peroxides
- release of inflammatory mediators
- release of cytokines
- leukocyte adhesion and chemotaxis
- activation of collagenase, elastase and hyaluronidase.

In order to understand the role of specific inflammatory reactions in the process of premature skin aging, it is necessary to develop a proper methodology to evaluate which is the most prevalent when the skin is exposed to a specific challenge.

Determination of lipid peroxidation

The peroxidation process in the skin results from direct interaction of free radicals with unsaturated lipids of the cell membrane.[16,17] Free radicals can have two origins. They can be generated during the interaction of UV light with specific proteins and lipids; this reaction takes place immediately when the skin is exposed to the sun. They can also be generated approximately 24 hours later, by cells of the immune system such as polymorphonuclear leukocytes.

Whatever the source, free radicals can induce significant damage to cell membranes. It is therefore important to detect their presence, and even more important to quantify the activity of free-radical scavengers and antioxidants in inhibiting their formation.

The first method to be reviewed here involves the determination of UV-induced lipid peroxides. This information is needed to evaluate the comparative efficacy of antioxidants and free-radical scavengers. Assays exist that can be used in vitro, ex vivo or in vivo.

In vitro, the liposome assay is an excellent screening tool to evaluate the activity of lipophilic and hydrophilic antioxidants.[4] This method is based on the measurement of the amount of thiobarbituric acid-reacting substances generated in phospholipid liposomes irradiated by UV light.

This method provides data that demonstrate a linear relationship between the dose of UV light and the extent of lipid peroxidation. In addition, it shows that well-known antioxidants such as vitamins E and C significantly reduce the amount of UV-generated free radicals, whether they are used separately or in combination (Figure 39.1).

The ex vivo method uses fibroblast and keratinocyte cocultures lifted to an air interface as a substrate to measure the amount of hydroperoxides generated by the exposure to UV light.[5] This method is one step closer to a real-life situation. Here the antioxidants tested must penetrate the cornified layers of

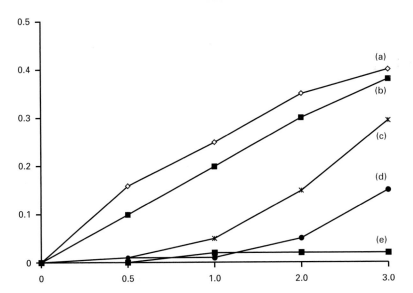

Figure 39.1 Inhibition of UVB-induced lipid peroxidation by a mixture of α-tocopherol and ascorbic acid: (a) no α-tocopherol; (b) 1 mol%; (c) 5 mol%; (d) 10 mol%; (e) covered control.

the epidermis in order to protect the unsaturated lipids of the cell membranes in the deeper layers of the artificial skin.

Results shown in Figure 39.2 indicate that increasing doses of UV light generate a linear increase in the amount of peroxides in the skin models. Treatment with antioxidant results in a significant reduction in UV-induced lipid peroxidation (Figure 39.3).

These two in vitro methods are quite useful for screening large numbers of antioxidants before they are tested in a more complex in vivo situation.

The in vivo method consists of the measurement of the amount of squalene hydroperoxide extracted from the forearm of human volunteers who treated their skin with an antioxidant composition during a defined

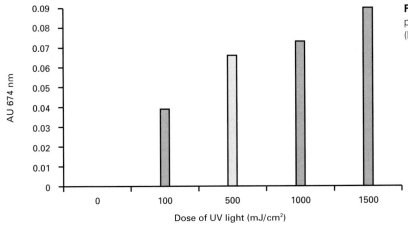

Figure 39.2 UVB-induced peroxidation in skin models (living-skin equivalent).

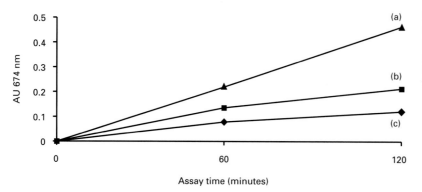

Figure 39.3 Effect of antioxidant on UVB-induced peroxidation (living-skin equivalent): (a) UVB; (b) UVB + antioxidant; (c) control.

period. By comparing the amount of peroxides extracted from treated and non-treated areas, we have been able to quantify the efficacy of the antioxidants in reducing the *endogenous* level of peroxides generated through casual exposure to the sun and environmental pollution (Figure 39.4).

Additional information relating to the efficacy of any antioxidant can be obtained by measuring the extent of peroxidation resulting from the additional irradiation of the skin lipids extracted with ethanol from the treated and non-treated areas. This method has the advantage of providing measurements of the activity of an antioxidant composition in redu-

cing the level of endogenous peroxides, as well as providing data on its efficacy in reducing the extent of peroxidation induced by an additional UV exposure.

The results shown in Figure 39.5 indicate that the same preparation is able to reduce both endogenous and UV-induced lipid peroxides after regular application of a test material containing a blend of antioxidants. However, the regression data shown in these figures also indicate that antioxidants lose their ability to reduce both the endogenous and UV-induced peroxidation as soon as the topical application is interrupted.

Similar methodologies can be used to mea-

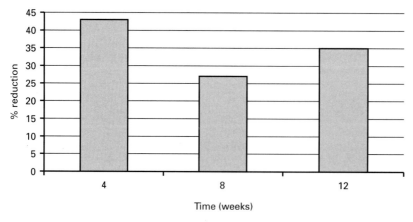

Figure 39.4 Reduction in lipid peroxides in vivo during treatment with antioxidants (endogenous lipid peroxides).

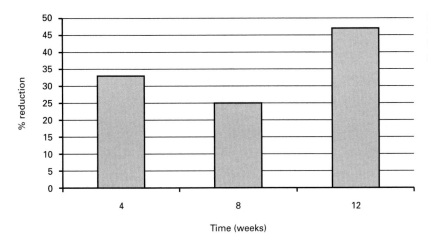

Figure 39.5 Reduction of UVB-induced lipid peroxides during treatment with antioxidants.

sure the extent of smoke-induced oxidation on the skin. Both the in vitro and in vivo methods are well adapted to measure the extent of lipid peroxidation after exposure to cigarette smoke. They can also provide an accurate estimate of the efficacy of antioxidants in controlling this process. The results shown in Figures 39.6 and 39.7 indicate that exposure to smoke can generate a significant amount of lipid peroxides both in air-lifted cocultures and in the in vivo situation. In both cases, pretreatment of the skin with an antioxidant preparation results in a significant reduction of the amount of lipid peroxides generated by exposure to cigarette smoke.

Measurement of UV-induced inflammatory mediators

One of the first events to take place after the cell membrane lipids have been oxidized by free radicals, is activation of the enzyme phos-

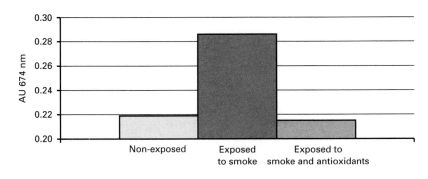

Figure 39.6 Evaluation of smoke-induced lipid peroxidation: In vitro (skin equivalent).

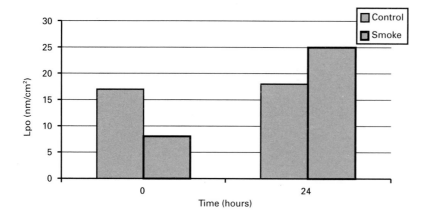

Figure 39.7 Evaluation of smoke-induced lipid peroxidation. In vivo evaluation of hydroperoxides extracted from smoke-exposed forearms (Lpo, lipid hydroperoxide).

pholipase A_2. This enzyme cleaves arachidonic acid from the cell membrane. This event is the first committed step leading to the development of the cascade of inflammatory reactions, which results in an increase in vascular permeability through leukotriene B_4 and an increase in blood flow through prostaglandin E_2.

Therefore it is quite important to be able to measure the activity of phospholipase A_2 in various situations in order to predict the extent to which inflammatory reactions may develop in the skin at a later stage. In vitro methods allow for precise quantification of the efficacy of a combination of various antioxidants in inhibiting the action of phospholipase A_2 in releasing arachidonic acid (Figure 39.8).

As a direct consequence of the inhibition of the activity of this enzyme by antioxidants, a correlative and significant reduction in the UV-induced release of arachidonic acid using

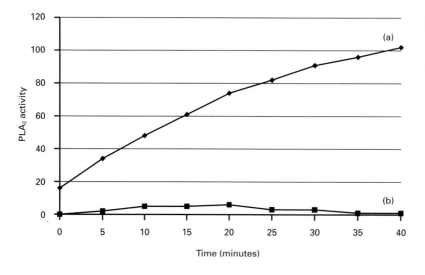

Figure 39.8 Evaluation of the release of inflammatory mediators. Inhibition of PLA_2 by antioxidants: (a) control; (b) antioxidant.

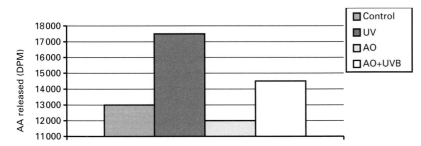

Figure 39.9 Evaluation of the UV-induced release of inflammatory mediators. Release of arachidonic acid (AA) from living-skin equivalent after irradiation with UVB (DPM, disintegrations per minute; AO = antioxidant).

a skin model has been observed (Figure 39.9).[7]

Based on these data, it seems clear that antioxidants can play a significant role in the prevention of inflammatory reactions in skin. This can occur through control of the initial phases of the process, i.e. free-radical-induced peroxidation of cell membrane lipids. Thus regular application of antioxidants should result in a significant reduction of the visible indications of inflammatory reaction within the skin, such as the delayed development of redness after sun exposure. Consequently, the efficacy of various blends of antioxidant compounds that do not absorb UV light directly has been evaluated for their ability to prevent UV-induced erythema.

After topical application of antioxidants, the reduction of erythema generated by UV light corresponded to a UV protection factor of 4 (SPF). Furthermore, the protection provided through the multiple applications of the same blend of antioxidants over a four-day time period provided an increase in protection corresponding to an SPF of 5.

Further investigation of the extent of protection provided by regular topical application of antioxidants has led to the evaluation of UV-induced sunburn cells. The results shown in Figure 39.10 clearly indicate that application of antioxidants results in a reduction in the number of sunburn cells by more than 50%.[18]

Similarly, the evaluation of the protective benefits of antioxidants at a molecular level revealed a 75% reduction in the amount of thymine–thymine dimers (T–T dimers) generated in the DNA after exposure to UV light (Figure 39.11).[6]

Taken together, these results show the

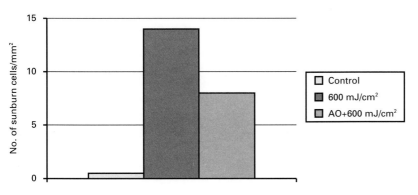

Figure 39.10 Prevention of epidermal cell damage by antioxidants (AO).

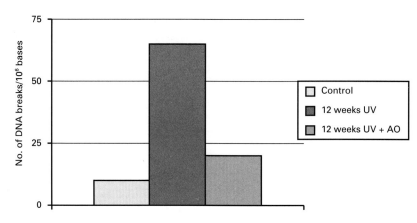

importance of controlling lipid peroxidation and other oxidative processes at the cellular level. This control can be provided by regular topical application of antioxidant blends. However, this protective technology is only the first step of a broader prevention therapy that can be provided by agents that control other inflammatory processes. These include release of cytokines, leukocyte adhesion, neutrophil chemotaxis, and activation of collagenase and elastase.

Release of cytokines

Although the field of research on cytokine release has become a science of its own, as new cytokines are identified regularly, two of the most frequently involved cytokines in inflammatory reactions are tumor necrosis factor alpha (TNF-α) and interleukin-1 (IL-1). There is now considerable evidence indicating that upon exposure to UV light, keratinocytes rapidly release these two cytokines into the intercellular milieu, resulting in the recruitment of leukocytes, and the concomitant activation of a more generalized immunological response.[9]

In such conditions, measurement of the release of these cytokines from the cells can provide a good indication of the development of other stages of the inflammatory reaction. Using standard ELISA techniques, it is possible to quantify the release of these two cytokines upon exposure to UV, as shown in Figures 39.12 and 39.13.

The pretreatment of keratinocytes with antioxidants such as vitamin E, before irradiation with UV, results in a significant reduction in the release of TNF-α (Figure 39.14). This effect could be explained by the fact that reduction of UV-induced lipid peroxidation by antioxidants has a direct influence on the release of cytokines by the cells. This supports the idea that cytokine release is generally due to oxidative stress occurring at the level of the cell membrane.

Evaluation of protease activity

The activation of polymorphonuclear leukocytes (PMNs) during acute inflammation and recruitment of T lymphocytes during chronic inflammation both result in the release of free radicals and metalloproteases such as collagenase, elastase and hyaluronidase. These enzymes are essential, since they aid in dissolution of the extracellular matrix to allow passage for various cells of the immune system to

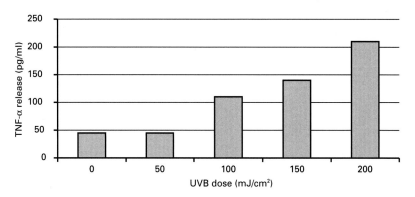

Figure 39.12 Release of inflammatory cytokines: UVB-induced release of TNF-α.

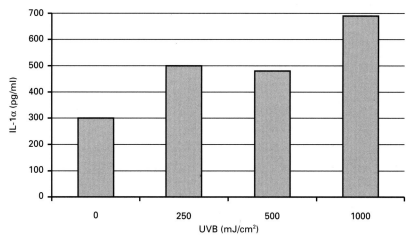

Figure 39.13 Release of inflammatory cytokines: UVB-induced release of IL-1α.

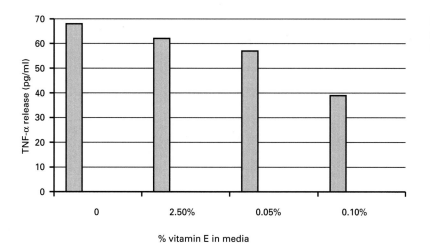

Figure 39.14 Effects of vitamin E on the UVB-induced release of TNF-α.

reach the site of activity. In doing this, they can induce structural perturbation in the dermis, since they are very effective in their ability to digest the three most important components of this part of the tegument.

The long-term consequence of the almost-permanent activity of these enzymes is what we believe leads to premature skin aging. Indeed, the skin may suffer somewhat from the damage caused by interactions of free radicals and cell membranes. In terms of aging, however, the indirect effect of free radicals involves activation of metalloproteases. The formation of lines and wrinkles, or the appearance of slacking skin, is not apparently caused by direct photochemical free-radical-controlled reactions, but rather by the indirect activation of the skin's own enzymes as a consequence of the activity of the immune system.

This conclusion is supported by observations that both collagenase and elastase can be activated in vitro, using air-lifted cocultures, through direct exposure to UV light (Figure 39.15).

At this stage, it seems that the activation of these enzymes is mediated through UV-generated free-radical interaction with cell membranes, resulting either in the release of prostaglandins and leukotrienes or in the direct activation of cytokines like IL-1, and TNF-α. This hypothesis has been explored using an in vitro cell culture assay, after a direct relationship was found between the release of IL-1α and collagenase activity (Figure 39.16).

The relationship between the different processes just discussed is summarized in Figure 39.17. Despite the complexity of the different pathways in skin, one thing is quite clear: whatever the mechanism of the inflammatory reactions, the end result is always the same – the premature degradation of the key structural components of the dermis due to increased activity by metalloproteases.

Leukocytes: adhesion and chemotaxis

One of the most exciting areas in the field of immunology is related to understanding adhesion and chemotaxis of lymphocytes during their migration to sites where an inflammatory reaction is taking place.

New therapies developed on this basis have been shown to be very effective in reducing both acute and chronic inflammation. The possibility now exists of controlling the attraction and adhesion of polymorphonuclear leukocytes and lymphocytes to endothelial cells.[19] In order to evaluate the efficacy of this new approach, in vitro assays have been developed that correlate with the clinical efficacy of the same agents in controlling the progress of inflammatory reactions in skin.

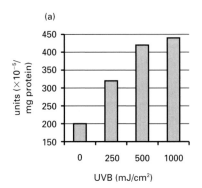
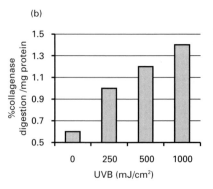

Figure 39.15 Evaluation of the UV-induced activation of proteases: (a) UVB-induced elastase activity in living-skin model; (b) UVB-induced collagenase activity in living-skin model.

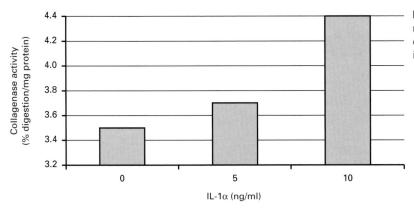

Figure 39.16 Role of cytokine release in protease activation: effect of IL-1α on collagenase in human fibroblasts.

The activity of an extract of the cola plant (*Cola nitida*) in inhibiting neutrophil adhesion to human endothelial cells was tested in vitro using standard ELISA techniques (Figure 39.18). The results show that in vitro cola extract was able to reduce the intensity of a neutrophil-driven acute inflammatory reaction in a dose-dependent manner. These results correlate with clinical data. Figure 39.19 demonstrates a dose dependence in the concentration of cola extract in reducing the balsam of Peru-induced and neutrophil-mediated erythemic response.[20]

Similar results were obtained for lymphocyte-controlled chronic inflammation. In this case, adhesion of lymphocytes to endothelial cells was reduced by pretreatment with a sialyl Lewis[x] mimic molecule, as shown in Figure 39.20. Here no increase in lymphocyte adhesion occurred over a broad range of phyto-

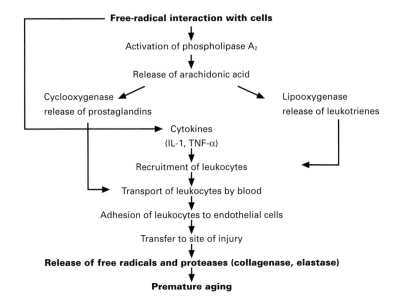

Figure 39.17 Summary of processes discussed in Figures 39.12–39.16.

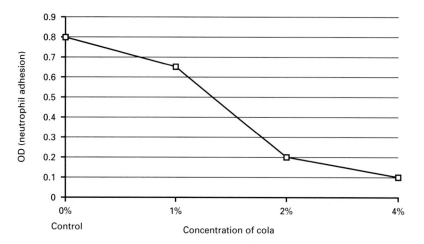

Figure 39.18 Reduction of chemically induced acute inflammation: inhibition of neutrophil adhesion to endothelial cells (OD, optical density).

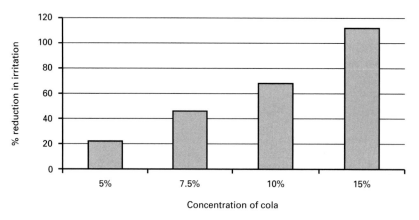

Figure 39.19 Clinical evaluation of the anti-irritant activity of cola.

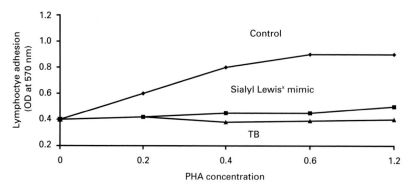

Figure 39.20 Reduction of chemically induced chronic inflammation: inhibition of lymphocyte (T cells) adhesion to endothelial cells by terbinafine (TB) and a sialyl Lewis^x mimic at 2%.

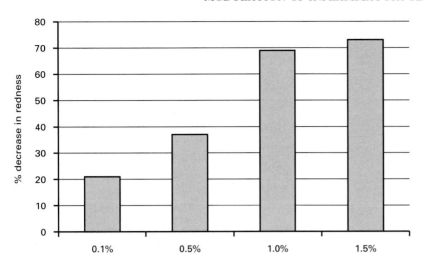

Figure 39.21 Clinical evaluation of the anti-irritant activity of a sialyl Lewis^x mimic.

hemagglutinin (PHA) used to activate the lymphocytes. These in vitro results also correlate with clinical observations made during the assessment of the efficacy of the sialyl Lewis^x mimic in reducing skin irritation, as seen in Figure 39.21.

Thus intervention in a variety of these inflammatory processes is quite appealing as a general approach in looking for ways of reducing the progression of inflammatory reactions. These intervene at a totally different level than classical anti-inflammatory therapies, which control lipid-peroxidation processes and release of inflammatory mediators. The combination of classical anti-inflammatory therapies with the utilization of new adhesion inhibitors is likely to provide a broader range of anti-inflammatory activity than in the past.

CONCLUSIONS

The role played by inflammatory reactions in the premature aging process is now becoming clear. It seems that there is no single agent that will suffice in providing broad enough

control of inflammatory processes in order to significantly reduce premature skin aging.

At this stage, the best therapy to effectively protect the skin from damage caused by the environment consists of the use of multiple agents. Useful therapy should control free-radical-induced peroxidation, activation of phospholipase A_2, release of various cytokines such as IL-1, IL-6 and TNF-α, activation of proteases such as collagenase and elastase, and finally adhesion and chemoattraction of lymphocytes.

Although antioxidants play a key role in the development of inflammatory reactions, since they are the first and a controlling step leading to the release of other inflammatory mediators, it is essential to add other materials that can have a more direct effect at the different stages of the inflammatory process.

Such treatments should be applied well in advance of the exposure to environmental challenge. Based on the very short lifetime of the various free radicals generated by UV light, antioxidants will have a beneficial effect only if they are given time to penetrate into the deeper layers of the skin, where they can scavenge free radicals as soon as they are generated, thus resulting in the control of the formation of lipid peroxides in the cell membranes.

Similarly, the activation of proteases by UV light occurs within a few minutes after irradiation with as little as 1/10 of an MED of UV.[21] As a result, protease inhibitors can have an effect in reducing premature degradation of the collagen and elastin in the dermis only if they are in place well in advance of exposure to UV light.

These data reinforce our conviction that effective anti-aging therapy starts with regular topical application of a blend of agents that can appropriately modulate the course of dermal inflammatory reactions. This is far better than just applying a layer of sunscreen on the skin. Although sunscreens are a necessary part of daily protection, they are far from being sufficient in providing complete protection from damage that can be caused by the environment. There are many more factors than UV, such as smoke, irritation and allergic reactions, that can induce inflammatory reactions in the skin.

Based on the information described here, the need to incorporate agents that provide the broadest possible protection from the damage generated by the environment is quite obvious. Although such technology still has a very limited appeal in the consumer's mind, it is a necessity to provide strong protection before any improvement of the skin's structure can be provided through 'repair technology'.

Therefore it is essential to educate the consumer about the need to use products that provide sufficient protection benefits through the utilization of 'protective technology', combined with the judicious use of sunscreens. Once 'protective technology' is incorporated systematically and combined with 'repair technology' in all skin care products, we can be assured that consumers will benefit from the most advanced technology available at this stage.

REFERENCES

1. Kligman LH, Akin FJ, Kligman AM, The contribution of UVA and UVB to connective tissue damage in hairless mice. *J Invest Dermatol* 1985; **84:** 272–6.

2. Kligman LH, Agin PP, Sayre RM, Broad spectrum sunscreens with UVA I and UVA II absorbers provide increased protection against solar-simulating radiation-induced dermal damage in hairless mice. *J Soc Cosmet Chem* 1996; **47:** 129–55.

3. Marenus K, Fthenakis C, Vallon P et al, Cigarette smoking. Effects on the barrier properties of the skin. Poster presented at the American Academy of Dermatology, San Francisco, 1992.

4. Pelle E, Maes D, Padulo G et al, An in-vitro model to test relative anti-oxidant potential: Ultraviolet induced lipid peroxidation in liposomes. *Arch Biochem Biophys* 1990; **283:** 234–40.

5. Pelle E, Marenus K, Maes D, Anti-oxidant protection against ultraviolet light-induced skin damage. In: *Oxidative Stress in Dermatology* (Fuchs J, Packer L, eds). New York: Marcel Dekker, 1993:127–40.

6. Marenus K, Muizzuddin N, Kasman K et al, The use of anti-oxidants in providing protection from chronic suberythemal UVB exposure. Presented at the 16th IFSCC Congress, New York, 1990.

7. De Leo VA, Hanson D, Weinstein IB, Harber LC, Ultraviolet radiation stimulates the release of archidonic acid from mammalian cells in culture. *Photochem Photobiol* 1985; **41:** 51–6.

8. Sondergaard J, Bisgaard H, Thorsen S, Eicosanoids in skin inflammation. *Photodermatology* 1985; **2:** 359–66.

9. Schwarz T, Luger TA, Effect of UV irradiation on epidermal cell cytokine production. *J Photochem Photobiol B: Biol* 1989; **4:** 1–13.

10. Ward AJI, Du Reau C, The essential role of lipid bilayers in the determination of stratum corneum permeability. *Int J Pharmaceutics* 1991; **74:** 137–46.

11. Feingold KR, A dermatological viewpoint of the permeability barrier. *Cosmetics and Toiletries* 1992; **107:** 42.

12. Muizzuddin N, Marenus K, Tonnesen M, Maes D, Factors defining sensitive skin and its treatment. Poster presented at the American Academy of Dermatology, Washington, February 1996.

13. Yarosh D, Bucana C, Cox P et al, Localization of

liposomes containing a DNA repair enzyme in murine skin. *J Invest Dermatol* 1994; **103:** 461–8.

14. Liou A, Elias PM, Grunfeld C et al, Amphiregulin and nerve growth factor expression are regulated by barrier status in murine epidermis. *J Invest Dermatol* 1997; **108:** 73–7.

15. Wood LC, Elias PM, Calhoun C et al, Barrier disruption stimulates interleukin-1 alpha expression and release from a preformed poll in murine epidermis. *J Invest Dermatol* 1996; **106:** 397–403.

16. Pathak MA, Stratton K, Free radicals in human skin before and after exposure to light. *Arch Biochem Biophys* 1968; **123:** 468–76.

17. Harman D, Free radical theory of aging: the 'free radical' diseases. *Age* 1984; **7:** 111–31.

18. Maes D, Marenus K, Smith WP, New advances in photoprotection. *Cosmetics and Toiletries* 1990; **105:** 45–52.

19. Groves RW, Allen MH, Barker JNWN et al, Endothelial leucocyte adhesion molecule-1 (ELAM-1) expression in cutaneous inflammation. *Br J Dermatol* 1991; **124:** 117–23.

20. Muizzuddin N, Marenus K, Maes D, Use of a chromameter in assessing the efficacy of anti-irritants and tanning accelerators. *J Soc Cosmet Chem* 1990; **41:** 269–78.

21. Fisher GJ, Subhash CD, Harvinder ST et al, Molecular basis of sun-induced premature skin ageing retinoid antagonism. *Nature* 1996; **379:** 335–9.

40

Menopause, skin and cosmetology

Claire Beylot

INTRODUCTION

The hormonal disorders of menopause cause changes in the whole organism requiring special management, and the skin is no exception. Today, thanks to better physiopathological knowledge of these disorders and to therapeutic advances, women can avoid or limit such undesirable side-effects of menopause, and are aware that they are not necessarily ineluctable. To this end, appropriate cosmetology can efficiently complement the favourable effects of hormonal replacement therapy.

WHAT HAPPENS IN MENOPAUSE?

Accentuation of skin aging by oestrogen deficiency

Cessation of ovarian oestrogen production around age 50
The plasma oestradiol level falls from a mean 100 pg/ml in a normal menstrual cycle to 25 pg/ml.[1] However, there exists an extra-ovarian oestrogen synthesis, especially in adipose tissue, owing to androstenedione aromatization in oestrone, which after menopause becomes the dominant oestrogen. Particularly in fat women, this may lead to a localized hyperoestrogenism, which is undetectable by plasma assays.[1] The drawback of this tissue hyperoestrogenism is an increase in the panniculus adiposus, and this is a risk factor for oestrogen-dependent cancers, especially breast cancer. On the other hand, it is rather beneficial for the skin, owing to its protective activity against skin aging. In fact, such skin aging is usually less marked in fat women than in thin ones, who are frequently more osteoporotic.

Apparent sudden aging in menopause
Insidious cutaneous signs accompany the dramatic climacteric flushing. So aging related to oestrogen failure adds to chronological aging, and photoaging suddenly increases the visible age of the menopausal woman. However, menopause-related skin changes are quite different in clinical and pathological terms from photoaging, and rather resemble chronological aging. Indeed, the skin becomes thin, shrivels and dries, particularly on the face, where oestrogen receptors are more numerous.

The targets of oestrogens are still not clearly identified in the skin, and only some groups of cells, such as fibroblasts, basal keratinocytes and probably melanocytes, seem to be really oestrogen-dependent.[1]

- Oestrogen deficiency particularly involves the fibroblasts of the dermis, and therefore all the components of extracellular matrix that it synthesizes, such as collagen and elastic fibres, and the ground substance.
  (i) The thinning of the skin is primarily related to a decrease in skin collagen content,[2] valued by Brincat et al[3] between 1% and 2% per year. This decrease is correlated with the decline in bone mineral content assessed by the metacarpal index and absorptiometry,[3] and with the decline in urethral collagen that is responsible for incontinence.[4] In Caucasian females, osteoporosis is correlated with skin colour, and fair complexion is a risk factor for low bone mineral density.[5]
  (ii) Skin elasticity decreases with age – but more in women than in men, and in early menopause there may occur degenerative changes of elastic fibres similar to those normally found in older women.[6]
  (ii) Finally, the decline in the fibroblastic synthesis of the dermis ground-substance macroproteins, particularly hyaluronic acid, which is able to bind water, is responsible for a decrease in dermal hydration.
- In the epidermis, menopausal oestrogen deficiency slows down the mitotic activity of basal keratinocytes, and consequently leads to epidermal atrophy, which is also noted in castration. A decrease in skin pigmentation may also be observed clinically and spectrophotometrically.[7]
- Oestrogen deficiency also changes the vulvar mucous membrane, which becomes atrophic and dry, and may lead to pruritus and dyspareunia.

This atrophic fragile skin is less protected by the surface hydrolipidic film, because of the usual decrease in sebum secretion. The stratum corneum barrier is less effective, and the skin may develop irritant or eczematic reactions, particularly if skin care is inadequate or too aggressive. However, this is not confirmed by other studies, which find a more intense irritant reaction with lauryl sodium sulfate[8] and a greater percutaneous absorption of hydrocortisone by vulvar and forearm skin in premenopausal women[9] than in postmenopausal women. Therefore a diminished barrier capacity of older skin is a misconception.

Cutaneous signs of virilization due to relative hyperandrogenism

Decrease in ovarian hormones

This leaves a clear field for androgens. Nevertheless, ovarian and adrenal androgen production does not increase, and even has a tendency to decrease in post-menopausal women. However, because of the sudden oestradiol decline in menopause and the more gradual progesterone decrease during the pre-menopausal years, the ovarian hormones no longer exert their antiandrogenic effect.

The oestradiol drop leads to a decrease in SHBG (sex-hormone-binding globulin) and consequently to an increase in available free testosterone on receptors. There is a deficiency in progesterone, whose antiandrogenic activity is greater than that of oestradiol, and it no longer plays its antiandrogenic role as a testosterone competitor in enzymatic alpha reduction on the level of the cutaneous receptors.

Finally, synthetic progestogens, usually prescribed in premenopausal women in order to avoid the risks of endogen progesterone deficiency on mammary and uterine targets, increase the spontaneous tendency to hyperandrogenism. By their antigonadotropic activity, they still decrease the ovarian natural progesterone production, without the offsetting advantage of an equivalent antiandrogenic effect. Some synthetic progestogens, particularly the 19-nortestosterone derivatives, are even hyperandrogenic.

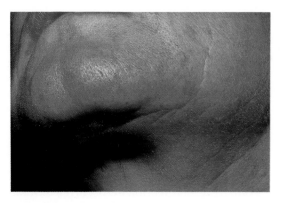

Figure 40.1 The hair grows stronger on the chin, needing frequent epilations.

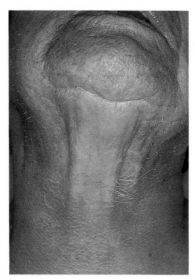

Figure 40.2 Post-menopausal hirsutism.

Progressive development of clinical cutaneous androgenization

The severity of the androgenization is highly variable, according to the genetic programming of cutaneous alpha-reductase activity. But, even if it is mild, this androgenization deeply affects women as a visible loss of their femininity.[10]

- The hair tends to grow stronger, particularly on the face, upper lip and chin (Figure 40.1). Sometimes, real hirsutism may become a hallmark in some older women (Figure 40.2). Although this hirsutism is pronounced on the face, the other androgen-dependent areas of the body are less involved than in young hyperandrogenic women. The ambosexual, axillary and pubic hair become scarce.
- On the other hand, an androgenetic alopecia slowly develops (Figure 40.3). As in younger women, the alopecia may spare the frontal border area of the scalp.[11] If such androgenetic alopecia was present before, it now becomes much more pronounced after menopause. However, in menopausal women, the alopecia is often of a male pattern, also involving the frontal area (Figure 40.4). This process is different from the recently described postmenopausal fibrosing alopecia, with an involvement of eyebrows, corresponding to a variant of lichen planopilaris.[12]
- The sebaceous glands are less influenced by menopause-related hyperandrogenism than

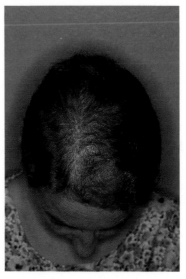

Figure 40.3 Post-menopausal androgenetic alopecia.

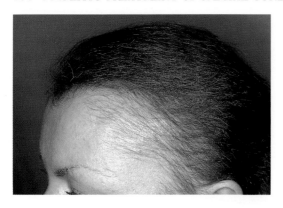

the hair. Even sebum secretion usually decreases, and in physiological conditions does not seem to be androgen dependent in menopausal women. In spite of this, rare post-menopausal acne may occur in darker-skinned, formerly oily-skinned, large-pored women, who usually did not experience adolescent acne. It is a low-grade, long-smouldering acne in which small closed comedones are dominant, and associated with scattered papulopustules.[13]

Sometimes, a mild seborrhoeic dermatitis also appears in post-menopausal women.

HORMONE REPLACEMENT TREATMENT

Above all, hormone replacement treatment (HRT) may prevent or limit aging and the signs of androgenization associated with oestrogenic deficiency. This in fact corresponds to clinical impressions, and in women given a hormone replacement treatment this sudden acceleration in aging and such undesirable signs of androgenization are not normally observed.

Positive effects

Studies based on measurable criteria have revealed positive effects in the various skin components.

- The most well documented work relates to collagen, notably the study of Brincat et al,[14] who found a significant increase in the collagen of menopausal women given various modalities of oestrogenic treatment, either percutaneously or by implant. In women whose menopause occurred several years previously, this increase is distinct above all during the first six months of treatment. The oestrogenic replacement is then therapeutic and prophylactic, whereas it is only prophylactic in women whose menopause is recent and who still have a subnormal level of skin collagen. Brincat et al demonstrated that the oestrogenic effect on skin collagen content is restricted to recovery of the pre-menopausal condition. There is therefore no point in giving oestrogen treatment to women who still present an oestradiol secretion, and cosmetics containing oestradiol, prescribed before menopause or for properly treated menopausal women, do not provide any additional benefit. Varila et al[15] confirmed the increase of collagen in the skin, particularly type I collagen. However Sauvas et al[16] demonstrated an increase in the proportion of type III collagen. The effect of HRT and of oestrogen cream can also be evidenced by non-invasive methods such as B-scan ultrasonography[17,18] showing an increase in skin thickness, and a computerized suction device[19] demonstrating that HRT limits the age-related increase in cutaneous extensibility, and so has a beneficial effect on the mechanical properties of the skin, with a preventive effect on skin slackness.

- Punnonen et al[20] have shown that local treatment with oestriol compared with a placebo improved the structure of the elastic fibres.

- The dermal hyaluronic acid content increases, according to Bentley et al,[21] seven- or eightfold following oestrogen treatment, and hydration of the dermis increases accordingly.
- Punnonen et al[20] have shown that oestrogens usually cause a cellular proliferation and a thickening of the epidermis.
- Using skin microrelief profilometry, Creidi et al[18] have shown a significant improvement of fine wrinkles, although others[17] have found no difference.

Other research, however, is less optimistic: in particular, Bolognia et al[6] failed to record any significant clinical difference in women given 17-β-oestradiol percutaneously for six months; moreover, others[17,22] noted no modification in epidermal hydration in women given the same treatment over a period of 50 days. However, using a plastic occlusion stress test, Pierard-Franchimont et al[23] demonstrated an improvement in skin water-holding capacity.

Oestrogen dose

Irrespective of hormone treatment modalities, for cutaneous effectiveness the oestrogen dose must be sufficient to ensure a plasma oestradiol level of 75 pg/ml, as in the prevention of osteoporosis. Excessively low doses of around 40–50 pg/ml only lead to the disappearance of hot flushes, but are ineffective on the skin and bone.

Oestrogen is prescribed in the form of subcutaneous implants, percutaneous gel or transdermal systems, or orally. In the latter case, β-oestradiol is preferred to ethinyloestradiol in order to avoid intestinal absorption, with the conversion of much of the oestradiol into oestrone. This would result in a greatly increased and non-physiological oestrone/oestradiol ratio, interference with the hepatic metabolism, and its inherent disadvantages for coagulation and the lipid level.

A progestogen is administered in combination over 7–10 days to prevent endometrial hyperplasia.

Hyperandrogeny

The signs of menopausal hyperandrogeny are generally prevented or corrected by the usual replacement therapy, provided that the progestogen is not androgenic.

At menopause, as in the pre-menopausal period, 19-nortestosterone derivatives must therefore be avoided, and a third-generation synthetic progestogen or natural progesterone must be chosen.

If there are already signs of hyperandrogeny, cyproterone acetate must be used. When androgenization is discreet, cyproterone acetate can be prescribed as a progestogen in the conventional replacement regimen. If cyproterone acetate is not available, one can prescribe spironolactones (100–200 mg per day).

COSMETOLOGICAL CARE

The quality of local and especially cosmetological care has an important role to play for the menopausal woman.

Pitfalls to be avoided

Excessively hot, over-frequent and over-long baths or showers, and excessively detergent soaps and foams are deleterious for the fragile skin, which tends to dehydrate and become easily irritated. A single bath, or even better a single shower, per day, taken quickly and without excessively hot water, is sufficient.

Local forms of care

Moisturizing creams

In the menopausal woman, dehydration of the stratum corneum greatly increases the impression of an old, atrophic skin. Extra-fatty soaps or soap-free agents are to be advised for the body. For the face, it is often preferable to use a cleansing milk.

A moisturizing cream is essential for the face. For it to be anti-dehydrating, it must be sufficiently occlusive to slow the loss of water in the stratum corneum, as is the case with a hydrophil/lipophil emulsion type. Certain patients do not like this type of cream, which they find too greasy and unpleasant, cosmetologically speaking. Instead, they can use creams of the lipophil/hydrophil emulsion type, which have proved to be effective thanks to progress in cosmetology, despite their lighter texture. They contain hygroscopic substances that enable the stratum corneum, whose plasticizer is water, to absorb a large quantity.

For the body, the use of a moisturizing cream or milk is desirable – especially in winter, when the skin tends to dehydrate and to dry more. The use of a bath oil, added to the water in the bath or applied to the body after a shower, is also beneficial.

Anti-aging bio-activators

Anti-aging bio-activators are often added to such moisturizing creams. Some of them, such as those containing small quantities of hormones, are on the borderline of cosmetology. In menopausal women following a proper replacement hormone treatment, the use for the face of creams containing oestradiol does not provide any additional benefit. On the other hand, in women presenting genuine contra-indications for replacement therapy, such creams (in which, in principle, the quantity of hormones is too small to have any undesired systematic effect) can be prescribed to slow cutaneous atrophy and in particular collagen loss. Their application must be strictly limited to the face and neck, to avoid any appreciable systemic passage of oestradiol. In certain creams, testosterone is added to the oestradiol. Even if the testosterone doses are still too low to alter the plasma level, and although topical testosterone plays a favourable trophic role on the dermal fibrob-

last and its production of collagen, it seems wise to avoid this input of androgen in menopausal women, who are already relatively hyperandrogenic, given the risk of accentuating the tendency to hirsutism.

Many creams contain collagen, elastin, DNA, various tissue extracts, and essential fatty acids. The penetration of these large molecules into the skin is uncertain, but can perhaps be helped by certain vehicles and especially by liposomes. Even if these substances or their fractions penetrate to where they are theoretically to be used, namely the epidermis and especially the dermis, there is still no clear-cut proof that they are correctly metabolized and integrated to play the anti-aging role they claim. On the other hand, collagen and elastin possess appreciable hydrating and filmogenic properties, and the essential fatty acids restore the integrity of the epidermal barrier, through their integration with membrane phospholipids.

Free-radical inhibitors

Compounds that inhibit the formation of free radicals are often included in the above preparations. While their action has been clearly evidenced when their input is systemic or in vitro and in experimental conditions, their anti-aging efficacy in topical use is much less well documented.

Sunscreen products

Sunscreen products (see Chapters 25 and 26) are obviously strongly recommended for the menopausal woman, to restrict or delay the photo-induced aging process that is associated with that age, to varying degrees.

Topical products considered as medicines

Tretinoin-containing products and *glycolic acid products* should be considered as medicines for which the indications and use are detailed in other chapters. These are intended more for photo-induced effects than for chronological aging or aging related to oestrogenic deficiency. In the menopausal woman, however, all these various causes of aging are closely interconnected, and, even in the case of aging due to hormone deprivation, the subepidermal neo-collagenesis and the epidermal thickening resulting from the use of topical tretinoin produce a very valuable cosmetic effect, with retinoic acid being superior to glycolic acid.[24] Any excessive irritation detrimental to the pursuit of the treatment is to be avoided by applications that increase in frequency according to the quality of the skin and the level of tolerance, and by the alternate application of an effective moisturizing cream.

For the rare cases of post-menopausal acne, topical tretinoin is an effective therapy.

Minoxidil lotions, which are a useful adjuvant for replacement hormone treatment in cases of menopausal androgenic alopecia, are also medicines that must be prescribed by a doctor.

Anti-androgenic topical products, such as progesterone or promestriene creams, have only a very slight transient action, and can never be claimed to attentuate the cutaneous signs of androgenization at menopause. Their prescription, even as a prophylaxis, seems pointless.

Oestrogenic hormone-based topical products are valuable for vulval mucosa only when a replacement therapy is contraindicated, as with the skin.

Techniques for improving the skin of the menopausal woman

Injections of collagen, deep and medium peelings, and above all resurfacing CO_2 laser, are designed more for photo-induced wrinkles and solar elastosis; a lifting is more for cutaneous ptosis of the face and neck.

Menopausal cutaneous atrophy can, however be slightly improved by other forms of peeling (see Chapter 51). Such operations – either very light with Jessner's solution, or more aggressive with resorcin at 50%, and with trichloroacetic acid (at 30% in such indications) – stimulate epidermal proliferation, fibroblastic activity and especially collagenesis.

Electric epilation and perhaps *ruby or Nd:YAG laser or epilight*, combined with replacement treatment and/or the anti-androgenic treatment of menopause, reduces or eliminates hirsutism.

Hair grafts are performed in women only in very pronounced cases of androgenic alopecia.

ENVIRONMENTAL FACTORS

Finally, during menopause, as at all ages, the environmental factors that favour cutaneous aging must never be forgotten. The harmful effects of the sun and the need for protective measures must always be underlined. Also, smoking is responsible not only for a greyish complexion and the accentuation of wrinkles due to deterioration in microcirculation, but also for bringing on an earlier menopause.

REFERENCES

1. Lignieres B. de, Hormones ovariennes et vieillissement cutané. *Gynécol Obstet* 1991; **86:** 151–4.
2. Castelo-Branco C, Pons P, Gratacos E et al, Relationship between skin collagen and bone changes during aging. *Maturitas* 1994; **18:** 199–206.
3. Brincat M, Kabalan S, Studd WW et al, A study of the decrease of skin collagen content, skin thickness and bone mass in the postmenopausal woman. *Obstet Gynecol* 1987; **70:** 840–5.
4. Versi E, Cardozo L, Brincat M et al, Correlation of urethral physiology and skin collagen in postmenopausal women. *Br J Obstet Gynaecol* 1988; **95:** 147–52.
5. May H, Murphy S, Khaw KT, Bone mineral density and its relationship to skin colour in Caucasian females. *Eur J Clin Invest* 1995; **25:** 85–9.
6. Bolognia JL, Braverman IM, Rousseau ME et al, Skin changes in menopause. *Maturitas* 1989; **11:** 295–301.

7. Jamin C, Phanères, peau, ménopause et oestrogénes. *Sém Hôp Paris* 1988; **64:** 1641–7.

8. Elsner P, Wilhelm D, Maibach HI, Sodium lauryl sulfate induced irritant contact dermatitis in vulvar and forearm skin of premenopausal and postmenopausal women. *J Am Acad Dermatol* 1990; **23:** 648–52.

9. Oriba HA, Bucks DAW, Maibach HI, Percutaneous absorption of hydrocortisone and testosterone on the vulva and forearm: effect of the menopause and site. *Br J Dermatol* 1996; **134:** 229–33.

10. Georgala S, Gourgiotou K, Kassouli S et al, Hormonal status in postmenopausal androgenetic alopecia. *Int J Dermatol* 1992; **31:** 858–9.

11. Venning VA, Dawber RP, Patterned androgenic alopecia in women. *J Am Assoc Dermatol* 1988; **18:** 1073–7.

12. Kossard S, Lee MS, Wilkinson B, Postmenopausal frontal fibrosing alopecia: a frontal variant of lichen planopilaris. *J Am Acad Dermatol* 1997; **36:** 59–66.

13. Kligman AM, Postmenopausal acne. *Cutis* 1991; **47:** 425–6.

14. Brincat M, Versi E, Moniz CF et al, Skin collagen changes in postmenopausal women receiving different regimens of oestrogen therapy. *Obstet Gynecol* 1987; **70:** 123–7.

15. Varila E, Rantala I, Oikarinen A et al, The effect of topical oestradiol on skin collagen of postmenopausal women. *Br J Obstet Gynaecol* 1995; **102:** 985–9.

16. Sauvas M, Bishop J, Laurent G et al, Type III collagen content in the skin of postmenopausal women receiving oestradiol and testosterone implants. *Br J Obstet Gynaecol* 1993; **100:** 154–6.

17. Vaillant L, Callens A, Traitement hormonal substitutif et vieillissement cutané. *Therapie* 1996; **51:** 67–70.

18. Creidi P, Faivre B, Agache P et al, Effect of a conjugated oestrogen (Premarin®) cream on aging facial skin. A comparative study with a placebo cream. *Maturitas* 1994; **19:** 211–23.

19. Pierard GE, Letawe C, Dowlati A et al, Effect of hormone replacement therapy for menopause on the mechanical properties of skin. *J Am Geriatr Soc* 1995; **43:** 662–5.

20. Punnomen R, Vaajalahti P, Teisala K, Local oestriol treatment improves the structure of elastic fibers in the skin of postmenopausal women. *Ann Chir Gynaecol* 1987; (Suppl 202): 39–41.

21. Bentley JP, Brenner RM, Linstedt BS et al, Increased hyaluronatic and collagen biosynthesis and fibroblast oestrogen receptors in macaque-sex skin. *J Invest Dermatol* 1986; **87:** 668–73.

22. Jemec GB, Serup J, Short-term effects of topical 17 beta-oestradiol on human post-menopausal skin. *Maturitas* 1989; **11:** 229–34.

23. Pierard-Franchimont C, Letawe C, Goffin V et al, Skin water-holding capacity and transdermal oestrogen therapy for menopause: a pilot study. *Maturitas* 1995; **22:** 151–4.

24. Pierard GE, Henry F, Pierard-Franchimont C, Comparative effect of short-term topical tretinoin and glycolic acid on mechanical properties of photodamaged facial skin in HRT-treated menopausal women. *Maturitas* 1996; **23:** 273–7.

FURTHER READING

Dunn LB, Damesyn M, Moore AA et al, Does estrogen prevent skin aging? *Arch Dermatol* 1997; **133:** 339–42.

Graham-Brown R, Dermatologic problems of the menopause. *Clin Dermatol* 1997; **15:** 143–5.

Mor E, Caspi E, Cutaneous complications of hormonal replacement therapy. *Clin Dermatol* 1997; **15:** 147–54.

PART SEVEN

SKIN CARE FOR SPECIAL GROUPS

41

Cosmetics for men

Robert Baran

INTRODUCTION

Cosmetic needs develop in cycles according to different cultures. They are at present far more limited in the male population than in the female. Dermatologists have now observed a change in male attitudes toward cosmetology, and commonly attribute that change to the combined influences of advertising, the introduction of new ranges of cosmetic products for men, and the influence of women. Men are taking more care of their appearance. They have been conditioned to do so gradually by the availability of a range of products directed toward men only and presented with a masculine orientation. The correct terminology would now appear to be *care* rather than *beauty* as the male market gradually enters the female domain, and male consumers, rather than their wives, become the targets of these products. The potential market comprises virtually all males over the age of 14. Shaving products and hair lotions usually represent a consumer's first contact with men's toiletries. Aftershave balms, emulsions and gels, eau de toilette and eau de cologne are likely to be the products most often sold in specialized departments. Deodorants, bath preparations and shower gels are also popular. Based on a survey by Frost and Sullivan,[1]

nearly half of the masculine grooming business consists of toilet soap (63% of sales are deodorant soaps, 25% are purifying soaps and the rest are specific products). Fitness, freshness, naturalness and, in particular, care are today's key terms for conveying the product message.

Cosmetics for men and women have traditionally been formulated differently. Products for men are usually characterized by the presence of alcohol, which has rarely been used in cosmetics for women. The appeal to the two groups is also distinct, with men seeking well-being and health and women pursuing health and beauty. Men treat their skin in response to a need, such as shaving, cleansing, and treating cuts and nicks. They are less prone to viewing skin care as an aging-prevention or appearance-enhancing practice. Analysts report, however, that this attitude is changing. Some men, they say, are already dipping into their partners' skin-care products. Some men do worry about aging (aging spots, for example) – probably to present an image compatible with their profession. That view is supported by the increasing number of men who seek cosmetic plastic surgery. Moreover, men ask for discreet products labelled 'For Men', which appeal to their virility.

Skin physiology shows differences between

women and men (see Chapter 2).[2] The influence of age and sex on skin thickness, skin collagen and density has been studied by Shuster et al.[3]

- The relationship of skin collagen to sex is obvious. There is a linear decrease in skin collagen with increasing age, and male forearm skin contains more collagen than female skin at the same site at all ages, but the rate of decrease is the same in both sexes, at 1% per year throughout adult life. Male skin is approximately 25% thicker than that of women.
- There is a gradual, but highly significant, thinning of male skin with increasing age. In female skin, however, thickness remains surprisingly constant until the fifth decade, after which there is also a significant thinning with increasing age. At the same age and following the same weathering conditions, wrinkles are more pronounced in male than in female skin.
- There is a highly significant relationship between skin thickness and collagen content in males at all ages. A similar and equally significant relationship has been found among females over 60 years of age, but is not evident in women under 60 years old.
- Collagen density, calculated as the ratio of skin collagen to thickness, is very significantly related to age in both males and females, but the density is consistently lower in females at all ages.

In adult skin, the clinical features of aging are closely related to the total collagen content. Lower initial skin collagen content is therefore the reason women appear to age earlier than men. As far as their skin is concerned, women are about 15 years older than men of the same age throughout their adult life. One reason for the sex difference in skin collagen content may be the difference in androgen production between men and women.[4–6] The packing of fibrils in the dermis is also influenced by age and sex. With increasing age, skin collagen decreases more rapidly than skin thickness, resulting in reduced collagen density. Skin collagen is packed less densely in females than males possibly because of the influence of androgen, since collagen density is increased in patients with primary cutaneous virilism.

The general aspect of the skin of a man is different from that of a woman. The texture is rougher and the stratum corneum thicker. There is a difference in the composition of the sebum. In males over 10, and females over 15 with no present or past acne, sebum excretion (primarily simulated by androgens) increases until the third or fourth decade, and then decreases, the rate of decrease being similar in both sexes.[7] After puberty, sebum production is significantly greater throughout life in males than in females.[7] Greater sebum production results in more severe and long-lasting acne in men. They present dilated pores, sometimes with blackheads.

Puberty also brings about the appearance of facial hair on men, which becomes the focus of their grooming habits.

There are differences in sweat secretion between the sexes. Men have fewer eccrine and apocrine sweat glands. Pubertal sweating is more pronounced on the hands and feet of girls than boys. Male eccrine sudoral secretion is more acid than female. Its pH is about 0.5 lower. Moreover, the rate of sweating in men is more than double that in women.[8] Male eccrine secretion is much greater when stimulated by cholinergic agents or thermogenically, although the difference seen in young adults is attenuated with age. The difference between male and female eccrine secretion is an effect of irreversible gene expression due to androgen at puberty and not to androgen modulation in adult life. The result is that a man's skin needs more rehydrating than a woman's. The lack of protection against weathering by creams and make-up accentuates these physiological differences, which are further aggravated by shaving and microtraumas. The differences between male and female skin becomes especially evident with the onset of puberty. Increased production of androgen is responsible for many of the differences.

Lastly, haircare differs greatly between the sexes. Men and women do not maintain the same standard of haircare – apparently because of psychological differences.

Product prescriptions should respond to masculine needs according to the use, if not the range, of specific preparation. The texture of the product should be light. Creams should be non-greasy, easy to spread and rapidly absorbed. The product should be invisible and not stain. Men's products are more pH-neutral, since their skin is naturally more acid. Men want easy to use products that are non-greasy, easy to spread and only lightly perfumed. Beauty masks and other care products requiring time and patience for application are not popular. Shaving creams containing soap and detergents remove lipids. Shaving itself adds to this process by removing the top layers of skin cells. Finally, lipid removal is further compounded by the use of high-alcohol-content aftershave lotions, which dissolve even more lipids. Skin cells also become temporarily over-hydrated because of the action of detergents and hot water during shaving. The cells later lose water, since they are depleted of the lipids that help them retain moisture, and the result can be dry, flaky cells and dull-looking skin. As a result, an uncomfortable tight-skin feeling frequently develops as the outer cells shrink owing to the water-loss, becoming, in turn, more sensitive to the irritant effects of sweating, sebum and the environment. Regular shaving also causes ingrown beard hairs in some men (see below).

There are several types of products providing cosmetic needs:

- alcoholic perfumery;
- shaving products;
- hair products;
- washing products;
- antiperspirants and deodorants;
- depilatories;
- products for the sun;
- beauty products.

TOILET WATER AND EAU DE COLOGNE

Several motives may play a role in the purchase and use of eau de cologne and shaving lotions by men: creating a personal identity, communicating with others, projecting an appearance of freshness and well-being, and looking neat and self-assured.

SHAVING PRODUCTS

Above all, masculine needs are concentrated on shaving. The importance of the beard is closely linked to a number of psychological factors. The beard has a sexual element, which develops with puberty. The first shave is one of the most important initiation rites whereby a boy becomes a man. Psychological states as diverse as nervous tension, anxiety and overwork can accelerate beard growth. Alcohol abuse can noticeably slow beard growth. Since the beard grows 2 mm a day, shaving is a daily necessity. It has been said that men spend six months of their lives shaving.

Shaving repeatedly injures the skin of the face and neck. It imposes a constant stress on male skin. The outer layers of the stratum corneum are removed by force before the cells are ready to desquamate spontaneously. This forced exfoliation induces an accelerated cell turnover (more than 35%) and exposes skin cells that have not yet been programmed to withstand the effects of the environment. The process of scraping with the razor also results in minute scratches to the outermost layer of the skin. Therefore shaving preparations are a logical answer to a man's main problem.

Pre-shaving products

The most important component in shaving (electric or manual) is the preparation of the skin and beard. The more the beard has been treated before being attacked by the blade, the easier it will be for the razor to slide over the skin. In wet shaving, the aim is to soften and engorge the beard with water so that the hairs offer the least possible resistance to cutting, thus avoiding trauma to the skin. The shaving products contain soaps, syndets and lubricants. Washing with hot water and soap before applying a shaving preparation makes wet shaving much easier. In the case of shaving with an electric razor, stiffness and hardening of the beard is favoured, along with drying and degreasing of the skin. To minimize the risk of irritation, the addition of lipids is indispensable, and the amount of alcohol in the preshave lotion is generally greater than in aftershave lotions. Astringents are added to stiffen the beard.

Special shaving products

Soaps for the beard are not washing soaps. They are more greasy and characterized by a more absorbent, long-lasting, non-drying compact foam. Shaving creams, sometimes called brushless, are especially adapted to dry and sensitive skin, since they provide a better lubricating action than foams. Foaming shaving creams are very soapy emulsions, consisting of 40–50% fatty acids. Aerosol shaving creams employ soaps that are very soluble in water to maintain their effectiveness at low temperatures.

Aftershave products

The use of an aftershave lotion and a warm towel removes all traces of cream and relaxes the skin. Lotions have generally replaced the shaving block, the haemostatic pencil and the vinegar bar – however, some skins are easily cut during shaving, so the use of styptics (alum, aluminium sulfate) is entirely appropriate. Lotions close the pores of the skin, which have been opened by hot water, relieve the burning sensation, stop bleeding from cuts and subtly perfume the skin. In theory, these alcohol-containing lotions should fight infections in cuts caused by the razor blade. The alcohol content is calculated to minimize any sensation of burning. No feeling of discomfort should remain after shaving.

Pathological skin problems related to beard

Shaving with razor blades increases the risk of perfume contact allergy in men[9] – probably because the fragranced lotion is a 'leave-on' product.

The five o'clock shadow observed in heavy dark beards, especially after early shaving, is a non-pathological inconvenience, and should be differentiated from excess skin pigmentation resulting from irritation due to shaving too closely and to a photoreaction caused by the perfume. Transparent facial powder dusted over the entire face is useful to lighten the dark areas.[10]

Existing skin problems may be worsened under beards, but the most common complaint in shaving is bacterial infection of the beard area (barber's itch),[11] usually following an injury to the skin (with any type of razor) or by pseudofolliculitis.

Folliculitis is most often due to staphylococcal infection involving the hair follicle.

Sycosis barbae most often refers to a superficial follicular involvement of the beard area as pustules or papules.

Antimicrobial soaps are effective in reducing the number of bacteria. With antimicrobial topical agents such as fusidic acid and mupirocine, the need for systemic antibiotics is greatly reduced.

Pseudofolliculitis (Figure 41.1) is a common inflammatory disorder of the follicles, most commonly occurring when tightly coiled or very curly hair is closely shaved and the tips of shaved hairs penetrate the follicular wall or grow back to re-enter the skin near the follicle, producing ingrowing hairs.[12] Pseudofolliculitis may also occur if the hairs are

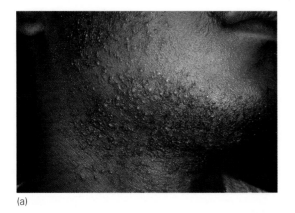

(a)

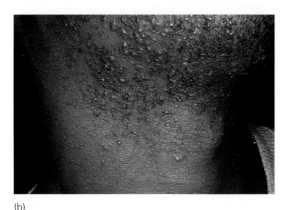

(b)

Figure 41.1 Pseudofolliculitis of the beard. (Courtesy L Dubertret.)

plucked. This condition is extremely common in negroid men, and presents as an eruption of follicular papules or pustules on the sides of the neck and over the angles of the jaw.

Men who cannot or will not stop shaving must, at least, avoid close shaving. A cortisteroid/antibiotic cream may be helpful in mild cases. Retinoic acid and ammonium lactate are very useful. A twice-daily application of 8% glycolic acid lotion is an effective therapy, and allows the patient to resume a daily shaving regimen.[13] The use of depilatory

creams every other day or every three days may be advisable if a topical corticosteroid is used to counteract the irritation caused by the chemical depilatories. Barium sulfide depilatories act rapidly (within 5 minutes). They are the most convenient to use and give the smoothest shave, but they are characteristically malodorous. Calcium thioglycolate depilatories have a mercaptan or sulfide odor, which can be masked with fragrances. However, they do not leave the skin as smooth as do barium sulfide products.[14]

HAIR PRODUCTS

Shampoos

The fundamental aim of any hair care product is to free the hair shaft from its static charge. Anti-dandruff shampoos make up the largest product group.

After-shampoo and hair-setting gels

These are used mainly by young people.

Brillantines

These have become obsolete.

Hair colouring products

Two of the trends currently seen on the United States male market are the tinting of grey hair and staying trim. Despite the attraction of looking 'distinguished', many men prefer the youthful look, and cover up grey areas. As a result, the male hair colouring market is growing.

Metallic gradual hair colours

'Gradual hair colour', often referred to as 'hair colour restorers', are particularly popular among men with grey hair. These products generally consist of an aqueous solution of lead acetate containing suspended sulfur. They are applied daily, as a hair dressing. They are very handy and safe to use.

Unfortunately, the final shade is difficult to control.[15]

Non-metallic progressive hair dye 'Equa ton Homme'

This product is based on the technology of tone-on-tone colouring, which means oxidation colouring without lightening or bleaching. It is a foaming fluid gel, which colours grey hair within 5 minutes, giving a shade similar to the natural shade of hair. It covers grey hair nicely when this averages up to 50% of the hair, always providing a very natural-looking result without any untoward highlights. It is a permanent colouring; that is, it resists shampoos until the next application, which is required only when grey hair has grown again.

'Equa ton Homme' involves the use of two components, which are mixed just prior to application on wet, but not shampooed, hair. One of the components is the gel containing the oxidation dyestuffs (combinations of primary intermediates, e.g. para-dyes such as PPD, and derivatives or analogue modifiers[16]) with foaming agent. The other component is an alkali. Tone-on-tone colouring requires only a mild alkali, in clear contrast with conventional oxidation colouring, which requires ammonia in a sufficient amount to generate enough active oxygen from hydrogen peroxide in order to lighten hair (to even the background shade of hair to which colouring is applied) or to bleach hair (when a lighter shade is desired). Tone-on-tone colouring neither requires nor involves lightening or bleaching of hair.

Repigmenting gel 'Progress Homme'

'Progress Homme' is a product whose colouring agent is a key intermediate in the natural biosynthesis of melanin, namely 5,6-dihydroxyindole (DHI). This is a very sensitive colourless material that reacts easily with oxygen to produce a black pigment that has been shown by electron paramagnetic resonance (EPR) and pyrochromatography to be similar to the natural eumelanin of hair.

DHI is a very unstable material: it is very easily oxidized when exposed to air at ambient temperature. Any trace of metallic impurity leads to rapid oxidization. Therefore it has taken several years to find appropriate conditions for manufacturing DHI and formulating a stable, reliable, marketable product on an industrial scale.

Composition of 'Progress Homme' gel

- DHI
- nonionic surfactant
- gelifier
- stabilizing system
- alcohol, 12% vol.

This product is designed for men with up to 50% grey hair. It gradually repigments grey hair by inducing the formation of natural-like pigment inside the hair. Grey hairs are progressively pigmented, restoring the natural shade of the hair. 'Progress Homme' is suitable for natural blond or brown hair. It is applied for 10–15 minutes (then rinsed) twice a week for approximately 2 weeks, and then every 2 or 3 weeks.

Despite this significant breakthrough and the opening of a new era in hair colouring, this progressive coloration of hair has not gained the popularity it deserves.

Hair thickeners

There has been a surge in the sale of 'thickeners', although these provide only cosmetic benefit and do not help hair restoration.[17]

Minoxidil

Minoxodil is a piperidinopyrimidine derivative and a potent vasodilator, effective orally, for severe hypertension. When applied topically, minoxidil has shown to change vellus to terminal hair. No beneficial effect has been observed in the frontal area of the scalp.

Topical minoxidil appears to be a safe therapy, with side-effects only of local irritation, which is increased with simultaneous use of topical 0.025% retinoic acid. Transitory hypertrichosis in unusual areas (forehead, temples and cheeks) is rare. The explosive eruption of pyogenic granuloma on the scalp due to a topical combination therapy of minoxidil and retinoic acid is exceptional.[18]

Patients should be informed that to maintain any beneficial effect, applications must continue twice daily for life.

Aminexil

Fibrosis of the connective sheath that surrounds the hair follicle has recently been identified as a factor associated with hair aging and loss in alopecic subjects. It may be responsible for shortening blood supply and hindering hair follicle anchoring in the deep dermis.

Perifollicular fibrosis is the result of abnormal changes in collagen production and maturation involving activation of an enzyme that generates collagen crosslinking. A new active ingredient, 2,4-diaminopyrimidine oxide (2,4-DPO or Aminexil), that inhibits the expression of the enzyme implicated lysyl hydroxylase, has been shown to efficiently prevent seasonal hair loss and to contribute to maintaining and improving hair density.

Scalp camouflage

Tattooing and dermopigmentation
These may sometimes improve the aspect of hair transplants.

Hairpieces
The traditional solution for the balding man has been the toupee. The main drawback of the wig has been its attachment. Partial baldness has often been camouflaged by the use of small hairpieces composed of synthetic or natural hair. These may be worn for as long as two months before being reset.

WASHING PRODUCTS

The man of today feels the need to care for his appearance, to stay young and athletic, and to maintain a refined, yet virile, image. He wants products that are pleasant, efficient and simple to use every morning.

Body hygiene products include soaps, soap bars, cleansing liquids, bubble baths (or foam baths), bath salts, body creams and bath oils (or body milks), although bath oils and body milks are rarely used by men. Bath salts are soluble sodium salts in crystalline form, which may be coloured. They soften the water.

These products have a dual role: to soften the skin and to make it supple. They are particularly recommended for athletes, whose skin suffers trauma from the sun, wind, seawater, snow and sweat.

Soaps are composed of fatty acid salts obtained by saponification. In 'soap cakes' (or soap bars), the soap has been replaced by non-ionic synthetic tensio-active ingredients called 'syndets'.

Cleansing liquids are aqueous (or watery) solutions containing tensio-active agents, of neutral or acid pH, which can be added to various substances.

ANTIPERSPIRANTS AND DEODORANTS
(See also Chapters 15 and 37)

Sweating is a very masculine concern, especially when there are malodorous consequences for the feet. Odours are due to

- the sweat constituents of apocrine glands in certain areas – principally the axillae;
- rarely, abnormal constituents in the sweat in metabolic diseases.

These odours result from the bacterial decomposition of the sweat produced by apocrine and eccrine glands. Eccrine bromhidrosis usually emanates from the feet. Excessive secretion produces softening of the stratum corneum, and bromhidrosis occurs as a result of bacterial action on the softened wet keratin. This explains its predilection for the soles of the feet and other intertriginous areas. Eccrine bromhidrosis tends to be maximal in young and middle-aged adults, and is increased by a raised ambient temperature; this contrasts with volar sweating, which is more responsive to emotional stimuli.

Athlete's foot results from the concomitant presence of bacteria, dermatophytes and hyperhidrosis. This latter should be treated along with the infection. Beside the use of fluffy tannic acid, antifungal powder may be very helpful in foot hygiene.

There are two main types of medical treatment: antiperspirants, which attempt to tackle the cause, and fragrances, which seek to mask the result. The distinction between antiperspirants and deodorants is usually confused by the consumer. This may explain some of his dissatisfaction with the results.

Antiperspirants, containing aluminium salts, tend to suppress the production of sweat. Deodorants, which may contain mild antibacterials such as benzethonium chloride or triclosan, are usually well perfumed. They work by masking the body odour (i.e. competing with it), destroying the smell (rare) or trapping the odour. For palmoplantar hyperhidrosis, tap water iontophoresis has been established as the most effective and inexpensive therapeutic modality.[19]

DEPILATORIES

At present, these are primarily used by athletes and transvestites.

There are four main types of hair removal.

- *Mechanical depilation* uses wax.
- *Chemical depilation* is used especially as a treatment for pseudofolliculitis of the neck (see above).
- *Electrolysis* is the only permanent method of hair removal, involving destruction of the hair root with an electric current. Today, a modified high-frequency electric current is used to destroy the hair by electrocoagu-

lation. This has the advantage that it requires less time than true electrolysis. This technique is not recommended for large areas such as arms and legs.
- *Lasers* may be a new tool in the near future.

PRODUCTS FOR THE SUN

See Chapters 25 and 26.

BEAUTY PRODUCTS

Apart from actors and transvestites using cosmetics designed for women, the market for make-up products is limited. It is restricted to bronzing gels, transparent facial powder and facial cover sticks designed to mask skin blemishes.[10] Green facial cover sticks camouflage a reddish complexion by producing a brown tone.

Colourless nail polish dermatitis is of little significance. Only four cases have appeared in the literature between 1925 and 1993.[20]

CONCLUSIONS

We are far from a return to 'Louis-XV-type' pampering by males, but with increased education of men with regard to the need for skin care beyond daily basic grooming, the male skin care market will experience the growth expansion that many have been predicting for years.

REFERENCES

1. Anon, The US male. *SPC* 1990; **63:** 29–31.
2. Tur E, Physiology of the skin – differences between women and men. *Clin Dermatol* 1997; **15:** 5–16.
3. Shuster S, Black MM, McVitie E, Influence of age and sex on skin thickness, skin collagen and density. *Br J Dermatol* 1975; **93:** 639–43.
4. Shuster S, Black MM, Bottoms E, Skin collagen and thickness in women with hirsuties. *Br Med J* 1970; **iv:** 772.

5. Black MM, Shuster S, Bottoms E, Osteoporosis, skin collegan and androgen. *Br Med J* 1970; **iv:** 773.

6. Burton JL, Johnson C, Libman L, Shuster S, Skin virilism in women with hirsutism. *J Endocrinol* 1972; **53:** 349.

7. Cunliffe WJ, Shuster S, Pathogenesis of acne. *Lancet* 1969; **i:** 685–7.

8. Rees J, Shuster S, Pubertal induction of sweat gland activity. *Clin Sci* 1981; **60:** 689–92.

9. Edman B, The influence of shaving method on perfume allergy. *Contact Dermatitis* 1994; **31:** 291–2.

10. Draelos ZK, *Cosmetics in Dermatology*, 2nd edn. Edinburgh: Churchill Livingstone, 1995.

11. Schoen LA, Lazar P, *The Look You Like*. New York: Marcel Dekker, 1990.

12. Rook A, Dawber RPR (eds), *Diseases of the Hair and Scalp*, 2nd edn. Oxford: Blackwell, 1991.

13. Pericone NV, Treatment of pseudofolliculitis barbae with topical glycolic acid. *Cutis* 1993; **52:** 232–5.

14. Halder RH, Pseudofolliculitis barbae and related disorders. *Dermatol Clin* 1988; **6:** 407–12.

15. Corbett JF, Hair care products. In: *Clinical Dermatology* (Demis J, ed.). Philadelphia: Lippincott-Raven, 1996:2–44.

16. Zviak C, *Science des Traitements Capillaires*. Paris: Masson, 1988:235–86.

17. Simpson NB, Barth JH, Hair patterns. Hirsuties and baldness. In: *Diseases of the Hair and Scalp*, 2nd edn (Rook AJ, Dawber RPR, eds). Oxford: Blackwell, 1991:71–135.

18. Baran R, Explosive eruption of pyogenic granuloma on the scalp due to a topical combination therapy of minoxidil and retinoic acid. *Dermatologica* 1989; **179:** 76–8.

19. Sloan JB, Soltani K, Iontophoresis in dermatology. *J Am Acad Dermatol* 1986; **15:** 671.

20. Hausen BM, Nagellack-Allergie. *Z Hautkr* 1994; **69:** 252–62.

42

Cosmetic dermatology in children

Danielle Marcoux, John Harper

INTRODUCTION

Skin hygiene practices vary within different cultures, and historically attitudes have changed. For centuries, soiled skin, scalp and hair were socially accepted. The causes for this lack of hygiene were partly neglect and lack of time, but more importantly lack of water in the home, the fear of making a child sick with a cold, or even superstitious and religious beliefs. For example, cradle cap was seen as a sign of good health, indicating that the child was taking all the benefits from breastmilk. Head lice were even believed at one time to clear the child's blood of detrimental humours or influences.

In comparison, at the end of the 20th century, in many households, a daily routine of washing and grooming is practised from the first days of life and reflects parental loving attention. Over the last decade, occidental countries have seen a booming market for baby products. In the United States, sales will soon reach 630 million US dollars and correspond to 2.5% of the total cosmetic and toiletries market.[1] The consumers of this market are a rising number of children with concerned parents financially able to buy the best and safest products for their offspring. Baby products are also widely used by older chil-

dren, teenagers and adults with sensitive skin seeking the safest products, which is what this market is claiming to offer.

The different categories of products that are used in infancy, childhood and the teenage years include detersion products such as shampoos and soaps, which are rinse-off products, and protection products, such as protective creams for diaper dermatitis, sunscreens and hydrating products, which are leave-on products.

A prospective study conducted by questionnaire in Illinois, USA, has shown that the average term newborn has 8 ± 3 skin care products applied, with a resultant exposure to 48 ± 18 different chemicals. The average one-month-old baby was bathed four times a week and was shampooed three times weekly.[2]

SKIN PERMEABILITY IN NEWBORN AND YOUNG CHILDREN

The full-term infant has a well-developed epidermis that possesses excellent barrier properties. By contrast, the infant who is born prematurely, particularly before 30 weeks gestation, has a thin epidermis with a poorly developed stratum corneum. Although rapid postnatal maturation occurs over the first two to three weeks of age, the preterm infant's skin is a poor barrier in the early neonatal period.[3,4] Two important effects of this are a high transepidermal water loss, leading to difficulties in fluid balance and temperature control, and absorption of topically applied agents. The latter has therapeutic and toxicological implications.[5] It is possible to administer drugs for systemic effect by the transdermal route (e.g. theophylline[6]), and it is possible for preterm infants to be inadvertently poisoned by agents that are in contact with the skin (e.g. aniline dyes, hexachlorophene, methylated spirits and neomycin).

In infants, care should be taken using topical agents because of the higher skin surface-to-weight ratio than adults and therefore the increased risk of toxicity from percutaneous absorption.

SAFETY ASPECTS AND TOXICITY TESTING[7]

Baby- and child-oriented toiletry products should have high requirements with regards to safety. Although, as of today, there are no government requirements for toxicity testing of baby care products, it is essential that manufacturers carry out appropriate toxicity tests on all new baby care or child products, and this is effectively done by responsible manufacturers. In some countries, mandatory listing of ingredients is enforced.

The repeated insult patch test (RIPT) performed over a six-week period will help predict an allergic sensitization. A 1% dilution of a shampoo or a full-strength conditioner or cleansing product is applied to the skin under occlusion for nine 24-hour induction tests over a three-week period. After a two-week rest, a final application is made. The site is scored for erythema and oedema. The test is applied on 100–200 volunteers. The cumulative irritation test (CIT) implies a two or three week repeated application of the tested product at the same cutaneous site. Phototoxicity and photoallergy testing are also performed to determine whether a product is a photoirritant or a photoallergen.

Another important safety consideration is that, because they frequently get into the eyes, products for babies and children should have a low eye and skin irritancy potential. Eye sting is an immediate but temporary pain sensation, while palpebral or conjunctival irritation is gradual and progressive.[1]

Ocular toxicity testing is therefore of prime importance for the manufacturer to select the ideal formulation with the least risk of ocular symptoms. The classic tests are the ocular sting test, in which one drop of either a diluted shampoo or cleansing product or an undiluted conditioner is instilled in one eye of the subject. One drop of distilled water or another test material is put into the second eye. Over a 1–2 hour period, the amount of sting is recorded. An ophthalmologist will also record the amount of ocular and palpebral irritation as well as lacrimation over the same period of time.

Of course, toiletry products should remain free of microbial contamination throughout their usage life.

DETERSION PRODUCTS

Shampoos[1,8,9]

In the United States, baby shampoos make up 14.5% of the baby care product category.[1] The main goal of shampoos is to cleanse the scalp and hair of sebum, keratin fragments and dust, and of cosmetic residues in older users. In older children, cosmetic benefits such as providing gloss, softness, combability, bounce and volume to hair might be desired. Also, some therapeutic benefits can be obtained, for example, with the use of anti-dandruff shampoos in teenagers.

Cleansing is achieved by surfactants whose chemical structure allows linking to fatty material by their hydrocarbon fatty chain, and water solubility and rinsibility by their hydrophilic polar group.

Surfactants are classified according to their ionic charges. Anionic surfactants, negatively charged, are widely used in shampoos. Lauryl sulfate, for example, has good cleansing and foaming properties, but can be irritating to the eye. Cationic surfactants are very substantive to hair because of their positive charge, but, although they provide good conditioning, they can also cause eye irritation and therefore are not used in baby shampoo formulations. Amphoterics, both positively and negatively charged, either betaine- or imidazoline-derived, are widely used in baby hair care products, since they are very well tolerated. Because of their anti-irritant effect, they are often associated with anionic surfactants, which otherwise would not be well tolerated by themselves. Non-ionic surfactants are also widely used in baby hair care products, while saponin still has not really found a niche in this market.

Eye irritancy and sting are greater with cationic than with anionic or non-ionic surfactants. Also, one must take into account the surface activity of the formulation, pH, wetting power, foaming power, and combinations of these. The pH of the shampoo should be close to lacrimal pH. Usually, skin irritation does not occur with shampoos that have a low eye-irritancy potential.

Baby shampoo formulations must have certain characteristics to minimize eye sting and irritation. They should avoid highly detersive or foaming agents. They usually include ingredients that act as anti-irritant or detoxifying agents. The industry has now developed modified surfactants that have a lower irritancy potential, such as alkylether sulfates. Also, combining certain surfactant mixtures will result in a lower irritancy level than the individual components would have by themselves.

The basic components of all shampoos are water, a mixture of principal cleansing surfactants, and secondary foam-producing surfactants. Thickeners, such as gums or salts, are added to increase the shampoo's viscosity, which makes hair and scalp application easier, and reduces the risk of the shampoo running into the eye. Conditioning agents, such as fatty materials or cationic polymers, will make hair easier to untangle and more glossy. This attribute is sought in shampoos for children over the age of five.

Preservatives have to be used in shampoos because of the high water content, to avoid bacterial or mould contamination.

Fragrances and colouring are used to make the product more attractive. Chelating or sequestering agents, such as ethylene diamine tetraacetic acid (EDTA) or citric acid, will prevent the formation of heavy metal precipitation, the discoloration of the product and the rancidity of oils. For example, shampoos may be processed in steel equipment, and chelating agents will keep the iron 'in solution'.

Pearlescents and opacifiers are found mostly in adult shampoos. Usually baby and children's shampoos are crystal-clear.

Special care ingredients, such as tar, salicylic acid, selenium sulfide and zinc pyrithione, may be added for seborrhoeic dermatitis.

It is not always clear what certain promotional additives do for shampoos, other than appealing to consumers, particularly if the additive is following the fashion of the moment. This can apply to a variety of 'natural' ingredients that are today included in the formulations of different shampoos and cosmetics.

Taking into account the wide range and number of baby and children's shampoos sold in a one-year period, it is clear that adverse reactions are rare. Eye sting or ocular irritation is the primary concern, and, in spite of thorough testing, it might still occur with certain products. Of course, it is to be expected with the use of products that are not formulated to minimize this risk. Hair dryness can occur because of the small quantity of conditioning agents used in the formulation. If parents wash a child's hair and rinse it, allowing the child to sit in the bathtub to play for a period of time, there is a prolonged contact of the sensitive mucosa with the surfactants, fragrance and other materials of the shampoo. This can lead to urethritis[10] or vulvovaginitis.[11] To remedy this, a change in the mode of hair washing is necessary.

Adverse reactions to shampoos on the skin are rare, because they are wash-off products that are used diluted and that remain in contact with the skin for only a short time. Contact urticaria or irritant dermatitis from inadequately rinsed shampoo are reported, although, as mentioned, skin irritation is rare with shampoos that have a low ocular irritancy potential. Allergic contact dermatitis has not, as far as we are aware, been reported in children.

Skin cleansing agents[9,12,13]

A daily bath in tepid water at a 37°C temperature at most is adequate to cleanse the newborn's soiled skin folds and perineal areas.

Skin cleansing agents include soaps, which are made from lipids and an alkaline base, forming fatty acid salts with detersion properties, or syndets, which are synthetic detergents usually formulated with lauryl sulfate derivatives. They are formulated as fatty or non-fatty bars of soaps or syndets, as liquids or as gels, in which different additives can be included. For example, lipids might be added for a superfatted soap, sugars or glycerol for a transparent soap, antimicrobials for a deodorant soap, and abrasive particles for exfoliating purposes.

With cleansing agents, delipidation and a secondary irritant contact dermatitis can occur. The factors in relation to the irritancy potential of soaps and syndets are the chemical structure with a short carbon chain, an alkaline pH and the detergency power.[9] The potential for irritancy is evaluated by the cutaneous irritancy chamber test,[14] and has been shown to be least with superfatted and neutral soaps and most severe with some antiseptic and abrasive soaps.

In recent years, with the growth of travel, the need to keep babies clean while away from home and their ease of use, baby wipes have become very popular. Wipes contain a blend of water-based cleansers, often with skin emollients to effectively remove faecal residues and leave a protective film on the skin. Some babies develop irritation secondary to fragrances in the wipes.

To cleanse babies' skin, a mild neutral pH soap or syndet, which can be superfatted, is appropriate. Gentle cleansing implies the use of a mild product and avoidance of overuse. The same applies for sensitive atopic skin. In adolescents with sebhorrhoea and acne, again a mild cleansing agent is indicated in cases of sensitive skin. At times, if tolerated, cleansing agents with additives such as oat, salicylic acid, sulfur or benzoyl peroxide might be useful to produce astringency and mild exfoliation of superficial acne lesions. Abrasive cleansers have not been shown to be of help in acne cases.[15] Furthermore, any cleansing agents that are too abrasive or irritant would decrease the tolerance to topical treatments. An antiseptic soap or cleansing agent might also be of help for body odours or for limited cases of folliculitis.

Skin cleansing of atopic eczema is often seen to be inadequate. The current recommendation would be a regular daily bath using an appropriate mild cleansing agent,[16] and for severe eczema twice-daily bathing. Improvement is attributed to gentle debridement of crusts and scales and to the reduction of *Staphylococcus aureus* colonization.[17] The addition of an oil bath additive can be useful, and is usually well tolerated.

SKIN PROTECTION

Protective creams for diaper dermatitis

An anatomical area of much concern in babies' skin protection is the diaper area.

Moist occlusion, increased coefficient of skin friction, maceration and primary irritant dermatitis due to constant wetness, faecal proteases, lipases, bile salts and an alkaline pH are most frequently responsible for diaper dermatitis.[18] Ammonia – once thought to be a major offender – will only cause an irritant dermatitis when in contact with an already damaged skin, and will also contribute to increase the pH. Diaper dermatitis can easily become superinfected by *Candida albicans* by *Staphylococcus aureus* and, more rarely, by *Streptococcus pyogenes*. There appears to be a correlation between the quantity of faecal *C. albicans* and the severity of diaper dermatitis.[19,20]

Prevention of diaper dermatitis is achieved by keeping the skin dry and promoting the evaporation of moisture. Frequent changes of cloth or cellulose core diapers can be adequate, although absorbent gelling material consisting of crosslinked sodium polyacrylate polymers in disposable diapers has been shown to be superior in absorbing more humidity and decreasing the prevalence of diaper dermatitis.[21,22] Protective preparations used include lotions, creams or ointments containing emollients, to which might be added kaolin, talc or zinc oxide. The pH is usually slightly acidic to approximate that of normal skin and to act as a buffer against the higher pH due to the presence of ammonia. If the diaper dermatitis is severe, an anti-*Candida*–hydrocortisone preparation might be necessary for five to seven days. The presence of peripheral desquamation and satellite papules and pustules is indicative of candidial superinfection and should be treated with oral and topical nystatin or imidazole. In addition, a severe seborrhoeic dermatitis during the first three months of life may affect the inguinal folds and the perineal area. Rarer causes of diaper dermatitis include tinea, psoriasis. Langherans cell histiocytosis and acrodermatitis enteropathica.

Baby powders

In spite of medical reports about the risks of aspiration,[23–25] baby powders are still used in 47%[2] to 69%[26] of households for infant care. Baby powders usually contain starch or talc in respective proportions of 23% and 87% of products on the American market. They are hygroscopic, will help absorb moisture, and will decrease friction and maceration. As lubricants, they spread easily and feel smooth on the skin. Talc is a powder of hydrous magnesium silicate ($Mg_3Si_4O_{10}\cdot H_2O$). Its chemical structure is similar to that of asbestos, which is also a mineral magnesium silicate. Both can be found in the same mineral deposits, and in the 1970s it was found that some talc samples were contaminated with asbestos.[27] Today, cosmetic-grade talc requires the major component to be mineral talc, free of asbestos. In an American study performed a few years ago, accidental baby powder inhalation accounted for approximately 1% of calls to poison control centres.[25] The inhalation of talc can result in an inflammation that may lead to granuloma formation and fibrosis, and in the most severe cases to pulmonary insufficiency and death. Today, because of the risk of baby powder inhalation, many pediatricians discourage the use of powders in infant care.

It has been shown that cornstarch and talc powder do not enhance the growth of yeasts on human skin and do provide protection against frictional injury.[28] Powders should be gently padded in intertriginous areas – not dusted or shaken, in order to avoid inhalation.

Sunscreens

The annual UVB dose received by children tends to be significantly greater than that received by adults, because of frequent exposure in outside activities.[29]

With the knowledge that we now have of the short- and long-term consequences of excessive sun exposure, ultraviolet radiation protection should be practised from an early age.[29,30] This requires adequate information and enforcement by parents, who should set an example. The message must be that children should be protected from overexposure to the sun from the day they are brought home from the hospital.[29] It would seem reasonable to use sunscreens on babies under the age of six months, although there is little toxicological data for this age group. Common sense should dictate that sun avoidance and physical protection with clothing should be practised in this age group. Children with a lighter phototype, with multiple naevi[31] or with a positive family history for skin cancer are those who most require protection. Surveys have shown that only a minority of children and teenagers use sunscreens consistently when exposed to ultraviolet radiation.[32,33] Some used plain emollient as sunscreens or used sunscreens to promote tanning.

A sunscreen agent with an SPF of 15 is usually adequate. The stronger sunscreens can be used in certain situations of extreme exposure (boating, beaching, high altitude, etc.), but are not necessary for everyday use. It has been estimated by a mathematical model that regular use of a sunscreen with an SPF of 15 during the first 18 years of life will decrease the risk of basal and squamous cell carcinoma by 78%.[33] It will also prevent immediate sunburns and accelerated photoaging, and possibly melanoma. Malignant melanoma is associated with intense, sporadic sun exposure and painful blistering sunburns in childhood.[34-36]

Sunscreen products have been developed specifically for children. The only differences between these and the adult products are that they do not contain *p*-aminobenzoic acid (PABA) or fragrances, and they are usually waterproof so that sweating or bathing do not remove them. Hypoallergenic formulations of sunscreens have similar characteristics.

Vitamin D deficiency has been a preoccupation, because it has been shown that the chronic application of a PABA sunscreen will decrease the photosynthesis of 17-dehydrocholesterol (17-DHC) in previtamin D.[37] Therefore it is suggested that elderly people take 200 IU of vitamin D daily.[38] However, no supplement is indicated for children, since their sun exposure is much greater and they consume dietary vitamin D supplements, particularly from dairy products.[29] Reported adverse effects are stinging or burning of the skin or eyes, often due to surfactants. Contact urticaria and allergic contact dermatitis occur rarely. Occasional irritant contact dermatitis is reported, which can aggravate a pre-existing dermatitis such as atopic dermatitis.

Avoidance of sun exposure between 10 am and 2 pm (11 a.m. to 3 p.m. daylight saving time) will reduce by up to 60% the total potential daily dose of sunlight that is received. Protective clothing such as a sunhat and shirt should be worn when exposed to the sun for a prolonged period of time. It has been shown that hats with a wide (>7.5 cm) brim provide reasonable protection factor around the nose and cheeks.[39] Furthermore, suntanning parlours and sun lamps, favoured by some youngsters, should be discouraged, since they increase the risk of skin cancers, photodamage and eye damage in the long term. Contrary to popular belief, the tan obtained in suntan parlours does not act as effective protection against sunburn from natural sun rays. In fact, it only provides an SPF of 3.[40]

Throughout the world, teenagers' lack of photoprotection remains a major health concern. In Australia, 70% of teenagers were exposed from two to eight hours a day without sun protection.[41] In the United States, only 9% used sun protection, and one-third had experienced severe sunburns during the two previous summers.[42] In France, two-thirds of teenagers were overexposed to the sun.[43] In Norway, although 90% used sunscreens, only one-quarter used products with an adequate SPF.[44] Teenagers expose themselves to the sun and use tanning salons to enhance their appearance. They perceive suntans as healthy and attractive.[45] They will seek protection if convinced that the sun's effects are deleterious to their appearance.[46] The fashion and cosmetic industries can be very influential on teenagers perception of the risks of unprotected and excessive sun exposure.

Children should be educated early as to the importance of sunscreen and sun protection, and are greatly influenced by parental attitudes. The American Academy of Dermatology with the American Cancer Society has developed a teaching programme called 'Children's Guide to Sun Protection', aimed at different age groups from kindergarten through elementary school. A similar programme is taking place in Canada and Australia. It is to be hoped that these educational programmes will increase awareness and practices for sun protection.

Hydrating agents

Dry skin is not uncommon in children. Exogenous causes of dry skin include environmental factors such as climate (particularly northern winters) and central heating dehydrating ambient air and consequently the epidermis. Dry skin can be secondary to certain treatments such as lindane, retinoic acid and benzoyl peroxide. Among the endogenous causes, atopic dermatitis and ichthyosis vulgaris are the most frequent. Over the past 20 years, the incidence of atopic dermatitis in infants has increased considerably in several western countries. Skin care creams and ointments that provide a high level of moisturization can restore barrier properties, and are useful in helping to manage atopic dermatitis.

To maintain a normal hydration to the stratum corneum, emollients, which are usually oleagenous and occlusive such as petrolatum and lanolin, are used, and will help to reduce transepidermal water loss and act as skin protectants. Humectants, such as lactic acid, urea and glycerol, will capture water from ambient air or the epidermis, and are used mostly in ichthyotic disorders. They can be poorly tolerated, causing a stinging sensation on inflamed skin. The classic formulation of a hydrating lotion comprises 60–80% water, 30–40% lipids, low quantities of surfactants, preservatives, fragrances and colourants.

ADVERSE REACTIONS

Cosmetics for children are generally safe, with only rare instances of reported adverse effects. On the skin, an irritant contact dermatitis can be observed, and rarely an allergic contact dermatitis. A Netherlands study[47] showed that in an overall-tested population only 2.5% of patients were younger than 16 years old. In only one-quarter of them was a positive epicutaneous test considered to be clinically relevant. Balsam of Peru, fragrance mix and colophony accounted for 6% each of positive reactions. Contact urticaria has also been reported, as well as photosensitivity reactions. Mucosal irritation of the genitalia or of the conjunctiva can also occur.

Brittleness and dullness of hair are reported with the use of baby shampoos – mostly on hair that was previously damaged and that required the use of conditioners. Residues occur secondarily to accumulated hair setting agents or soap shampoos.

Systemic intoxication can occur owing to accidental ingestion of cosmetic products. Depending on the country, intoxication by cosmetic products represents 2.3–6% of all systemic intoxications recorded by different poison control centres (France, Belgium, Switzerland, Italy, the United States and the United Kingdom). In France, cosmetics are sixth on the list of categories of products responsible for accidental systemic intoxication.[48] Children, mostly boys, aged 18 months to 3 years account for 84% of intoxication cases. One out of forty require medical attention. At the Centre Anti-Poison de Paris in 1989, foaming agents such as shampoos accounted for 35% of the products responsible for intoxication in the cosmetic category, alcoholic fragrances for another 24%, and nail solvents for 12%. Systemic toxicity from topically applied cosmetics is exceptional, but sad historic cases of hexachlorophene poisoning can be recalled, as well as lead or mercury poisoning from topicals used culturally by some immigrants from developing countries.[49]

Applying the following recommendations should help to prevent occurrences of adverse effects in children from cosmetics. At home, parents should dispose of toiletries safely and educate children early not to put them into their mouths. Users should always follow the instructions for use. Manufacturers should devise safe packaging to avoid misuse by infants or children, with precautions clearly printed when required. Listing of ingredients should also be mandatory, and pressure should be put on governments to enforce this.

Of course, poison control centres should have easily available databanks on previous incidents of intoxication, as well as toxicity profiles of all product ingredients.

CONCLUSIONS

Cosmetic products for infants, children and teenagers are useful and effective for hygiene and detersion and for skin protection from environmental factors. Proper care and grooming will help maintain the integrity of skin and its appendages, and can prevent the deterioration of certain skin disorders and, in the long term, more deleterious effects, particularly those due to ultraviolet radiation exposure.

REFERENCES

1. Lindemann MKO, The design of baby care products. *Happi* Oct 1991; 44–50.
2. Cetta F, Lambert GH, Ros SP, Newborn chemical exposure from over-the-counter skin care products. *Clin Pediatr* 1991; **30:** 286–9.
3. West DP, Halkett JM, Harvey DR et al, Percutaneous absorption in preterm infants. *Pediatr Dermatol* 1987; **4:** 234–7.
4. Barker N, Hadgraft J, Rutter N, Skin permeability in the newborn. *J Invest Dermatol* 1987; **88:** 409–11.
5. Rutter N, Percutaneous drug absorption in the newborn: hazards and uses. *Perinatal Pharmacol* 1987; **14:** 911–30.
6. Evans NJ, Rutter N, Hadgraft J, Parr G. Percutaneous administration of theophylline in the preterm infant. *J Pediatr* 1985; **107:** 307–11.
7. Harrison Research Laboratories, Inc, Personal Communication, May 1992.
8. Zviak C, Vanlerbergh E, Scalp and hair hygiene. Shampoos. In: *The Science of Hair Care* (Zviak C, ed.). New York: Marcel Dekker, 1986:49–86.
9. Morelli JG, Weston WL, Soaps and shampoos in pediatric practice. *Pediatrics* 1987; **80:** 634–7.
10. Rogers WB, Shampoo urethritis (letter). *Am J Dis Child* 1985; **139:** 748–9.
11. Brown JL, Hair shampoo technique and pediatric vulvovaginitis. *Pediatrics* 1989; **83:** 146.
12. Willcox MJ, Crichtow WP, The soap market. A review of current trends. *Cosmetics and Toiletries* 1989; **104:** 61–3.
13. Duke Strube D, The irritancy of soaps and syndets. *Cutis* 1987; **39:** 544–5.
14. Frosh PJ, Kligman AM, The soap chamber test. A new method for assessing the irritancy of soaps. *J Am Acad Dermatol* 1979; **1:** 35–41.
15. Mills OH, Kligman AM, Evaluation of abrasives in acne therapy. *Cutis* 1979; **23:** 704–5.
16. Rasmussen JE, Advances in non dietary management of children with atopic dermatitis. *Pediatr Dermatol* 1987; **6:** 210–15.
17. Uehara M, Takada K, Use of soap in the management of atopic dermatitis. *Clin Exp Dermatol* 1985; **10:** 419–25.
18. Berg RW, Etiologic factors in diaper dermatitis: a model for development of improved diapers. *Pediatrician* 1987; **14** (Suppl 1): 27–33.
19. Aly R, Shirley C, Cunico B et al, Effect of prolonged occlusion on the microbial flora, pH, CO_2 and transepidermal water loss. *J Invest Derm* 1978; **71:** 378–81.
20. Jordan WE, Lawson KD, Berg RW et al, Diaper dermatitis. Frequency and serverity among a general infant population. *Pediatr Dermatol* 1986; **3:** 198–207.
21. Lane AT, Rehder PA, Helm K, Evaluation of diapers containing absorbent gelling material with

conventional disposable diapers in newborn infants. *Am J Dis Child* 1990; **144**: 315–18.

22. Campbell RL, Seymour JL, Stone LC et al, Clinical studies with disposable diapers containing absorbent gelling materials: evaluation of effects on infant skin condition. *J Am Acad Dermatol* 1987; **17**: 978–87.

23. Reyes de la Rocha S, Brown MA, Normal pulmonary function after baby powder inhalation causing adult respiratory distress syndrome. *Pediatr Emerg Care* 1989; **5**: 43–8.

24. McCormick MA, Lacouture PG, Gaudreault P et al, Hazards associated with diaper changes. *J Am Med Assoc* 1982; **248**: 2159–60.

25. Mofenson HC, Greensher J, Ditomasso A et al, Baby powder – a hazard. *Pediatrics* 1981; **68**: 265–6.

26. Hayden GF, Sproul GT, Baby powder use in infant skin care. Parents' knowledge and determinants of powder usage. *Clin Pediatr* 1984; **23**: 163–5.

27. Natow AJ, Talc: Need we beware? *Cutis* 1986; **37**: 328–9.

28. Leyden JJ, Cornstarch, *Candida albicans* and diaper rash. *Pediatr Dermatol* 1984; **1**: 322–5.

29. Hurwitz S, The sun and sunscreen protection: recommendations for children. *J Dermatol Surg Oncol* 1988; **14**: 657–80.

30. Marks R, Skin cancer – childhood protection affords lifetime protection. *Med J Aus* 1987; **147**: 475–6.

31. Holman CDJ, Armstrong BK, Heenan PJ, Relationship of cutaneous malignant melanoma to individual sunlight-exposure habits. *J Natl Cancer Inst* 1986; **76**: 403–14.

32. Sherertz EF, Pupo RA, Russin NM, Sun protection for children: practices of mothers and pediatricians. *Skin Cancer Found J* 1986; **4**: 3785.

33. Stern RS, Weinstein MC, Baker SS, Risk reduction for non melanoma skin cancer with childhood sunscreen use. *Arch Dermatol* 1986; **122**: 537–45.

34. Elwood JM, Gallagher RP, Hill GB, Pearson JC, Cutaneous melanoma in relation to intermittent and constant sun exposure. The Western Canada Melanoma Study. *Int J Cancer* 1985; **35**: 427–33.

35. Urbach F, Bailar JC, Demopoulos H et al, Ultraviolet radiation and skin cancer in man. *Prev Med* 1980; **9**: 227–30.

36. Fitzpatrick TB, Sover AJ, Editorial: Sunlight and skin cancer. *N Engl J Med* 1985; **313**: 818–20.

37. Matsuoka LY, Wortsman J, Hanifan N et al, Chronic sunscreen use decreases circulating concentrations of 25-hydroxyvitamin D. A preliminary study. *Arch Dermatol* 1988; **124**: 1802–4.

38. Prystowsky JH, Photoprotection and the vitamin D status of the elderly. *Arch Dermatol* 1988; **124**: 1844–8.

39. Diffey BL, Cheeseman J, Sun protection with hats. *Br J Dermatol* 1992; **127**: 10–12.

40. Rivers JK, Norris PG, Murphy GM et al, UVA sunbeds: tanning, photoprotection, acute adverse effects and immunological changes. *Br J Dermatol* 1989; **120**: 767–77.

41. Fritschi L, Green A, Solomon PJ, Sun exposure in Australian adolescents. *J Am Acad Dermatol* 1992; **27**: 25–8.

42. Banks BA, Silverman RA, Schwartz RH, Tunnesen WW Jr, Attitudes of teenagers towards sun exposure and sunscreen use. *Pediatrics* 1992; **89**: 40–2.

43. Grob JJ, Guglielmina C, Gouvernet J, Study of sunbathing habits in children and adolescents: application to the prevention of melanoma. *Dermatology* 1993; **186**: 94–8.

44. Wichstrom L, Predictors of Norwegian adolescents' sunbathing and use of sunscreen. *Health Psychol* 1994; **13**: 412–20.

45. Broadstock M, Borland R, Sason R, Effects of suntan on judgements of healthiness and attractiveness by adolescents. *J Am Soc Psychol* 1992; **22**: 157–72.

46. Jones JL, Leary MR, Effects of appearance-based admonitions against sun exposure on tanning intentions in young adults. *Health Psychol* 1994; **13**: 86–90.

47. Kuiters GRR, Sillevis Smitt JH, Cohen EB et al, Allergic contact dermatitis in children and young adults. *Arch Dermatol* 1989; **125**: 1531–3.

48. Riboulet-Delmas G, Toxicité des produits cosmétiques chez l'enfant. L'Expérience du Centre Anti-Poisons de Paris. In: *Journées Européennes de Dermocosmétologie. La Cosmétologie et l'Enfant. Bruxelles, 1990*; 8a–8c (abst).

49. Song M, De Berdt PA, Toxicity problems of cosmetics products in children. *Pediatr Dermatol* 1992; **9**: 194 (abst).

43

Ethnic cosmetics: Blacks, Hispanics and Orientals

Alessandra Pelosi, Enzo Berardesca, Howard I Maibach

Racial differences in skin physiology and function have been minimally investigated. The quantitative and qualitative ability of Black skin to react to physical or chemical injury appears controversial.[1,2] It is often stated that dark skin is less susceptible than light skin to cutaneous irritants, but the paucity of objective investigations of chemical exposure and of interpretable epidemiologic data makes it difficult to compare the potentially different behavior of Black, White and Oriental skin precisely. If such a difference exists, the mechanism might involve either stratum corneum, epidermal, dermal or appendageal structural or functional variation. It is therefore relevant to review data on skin structure and function as well as the specific studies of reactivity. Experimental human models usually refer to Caucasians, and data are discussed on the basis of the known functional, physical and biochemical properties of White skin. Blacks are reported to have increased stratum corneum cell cohesion and resistance to stripping,[3] and an increased lipid content[4] (Table 43.1). Sugino, Imokawa and Maibach found that ceramide levels were inversely correlated with transepidermal water loss (TEWL) and directly correlated with water content, and demonstrated a significant difference in the amount of ceramide – with the

Table 43.1 Racial differences in stratum corneum: Blacks versus Caucasians[a]
Equal thickness
Increased number of cell layers
Increased resistance to stripping
Increased electrical resistance
Increased lipid content

[a] Reproduced from Berardesca E, Maibach HI, Physical anthropology and skin: a model for exploring skin function. In: *Models in Dermatology 4* (Maibach HI, Lowe N, eds). Basel: Karger, 1989:202–8.

lowest levels in Blacks, the next lowest in Whites, followed by Hispanics and Asians.

Functionally, Black skin is believed to behave differently from White: experimental irritant dermatitis results in lower visual scoring in Blacks,[5,6] with decreased minimal perceptible erythema after chemical irritation, suggesting a decreased susceptibility of Black skin to develop irritation. The difference has been stated as being due to a different permeability of the stratum corneum, since cellophane tape stripping in both races produces a homogeneous response.[6]

As early as 1919, Marshall and associates

investigated cutaneous reactions to bis(2-chloroethyl) sulphide ('mustard gas') in Whites and Blacks.[5] A drop containing a 1% concentration in mineral oil on the arm elicited erythema in 58% of the Whites but only 15% of the Blacks, suggesting a decreased susceptibility to cutaneous irritants in Blacks.

Weigand and Mershon[7] studied patch test reactions to o-chlorobenzylidene malononitrile ('CS gas') with occlusive plastic patches applied for 24 hours to the backs of volunteers. The results confirmed that Blacks are more resistant and required a significantly longer exposure to develop an irritant reaction. Subsequently, Weigand and Gaylor[6] measured minimal perceptible erythema in Blacks and Whites by applying a measured amount of dinitrochlorobenzene on the back both in normal skin and in skin with the stratum corneum largely removed by tape stripping.[6] The results confirmed the view that Blacks are generally less susceptible to cutaneous irritants, even if the difference is not great. Furthermore, this difference was not detectable when the stratum corneum was removed. These investigators observed that the range of reactions in normal skin in both races is wider than of stripped skin: that is, the stratum corneum may modulate the different racial responses to skin irritants.

Racial differences in transcutaneous penetration of chemicals may exist, and are presumably related to the nature of the compound.

Penetration of diflorasone acetate does not reveal differences between Whites and Blacks.[8] Penetration of nicotinates and dipyrithione is decreased in Black skin,[9,10] whereas it does not differ significantly between Orientals and Whites.[11] In 1989, Gean et al[12] found that, at the higher concentrations of methyl nicotinate studied (0.3–1.0 M), the area under the LDV response-versus-time curve (AUL) is significantly higher for Orientals than for Caucasians.

Furthermore, in 1993, Lotte et al[13] studied percutaneous penetration with benzoic acid, caffeine and acetylsalicylic acid at a dose of 1 mM/cm². The data confirmed that there is no difference between Whites, Blacks and Orientals.

Several parameters (skin thickness, transepidermal water loss, water content of the stratum corneum, and skin biomechanics) have been measured using non-invasive tools in Whites, Hispanics, Blacks and Asians to assess whether the melanin content could induce changes in skin biophysical properties.[14] Marked differences between races appear in stratum corneum water content and in skin extensibility, recovery and elastic modulus. Measurements done in different sun-exposed sites highlight the effects of solar irradiation on the skin and the role of melanin in preventing skin damage. The study shows that racial differences in skin physiology exist and are mainly related to the protective role of melanin present in races with darker skin (Table 43.2).

The melanocyte plays the primary, although not the only, role in distinguishing the Black races. The major differences between Black, Oriental and White melanocytes are the type and amount of melanosomes produced and their distribution to the keratinocytes.[15] In Orientals, the melanosomes are approximately

Table 43.2 Differences in some biophysical parameters between volar (unexposed) and dorsal (exposed) forearm (Y = significant difference); less difference is detectable when the color is dark[14]

	Blacks	Hispanics	Whites
Water content	Y	Y	Y
Skin thickness	Y	Y	Y
Extensibility	N	Y	Y
Elastic modulus	N	N	Y
Elastic recovery	N	Y	Y
Viscoelasticity	N	Y	Y
Elasticity	N	N	N
TEWL	N	N	N

0.6 nm × 0.3 nm in size, mostly in stage 3 and 4 in melanocytes, and are distributed as a mixture of single and complex forms of melanosomes.

In negroid Black skin, the melanosomes are larger (approximately 1.0 nm × 0.5 nm), heavily pigmented in stage 4 in melanocytes, and singly distributed in keratinocytes, whereas in Caucasian White skin they are small (0.5 nm× 0.3 nm), less-melanized in stage 2 or 3 in melanocytes, and distributed as aggregates (melanosome complex) in keratinocytes.[16]

Melanosomes in Australian aborigines, in normal Blacks, and in deeply tanned Whites may be dispersed singly throughout the epidermis and even the stratum corneum.[17,18] In American Indians and dark-skinned American Blacks, they are also complexed in keratinocytes in lysosomal structures containing two or three heavily melanized melanosomes, whereas Whites have complexes of five to seven variably melanized melanosomes. American Blacks with light and medium complexions have both types of complexes.

The subcellular processes for melanin synthesis in Oriental skin are different from those of negroid Black and Caucasian White skin.[19]

Some pigmentary disorders are frequently and characteristically seen in Orientals: café-au-lait macules, Becker's melanosis, naevus of ota, melasma, ceruloderma. 'Mongolian spots' are typical blue pigmentations: the term refers to a blue-black pigmented macule observed first at birth in more than 90% of Orientals (Asiatic races and American Indians), less frequently in Blacks and in less than 10% of Whites.[20] The congenital pigmentary disorders in Oriental skin are numerous, and some of them take a distribution following Blaschko's lines (e.g. naevus depigmentosus, incontinentia pigmenti and incontinentia pigmenti achromians).[19]

SKIN IRRITABILITY

Transepidermal water loss (TEWL) is a useful method for assessing the damaging effects of irritants on the skin. It is also useful to differentiate allergic and irritant reactions.[21,22] No differences in baseline TEWL between race or site have been detected.[14]

Goh and Chia[23] studied skin irritability of different Oriental groups: Chinese, Malays and Indians. This study showed that the mean TEWL of unirritated skin in female volunteers was significantly lower than in male volunteers. The irritation index was significantly lower in males than females (Figure 43.1). There were no significant differences in the mean TEWL values of unirritated and irritated skin among different races. Similarly, the mean irritation indices among the different races were not significantly different (Figure 43.2).

Berardesca et al[14] reported no difference in baseline TEWL on the back among Whites, Blacks and Hispanics.[24,25] Moreover, TEWL revealed a different pattern of reaction in

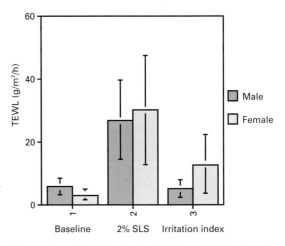

Figure 43.1 TEWL levels after irritation of Oriental male and female skin with sodium lauryl sulfate (SLS). (Modified from Goh and Chia.[23])

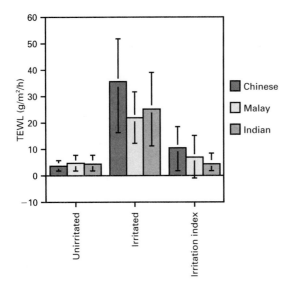

Figure 43.2 TEWL values of unirritated and irritated skin of volunteers of different Oriental ethnic groups. (Modified from Goh and Chia.[23])

Whites after chemical exposure to sodium lauryl sulphate. Blacks and Hispanics developed stronger irritant reactions (as measured by TEWL) after exposure to 2.0% sodium lauryl sulfate proportional to the individual's TEWL basal level (Figure 43.3).

Furthermore, Hispanics showed a higher (even though not significant) water content on the site investigated (the back); the data confirm that no racial differences in TEWL exist on either the volar or the dorsal forearms.

Interestingly, water content is increased on the volar forearm in Hispanics, and decreased on the dorsal forearm in Whites (compared only with Blacks). These findings partially confirm previous observations.[24,25] Racial differences in skin conductance are difficult to interpret in terms of stratum corneum water content, because some other physical factors, such as skin microrelief or the presence of

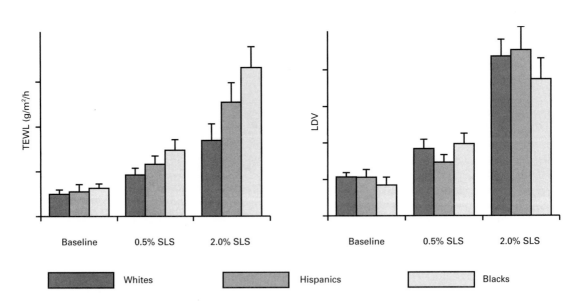

Figure 43.3 TEWL and blood flow measured by laser Doppler velocimetry (LDV) after irritation with SLS. The response is higher in dark skin.

hair on the measuring site, can modify the quality of the skin–electrode contact. Significant differences exist between the volar and dorsal forearm in all races. The race–site interaction is significant, and consequently on dorsal sites Whites are different from Blacks and Hispanics. Besides, it was evident that the White group was much hairier than the others, and the trend between dorsal and volar sides was different in Blacks compared with the other races.

The results are in apparent contrast with TEWL recordings. Indeed, the higher the stratum corneum water content, the higher the TEWL that may be expected.[26] The data may be explained on the basis of the different intercellular cohesion or lipid composition. A greater cell cohesion with a normal TEWL could result in increased skin water content. Weigand et al,[3] in stripping experiments, reported increased intercellular cohesion, while Reinertson and Wheatley[4] noted a higher lipid content in Black stratum corneum.

In vivo TEWL studies are characterized by large interindividual variability and biased by environmental effects and eccrine sweating. An in vitro technique for measuring TEWL was used to compare transepidermal water loss in the two racial groups of Blacks and Whites.[27] A significant correlation between skin temperature and increased TEWL was found in both groups. Furthermore, Black skin had a significantly higher mean TEWL than White skin. The difference in TEWL between the groups has been recorded in the absence of eccrine sweating and other vital functions; the higher TEWL in Black skin could be explained on the basis of a thermoregulatory mechanism.

According to this observation, there might be a different behavior of blood vessels between Blacks and Caucasians: Blacks develop less erythema than Caucasians (detected as an increase of blood flow) after exposure to the same amount of sodium lauryl sulfate.[24]

Reactive hyperemia before and after a vasoconstrictive stimulus (topical application of clobetasol propionate 0.05% ointment) has been investigated.[28] The reaction before and after a single one-hour application of the corticoid was recorded by means of laser Doppler velocimetry in order to elucidate different racial responses in skin vasoconstriction. Reactive hyperemia was recorded after four minutes of occlusion of the forearm blood flow.

Different responses were recorded in Black subjects after the vasoconstrictive stimulus compared with Caucasians: decreased area under the curve response ($P < 0.04$), decreased peak response ($P < 0.01$) and decreased decay slope after peak blood flow ($P < 0.04$). These data are consistent with a different reactivity of blood vessels in Black skin, and possibly are not related to the transcutaneous penetration of the chemical compound.

CONTACT DERMATITIS

Controversial findings have been reported about the incidence of allergic contact dermatitis in Blacks. Kenney[29] reported a decreased rate, which was 5% in Black patients in his own private practice. Marshal and Heyl[30] reported that the incidence of industrial contact dermatitis in South Africa was less in darkly pigmented blacks. According to Dogliotti,[31] Bantus show a 7.4% prevalence. Scott[32] noted that contact dermatitis was less frequent in Bantus handling detergents, waxes and fuels. Despite a previous report describing an increased sensitization rate in Whites, Kligman and Epstein[33] in 1975 found no significant difference in the two races when testing a wide spectrum of materials for topical use.

Fisher[34] reported an approximately equal incidence of contact dermatitis in Blacks and Whites. *p*-Phenylenediamine (used in hair dyes by elderly black women), nickel and potassium dichromate appeared to be the most common allergens. 'Rhus'-type dermatitis and other similar oleoresin types of dermatitis are not frequent. In a review of contact dermatitis in Nigeria,[35] nickel was the most important sensitizer, with an incidence of 12.3% compared with 11% in North America.[36] In Lagos, the female-to-male ratio is about 1:1, whereas Fregert et al[37] recorded a ratio of 6:1. In North America, the ratio is 3:1 and in Stockholm 7:3. The principal source of sensitization in men was cheap plated wristwatches, watch straps, and belt buckles. Also, Nigerian coins contain nickel. Chromate, the next most common allergen, is contained in cement and shoes. Housewife dermatitis was reported to be uncommon, whereas wood tars, fragrance mix and balsam of Peru seem to be important sensitizers. The clinical pattern in these patients was either exfoliative dermatitis or photodermatitis.

From a clinical viewpoint, acute contact dermatitis with exudation, vesiculation or bullae formation is more common in Whites, whereas Blacks more easily develop disorders of pigmentation and lichenification. Hypopigmentation is described from contact with phenolic detergents,[38] alkylphenols and the monobenzyl ether of hydroquinone.[39]

Hyperpigmentation occurs more readily in Black patients after contact with mild irritants. Keratolytics and other chemicals used in acne therapy often cause hyperpigmentation that is more distressing than the acne itself.

Considering the importance of this information to therapeutics and toxicology, we clearly need more experimental data on the various mechanisms (irritation, sensitization, subjective sensory irritation, etc.), as well as a variety of related and unrelated chemicals of different physical and chemical properties. Until the hardness of the data and the variety of experiments increase, we cannot, with veracity, answer the question of how resistant Black skin is compared with White. Nevertheless, the current data demonstrate sufficient differences in reactivity to suggest the utility of race-related skin care products.

REFERENCES

1. Marshall J, New skin diseases in Africa. *Trans St John's Hosp Dermatol Soc* 1970; **56:** 3.
2. Schwartz L, Tulipan L, Birmingham DJ, In: *Occupational Diseases of the Skin*, 3rd edn. Philadelphia: Lea & Febiger, 1957:31.
3. Weigand DA, Haygood C, Gaylor JR, Cell layers and density of negro and Caucasian stratum corneum. *J Invest Dermatol* 1974; **62:** 563–8.
4. Reinertson RP, Wheatley VR, Studies on the chemical composition of human epidermal lipids. *J Invest Dermatol* 1959; **32:** 49–59.
5. Marshall EK, Lynch V, Smith HV, Variation in susceptibility of the skin to dichloroethylsulphide. *J Pharmacol Exp Ther* 1919; **12:** 291.
6. Weigand DA, Gaylor JR, Irritant reaction in Negro and Caucasian skin. *South Med J* 1974; **67:** 548–51.
7. The cutaneous irritant reaction to agent *o*-chlorobenzylidene malonitrile (CS). Quantitation and racial influence in human subjects. *Edgewood Arsenal Tech Rep* 4332 (Feb 1970).
8. Wickema Sinha WJ, Shaw SR, Weber OJ, Percutaneous absorption and excretion of tritium labelled diflorasone acetate, a new topical corticosteroid in the rat, monkey and man. *J Invest Dermatol* 1978; **71:** 372–3.
9. Berardesca E, Maibach HI, Racial differences in percutaneous penetration of nicotinates in vivo in human skin: black and white. *Acta Dermatol Venereol (Stockh)* 1990; **70:** 63–6.
10. Wedig JH, Maibach HI, Percutaneous penetration of dipirithione in man: effect of skin color (race). *J Am Acad Dermatol* 1981; **5:** 433–8.
11. Lin S, Ho H, Chien YW, Development of a new nicotine transdermal delivery system: in vitro kinetics studies and clinical pharmacokinetic evaluations in two ethnic groups. *J Contr Rel* 1993; **26:** 175–93.
12. Gean CJ, Tur E, Maibach HI, Guy RH, Cutaneous responses to topical methyl nicotinate in Black, Oriental and Caucasian subjects. *Arch Dermatol Res* 1989; **281:** 95–8.
13. Lotte C, Wester RC, Rougier A, Maibach HI, Racial differences in the in vivo percutaneous absorption of some organic compounds: a comparison between Black, Caucasians and Asian subjects. *Arch Dermatol Res* 1993; **284:** 456–9.

14. Berardesca E, de Rigal J, Léveque JL, Maibach HI, In vivo biophysical characterization of skin physiological differences in races. *Dermatologica* 1991; **182:** 89–93.

15. Gawkrodger DJ, Racial influences on skin disease. In: *Rook, Wilkinson, Ebling: Textbook of Dermatology*, 5th edn, Vol 4 (Champion A, Burton DS, Ebling FJG, eds). Oxford: Blackwell, 1992:2859–75.

16. Jimbow K, Fitzpatrick TB, Quevedo WC Jr, Formation, chemical composition and functions of melanin pigments in mammals. In: *Biology of Integument*, Vol 2 (Matoltsy AG, ed.). New York: Springer-Verlag, 1986:278–91.

17. Olson R, Skin color, pigment distribution and skin cancer. *Cutis* 1971; **8:** 225–31.

18. Szabo G, Gerald A, Pathak M et al, Racial differences in the fate of melanosomes in human epidermis. *Nature* 1969; **222:** 1081–2.

19. Jimbow M, Jimbow K, Pigmentary disorders in oriental skin. *Clinics Dermatol* 1989; **7**(2): 11–27.

20. Kikuchi I, Mongolian spots remaining in school children: a statistical survey in central Okinawa. *J Dermatol* 1980; **7:** 213–16.

21. van der Valk PGM, Nater JP, Bleumink E, The influence of low concentrations of irritants on skin barrier functions as determined by water vapour loss. *Dermatosan in Beruf und Umwelt* 1985; **33:** 89–91.

22. Serup J, Staberg B, Differentiation of allergic and irritant reactions by transepidermal water loss. *Contact Dermatitis* 1987; **16:** 129–32.

23. Goh CL, Chia SE, Skin irritability to sodium lauryl sulphate as measured by skin water vapour loss by sex and race. *Clin Exp Dermatol* 1987; **13:** 16–19.

24. Berardesca E, Maibach HI, Racial differences in sodium lauryl sulphate induced cutaneous irritation: black and white. *Contact Dermatitis* 1988; **18:** 65–70.

25. Berardesca E, Maibach HI, Sodium lauryl sulphate induced cutaneous irritation. Comparison of White and Hispanic subjects. *Contact Dermatitis* 1988; **19:** 136–40.

26. Rietschel RL, A method to evaluate skin moisturizers in vivo. *J Invest Dermatol* 1978; **70:** 152–5.

27. Wilson D, Berardesca E, Maibach HI, In vitro transepidermal water loss: differences between Black and White human skin. *Br J Dermatol* 1988; **119:** 647–52.

28. Berardesca E, Maibach HI, Cutaneous reactive hyperaemia: racial differences induced by corticoid application. *Br J Dermatol* 1989; **120:** 787–94.

29. Kenney J, Dermatoses seen in American negroes. *Int J Dermatol* 1970; **9:** 110–13.

30. Marshall J, Heyl T, Skin disease in Western Cape Province. *S Afr Med J* 1963; 1308.

31. Dogliotti M, Skin disorders in the Bantu: a survey of 2000 cases from Baragwanath Hospital. *S Afr Med J* 1970; **44:** 670–2.

32. Scott F, Skin diseases in the South African Bantu. In: *Essays on Tropical Dermatology* (Marshall J, ed.). Amsterdam: Excerpta Medica, 1962; **38:** 561.

33. Kligman AM, Epstein W, Updating the maximization test for identifying contact allergens. *Contact Dermatitis* 1975; **1:** 231–9.

34. Fisher AA, Contact dermatitis in Black patients. *Cutis* 1977; **20:** 303–9.

35. Olumide YM, Contact dermatitis in Nigeria. *Contact Dermatitis* 1985; **12:** 241–6.

36. Rudner J, North American Group Result. *Contact Dermatitis* 1977; **3:** 208–9.

37. Fregert S, Hjorth N, Magnusson B et al, Epidemiology of contact dermatitis. *Trans St John's Hosp Dermatol Soc* 1969; **55:** 17–35.

38. Fisher AA, Vitiligo due to contactants. *Cutis* 1976; **17:** 431–48.

39. Kahn G, Depigmentation caused by phenolic detergent germicides. *Arch Dermatol* 1970; **102:** 177.

PART EIGHT

NON-INVASIVE ASSESSMENT TECHNIQUES IN COSMETOLOGY

44

Measurement of blood flow in the cutaneous microvasculature

Maria Beatriz Lagos, Andreas J Bircher, Howard I Maibach

INTRODUCTION

In human skin, particularly with increasing age, considerable biochemical and physiological changes take place. These include a wide range of functional and structural alterations – for example, decrease in glandular functions, significant modifications in the cutaneous microvasculature, and alterations in the epidermal barrier structure and functions as well as in the immunological defences.[1] One particular aim of cosmetology is the prevention or reversal of such changes. To objectify the cutaneous effects of agents used in cosmetics, modern non-invasive techniques are available, with which the influence can be measured in an objective and frequently semi-quantitative way. The determination of dynamic changes in the cutaneous microvasculature is one approach to the evaluation of the effect of chemical agents applied to the skin. Several techniques are in use that measure cutaneous blood flow (CBF) either in a direct (venous occlusion plethysmography, ^{133}Xe clearance) or an indirect (skin temperature, transcutaneous pO_2) manner (Table 44.1). Recently, non-invasive technologies based on optical principles that allow direct measurement of red blood cell movements have been increasingly employed. Of these, photopulse plethysmography (PPG) and laser Doppler flowmetry (LDF) have been the most widely used. Both techniques operate using an optical principle, and are therefore completely non-invasive.

OPTICAL TECHNIQUES

In PPG, infrared radiation (800–940 nm) from a light-emitting diode is directed into the skin. The incident radiation is scattered, absorbed and reflected by tissue components – at this wavelength primarily by the hemoglobin of the erythrocytes. A phototransistor, positioned either on the opposite side or adjacent to the diode, collects the backscattered radiation. The change of blood volume in the illuminated tissue is correlated with the amount of light absorbed by the blood.[2]

In LDF (Figure 44.1), the radiation emitted from a helium–neon laser ($\lambda = 632.8$ nm), enters the skin and is reflected by stationary and moving tissue components. Stationary tissue scatters and reflects the incident radiation at the same frequency. Red blood cells moving with a certain speed reflect the light with a shifted frequency (Doppler effect). Thus

Table 44.1 Non-invasive bioengineering techniques used to study skin microcirculation

Bioengineering technique	Parameter evaluated	Clinical correlate	Main applications
Laser Doppler flowmetry	Erythrocyte flux	Blood flow, erythema	Skin pharmacology, irritation, skin and vascular disease
Photopulse plethysmography	Blood flow volume	Blood flow, erythema	Skin pharmacology, vascular disease
Transcutaneous oxygen pressure	Transcutaneous oxygen	Blood flow, arterial oxygen	Vascular disease
Infrared thermography	Infrared photon flux	Skin temperature, blood flow	Skin pharmacology, vascular disease
Contact thermometry	Heat flow	Skin temperature, blood flow	Vascular disease
Capillary microscopy	Skin capillaries	Superficial capillaries	Skin and vascular disease
Colorimetry	Skin colour	Erythema, pigmentation	Irritation and pigmentation

the light returning to the instrument is composed of two components: the frequency-modulated, spectrally broadened light, which is directly related to the number of erythrocytes times their velocity (flux), and the non-shifted fraction, which has been reflected from non-moving tissue.[3]

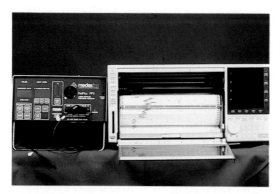

Figure 44.1 Laser Doppler flowmeter PF 3 interfaced to a four-channel chart recorder.

In both techniques, the CBF data are collected via a probe held to the skin surface by double-sided adhesive tape. Both PPG and LDF permit fast and semiquantitative measurement of CBF. LDF, however, has been used more frequently because of the sophisticated technology and ease of handling.

Another frequently used non-invasive method is based on the measurement of the transcutaneous oxygen pressure ($tcpO_2$). In this technique, a cathode and a ring anode are combined with a heating element. Under normal conditions, $tcpO_2$ is practically not measurable on the skin surface. The measurable level of $tcpO_2$ is closely related to the electrode temperature. At a temperature of 45°C, $tcpO_2$ reflects the level of the arterial oxygen tension, which has been used, for example, in the monitoring of neonates and in the evaluation of arterial vascular disease. At an electrode temperature close to the temperature of the skin surface, investigations of the functions of the cutaneous microcirculation can be performed. It must be taken into consideration, however, that numerous factors, local and systemic, influence the level of $tcpO_2$.[4,5]

APPLICATIONS IN COSMETOLOGY

In cosmetology there are several topics of interest concerning the function of the skin microvasculature:

- the influence on and the permanent modification of the cutaneous microcirculation by cosmetic agents;
- the protective properties of cosmetic products (e.g. the effect of ultraviolet-absorbing chemicals or the prevention of skin irritation);
- the examination of an irritating or sensitizing potential of cosmetic ingredients themselves or the evaluation of individuals with 'sensitive' skin.

Some examples of the application of non-invasive techniques to such questions are given below.

Photoaging

It has been observed that topical tretinoin may reverse – at least partly – the structural and functional changes in photoaged skin. Since one factor involved in photoaging is change in cutaneous microvasculature, the long-term effects of topically applied tretinoin on skin vessels have been studied.[6] Monitoring of baseline blood flow indicated that in the tretinoin-treated areas the concentration of red blood cells was increased, although the erythrocyte flux was not elevated. After CBF stimulation by administration of a vasoactive compound, the flux and the concentration of erythrocytes were both significantly increased in the tretinoin-treated sites. The LDF measurements correlated well with the visual grading of the clinically observed effect. Another study performed using LDF to assess the effects of topical retinoic acid in photoaging likewise showed an increase in blood flow through the skin.

However, this increase is not a specific retinoid effect, and does not indicate angiogenesis.[7]

Protection from irritation

Protection of the skin against environmental threats is a new challenge that may also influence the development of cosmetics. On the one hand, air pollution – particularly airborne particles – stresses or damages the skin, while, on the other, prevention of ultraviolet-induced skin alterations has become and will be increasingly important in the future. One approach to evaluating the protective effect of barrier creams involves the application of irritants such as the anionic surfactant sodium lauryl sulfate (SLS) or the alkali sodium hydroxide (NaOH) as indicator agents of skin irritation. Using LDF measurements, the considerable protective effect of a barrier cream against the skin irritation elicited by NaOH has been demonstrated.[8] The irritant potency of SLS was also considerably decreased by the application of a protective agent in comparison with an unprotected skin site. In measurements made by bioengineering methods, however, there were no significant differences between the barrier agent with and without silicone, indicating that the physical barrier is more important than the alleged protective effect of silicone.[9] In a comparison of eight moisturizers applied after washing, prevention of skin irritation as measured by transepidermal water loss (Evaporimeter) and LDF could be demonstrated. Washing alone induced visible dermatitis in some individuals, together with significant increases in water loss and CBF. There were, however, no differences in the preventive effects of the different moisturizers used. Therefore, as determined using this model, the particular composition of such creams seemed to play a minor role in the prevention of skin irritation.[10] Recently, two test models have been developed to assess the efficacy of protective creams or gels: the repetitive irritant test (RIT) in guinea pigs and the RIT in humans with a set of four standard irritants (10% sodium lauryl sulfate, 1% sodium hydroxide, 30% lactic acid and pure toluene).

Both tests used low, subtoxic doses of irritants, short-time repetitive applications for two weeks and quantification of the cutaneous irritant reaction by modern biophysical instruments such as TEWL by evaporimetry, skin blood flow volume by the Periflux laser Doppler, stratum corneum hydration by skin capacitance or corneometry, and scoring of erythema on a 5+ scale. The protective effect of several creams and gels available on the German market were studied, and the results showed that protection against chemical irritants may be quite specific, with protection varying widely when various irritants are used.[11–14]

Protection from ultraviolet light

Ultraviolet (UV) protection of the skin has become increasingly important. Since UV-induced erythema is partly caused by increased cutaneous blood flow, it can be quantified by LDF. In a large study, the protective potency of the sunscreen agent 2-ethylhexyl cinnamate and a pigmentation-enhancing furocoumarin (5-methoxypsoralen) were tested. Skin sites were irradiated with a single dose of the complete natural UV spectrum (UVA 15 J/cm² plus four minimal erythema doses (MED) of UVB and UVC). Only the cinnamate protected against UV, whereas 5-methoxypsoralen had no demonstrable protective effect. In a multiple-exposure experiment to test skin protective mechanisms, five daily doses of UV (10 J/cm² UVA and one MED UVB/UVC) were administered, followed by a challenge dose (UVA 15 J/cm² plus four MED UVB/UVC). A smaller CBF response was obtained, thus demonstrating the shielding effect of tanning and epidermal thickening.[15] The UV photoprotective effect of topically applied vitamin C has also been studied. Using the porcine model, 10% aqueous vitamin C was applied to the animal's skin, irradiated with 400 mJ/cm² UVB, and sampled 24 hours later. UVB-induced erythema measured by laser Doppler velocimetry after a 2–3 MED dose of UVB had been applied to intact skin showed a significant reduction in the vitamin C-treated skin.[16]

Skin irritation

The irritant potential of cosmetic compounds themselves can be investigated by non-invasive techniques. As in the evaluation of the protective quality of barrier agents, SLS has frequently been used to determine the sensitivity of human skin. Defined stimuli with different model skin irritating agents were studied using a series of bioengineering methods, and were compared with visual scoring.[17] Independently of the irritant used, LDF for CBF and ultrasound for the skin thickness were the most helpful in the quantification of the irritant reaction. The classification of the irritant response was better done by bioengineering techniques, which measure the extent of the epidermal damage by increased transepidermal water loss. A study using LDF to assess reactions caused by finished products like shampoos was done. To determine the skin irritant potential of several commercial shampoos, cultured human keratinocytes as an in vitro model was employed using the MTT (3-(4,5-dimethylthiazol-2-yl)-2,5-diphenyltetrazolium bromide) test and the LDH (lactic dehydrogenase release) test to document cell toxicity. Volunteers in the study were patch-tested, and their reactions were evaluated using LDF and compared with the in vitro data. Patch-test reaction, especially at high concentrations, correlates relatively well with the in vitro test, especially with shampoos of strong and weak irritancy.[18] In a recent study, irritant effects of 0.05% and 0.1% retinoic acid in ethanol on normal skin compared with 1% sodium lauryl sulfate in water as a model irritant in a 24-hour occlusive patch test assay was quantified using measurements of TEWL, stratum corneum hydration and cutaneous blood flow. Retinoic acid caused more intensive scaling than sodium lauryl sulfate, while other skin responses to retinoic acid were significantly weaker than those due to SLS. Results demonstrated that RA, like SLS, is capable of impairing stratum corneum water barrier function, which may be responsible in part for the irritation associated with its topical use.[19] Evaluation of allergic patch test reactions to a panel of 31 contact allergens in 18 patients revealed a significant correlation between the visual score and the CBF values measured by LDF. It was possible to discriminate between negative, doubtful and clearly positive reactions, which also pose the greatest challenge in visual scoring. Discrimination between the weak and strong positive reactions, however, was not possible, and therefore quantification of these tests based on LDF measurements could not be done.[20] Another study measured responses to a range of doses of common contact allergens using a novel scanning Doppler velocimeter. In contrast to the conventional laser Doppler velocimeter, measurement error was less, and it has the added advantage of being able to measure areas of reaction without contact with the skin surface and to measure reactions at all skin sites.[21]

CONCLUSIONS

All bioengineering methods currently in use have some limitations. Measurements of cutaneous microcirculation are particularly prone to influence by environmental and, even more importantly, individual factors.[3] Some of the measurable differences in the LDF-determined CBF as compared with other methods may also be explained by the technical limitations of this technique – for example the small (1 mm^3) tissue volume in which the LDF measurement is made. In such a small measurement volume, the heterogeneity of the cutaneous microvasculature has a greater influence, and therefore it is more likely that

high intra- and interindividual variations in blood flow are present.[22] Some of these inconsistencies in LDF blood flow measurements may be overcome by technical modifications, such as the acquisition of multiple standardized readings through the use of special probe holders or the application of a scanning laser Doppler instrument.[3,21] The standardization group of the European Society of Contact Dermatitis has provided guidelines for the measurement of cutaneous blood flow by LDF.[23] Depending on the problem to be investigated, the application and combination of several bioengineering methods, such as LDF, colorimetry, thermometry (Table 44.1), transepidermal water loss, skin conductivity and ultrasound measurements,[24] have to be carefully considered. With such techniques, different reaction patterns of the skin, such as erythema, blood flow, skin temperature, changes in the epidermal barrier function, hydration, infiltration and edema, can be measured objectively. Only this comprehensive approach allows circumvention of the technical and other limitations inherent in every measuring device. Synthesis of the data generated by several measuring techniques allows detailed and accurate interpretation with regard to the problem under investigation.

REFERENCES

1. Kligman A, Takase Y, *Cutaneous Aging*. Tokyo: University of Tokyo Press, 1988.
2. Challoner A, Photoelectric plethysmography for estimating blood flow. In: *Non Invasive Physiological Measurements*, Vol 1 (Rolfe P, ed.). New York: Academic Press, 1979:125–51.
3. Shepherd A, Öberg P, *Laser Doppler Flowmetry*. Boston: Kluwer, 1990.
4. Stüttgen G, Ott A, Flesch U, Measurement of skin circulation. In: *Cutaneous Investigation in Health and Disease* (Leveque J, ed.). New York: Marcel Dekker, 1989; 359–84.
5. Franzeck U, Nichtinvasive Messmethoden zur Beurteilung der kutanen Mikrozirkulation. *Phlebol Proctol* 1988; **17**: 122–30.

6. Grove G, Grove M, Zerweck C et al, Determination of topical tretinoin effects on cutaneous microcirculation in photoaged skin by laser Doppler velocimetry. *J Cutan Aging Cosmet Dermatol* 1988; **1:** 27–32.

7. Marks R, Methods for the assessment of the effects of topical retinoic acid in photoaging and actinic keratoses. *Int Med Res* 1990; **18**(Suppl): 29C–34C.

8. Marks R, Dykes P, Hamami I, Two novel techniques for the evaluation of barrier creams. *Br J Dermatol* 1989; **120:** 655–60.

9. Nouaigui H, Antoine J, Masmoudi M et al, Etudes invasive et non invasive du pouvoir protecteur d'une crème siliconée et de son excipient vis-à-vis de l'irritation cutanée induite par le laurylsulfate de sodium. *Ann Dermatol Venereol* 1989; **116:** 389–98.

10. Hannuksela A, Kinnunen T, Moisturizers prevents irritant dermatitis. *Acta Derma Venereol (Stockh)* 1992; **72:** 42–4.

11. Frosch PJ, Schulze-Dirks A, Hoffmann M et al, Efficacy of skin barrier creams. I. The repetitive irritation test (RIT) in the guinea pig. *Contact Dermatitis* 1993; **28:** 94–100.

12. Frosch PJ, Schulze-Dirks A, Hoffmann M et al, Efficacy of skin barrier creams. II. Ineffectiveness of a popular skin protector against various irritants in the repetitive irritation test in the guinea pig. *Contact Dermatitis* 1993; **29:** 74–7.

13. Frosch PJ, Kurte A, Pilz B, Efficacy of skin barrier creams. III. The repetitive irritation test in humans. *Contact Dermatitis* 1993; **29:** 113–18.

14. Frosch PJ, Kurte A, Efficacy of skin barrier creams. IV. The repetitive irritation test (RIT) with a set of 4 standard irritants. *Contact Dermatitis* 1994; **31:** 161–8.

15. Drouard V, Wilson D, Maibach H et al, Quantitative assessment of UV-induced changes in microcirculatory flow by laser Doppler velocimetry. *J Invest Dermatol* 1984; **83:** 188–92.

16. Darr D, Combs S, Dunston S et al, Topical vitamin C protects porcine skin from ultraviolet radiation-induced damage. *Br J Dermatol* 1992; **127:** 247–53.

17. Agner T, Serup J, Skin reactions to irritants assessed by non-invasive bioengineering methods. *Contact Dermatitis* 1989; **20:** 352–9.

18. Eun HC, Jung SY, Comparison of irritant potential of shampoos using cultured epidermal keratinocytes model and patch test reactions measured by laser Doppler flowmetry. *Contact Dermatitis* 1991; **30:** 168–71.

19. Effendy I, Weltfriend S, Patil S, Maibach H, Differential irritant skin responses to topical retinoic acid and sodium lauryl sulfate: alone and in a crossover design. *Br J Dermatol* 1996; **134:** 424–30.

20. Staberg B, Klemp P, Serup J, Patch test responses evaluated by cutaneous blood flow measurements. *Arch Dermatol* 1984; **120:** 741–3.

21. Quinn AG, McLelland J, Essex T, Farr PM, Quantification of contact allergic inflammation: A comparison of existing methods with a scanning laser Doppler velocimeter. *Acta Derm Venereol (Stockh)* 1993; **73:** 21–5.

22. Braverman I, Keh A, Goldminz D, Correlation of laser Doppler wave patterns with underlying microvascular anatomy. *J Invest Dermatol* 1990; **95:** 285–6.

23. Bircher A, de Boer E, Agner T et al, Guidelines for measurement of cutaneous blood flow by laser Doppler flowmetry: a report from the Standardization Group of the European Society of Contact Dermatitis. *Contact Dermatitis* 1994; **30:** 65–72.

24. Duteil L, Queille-Roussel C, Czernielewski J, Inflammations provoquées en peau saine chez l'homme. *Ann Dermatol Venereol* 1991; **118:** 339–46.

45

Stratum corneum water content and TEWL

Enzo Berardesca, Howard I Maibach

INTRODUCTION

Skin bioengineering is a rapidly growing field. The need for objective data, not biased by subjective assessment, and discerned non-invasively, has stimulated engineers and physicists to develop instruments capable of reliably monitoring some parameters of skin function that are useful in evaluating, understanding and quantifying pathophysiological skin mechanisms.

Although some researchers still reject the valuable data obtained non-invasively in vivo, trusting only subjective and visual judgements, the usefulness of bioengineering tools in the assessment of skin function has been increasingly documented.[1-4] Objective bioengineering techniques may provide important information concerning skin diseases, as well as supporting the investigator in the evaluation of 'non-visible' or 'clinically non-quantifiable' pathologies, such as uninvolved healthy skin in patients affected by various dermatoses and/or 'dry skin'.

One common aspect of this problem is the assessment of visually damaged stratum corneum function in the above-mentioned conditions. The stratum corneum is a primary barrier against the physical and biological environment; monitoring the parameters related to its efficiency may prevent exacerbation of skin disease and help evaluate the effectiveness of skin treatments.

Hydration and transepidermal water loss (TEWL) are important factors influencing the biophysical properties of the stratum corneum; these parameters are both narrowly as well as strictly and sometimes inversely related (see Figure 45.1 below).

Understanding their behavior in different conditions reveals a new approach to the non-invasive monitoring of skin pathophysiology.

SKIN PHYSIOLOGY

Transepidermal water loss reflects the integrity of the stratum corneum water barrier. Functionally, TEWL represents the water vapor evaporating from the skin surface; occlusion of the skin surface increases stratum corneum water content, and, when the occlusion is removed, the trapped water evaporates, increasing TEWL, which, in this case, is proportional to hydration.[5] One of the characteristics of healthy skin is that the relationship between TEWL and hydration remains directly proportional. Following skin damage, or a decrease in the efficiency of the water barrier, a dissociation of hydration (or water-holding capacity) and TEWL appears.

In vivo, TEWL can be measured according to three different water-sampling techniques.[3]

- The *closed-chamber method* uses a capsule applied to the skin to collect the vapor lost from the skin surface. The relative humidity inside the capsule is recorded with an electronic hygrosensor. The change in vapor loss concentration is initially rapid, and decreases proportionally as the humidity approaches 100%. The closed-chamber method does not permit recording of continuous TEWL, because skin evaporation ceases when the air inside the chamber is saturated.

- In the *ventilated chamber method*, a chamber through which a gas of known water content passes is applied to the skin. The water is picked up by the gas and measured using a hygrometer. This method allows the measurement of transepidermal water loss continuously, but, if the carrier gas is too dry, it artificially increases evaporation.

- The *open-chamber method* utilizes a skin capsule that is open to the atmosphere. TEWL is calculated from the slope provided by two hygrosensors precisely oriented in the chamber. Air movement and humidity are the greatest drawbacks of this method when in vivo studies are performed.[6]

TEWL is lower in infants,[7] suggesting a more efficient stratum corneum. TEWL is related to gestational age. Infants of 37 weeks gestation or more show low skin water losses, indicating an effective barrier.[8] In contrast, infants of 32 weeks gestation or less have high water loss in the early neonatal period. The varying barrier properties can be explained by the incomplete development of the stratum corneum in the first days of life. Hammarlund et al[9] reported regional variation in newborns in the rate of TEWL measured with an evaporimeter. Comparing the abdomen, forearm and buttocks, they found twofold TEWL on the buttocks. The findings were partially confirmed by Osmark et al[10] using a Meeco analyzer to detect TEWL. The technique allowed more precise measurements, not biased by air turbulence and ambient relative humidity over the probe. They recorded similar TEWL on these three sites, but found a lower hydration level (obtained by inducing skin occlusion with plastic film for one hour) on the abdomen, confirming that the stratum corneum on this site has a decreased water-holding capacity.

Regional variations of moisturization reflecting differences of thickness and function of the corneum occur in adults too. Tagami et al,[11] using high-frequency electrical measurements to evaluate hydration of the uppermost corneum layers, reported drier skin on the extremities than on the trunk. This correlates with the fact that clinically dry skin tends to develop more frequently on the limbs during winter.

Regional variations in hydration were confirmed using impedance techniques.[12]

Skin aging – more or less a physiological event – is characterized by several biological and histopathological changes. TEWL and skin hydration both decrease during the aging process, while maintaining their directly proportional relationship (see Figure 45.1).

The decrease in TEWL during life is conspicuous after the age of 60.[13] Several factors may be responsible for this. The increased size of corneocytes and the increased thickness of the stratum corneum due to the greater accumulation of corneocytes related to an impaired desquamation[14] are factors that should be considered. Similarly, corneum hydration is decreased in elderly subjects. Reduction in moisture content is more noticeable in exposed areas, where action damage is the predominant factor accentuating aging.[12]

The simultaneous decreases in TEWL and water content of the corneum are distinct features of elderly skin. They confirm the decreased corneum hydration without impairment of barrier function. Accordingly, dry skin in the elderly may be differentiated from pathologically dry skin, since in the latter the barrier function is defective.

One of the sites where xerotic changes occur more frequently in aged skin is the extensor aspect of the lower legs. Tagami et al,[15] using an evaporimeter to measure TEWL and a skin surface hygrometer[16] to evaluate the hydration state of the skin, compared hydration of the lower legs in young and aged subjects. They found lower TEWL in elderly subjects, confirming previous findings.[13]

SKIN PATHOLOGY

The correlation between TEWL and corneum water content shows an inverse relationship in pathological skin. The lower the skin hydration, the higher the TEWL: this is due to the damage of the skin barrier and/or the alteration of keratinization that are often present in scaly dermatoses. Water loss in these conditions is increased,[17] and the low water content recorded indicates a defective stratum corneum water-holding capacity.

Tagami et al,[16] employing the sorption–desorption test, evaluated the water-holding capacity in vivo in several scaly skin conditions. They found a good correlation between clinical scaling in psoriasis and chronic eczema and reduced water-holding capacity of the corneum (thicker scaling, lower water-holding capacity). A similar correlation was observed in the same lesions during successful treatment. Lesion clearing was associated with a return to normal levels of water-holding capacity. Hydration and water-retention capacity of stratum corneum have been investigated in uninvolved psoriatic and atopic skin, and compared with those of healthy controls.[18] Hydration was evaluated by means of TEWL and skin-capacitance measurements. Water-retention capacity was investigated using the plastic occlusion stress test. Atopic skin differed significantly from uninvolved psoriatic and control skin, which had a reduced water content and an increased TEWL.

Furthermore, the skin surface water-loss profile representing the stratum corneum water-retention capacity was significantly lower in normal atopic skin. The data suggest that clinically normal skin may be functionally abnormal, resulting in a defective barrier that could lead to a higher risk of irritant or contact dermatitis.

It is noteworthy that inconspicuous eczematous lesions showed defective water-holding capacity. The inverse relationship existing in pathological skin between TEWL and stratum corneum water content was examined by Tagami and Yoshikuni.[19] By performing simultaneous measurements of TEWL with an evaporimeter and of cutaneous conductance to record skin hydration, they assessed the stratum corneum of psoriatic patients with varying grades of disease severity. The data obtained indicated both the existence of an inverse relationship between these two parameters and the presence of a reduced water-holding capacity associated with increased TEWL.

Serup and Blichmann[20] confirmed these results in psoriasis using the same technique, stressing that this inverse pattern is a common feature in scaly dermatoses. They suggested that low conductance in psoriasis is not strictly related to low hydration, but might reflect abnormal keratinization. Indeed, visual scoring was not correlated with TEWL or electrical-conductance measurements. If scaling in psoriasis is a consequence of decreased hydration then plaques with glossy appearance should show higher conductance, which was not the case. Subsequently, the same findings were described in eczematous skin[21] and in atopic dermatitis.[22] Both eczematous skin and uninvolved skin of atopic subjects have higher TEWL compared with healthy skin of non-atopic individuals.[23] Differences between uninvolved skin and normal skin occur in psoriasis.[24] These results indicate that, while the intact stratum corneum of normal skin hampers the passage of water from the body to the environment, resulting in a low TEWL, the pathological horny layer has a low water content and high TEWL.[19]

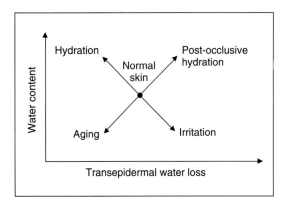

Figure 45.1 Relationship between TEWL and skin hydration in several skin conditions (see the text for details).

Figure 45.1 shows the different behavior of TEWL and water content of the stratum corneum in different skin conditions. By monitoring both parameters, it is possible to define non-invasively the functional pattern of the skin. Dry pathological skin presents increased TEWL and decreased hydration. Unfortunately, we are currently unable to differentiate among different dry pathological skins (eczema, psoriasis, atopic dermatitis and irritation), but future developments in techniques and methods may provide new approaches to the problem.

IRRITATION

Irritated skin behaves functionally like other pathological conditions.[25] TEWL and soap irritancy was evaluated by van der Valk et al[26] on 33 subjects exposed to solutions of 13 brand-name soaps in Finn chambers. The measurements were performed with an evaporimeter. All products caused a significant increase in water-vapor loss compared with the controls. The differences among the products were small; however, analyzing the data by means of a Neumann–Keuls test permitted the detection of significant differ-ences. A more precise attempt to correlate TEWL and visual scoring in assessing skin irritancy was made by the same group in 1985.[6] The skin of the volar forearm was exposed to 5% nickel sulfate, 5% sodium lauryl sulfate (SLS), 50% dimethyl sulfoxide (DMSO) and 5% phenol for 48 hours. Twenty-three subjects entered the study, 14 of whom had positive skin reactions to nickel sulfate. The correlation between the erythema and increase in water-vapor loss varied from substance to substance. The best correlation was found for 5% SLS, suggesting that cytotoxic damage of viable cells of the epidermis parallels impairment of barrier function. These data confirm those reported by Malten and Den Arend.[27] Thus TEWL measurements seem to correlate with impairment of barrier function, but, besides a great individual variability, the elicited responses vary from irritant to irritant, and do not allow comparison between different compounds. The stratum corneum is believed to form a uniform layer, which constitutes the main skin barrier against water diffusion. Acute or chronic exposure to surfactants may cause irritant dermatitis, leading to the development of dry or rough skin. From the biophysical point of view, this disorder is characterized by an increased TEWL, due to the defective water barrier and decreased stratum corneum water content. A study by Berardesca et al[28] shows that treatment with ceramides increases skin hydration and leads to rapid restoration of the barrier function, preventing prolonged water loss from the skin and thus contributing to improving the skin condition in the course of irritant contact dermatitis.

Skin surface water loss (SSWL) represents the evaporation of water from the skin surface after occlusion. When all the excess of water present in the corneum after occlusion has evaporated, SSWL is equal to TEWL.

SSWL and TEWL were studied after a plastic occlusion stress test (POST) in visually non-damaged skin treated with 7% SLS for three days in open application.[29] After removal of the 24-hour plastic occlusion, SSWL and TEWL were recorded continuously for 25 minutes. SSWL decay curves show significant differences between control and treated areas. The total amount of water trapped within the stratum corneum and released after one minute is significantly reduced in the treated site. Higher TEWL in visually non-irritated skin is noticeable in the terminal part of the curve, reflecting the damage to the water barrier in irritated skin. The data suggest that clinically normal skin exposed to subliminal irritant stimuli is less capable of storing water within the stratum corneum, resulting in decreased hydration. The POST appears to be a simple and reliable tool to investigate non-visible but biologically relevant changes in stratum corneum function.

TEWL may provide important information regarding the nature (allergic or irritant) of the skin response. Indeed, allergic and irritant reactions may be differentiated by TEWL. Some allergic reactions show a normal TEWL after 24 hours of application, in contrast with irritant reactions, where TEWL is increased after one day. Indeed, in allergic reactions, the deficiency in the water barrier is secondary to the inflammatory reaction, and occurs later than in primary irritant insult.[30]

Stripped skin shows both high TEWL and high hydration values, because the water-saturated epidermis is directly exposed.[11] The progressive restoration of the stratum corneum produces a normalization of TEWL levels in approximately two weeks and a reduction in the water content measurable at the skin surface, because of the deficiency of new parakeratotic horny layer to hold water.[11,31]

Monitoring and plotting TEWL and skin water content simultaneously is an easy and useful way to further define skin function. It permits discrimination between young and old, physiological and pathological skin, and provides information on skin behavior not understandable using only one technique.

There is good evidence that involved pathological skin differs from normal skin, but further work remains to be done to document differences between uninvolved skin of subjects prone to some pathological conditions (such as atopic dermatitis and psoriasis) and healthy skin of normal subjects. The detection of these differences and of other 'non-visible' pathological conditions (subliminal irritation) seems possible by standardizing and improving the available techniques and methods. It is likely that these bioengineering approaches will lead to greater sophistication in skin care regimens.

COSMETIC EFFICACY TESTING

TEWL and stratum corneum water content can be used to assess and compare the efficacies of different products applied to the skin – in particular, moisturizers.[32] Careful choices of instrumentation and calibration are recommended.[33,34] Guidelines have recently been

---

Table 45.1 Study designs for evaluating moisturizing properties of topical products, with their drawbacks and advantages (from Berardesca[36])

Single application (4–6 hours)
- Measurements start after 30 minutes from application
- Predictive for product efficacy
- Easy standardization of environment
- Effects of non-adsorbed material ('wiping')

Repeated application (3–4 weeks)
- Difficult standardization of climatic variables
- Improvement of hydration and/or skin condition expected
- Difficult discrimination between products
- More subjects may be needed

All studies
- Use always a reference control (e.g. glycerol in water)
- Standardize skin sites and environmental variables
- Combine different techniques with visual and tactile evaluation

published to allow correct experimental approaches to such studies.[35,36] In general, two different designs can be used in testing moisturizers: single and repeated application (Table 45.1). Short-term studies are less biased by environmental factors, while long-term studies give more information about the lasting effects of the products.

REFERENCES

1. Nilsson EG, Tenland T, Oberg PA, Evaluation of a laser Doppler flowmeter for measurement of tissue blood flow. *IEEE Trans Biomed Eng* 1980; **27:** 597–604.

2. Alexander H, Miller DL, Determining skin thickness with pulsed ultrasound. *J Invest Dermatol* 1979; **72:** 17–19.

3. Maibach HI, Bronaugh R, Guy R et al, Noninvasive techniques for determining skin function. In: *Cutaneous Toxicity* (Drill VA, Lazar P, eds). New York: Raven Press, 1984:63–97.

4. Berardesca E, Maibach HI, Bioengineering and the patch test. *Contact Dermatitis* 1988; **18:** 3–9.

5. Rietschel RL, A method to evaluate skin moisturizers in vivo. *J Invest Dermatol* 1978; **70:** 152–5.

6. van der Valk GM, Kruis-de Vries MH, Nater JP et al, Eczematous (irritant and allergic) reactions of the skin and barrier function as determined by water vapour loss. *Clin Exp Dermatol* 1985; **10:** 185–93.

7. Cunico RI, Maibach HI, Kahn H, Bloom E, Skin barrier properties in the newborn, transepidermal water loss and carbon dioxide emission rates. *Biol Neonate* 1977; **32:** 177.

8. Harpin VA, Rutter N, Barrier properties of the newborn infant's skin. *J Pediatr* 1983; **102:** 419–25.

9. Hammarlund K, Nilsson G, Oberg A, Sedin G, Transepidermal water loss in newborn infants. Relation to ambient humidity and site of measurement and estimation of total transepidermal water loss. *Acta Paediatr Scand* 1979; **68:** 371.

10. Osmark K, Wilson D, Maibach HI, In vivo transepidermal water loss and epidermal occlusive hydration in newborn infants: anatomical regional variations. *Acta Derm Venereol (Stockh)* 1980; **60:** 403–7.

11. Tagami H, Masatishi O, Iwatsuki K et al, Evaluation of skin surface hydration in vivo by electrical measurement. *J Invest Dermatol* 1980; **75:** 500–7.

12. Borroni G, Berardesca E, Bellosta M et al, Evidence for regional variations in water content of the stratum corneum in senile skin: an electrophysiologic assessment. *Ital Gen Rev Dermatol* 1982; **19:** 91–6.

13. Leveque JL, Corcuff P, de Rigal J, Agache P, In vivo studies of the evolution of physical properties of the human skin with age. *Int J Dermatol* 1984; **23:** 322–9.

14. Nicholls S, King CS, Marks R, The influence of corneocytes area on stratum corneum function. In: *Abstracts ESDR Annual Meeting, Amsterdam, 1980*.

15. Tagami H, In: *Cutaneous Aging* (Kligman AM, Takase Y, eds). Tokyo: University of Tokyo Press, 1988; 99–109.

16. Tagami H, Kanamaru Y, Inoue K et al, Water sorption–desorption test of the skin in vivo for functional assessment of the stratum corneum. *J Invest Dermatol* 1982; **78:** 425–8.

17. Grice K, Bettley FR, Skin water loss and accidental hypothermia in psoriasis, ichthyiosis and erythroderma. *Br Med J* 1967; **iv:** 195–8.

18. Berardesca E, Fideli D, Borroni G et al, In vivo hydration and water-retention capacity of stratum corneum in clinically uninvolved skin in atopic and psoriatic patients. *Acta Derm Venereol (Stockh)* 1990; **70:** 400–4.

19. Tagami H, Yoshikuni K, Interrelationship between water barrier and reservoir functions of pathologic stratum corneum. *Arch Dermatol* 1985; **181:** 642–5.

20. Serup J, Blichmann C, Epidermal hydration of psoriasis plaques and the relation to scaling. *Acta Derm Venereol (Stockh)* 1987; **67:** 357–66.

21. Blichmann C, Serup J, Hydration studies on scaly hand eczema. *Contact Dermatitis* 1987; **16:** 155–9.

22. Werner Y, The water content of the stratum corneum in patients with atopic dermatitis. Measurements with the Corneometer CM 420. *Acta Derm Venereol (Stockh)* 1986; **66:** 281–4.

23. Werner Y, Lindberg M, Transepidermal water loss in dry and clinically normal skin in patients with atopic dermatitis. *Acta Derm Venereol (Stockh)* 1985; **65:** 102–5.

24. Borroni G, Berardesca E, Gabba P, Rabbiosi G, Skin impedance in psoriatic epidermis. *Bioeng Skin* 1988; **4:** 15–22.

25. Lammintausta K, Maibach HI, Wilson D, Irritant reactivity in males and females. *Contact Dermatitis* 1987; **17:** 276–80.

26. van der Valk PM, Crijns MC, Nater JP, Bleumink E, Skin irritancy of commercially available soap and detergent bars as measured by water vapor loss. *Dermatosen* 1984; **32:** 87–90.

27. Malten KE, Den Arend J, Topical toxicity of various concentrations of DMSO recorded with impedance measurements and vapour loss measurements. *Contact Dermatitis* 1978; **4:** 80–92.

28. Berardesca E, Vignoli GP, Borroni G et al, Surfactant damaged skin: which treatment? In: *The Environmental Threat to the Skin* (Marks R, Plewig G, eds). London: Martin Dunitz, 1991:283–385.

29. Berardesca E, Maibach HI, Monitoring the water-holding capacity in visually non-irritated skin by plastic occlusion stress test (POST). *Clin Exp Dermatol* 1990; **15:** 107–10.

30. Serup J, Staberg K, Differentiation of allergic and irritant reactions by transepidermal water loss. *Contact Dermatitis* 1987; **16:** 129–32.

31. Spruit D, Malten KE, Epidermal water barrier formation after stripping of normal skin. *J Invest Dermatol* 1965; **45:** 6–14.

32. Loden M, Lindberg M, Product testing – testing of moisturizers. In: *Bioengineering and the Skin: Water and the Stratum Corneum* (Elsner P, Berardesca E, Maibach H, eds). Boca Raton, FL: CRC Press, 1994:275–89.

33. Distante F, Berardesca E. Transepidermal water loss. In: *Bioengineering and the Skin: Methods and Instrumentation* (Berardesca E, Elsner P, Wilhelm K, Maibach H, eds). Boca Raton, FL: CRC Press, 1995:1–4.

34. Distante F, Berardesca E, Hydration. In: *Bioengineering and the Skin: Methods and Instrumentation* (Berardesca E, Elsner P, Wilhelm K, Maibach H, eds). Boca Raton, FL: CRC Press, 1995:5–12.

35. Pinnagoda J, Tupker RA, Agner T, Serup J, Guidelines for transepidermal water loss (TEWL) measurements. *Contact Dermatitis* 1990; **22:** 164–78.

36. Berardesca E, EEMCO guidance for the assessment of the stratum corneum hydration: electrical methods. *Skin Res Technol* 1997; **3:** 126–32.

46

Non-invasive techniques for cutaneous investigation

Jean Luc Lévêque

INTRODUCTION

The first congress dealing with measurement of the skin's physical properties was organized by H Blank and R Marks in 1976. Since then, scientists from various fields (including dermatology, physics and biology) regularly meet during congresses organized by the International Society of Bioengineering and the Skin. They discuss the latest technical advances in skin research and also consider the progress in the knowledge of the skin brought by these new technologies.

Twenty-one years later, while numerous original techniques have been proposed, only those providing simple, reproducible parameters, easily interpretable in terms of skin structure and skin physiology, have been retained.

A book reviewing most of these new technologies and their use in dermatology and cosmetics has been published.[1] This chapter presents only some essential data on the topics of skin microrelief, skin colour, surface lipids, viscoelastic properties of the skin in torsion, and skin imaging by ultrasonography.

SKIN MICRORELIEF

A simple magnifying glass is sufficient to reveal the complexity of the human skin and the extensive variations from one anatomical site to another. The different types of relief are generally classified according to the depth of primary and secondary lines (respectively very deep and deep), tertiary lines (edges of corneocytes) and quaternary lines (trabecular network on the corneocyte itself). The arrangement of these lines (orientation and depth) differs according to the site, and changes with age and/or under the influence of environmental factors.

Studies of the skin microrelief in cosmetology are justified by the fact it conditions such factors as the softness of the skin and its macroscopic aspect. In both physiological and pathological states, the microrelief depends on the organization of collagen bundles in the upper dermis.

At present, there are two types of technique used to study the microrelief of the human skin:

- mechanical and profilometric methods;
- optical methods (densitometry, image analysis, laser-based techniques etc).

As we shall see, these methods have different sensitivities, but their main difference is their suitability for routine use. All, however, are based on replicas or counter-replicas of the skin surface.

Methods of measurement

Mechanical and profilometric techniques

These methods are derived from techniques developed in the metallurgical industry for examining the surfaces of metallic objects. A very fine, hard probe is used to scan the surface, and the data are then converted electronically into profiles that can be amplified and quantified. The parameters chosen to represent the surface include the mean interpeak distance and the mean (or maximum) peak height. Several devices for quantifying the skin surface have been developed, and include the Talysurf,[2] Anaglyphograph[3] and the Perth-O-Meter.[4] The main difficulty in this type of study is the time required to analyse every direction on a given surface.

Optical methods

Image analysis of skin replicas under low-angle lighting was first proposed in 1981 by Corcuff et al.[5] This technique, which has since been adapted by other workers in this field, uses a computer to quantify the various shades of grey on the image. A simple program enables the characteristic parameters of the relief (mean line depth, density, etc.) to be reconstituted.

Other optical methods have also been described, including photographic densitometry,[6] laser profilometry,[7] microscopic focalization and interferometry.[8] Needless to say, these methods can be used to quantify wrinkles.

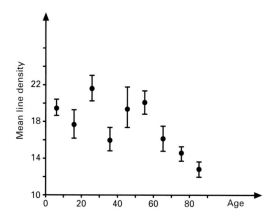

Figure 46.1 (a) Mean line depth as a function of age. (b) Mean line density as a function of age.

Main results

The great versatility of these techniques has allowed a number of changes in the skin surface with age to be described, including modifications due to environmental factors, and the effects of cosmetics and topical medication.

Numerous sites have been studied with regard to the effect of aging; these include the upper arm,[9] forearm,[5] leg,[10] abdomen[11] and face.[12] For instance, it has been shown that the mean relief on the arm increases after the fifth decade of life, whereas the density of the lines diminishes (Figure 46.1). These results have been confirmed by other techniques for the face.[13] Such variations could be explained by the reorganization of the collagen bundles in the papillary dermis. By way of an example, facial wrinkles vary greatly from person to person, mainly as a function of lifestyle and personality.[12]

With regard to the effect of topical agents, it has been shown that cosmetics[13,14] and retinoic acid-based lotions[15] can have a certain action on wrinkles.

SKIN COLOUR MEASUREMENTS

Skin colour can be measured using various types of apparatus that break down colour into its three principal components.[16] The most frequently-used apparatus is now the Minolta Colorimeter, which provides luminance (L) and chromaticity (a, b), in accord with the Commission Internationale de l'Éclairage (CIE-1976). The response of the system is similar to that of the human eye. Luminance represents the shade of grey (between white and black), while the chromaticity parameters a and b measure the colour of the object in the red/green and yellow/blue axes respectively. This highly integrated and precise apparatus can be used to obtain an objective determination of skin colour in various conditions.

The main applications of this technique are in studying the effects of sunlight, in terms of the minimal erythemal dose (MED)[17] – and thus the protection provided by sunscreens[18] and tanning.[17,19] It has therefore been possible to obtain a more objective classification of phototypes on the basis of skin colour measurements.[20]

The standardized measurement of immediate pigmentation darkening (IPD) has led to an objective method for measuring the protective index of UVA filters (Figure 46.2).[21]

Other applications concern inflammatory phenomena following treatment with topical irritants, vasodilators and anti-inflammatory drugs (skin blanching due to corticosteroids).[22] The pressure exerted on the skin by the device can slightly modify the colour, and this should be taken into account.

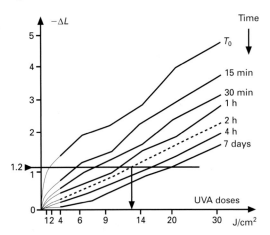

Figure 46.2 Darkening of the skin versus UVA dose as a function of time. The dotted line (- - -) indicates the optimum time, from a practical point of view, to measure IPD.

QUANTIFICATION OF SURFACE LIPIDS

Surface lipids consist of a mixture of molecules of sebaceous origin (the 'marker' is squalene) and epidermal origin (cholesterol and, in particular, the ceramides are characteristic).

Depending on the site, the lipid mixture at the skin surface is more or less rich in sebaceous and epidermal lipids. The forehead, the rest of the face, the thorax and the shoulders are very rich in sebaceous lipids, while epidermal lipids are predominant in the extremities. Sampling methods must be adapted to the quantities of lipids present on the skin surface. On the face, for example, these quantities are of the order of tens or hundreds of micrograms, whereas there are only a few micrograms per square centimetre on the limbs. The methods used are therefore very different.

Methods for quantifying sebum

The first method used was the 'cigarette paper' technique developed by P Pocchi in 1961. It was very difficult to use, and is rarely employed these days. It has been replaced by two more rapid methods, which are also more precise.

The first of these was the 'ground glass' technique presented in 1970 by Schaefer and Kuhn-Büssius,[23] which is based on the fact that a ground glass surface becomes transparent when lipids are applied to it. This principle gave rise to an automated device, the Lipometre, the practical use of which was described by Saint-Léger and Cohen.[24] All the lipids present at the skin surface can be removed by successive applications of the ground glass surface. The quantities of lipids (in $\mu g/cm^2$) are quantified directly by the apparatus following prior calibration of the ground glass plates. This method was validated in 1980 by Cunliffe et al[25] by comparison with the recognized 'cigarette paper' technique. The method has been used in numerous studies concerning, for example, the physiology of the sebaceous gland and the effect of various treatments. A device based on a similar principle is marketed under the tradename Sebumeter.

In 1986 an even simpler system was presented by Professor Kligman's team. It is based on the use of a special adhesive that is applied to the surface of the skin following delipidation. After about an hour, one observes shiny points on the adhesive, which correspond to the orifices of the hair follicles. The sebum secreted is thus progressively absorbed by the paper. Once the 'Sebutape' has been removed, the number of points and their surface area can be measured using a simple image-analysis system.[26] The results provided by this method have been correlated with those of the 'lipometric' technique (Figure 46.3).[27]

Methods for quantifying epidermal lipids

Epidermal lipids can only be harvested by applying to the skin a mixture of solvents suf-

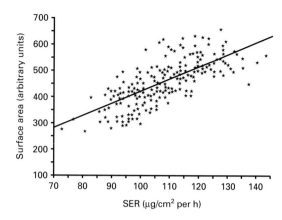

Figure 46.3 Linear correlation between surface area of dots and sebum excretion rate (SER) ($\mu g/cm^2$ per hour).

ficiently polar to extract the ceramides. Chloroform–methanol cannot be used as it injures the skin, but a hexane–methanol mixture is suitable. If quantitative data are to be obtained, the solvent must be applied in a standardized fashion. With this aim in mind, Saint-Léger et al developed a small stainless-steel turbine that can be dismantled.[28] After their removal, the lipids are concentrated and analysed by means of thin-layer chromatography. Various studies have been carried out using this system.[29,30]

MEASUREMENT OF THE VISCOELASTIC PROPERTIES OF THE SKIN: THE 'TWISTOMETER'

There are numerous physical systems that can be used to measure the viscoelastic properties of the human skin in vivo.[1] When measurements are made parallel to the skin surface – a method that has the advantage of minimizing the effect of the links between the dermis and the hypodermis – measurements of extensibility and torsion recovery are the most often used. In the Twistometer technique a given torsion couple is applied to the skin via a disc, and the rotational angle of the latter is determined as a function of time. The resulting curve shows an immediate rotation corresponding to immediate extensibility, followed by a slow increase corresponding to a phenomenon of creeping, which represents the viscous and plastic characteristics of the skin. The curve was modelled by de Rigal et al, and is expressed by the equation

$$U = U_E + U_V(1 - e^{-t/\tau})$$

where U is the rotational angle at each time, U_E is the instantaneous rotation angle, U_V is the final rotation angle and τ is the relaxation time. At a given time t the torsion couple is cancelled out, and the return of the skin to its initial deformation can be recorded. The immediate return is denoted by U_R, and the ratio U_R/U_E, which is independent of skin thickness, is called the elastic return or skin elasticity. As mentioned above, the couple is applied to the skin via a disc with double-sided adhesive tape. The rest of the skin is held in position by a guard ring, which is itself stuck to the skin. The work of de Rigal et al has shown that, for a given torsion couple, the greater the distance between the central disc and the guard ring, the deeper the deformation of the skin during the torsion.[31] By way of an example, for a distance of 2 mm and a couple of 0.6 N m, it was shown that the dermis was relatively undeformed and that, under these circumstances, only the epidermis and stratum corneum were involved. This apparatus has therefore been (and continues to be) used for testing the efficacy of cosmetic treatments.[32]

In addition to its applications in cosmetology, this apparatus can also be used to study the properties of the dermis when a suitable guard ring is employed. In this way, variations in the mechanical properties of the skin with age have been described.[33] During the aging process, the most strongly affected mechanical parameter is the elastic return of the skin, which decreases linearly when adulthood is

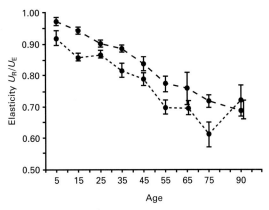

Figure 46.4 Skin elasticity as a function of age for a high torque (- - -) and a low torque (· · · ·).

reached (Figure 46.4). Similarly, the effects of the sun on the skin have also been described.[34] Finally, the effects of various types of scleroderma have been described using the apparatus.[35]

CUTANEOUS ULTRASOUND ECHOGRAPHY

In 1979 Alexander and Müller[36] adapted an apparatus designed for measuring certain geometrical parameters of the eye to determine skin thickness; this opened the way to the use of ultrasound techniques in dermatological research. There are now two main applications:

- ultrasound echography (A model – 'A' for amplitude), which can be used to measure the thickness of the various skin layers;
- ultrasound echography (B model – 'B' for brilliance), which allows the skin to be visualized in two dimensions.

A-mode ultrasonography

Principle
A-mode ultrasonography was developed on the basis of the experimental observation

(predicted theoretically) that the air/stratum corneum and derm/hypoderm interfaces generated echoes, whose amplitude could be measured simply.

Given the speed of ultrasound waves in the skin ($v = 1605$ m/s)[37] and the time t taken by an ultrasound impulse to cross the skin and be partially reflected by the derm/hypoderm junction, skin thickness can be calculated from the simple equation

$$\text{thickness} = \frac{v \times t}{2}$$

Implementation

The experimental device that enables this type of measurement to be made uses a strongly damped high-frequency ultrasound detector; the duration of the impulse must be as short as possible in order to detect the echoes generated by as many interfaces as possible. This is done by using certain transducers made of either ceramics or piezoelectric polymers. A rapid-response (about 10^{-9} seconds), high-tension electric impulse generator is used to excite the ultrasound detector. Finally, the receptor comprises a device protecting against emitter overcharge, a wideband radio-frequency amplifier and a detector of the radio-frequency signal envelope.

The signals generated by the skin are visualized using an oscilloscope. The two main echoes delimit the thickness of the skin. As the timescale follows the horizontal axis, the time interval between the echoes can be transformed into a distance, i.e. skin thickness.

Manufacturers are now marketing models that automatically measure the time interval between the echoes and thus the skin thickness.

B-mode ultrasonography (images)

Principle
The acquisition of a succession of signal lines in the A mode permits a cross-sectional image of the skin to be reconstructed, which is representative of the cutaneous echostructure.

Implementation
In contrast with the other organs of the human body, the thinness of the skin (about 1 mm) precludes the use of conventional echographs, since their spatial resolution is inadequate. It is therefore necessary to design a device specifically for skin imaging, taking into account the corresponding dimensions.

Such devices provide real-time observation of the skin in virtually all anatomical sites. An image of the skin of the arm, obtained using a prototype constructed in the research laboratories of L'Oréal, is shown in Figure 46.5. The various elements of this type of image are interpreted on the basis of comparative studies with histometric data.

In dermatology the value of A-mode and B-mode ultrasonography is that skin thickness can be measured in a non-invasive manner, in order to follow the effects of aging,[33] sunlight,[34] pharmacological agents (e.g. atrophy due to steroids)[38] and disease (e.g. scleroderma).[35]

B-mode ultrasonography provides images that are extremely useful, for example in skin

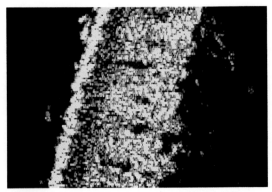

Figure 46.5 Ultrasonic imaging of the forearm skin.

cancers, by indicating the depth of the lesions. It has been shown that during the aging process, a non-echogenic band appears in the upper dermis. The amplitude of this band would be a far more sensitive marker of skin aging at the dermal level than is the measurement of skin thickness.[39] Variations in the images with time following a patch test can enable the physician to distinguish between an irritant and an allergic reaction to the product applied.

In the future the quality of these images will no doubt improve still further, and the epidermis, which is difficult to visualize because of its extreme thinness in certain sites, should be easier to study. In addition, the ultrasound waves reflected by the various elements of the skin carry information on the quality of the tissue in terms, for example, of its elastic properties. At present, this information cannot be interpreted, but when sufficient progress has been made, the qualitative parameters it carries will prove invaluable in the diagnosis of skin diseases.

REFERENCES

1. Lévêque JL (ed), *Cutaneous Investigation in Health and Disease.* New York: Marcel Dekker, 1989.
2. Makki S, Barbenel JC, Agache P, A quantitative method for the assessment of microtopography of human skin. *Acta Derma Venereol (Stockh)* 1979; **59:** 285–91.
3. Aubert L, Brun A, Grollier JF et al, A method to show the influence of cosmetic products on the cutaneous microrelief. *Cosmet Technol Sci* 1982; **3:** 265–70.
4. Kadner H, Biesgold C, Zur Technik der Rannhigkutsmessung der Hautoberflache mit dem Perth-O-Meter. *Derm Mschr* 1971; **157:** 758–9.
5. Corcuff P, de Rigal J, Lévêque JL et al, Skin relief and aging. *J Soc Cosmet Chem* 1983; **34:** 177–90.
6. Barton SP, Marshall RJ, Marks R, A novel method for assessing skin surface topography. *Bioeng Skin* 1989; **3:** 93–107.
7. Gormley DE, Automated optical profilometry. Bioengineering and the Skin Congress, San Francisco, September 1985.
8. Kim JI, Lee JH, Lee YY et al, New evaluation system of cosmetic effects on morphology of skin surface using TSRLM with image analyser. *Cosmet Toiletries* 1991; **106;** 156–71.
9. Hoppe U, Topologie der Hautoberfläche. *J Soc Cosmet Chem* 1979; **30:** 213–39.
10. Corcuff P, Lévêque JL, Grove GL et al, The impact of aging on the microrelief of periorbital and leg skin. *J Soc Cosmet Chem* 1987; **82:** 145–52.
11. Agache P, Mignot J, Makki S, Microtopography of the skin and aging. *Cutaneous Aging* 1988; **1:** 475–99.
12. Corcuff P, Chatenay F, Lévêque JL, A fully automated system to study skin surface patterns, *Int J Cosmet Sci* 1964; **6:** 167–76.
13. Meybeck A, Chanteloube F, Cosmetic wrinkle smoothing. In: *New Look at Old Skin* (Morganti P, Montagna W, eds). Rome: Int Ediemme, 1986:243–59.
14. Corcuff P, Chatenay F, Brun A, Evaluation of anti-wrinkle effects on humans. *Int J Cosmet Sci* 1985; **7:** 17–26.
15. Grove GL, Grove MJ, Optical profilometry: an objective method for quantification of facial wrinkles. *J Am Acad Dermatol* 1989; **3:** 631–7.
16. Lévêque JL, Physical methods to measure the efficiency of cosmetics in humans. *Cosmet Toiletries* 1984; **99:** 43–51.
17. Leitz JL, Whitmore CG, Measurement of erythema and tanning response in human skin using a tri-stimulus colorimeter. *Dermatologica* 1988; **177:** 70–5.
18. Chardon A, Dupont G, Moyal D et al, Colorimetric determination of sun protection factors. 15th IFSCC Conference, London, September 1988.
19. Chardon A, Crétois I, Hourseau C, Skin colour typology and sun tanning pathways. *Int J Cosmet Sci* 1991; **13:** 191–208.
20. Merot F, Masson Ph, Phototype and skin colour as predictive parameters for determination of minimal erythemal dose. IFSCC Conference, Helsinki, September 1991.
21. Chardon A, Moyal D, Hourseau C, *Skin Immediate Pigment Darkening Applied to UVA Protection Assessment.* San Antonio: American Society for Photobiology, 1991.

22. Queille-Roussel C, Poncet M, Schaefer H, Quantification of skin colour changes induced by topical corticosteroid preparations using the Minolta Chromameter. *Br J Dermatol* 1991; **124:** 264–70.

23. Schaefer H, Kuhn Büssius H, Methodik zur quantitativen Bestimmung der menschlischen Talgsekretion. *Arch Klin Exp Dermatol* 1970; **238:** 429–34.

24. Saint-Léger D, Cohen E, Practical study of qualitative sebum excretion on the human forehead. *Br J Dermatol* 1985; **113:** 551–7.

25. Cunliffe WJ, Kearney JN, Simpson NB, A modified photometric technique for measuring sebum excretion rate. *J Invest Dermatol* 1980; **77:** 394–5.

26. Nordstrom KM, Schmes HG, McGinley K et al, Measurement of sebum output using a lipid absorbent tape. *J Invest Dermatol* 1986; **87:** 260–3.

27. Lévêque JL, Pierard-Franchimont G, de Rigal J et al, Effect of topical corticosteroids on human sebum production assessed by two different methods. *Arch Dermatol Res* 1991; **283:** 372–6.

28. Deffond D, Saint Léger D, Lévêque JL et al, In vivo measurement of epidermal lipids in man. *Bioeng Skin* 1986; **2:** 71–85.

29. Saint Léger D, François AM, Lévêque JL et al, Stratum corneum lipids in skin xerosis. *Dermatologica* 1989; **178:** 151–5.

30. Chatenay F, Corcuff P, Saint Léger D et al, Alteration in the composition of human stratum corneum lipids induced by inflammation. *Photo Dermatol* 1990; **7:** 119–22.

31. de Rigal J, Lévêque JL, In vivo measurements of the stratum corneum elasticity. *Bioeng Skin* 1985; **1:** 13–17.

32. Aubert L, Anthoine P, de Rigal J et al, An in vivo assessment of the biomechanical properties of human skin modifications under the influence of cosmetic products. *Int J Cosmet Sci* 1985; **7:** 51–9.

33. Escoffier C, de Rigal J, Rochefort A et al, Age related mechanical properties of human skin: an in vivo study. *J Invest Dermatol* 1989; **93:** 353–7.

34. Lévêque JL, Porte G, de Rigal J et al, Influence of chronic sun exposure on some biophysical parameters of the human skin. An in vivo study, *J Cut Aging Cosmet Dermatol* 1987; **1:** 123–7.

35. Kalis B, de Rigal J, Léonard F et al, In vivo study of scleroderma by non invasive techniques, *Br J Dermatol* 1990; **122:** 785–91.

36. Alexander H, Müller DL, Determining skin thickness with pulsed ultrasound. *J Invest Dermatol* 1979; **72:** 17–19.

37. Escoffier C, Querleux B, de Rigal J et al, In vitro study of the velocity of ultrasound in the skin, *Bioeng Skin* 1986; **2:** 87–94.

38. Dykes PJ, Hill S, Marks R, In: *Topical Corticosteroid Therapy: A Novel Approach to Safer Drugs* (Christophers E, Kligman AM, Staughton RB, eds). New York: Raven Press, 1988:111–18.

39. de Rigal J, Escoffier C, Querleux B et al, Assessment of aging of the human skin by in vivo ultrasonic imaging. *J Invest Dermatol* 1989; **93:** 621–5.

47

The phototrichogram

Monique Courtois

This non-invasive technique was developed for the study of the principal parameters of hair growth.[1] It is of value both in research into the phenomena related to hair cycles and in the diagnosis and treatment of alopecia.

BACKGROUND: HAIR CYCLES

The hair cycle comprises three successive phases. The first, known as *anagen*, lasts several years, and is characterized by a growth rate of hair between 1 and 1.5 cm per month. The *catagen* phase is transitional, lasting a few weeks during which biological activity slows down. It leads to the final phase, known as *telogen*, a resting period during which hair growth terminates and the base of the bulb moves up towards the surface of the epidermis. At the end of the period in telogen, the hair is pushed outwards and is shed. A new cycle is then triggered at the same site.

Human hair growth takes on what is known as a mosaic pattern, in which individual hairs grow and are shed in a random and independent fashion. A permanent process of physiological hair renewal on the human scalp ensures a relatively constant density and ratio of anagen to telogen of about 90% anagen to 10% telogen in a healthy head of hair.

Common alopecia begins with a decrease in the duration of the growth phases, as a consequence of which the proportion of hairs in telogen increases and hair fall is accelerated. Progressively, hairs become finer and their number diminishes, allowing areas of sparse growth to appear on the scalp.

THE PHOTOTRICHOGRAM

This photographic technique, developed from that described by Saitoh et al[2] for the observation of body hair, is based on the following principle: after shaving an area of the scalp, it is possible to distinguish between the hairs in anagen, which lengthen by about 0.35 mm/day, and the resting hairs in telogen.

Equipment

The photographic apparatus used is a 35 mm camera equipped with a lens for macrophotography and a ring flash.

The camera is mounted on a rigid frame, which serves to establish a fixed distance between lens and scalp area. The section of the frame in contact with the scalp contains a window equipped with a non-reflective glass slide that delineates the field of view.

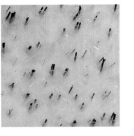
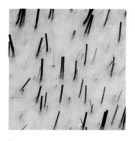

D$_0$ D$_2$

Figure 47.1 The principle of the phototrichogram: 250 hairs/cm^2; 26% telogen hairs.

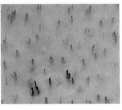
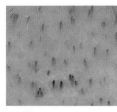

26.6.89   11.9.89

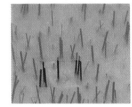
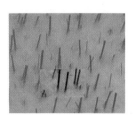

28.6.89   13.9.89

Figure 47.2 Phototrichogram: the regular study of an individual scalp area.

Methodology

- At the region of the scalp to be studied, an area measuring 0.5–1 cm^2 is selected. The hairs are shaved and the area photographed. Two to three days later, this zone is again photographed.

  On the basis of the two photographs (Figure 47.1), it is possible to calculate
  - the number of hairs/cm^2;
  - the anagen/telogen ratio;
  - the rate of growth;
  - the diameter of each hair.

- Regular observation of a precisely identified individual area shows that the inplantation of hairs and grouping of hairs are characteristic of that area; each hair can be identified. Hence it is feasible to monitor the renewal of hairs and to calculate the duration of hair cycles in a particular zone (Figure 47.2).

- Evaluation of the phototrichograms, usually performed by a trained technician, can be carried out by image analysis.[3]

PHOTOTRICHOGRAM APPLICATIONS

The phototrichogram allows the investigation of a number of aspects of hair growth, such as the following.

- *Study of the duration of hair cycles:*[4,5] alopecia and ageing lead to a decrease in the duration of anagen phases.
- *Diagnosis and treatment of alopecia:*[3,4] the parameters of hair growth can be followed over several months or years.
- *Periodicity in the growth and shedding of hair* can be studied[6] (Figure 47.3).

CONCLUSIONS

The phototrichogram is a precise and non-invasive technique that provides specific data on the main parameters of hair growth. Currently, it appears to be the most reliable and comprehensive method available for the study of hair life and of alopecia and its treatment.

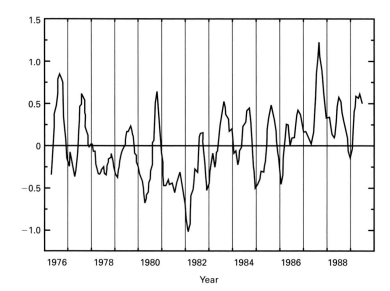

Figure 47.3 Mean evolution (10 subjects) of the monthly telogen percentage from 1976 to 1989.

REFERENCES

1. Fiquet C, Courtois M, Une technique originale d'appréciation de la croissance et de la chute des cheveux. *Cutis* 1979; **3:** 975–84.
2. Saitoh M, Uzuka M, Sakamoto M, Human hair cycle. *J Invest Dermatol* 1970; **54:** 65–81.
3. Chatenay F, Courtois M, Loussouarn G, Hourseau C, Phototrichogram: an entirely automated method of quantification by image analysis. In: *Hair Research for the Next Millennium* (Van Neste DJJ, Randall VA, eds). Amsterdam: Elsevier, 1996:105–8.
4. Courtois M, Loussouarn G, Hourseau C, Grollier JF, Hair cycle and alopecia. *Skin Pharmacol* 1994; **7:** 84–9.
5. Courtois M, Loussouarn G, Hourseau C, Grollier JF, Ageing and hair cycles. *Br J Dermatol* 1995; **312:** 86–93.
6. Courtois M, Loussouarn G, Hourseau C, Grollier JF, Periodicity in the growth and shedding of hair. *Br J Dermatol* 1996; **134:** 47–54.

48

Thermal sensory analysis

Gil Yosipovitch

INTRODUCTION

Skin care products contain complex ingredients that produce a variety of sensory stimuli. Many topical agents, especially those applied to the face, may produce strong disagreeable sensations such as stinging, burning or itching. Evaluation and product testing of cosmetics require carefully conducted experiments in order to provide definite information. Instrumental evaluation of the produced skin changes enables us to obtain objective and reproducible data. However, many topical agents produce disagreeable sensations without causing any skin changes of dermatitis as traced by these sensitive instruments. It is therefore of prime importance to include sensory evaluation in consumer testing of topical skin care products. A major limitation is the lack of objective criteria in evaluating symptoms such as itching, stinging and burning. Psychophysical objective measurements of the nature and degree of sensory disturbance are needed to trace patients with sensitive skin and to evaluate the effect of topical medications on sensation.

The superficial layers of the skin are essential for the induction of the sensations of pain, temperature, itching and burning. The skin is richly provided with sensory nerve fibers. These fibers are connected with various specialized receptor structures such as corpuscles and hair follicles, or end up as free, naked nerve endings. Two types of fibers are generally recognized as mediating the sensation of pain, itching, stinging and temperature:

- A-delta fibers are small myelinated fibers that mediate the sensation of cold and the first component of the sensation of pain at a conduction velocity between 2 and 30 m/s;
- C fibers are small non-myelinated fibers, mediating the sensation of warmth and the main component of the pain sensation, as well as of itch, at a conduction velocity less than 2 m/s.

Thermal sensation testing enables us to assess the function of these small fibers.

QUANTITATION OF CUTANEOUS THERMAL SENSATION

Since the C fibers and A-delta fibers transmit temperature, pain, itching and burning sensations, a sensitive thermal sensory testing device may enable us to trace chemosensory effects of substances on skin and patients who suffer from 'sensitive skin'.

In recent years, methods of thermal sensory testing have increasingly been utilized in clinical medicine, especially in neurology.[1,2] The thermal threshold is the function that can be measured most easily and conveniently. All modern automated thermal testing instruments have a thermode that is capable of heating or cooling the skin.[2] It consists of semiconductor junctions of dissimilar metals. Cooling will occur on one side of the junction and warming on the other, depending on the polarity of the electrical current. The thermode consists of a Peltier device, and a thermocouple fixed to the center of the thermode records the temperature. There are several commercially available units. The most advanced apparatus is the thermal sensory analyzer TSA 2001, which is a portable device, fully computerized and manufactured by Medoc (Ramat Yishai, Israel). It operates between 0°C and 54°C, with a linear and accurate temperature change. It features several algorithms for threshold measurement in order to minimize subjective variation and make the result as objective as possible. In addition, it can be used for measuring heat or cold pain thresholds and suprathreshold pain magnitude by applying stimuli of fixed temperature for various application times. There are two basic methods for measuring thermal thresholds:[2,3] the method of limits and the use of constant stimuli.

In the first method, the subject is exposed to a stimulus of changing intensity until he or she perceives a sensation. The subject then halts the stimulus increase by pressing a button. Several stimuli are given in succession, and a mean value provides a threshold. In this method, there is a reaction-time artifact, due to the time lapse between the moment at which sufficient energy has been administered to the stimulation site to induce the sensation and the moment at which the signal reaches the brain. This artifact can be minimized by using relatively slow rates of increase of stimulus.

In the second method, the stimulus is increased stepwise, and the subject is asked to respond with a 'yes' or 'no' as to whether or not the stimulus was felt. After the first 'yes' response, the stimulus is decreased by one-half of the value evoking a response, and then by half of this value, and so on until a 'no' is given. The subject's response determines the intensity of the next stimulus. The major disadvantage of this method is the longer performance time.

USEFULNESS OF THERMAL SENSORY TESTING

Thermal sensory testing is a relatively simple procedure that is both non-invasive and non-aversive. The data obtained by the thermal sensory analyzer can be used to detect subtle sensory loss and cutaneous hypersensitivity states, and can also be used in parametrical longitudinal evaluation. The clinical usefulness of any thermal testing device must be based on several factors.

1. *Sensitivity:* for diagnostic purposes, the device should be sufficiently sensitive to detect abnormality. For this purpose, smaller Peltier devices have been developed for specific body areas such as the face (Figure 48.1).
2. *Defined control range:* for recognition of a sensory deficit, the main requirement imposed upon the thermal testing device is that the control range should be defined, taking into account that detection thresholds in healthy subjects vary with site, age and gender.[1]
3. *Reproducibility/reliability:* the test–retest reproducibility of measurements is an important factor in the clinical usefulness of the thermal testing apparatus, especially for longitudinal studies. Yarnitsky et al[4] have published their normative data, including a repeatability factor, expressing the amount of inter-session change in threshold in normals. Knowledge of such factors allows for longitudinal studies of threshold measure-

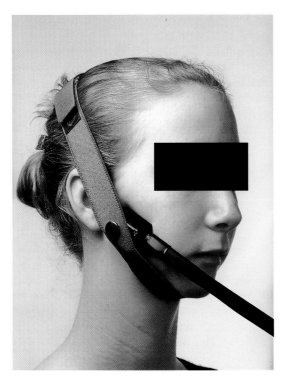

Figure 48.1 Thermal testing with a Peltier thermode on the face.

ple, in patients with postherpetic neuralgia (PHN), the use of thermal testing demonstrates significant changes in thermal thresholds in the acute phase for patients who later developed PHN, while patients who had recovered from shingles without PHN had no evidence of abnormal thresholds.[6] The average of the cool, warm and heat pain deficits in PHN skin measured with a thermal testing device has been shown to be significantly and positively related to cutaneous innervation density at the dermal–epidermal junction.[7]

APPLICATIONS OF THERMAL SENSORY TESTING IN DERMATOLOGY

We have recently demonstrated that warm sensation thresholds – a C-fiber-mediated sensation – are significantly elevated during histamine-induced itching, while cold sensation and thermal pain thresholds are not affected.[8,9] These results provide further support to the essential role of C fibers in itch transmission. This technique may enable us to examine the effect of various skin irritants on itching, burning and cold and warm sensations.

We have used this technique with several compounds, and have shown that alcohol, which is commonly used in cosmetic and antipruritic compounds, has a significant increase on cold-sensation thresholds.[10] Several topical counter-irritants, analgesics and anesthetics have been examined. Compounds such as capsaicin, menthol, pramoxine, topical aspirin and EMLA (a eutectic mixture of local anesthetics) have shown significant specific effects on thermal and pain thresholds.[9–11]

ments. Threshold measurement is a subjective test, and judgement based on test results may therefore be incomplete. Yarnitsky et al[5] have suggested a model for better interpretation of threshold measurement findings, based on the interplay of thresholds and their variances. According to this model, a normal mean threshold with small variance is regarded as a normal result, and a high mean threshold with small variance is suggestive of pathology. A normal mean threshold with high variance probably indicates inattention, and a high threshold with a high variance suggests feigning.

The thermal sensory analyzer enables early diagnosis of painful neuropathies. For exam-

THE FUTURE OF THERMAL SENSORY TESTING IN COSMETOLOGY

Utilizing the thermal testing analyzer may enable us to trace patients who suffer from 'problem sensitive skin'. It would be important to perform measurements with the thermal sensory analyzer during application of the lactic acid test of Frosch and Kligman[12] to identify members of the 'delicate skin club'.

Thermal sensory testing devices may be added to the battery of sensory subjective analyses to be performed before launching new cosmetic products.

REFERENCES

1. Dyck PJ, Karens JK, O'Brien PC, Zimmerman IR, Detection thresholds of cutaneous sensation in humans. In: *Peripheral Neuropathy*, 3rd edn (Dyck PJ et al, eds). Philadelphia: WB Saunders, 1993:706–28.

2. Yosipovitch G, Yarnitsky D, Quantitative thermal testing. In: *Dermatotoxicologic Methods: The Laboratory Worker's Vade Mecum* (Maibach HI, Marzulli FN, eds). New York: Taylor & Francis, 1997:315–20.

3. Maurissen JP, Quantitative sensory assessment in toxicology and occupational medicine, applications, theory, and critical appraisal. *Toxicol Lett* 1988; **43:** 321–43.

4. Yarnitsky D, Sprecher E, Tamir A et al, Thermal testing normative data and repeatability for various algorithms. *J Neurol Sci* 1994; **125:** 39–45.

5. Yarnitsky D, Sprecher E, Tamir A et al, Variance of sensory threshold measurements: discrimination of feigners from trustworthy performers. *J Neurol Sci* 1994; **125:** 186–9.

6. Nurmikko T, Bowsher D, Somatosensory findings in postherpetic neuralgia. *J Neurol Neurosurg Psychiatry* 1990; **53:** 135–41.

7. Rowbotham G, Yosipovitch G, Connolly K et al, Cutaneous innervation density in the allodynic form of post herpetic neuralgia. *Neurobiol Dis* 1996; **3:** 205–14.

8. Yosipovitch G, Szolar C, Hui XY, Maibach H, High potency corticosteroid rapidly decreases histamine induced itch but not thermal sensation and pain in man. *J Am Acad Dermatol* 1996; **35:** 118–20.

9. Yosipovitch G, Ademola J, Ping Lui, Maibach H, Effect of topically applied aspiring on thermal, pain and itch sensations. *Acta Derm Venereol (Stockh)* 1997; **77:** 46–8.

10. Yosipovitch G, Szolar C, Hui XY, Maibach H, Effect of topically applied menthol on thermal, pain and itch sensations and biophysical properties of the skin. *Arch Dermatol Res* 1996; **288:** 245–8.

11. Yosipovitch G, Maibach H, Effect of topical pramoxine on experimentally induced itch in man. *J Am Acad Dermatol* 1997; **37:** 278–80.

12. Frosch PJ, Kligman AM, Recognition of chemically vulnerable and delicate skin. In: *Principles of Cosmetics for the Dermatologist* (Frost P, Horwitz S, eds). St Louis, MO: CV Mosby, 1982:287–96.

PART NINE

TECHNIQUES IN COSMETOLOGICAL TREATMENT

49

Reduction syringe liposculpturing

Pierre F Fournier

INTRODUCTION

Reduction liposculpturing has made many advances in the past 15 years. At first only small localized adiposities were treated under local anaesthesia and as an ambulatory procedure. Today, most major adiposities can also be treated in this way, without the risk of blood transfusion.

Such advances are due to the use of the Klein formula, which ensures a bloodless operation, no shock and a shorter recovery period. Another reason for these advances is the use of the syringe instead of the suction machine, which makes the operation simpler and safer, and offers many other advantages, including the possibility of removing six or more litres of adipose tissue (Figure 49.1). These two factors have led to the procedure becoming popular with all surgical specialists. Liposculpturing does not belong to any one specialty, although cosmetic surgeons have been responsible for all of the major advances since the first demonstration of this technique in Paris by its inventor, Giorgio Fischer, in March 1977.

SURGICAL TECHNIQUE

For the past 12 years, in all cases of reduction liposculpturing, I have used only plastic syringes on which common cannulas are mounted. Cannulas and syringes are selected according to the volume of the adiposity.

Equipment

Cannulas (or lipodissectors)
Cannulas are classified according to their outside diameter and are made of metal. Those with a very small outside diameter (microcannulas) measure 1.5, 2 or 2.5 mm. Their useful length is 4–8 cm. They have a blunt opening

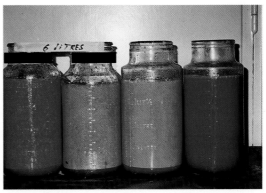

Figure 49.1 Six or more litres can be removed with a syringe without a blood transfusion.

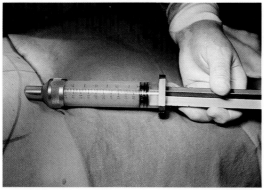

(a)

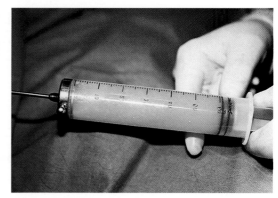

Figure 49.3 The French cannula.

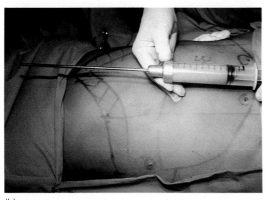

(b)

Figure 49.2 The tulip cannula (created by John Johnson): (a) with and (b) without lock on the syringe.

and a blunt tip, which can be round or bullet shaped. Those with an average outside diameter (minicannulas) measure 3, 3.5 or 4 mm. Their useful length is 8–14 cm, and they can either have a round or bullet-shaped tip with a blunt opening. Those with an outside diameter greater or equal to 5 mm (macrocannulas) measure 5, 5.5, 6, 7 or 8 mm. Their useful length is 15–24 cm or 29–35 cm. The cannulas are mounted in the syringe either externally (tulip; Figure 49.2) or passed through the syringe (French model; Figure 49.3).

Syringes

Average-size syringes (10 or 20 cm^3) are made of plastic, and are sterile and disposable. They are used with microcannulas or minicannulas.

Large-volume syringes are used with macrocannulas (50 or 60 cm^3). They are used by urologists as well as gynaecologists (for abortions). These syringes are plastic, sterile, and disposable. They should have a large opening: 5 mm or more outside diameter. The implantation of a hub on the syringe has an 8–10 mm external diameter (tumey tip). Some syringes have a lock to immobilize the plunger with the right hand throughout the liposculpturing procedure. The screw-type lock is useful only for 50–60 cm^3 syringes. Small or average syringes do not need one.

It is best to prime the syringe with a few cubic centimetres of normal saline before the extraction to avoid any dead space. After a small amount of saline has been aspirated into the syringe, pulling on the plunger with the right hand and operating the screw lock will be very easy. If a small amount of normal saline has been aspirated into a 60 cm^3 syringe, a lock is unnecessary. We have not used one for any of our cases of liposculpturing. If the surgeon believes a lock is needed, small holes can be drilled in the plunger of the plastic syringe and a needle can be passed through one of them to act as a lock on the plunger.

The awl or ice pick

We do not use the scalpel for any of our cases. To avoid incision scars, punctures are made through the skin with an awl. This opening can be dilated with a haemostat to allow entry of the cannula. The puncture of the skin made by the awl heals better than an incision with a scalpel, and is almost invisible. It must be made wide enough to avoid friction of the cannula on the skin and pigmentations.

When cannulas are reused, metal cleaners should be used before sterilization. Future cannulas will be made of hard plastic. They will be sterile, disposable, and in many lengths and diameters. It would be ideal to have a sterile, disposable cannula and syringe made in one piece.

The liposuction surgeon should be aware of the following.

The larger the diameter and capacity of the syringe, the less it is suited to transporting the fat. This is why *it is much better to use a syringe adapted to the volume of the adiposity and to the volume of fat to be extracted* (Figure 49.4). The outside diameter of the syringe should be as small as possible. This is why a 2 cm^3 syringe for insulin injections is better than the standard 2 cm^3 syringe, which is much shorter.

The cannulas should also be chosen according to the volume of the adiposity. If custom-made cannulas are not available to mount on the plastic syringes, it is easy to use the standard machine cannula. First the handle is sawn off, then the cannula is passed through the barrel of the plastic syringe and pushed with long scissors in a screw-type motion through the plastic hub after the opening has been cut appropriately. It may be necessary to use an ice pick or haemostat to further dilate the plastic hub. The cannulas have to be perfectly adapted to the hub and syringe (Figure 49.5).

This equipment is as useful as any manufac-

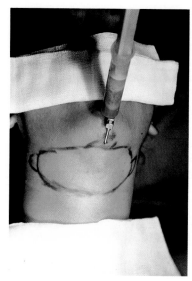

Figure 49.4 A 14-gauge cannula mounted on a 10 cm^3 syringe.

tured lipodissector for syringe-assisted liposculpturing. The equipment is tight, waterproof and airproof. Surgeons who choose to make their own equipment can obtain the syringes in medical, dental or veterinary supply stores. Cannulas of 2, 2.5 and 3 mm can be mounted externally, since their inside diameter corresponds to the inside diameter of the small syringes (Luer lock).

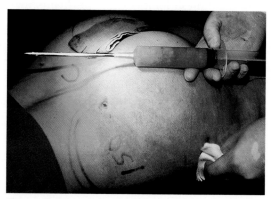

Figure 49.5 Makeshift equipment.

If the surgeon performing a liposculpture procedure does not have a cannula that can be mounted on a syringe, a Karman cannula (used by gynaecologists for abortions with an aspirator) can be used. A transparent and rigid tube about 50 cm long will connect the handle of the Karman cannula to a 60 cm^3 syringe.

If the surgeon works alone, the syringe plunger can be blocked with a lock, a haemostat or any other instrument after making a hole through the syringe's plunger. An assistant can pull on the plunger while the surgeon works. In both cases, it is necessary to prime the system with a certain amount of saline solution. In all systems described, suction is as fast as with the machine, but provokes less shock and less bleeding, and is less tiring for the surgeon.

The goal of the procedure

This is to perform a partial lipectomy in the localized adiposity. Four steps are required:

1. removal of the excess adipose tissue through a criss-cross dissection/extraction (lesional lipectomy or mesh lipoextraction);
2. remodelling of the remaining criss-crossed adipose tissue;
3. redistribution of the skin after a wide peripheral mesh undermining of the neighbouring normal adipose tissue (perilesional mesh lipoplasty) – this manoeuvre (performed with a cannula without suction) will sever many retinaculum cuti connecting the skin to the deep fascia, and will allow better remodelling of the tissues;
4. adequate immobilization of the treated area until shrinkage and healing proceed satisfactorily.

In some cases, after performing reduction liposculpturing on one of several adipose regions, it is worth using the harvested fat to fill in the neighbouring depressions. The final result will be improved.

The surgeon must keep in mind that closed liposculpturing is an artistic, three-dimensional architectural technique of body contouring. It is essentially a tactile operation, with the surgeon working almost blindly. We are dealing with a volume of space occupied by adipose tissue and a surface-covering tissue (the skin). Fat is highly vascularized; consequently, a lipectomy has to be performed using a blunt cannula to create criss-crossed dissection/extraction channels. It is imperative to avoid excessive bleeding by using vasoconstrictors. It is also crucial to reposition the skin and underlying fat using the shrinking properties of the skin and the technique of peripheral mesh undermining. Finally, adequate immobilization for one week is important to obtain good results.

Basic principles

The following are some of the basic principles in reduction syringe liposculpturing.

- A criss-crossed lipectomy (tunnels, columns of fat, lattice, and mesh lipectomy) has to be performed.
- A peripheral mesh-undermining technique is usually part of the operation, and is performed with a cannula without suction.
- Dissecting hydrotomy with vasoconstrictors (chilled normal saline at 2°C and adrenaline 1 mg/litre) is necessary (unless local anaesthesia is used).
- The required instruments include a small blunt-tipped cannula with one blunt opening, ice pick and syringes.
- The shrinking properties of the skin should be utilized after repositioning and immobilizing.

Pre-estimation of the quantity to be resected

The amount of adipose tissue to be resected during liposculpturing must be calculated during the patient's different preoperative examinations. This is a matter of experience and judgement, acquired only with time after assisting the operations performed by other surgeons. Only then can an accurate estimate be made.

During the operation, this estimate can be more or less modified, but overall the surgeon has a relatively good idea of the amount of tissue to be resected.

Pre-estimation requires the same kind of judgement that is necessary for other aesthetic operations. The eye will examine the state of the skin (thick, with or without stretch marks); the fingers will test the tonicity of the areas to be treated by using the pinch test in a standing position, lying down while the underlying muscles are contracted, and while walking.

The pre-estimation in a region such as the saddlebag area can be done only after a careful study of the neighbouring adipose areas that can play a role in the origin of the saddlebags: hips, buttocks and the lower buttocks fold. One must therefore differentiate between true saddlebags, false saddlebags and mixed cases.

Xerographies, echographies, scanner or other complementary examinations can be useful, but are never demanded because the pre-estimation is mainly done during the physical examination. The pre-estimation is noted on the patient's card, on special diagrams, or on the Polaroid photos made on the first visit.

General remarks

We must insist once more that the surgeon needs to know the approximate amount of adipose tissue to be resected before the operation (to put it bluntly: it is not a 'suck as you go procedure'). The following things depend on the quantity to be resected:

- whether the operation can be performed all at once or in several stages;
- whether local, general or epidural anaes-

thesia is to be used (the dose of local anaesthetic also needs to be estimated);
- the amount of intravenous fluids and electrolytes needed;
- the length of hospitalization (whether or not the patient is ambulatory);
- whether a blood transfusion needs to be considered;
- the approximate length of convalescence.

All of this requires experience and good judgement.

Steps of the operation

Marking the patient
Marking the patient is done in the standing position, just before the operation. We use a green Pentel pen; the skin marker must be of good quality to resist the preparations. We mark:

1. the adiposity by encircling it;
2. another circle 1–1.5 cm around the previous circle (the tip of the cannula will be pushed up to the second marking so there will be no stair-step deformity);
3. beyond the adiposity between 2 and 8 cm from the second marking – this corresponds to the extent of the peripheral mesh undermining;
4. finally, the openings (or incisions) are marked by a circle to avoid any permanent or transient tattooing from the ink of the marking pen.

All the adipose regions are marked before the operation, as is the site of the intended incisions or openings. The approximate amount of resection is marked in the middle of the adiposity (Figure 49.6).

Anaesthesia
Reduction liposculpturing can be done according to the type of anaesthesia that the patient desires – general, twilight, epidural, local or cryoanaesthesia. Local anaesthesia is the preferred method. For the past few years,

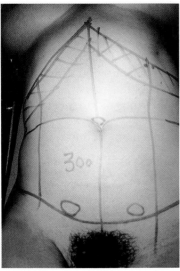

Figure 49.6 The abdomen is squared off.

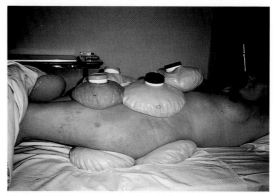

Figure 49.7 Cryoanaesthesia with ice cubes.

we have used the tumescent technique as described by Klein: chilled saline at 2°C is used instead of saline at room temperature. The Klein formula is

- normal saline   1 litre
- lidocaine (Xylocaine)   500 mg
- adrenaline   1 mg
- sodium bicarbonate   12.5 mmol (or 12.5 cm^3 of an 8.4% NaHCO$_3$ solution)

A great deal has been written on this topic, which should be used as a reference when using the tumescent technique.

External cryoanaesthesia can be used in addition to local anaesthesia. Ice packs will improve the anaesthesia and decrease the bleeding. If refrigerated bags are used, the patient should be closely monitored because the bags can cause skin burns or pigmentation. This does not occur with ice cubes (Figure 49.7).

Preparation of the operating area

In all cases of reduction liposculpturing, the area should be injected to decrease bleeding as well as to enhance the procedure. During general anaesthesia, we use the following solution: 1 litre of chilled normal saline at 2°C and 1 mg adrenaline. The amount injected is roughly one-half of the estimated fat to be removed. This solution is injected deep into the fatty layer to obtain a spasm of the vessels at this level. After 15 minutes, another injection of chilled saline at 2°C, without adrenaline, is administered in the upper layer before starting the procedure. This second step, however, is not absolutely necessary. There are no special recommendations when the area is prepared with conventional local anaesthesia.

Approaches in liposculpturing

The planned approach has to allow for easy, efficient work in the adiposity to obtain the best possible result. Approaches used at the beginning of the procedure that are concealed far from the adiposity must be avoided if they interfere with proper working conditions. There will be a minimum of two approaches for criss-cross work: one must use as many approaches as necessary to perform a

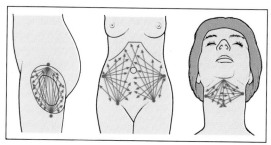

Figure 49.8 Approaches and criss-cross work.

good criss-cross mesh (Figure 49.8). Puncturing the skin is always done in the right tension line, and is better than incising it. For the past few years, we have used an awl or ice pick to make the openings in all of our approaches. Should the awl or ice pick puncture be too small to pass the cannula, the hole can be dilated by first passing one branch and then the other of a haemostat, which are then separated very gently. Since there is no incision in the skin, the wound heals much better than a standard incision, and is almost invisible. In most cases, the wounds need to be closed with a fine nylon 5–0 suture or by an inverted stitch of resorbable material. It can also be left unsutured if it is not too large.

Positioning the patient

The position of the patient will, of course, be that which is the most convenient for the surgeon. Choices include the supine, prone and lateral positions. With all of these positions, arms or legs to be moved during the operation should be prepared according to the needs of the surgeon. Under local anaesthesia, with the legs apart and feet together (frog position), there is no problem, since the patient can move or be moved if necessary. This also holds if epidural anaesthesia is used. However, during general anaesthesia, the patient is supine, and it is necessary to elevate a side of the patient to permit the surgeon to

work on the waist, the hip or the lateral chest roll. Other localizations are within easy reach, for example, thighs, knees, and double chin. If the patient is in a supine position, it is also possible to work on the buttocks or to create an infragluteal fold, although this is not as easily done as in the prone position. By moving a patient who has been specially prepared, it is possible to work on almost all localized adiposities of the pelvis in the supine position.

Turning the patient from the prone to the supine position or vice versa during a liposculpturing procedure under general anaesthesia should be avoided whenever possible. Nevertheless, it is sometimes necessary, and special precautions should be taken by the surgeon and the anaesthesiologist. For safety reasons, it is much better to do the requested procedures in two stages instead of taking risks with the patient when a change of position is needed.

A word of caution is in order here: positioning the patient is important – the surgeon should not be working under difficult conditions. The surgeon should always have easy access to the different approaches needed during the procedure in order to do the best work possible (Figure 49.9).

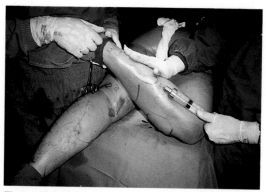

Figure 49.9 The surgeon has to work with ease.

Technique of liposculpturing

We shall use the work on a hip with a 5 mm cannula and a 60 cm³ syringe as an example to describe surgical technique. Incisions or openings are made at the previously marked sites (we prefer the puncture), and are dilated with a haemostat. Pretunnelling is not absolutely necessary, but is recommended if the fat is hard. Before liposculpturing begins, to-and-fro movements without suction are made with the cannula in a fan-shaped area from the penetrating point. Before starting, one should fill the syringe with 5 or 10 cm³ of chilled saline to eliminate all dead space in the cannula; the saline will then act as a buffer. The cannula is then passed through the opening while the left hand folds the skin.

The plunger is withdrawn and kept that way with the surgeon's right hand. The manoeuvre is not difficult, and can be facilitated by using a lock. The cannula is moved in a fan-shaped way, approximately five times in the same direction (we do not recommend staying in the same tunnel). The strength of the surgeon is exerted when pushing the cannula into the adipose tissue, not when pulling it. The opening of the cannula will face down during this manoeuvre. After 60 cm³ of fat has been collected in the barrel, the syringe is emptied into a basin on the operating table. The same procedure is followed until half of the pre-estimated amount of fat has been removed.

When half of the pre-estimated amount of fat has been removed from the localized adiposity, the cannula is inserted into another opening at right-angles or opposite to the first one, and tunnels are made in a criss-cross fashion. The left hand still guides and follows the work of the right hand. The work of the hands is summarized in Table 49.1. Liposculpturing is a tactile operation.

The division of labour between the two hands is opposite to that in standard surgery, in which the right hand is the dominant one. In liposculpturing, the left hand is the 'brain hand' and the right one is a mere piston.

Table 49.1 Functions of the left and right hands during liposculpturing

Left hand	Right hand
Stabilizes	Pushes
Grasps	Pulls
Lifts	Dissects
Hardens	Fills syringe
Guides	Empties syringe
Localizes	Pulls on plunger and locks it
Palpates	Measures fat extracted
Does pinch test	
Monitors	

In some circumstances, one may use a smaller cannula (No. 3) to do the criss-crossing at a different level. At intervals, the left hand will pinch the skin (pinch test) between the index and the thumb to elevate the thickness of the fold. The surgeon will usually monitor the modification of the contour of the area treated to avoid an overcorrection, and will also check the volume of fat removed against the pre-estimate.

A 1 cm uniform thickness of fat covering the area should be left; this is controlled by a pinch test done with the left hand. Should the fat in the syringe show too much blood, the surgeon must stop suctioning the area and work on another part of the adiposity. Should the patient complain under local anaesthesia, the surgeon should inject more of the anaesthetic solution.

It should be noted that the skin has to be grasped in order to put the cannula in the right place. The left hand should be flat during the whole operation, and should exert some pressure on the tissues to stabilize the skin. The surgeon will work at all levels of the adiposity except in the first centimetre below the skin.

When the lipectomy is complete, the surgeon performs a peripheral mesh undermining using the same openings and instruments. No suction is done during this procedure. The cannula is pushed in a fan-shaped motion until it reaches the marked line of the mesh undermining. This mesh is also done in a criss-cross fashion through the area already lipectomized. The peripheral mesh undermining allows the excess skin that is covering the criss-cross lipectomized adiposity to fit better in its new bed; less resistance will be encountered in the neighbouring tissues because many retinacula cutis will have been severed. The peripheral mesh undermining must be proportional to the amount of fat removed and also the quality of the skin.

When one area has been completely treated, the surgeon will work on the opposite paired adiposity unless another well-trained lipoplastic surgeon has already done the second side (Figure 49.10). When a neighbouring depressed area has to be grafted, part of the fat that has been harvested will be washed with normal saline and reinjected in a criss-cross manner. This area will be remodelled with the surgeon's left hand and immobilized together with the other treated areas. Remodelling of the adipose area is done with the surgeon's left hand.

Dressing

After suturing the skin openings, the surgeon will do the dressing using Elastoplast, unless a special garment is used. Several layers have to be used because the dressing acts as an external splint. This dressing will be kept on for one week in most cases. Afterwards, it is recommended to use a binder during the day for six weeks, however, no binder is necessary if the Klein formula has been used.

Fluid and electrolyte balance

The anaesthesiologist will take care of the problem of fluid and electrolyte balance. Roughly double the amount of fat removed has to be given to the patient in fluids. Most of the time, when using the tumescent technique, no fluids are used intravenously.

TECHNICAL CONSIDERATIONS

The quantity of fat to be removed is the visible resection. The to-and-fro movements of the cannula devitalize a certain amount of adipose tissue, which is later resorbed by the body: this is the invisible or biological resection. During the procedure, there is adipose tissue extraction – but there is also adipose tissue destruction. Therefore fat reduction is obtained in two ways: through mechanical disruption as well as suction friction scraping.

The visible resection is the one obtained by the scraping motion of the cannula, which also removes part of the fat that has been mechanically disrupted. The invisible resection is mostly made up of devitalized fat obtained by the friction of the cannula and some of the mechanically disrupted fat. Irrigation of the tissues with normal saline always removes small fragments of fat. After a certain lapse of time, the procedure will create scar tissue, which will be followed by contraction, as is true for any operation on or below the skin. This consideration enhances the prognosis for a thorough and even lipectomy. The purpose of the peripheral mesh undermining in the whole area treated is to obtain homogeneous contraction of the scar tissue.

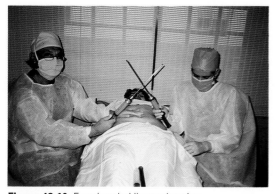

Figure 49.10 Four handed liposculpturing.

The skin will be affected by the primary contraction of the muscular fibres (immediate, active process). The adipose tissue will be modified by the contraction of the fibrous tissue (passive contraction, delayed). After a liposculpturing procedure, there is an immediate improvement in contour due to the biological resection. The skin will also be modified immediately by the primary contraction of elastic fibres, and later by the contraction of the underlying fibrous scar tissue.

Surgeons performing liposculpturing should remember that *the most important consideration is not what is removed, but what is left and how it is left* (as in rhinoplasty). If too much blood is in the aspirate, one should stop working in the area and work on another part of the adiposity or on another adiposity. Under no circumstance should windshield-wiper movements be made, since they will cut the adipose columns that harbour blood vessels, nerves and lymph vessels. When lumps are felt under the skin, one should work on them with a smaller cannula (decreasing work).

The following points should be kept in mind.

- Small lipodissectors (cannulas) with one opening should be used.
- Blunt tip and blunt openings should face downwards.
- The syringe should be used for extraction and hydrocryodissection.
- An atraumatic technique with no windshield-wiper movements should always be used.
- Tunnels should be fan-shaped, starting from the puncture wound.
- Dissection should be blunt and deep, leaving one centimetre of fat layer under the skin. The approach should be direct and the puncture made with an ice pick.
- Criss-crossing (tunnels and fat columns, lattice work) should be done. Two or more approaches have to be made.
- The left hand should direct the operation.

- Peripheral mesh undermining should be performed.
- Remodelling and immobilization are necessary.
- Grafting the neighbouring depressed areas has to be considered.

WARNINGS IN LIPOSCULPTURING

The following warnings should be kept in mind.

- Never use sharp cannulas.
- The opening should always look down opposite to the syringe's scale.
- Never make windshield-wiper movements.
- Decreasing work may be useful in certain circumstances; for example a smaller cannula may be used after a larger one.

Pushing the cannula below the skin and waiting, without moving it, does not remove fat; when using a suction machine or syringe, it is necessary to move the cannula in the fat to see the fat flow in the syringe. This is why 'liposuction' is not a good term for the procedure: 'lipoextraction' is more accurate. Lipoextraction carried out artistically is liposculpturing. 'Liposuction' makes one think of a passive act without possible complications, whereas liposculpturing makes one think of an active procedure with possible complications.

Larger-diameter cannulas produce more damage to the fat. A large contour defect can be created very quickly, and is difficult to treat. Smaller cannulas (4–6 mm outside diameter) are recommended. Because 1 cm of fat has to be left below the skin, all contour defects, such as cottage cheese deformity, can be treated later in a separate procedure (for example, by cutting the subcutaneous connections with a 14-gauge needle and grafting a certain amount of autologous fat, i.e. superficial liposculpturing).

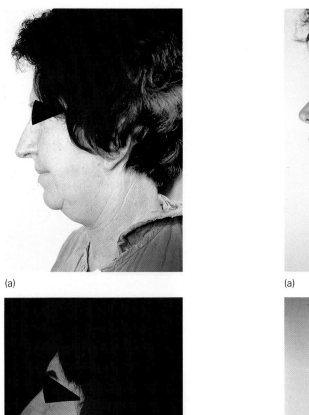

(a)

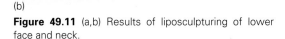

(b)

Figure 49.11 (a,b) Results of liposculpturing of lower face and neck.

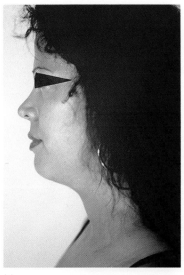

(a)

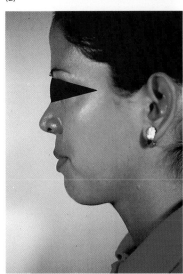

(b)

Figure 49.12 (a,b) Results of a double-chin operation.

COMPLICATIONS

There are very few surgical complications with syringe reduction liposculpturing in trained hands. The complications that have been encountered are mostly aesthetic (insufficient resection, a resection that is too large or irreg- ular, or cutaneous waves due to a bad skin tonicity). A good selection of candidates and a rigorous technique following a lengthy practical and theoretical training will help avoid most complications. Most complications occur with 'beginners'.

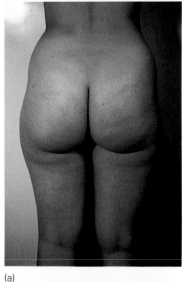

(a)

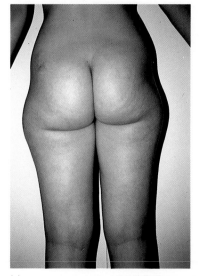

(a)

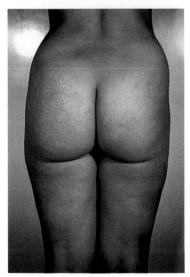

(b)

Figure 49.13 (a,b) Results of treatment of small saddle-bags only.

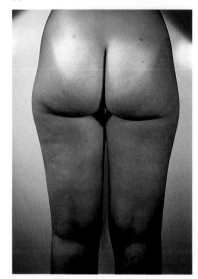

(b)

Figure 49.14 (a,b) Results of treatment of hips and mild saddlebags.

RESULTS

Examples of the results of reduction syringe liposculpturing are shown in Figures 49.11–49.19: (a) before and (b) after treatment in each case.

SUMMARY

The use of the syringe has been an advance in reduction and incremental liposculpturing. A real democratization in the medico-surgical field has been possible owing to the simplifi-

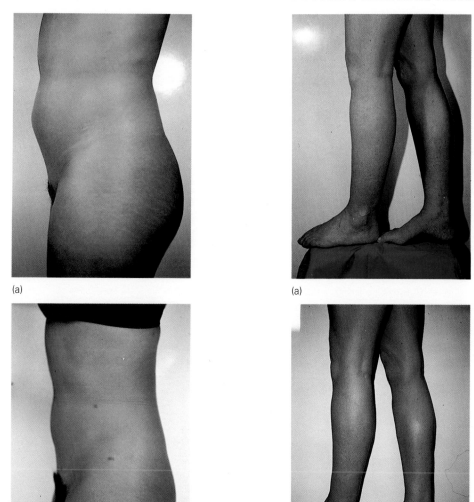

(a)

(b)

Figure 49.15 (a,b) Results of treatment of a fatty abdomen.

(a)

(b)

Figure 49.16 (a,b) Calves and ankles.

cation of the equipment. The shock-absorbing action of the syringe makes the operation safer, and allows more fat to be removed and better results to be obtained because one does perfectly symmetrical work. The syringe is a unit of measurement in this surgery of volume. The use of the tumescent technique allows the surgeon to perform most average cases on an out-patient basis and simplifies the operation considerably.

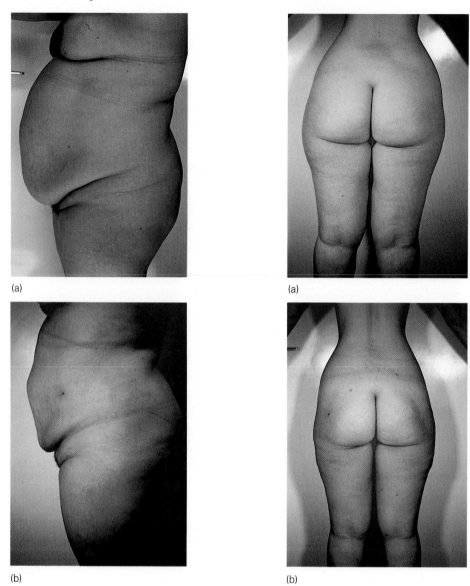

(a)

(b)

(a)

(b)

Figure 49.17 (a,b) Abdomen: three litres were removed (after filtration), followed by a weight loss of 18 kg post-operatively. Weight loss was impossible before the operation. The results were unchanged after three years.

Figure 49.18 (a,b) Liposculpturing of hips, buttocks, saddlebags, inner thigh, knees. Four litres were removed (after filtration). There was no post-operative weight loss.

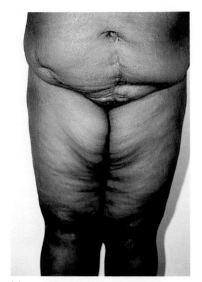

(a)

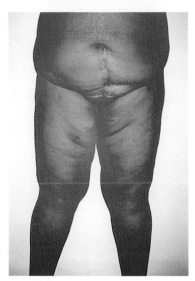

(b)

Figure 49.19 (a,b) Inner thigh: five litres were removed (after filtration). Abdomen: six litres were removed (after filtration) six months later. There was a post-operative weight loss of 10 kg. The results were unchanged after five years.

RECOMMENDED READING

Fournier PF, *Liposculpture: The Syringe Technique.* Paris: Arnette Blackwell, 1991.

Fournier PF, *Liposculpture: Ma Technique.* Paris: Arnette, 1989.

Fournier PF, *Body Sculpturing through Syringe Liposuction and Autologous Fat Re-injection.* Corona del Mar, CA: Samuel Rolf International, 1987.

Fournier PF, Why the syringe and not the suction machine? *J Dermatol Surg Oncol* 1988; **14:** 1062–71.

Fournier PF, Reduction syringe liposculpturing. *Dermatol Clin* 1990; **8:** 539–51.

Fournier PF, *Liposculpture: Ma Technique.* Paris: Arnette Blackwell, 1996.

Gasparotti M, Lewis CM, Toledo SM, *Superficial Liposculpturing: Manual of Technique.* Berlin: Springer Verlag, 1993.

Lewis CM, Comparison of the syringe and pump aspiration methods of lipoplasty. *Aesth Plast Surg* 1991; **15:** 203.

50

Syringe fat transfer

Pierre F Fournier

INTRODUCTION

In 1985, we demonstrated that it was possible to harvest fat with a syringe and the situation changed drastically. It was then possible to harvest fat (or even to process and store it) in order to reinject it in a completely closed manner. The ease and safety of this new technology totally changed the fat grafting procedure, since the advantages of the open technique still held, but its disadvantages and complications were eliminated. The syringe fat grafting technique spread rapidly, becoming popular very quickly, especially in aesthetic surgery.

The specimen of fat obtained with a 2 mm needle (14-gauge) and a syringe is different from that obtained with a machine. It is made up of cores and adipose tissue, and even though the peripheral part of this sliver of fat is damaged, the central fat is not and contains undamaged fat lobules (Figures 50.1–50.3). Damaged lobules do not take – only those with their vessels and septi intact can do so. This is a closed technique that keeps the removal sterile and whole, and the fat tissue can logically be used for a transfer. This technique is an innovation in aesthetic plastic surgery, since it permits closed removal and implantation with no scars or overcorrection.

It has thus been possible to perform fat transfers safely since syringe extraction was developed. The ease of the transfer and lack of scarring in the extracted and injected areas have made this procedure possible. Gentle vacuuming in the syringe may reduce the risk of lysis. The buffering action of the normal

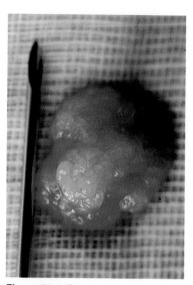

Figure 50.1 Fat slivers harvested with a 14-gauge needle (three-dimensional specimen).

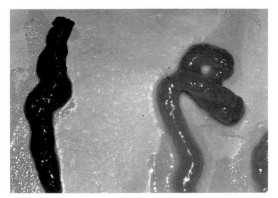

Figure 50.2 Low magnification of fat slivers.

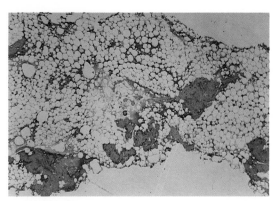

Figure 50.3 High magnification of fat sliver: undamaged adipose tissue.

saline decreases the impact of the adipose tissue fragments into the syringe, and their transportation is carried out without damage since the whole operation is performed in a fluid medium and not in a vacuum as with the machine. The less non-viable tissue that remains in the sample, the less resorption is expected. The syringe allows the surgeon to aspirate, process, expel and store adipose tissue using conventional plastic syringes. Overcorrection is still necessary – as it has been since the procedure started being used 100 years ago – except that today it is no longer necessary to disfigure the patient. It is now possible to use several injections, spread through time. As in any tissue transplant, the smaller the amount concerned, the more chances it has to take. The result of small and repeated implantations is that the patient can lead a normal social life a few days after the operation, and will readily accept this treatment in several stages.

Classical experimentation has been put into practice. The overcorrection necessary to obtain the final result can be accomplished with repeated injections, and is no longer performed in one operation. Patients are thus overcorrected over time and not in space. Progress has also been made in the instruments used, but this is not due to new scientific data. One of the basic principles of general surgery and general plastic surgery, 'respect of the tissues', is accomplished more efficiently with the use of the syringe.

In the history of fat grafting, we must note that the syringe technique has been used in the past – but it was a half-closed technique (or half-open). It was used by Brunnings in 1911 and later by Willy and Sava.

Charles Willy, a British aesthetic surgeon, wrote and published a book in 1925 showing photographs of him injecting fat into the face with a syringe for aesthetic reasons. In this procedure the fat was finely chopped with scissors from a block of tissue removed with a scalpel, placed in a syringe and reinjected. This semi-closed technique involving external manipulations and possible risks was in any case an improvement over the purely open technique.

George Sava, another British aesthetic surgeon, used the same procedure to modify the faces of Allied spies sent to the occupied territories during the Second World War. Whenever he desired a temporary face change, he used fat taken from another individual. When he desired a permanent result, he took the fat from the same person but from another part of the body.

OUR CLINICAL EXPERIENCE[1-3]

After a full twelve years of experience using the closed technique of syringe fat grafting, let us examine our present concept, the details of the actual procedure, its results and our conclusions.

We have performed about 35 000 injections in 3800 patients (faces mostly, body defects, breast augmentations, sequelae of reduction liposculpturing, and routine reinjections after reduction liposculpturing), and we are positive that syringe fat grafting is efficient.

Indications for syringe fat grafting

Facial recontouring

In many cases, one procedure is not enough, and several injections have to be given three months apart when there is a beautifying indication (building up a chin, or in the cheekbone area).

In the case of a rejuvenation indication, the older the patient the more injections are needed, since the face's fat reserve decreases considerably with time.

In young people who have 'weak points' in the face, fewer injections are needed. A maximum of four or five injections are necessary to have a permanent result or at least a long-term result. This is why fat grafting should be used as a preventive step in facial recontouring, as soon as it is needed, and not only as a treatment when the aging process is advanced. We have many long-lasting results (ten years) in young patients who came for repeated injections, and the result is obvious clinically as well as on xerographies.

In the face, the results are better in the glabella, forehead, cheekbone area, cheeks, nasolabial furrows and chin. The least satisfying results are in the lips.

Body contouring

This has unpredictable results – sometimes only one injection gives long-lasting results, especially where there is scar tissue. In other cases, the injections have to be repeated every six months.

Legs

We have had long-lasting results five years after one or two injections were done in cases involving poliomyelitis.

Breasts

We have injected large amounts of fat in the submammary space: 150, 200 or 250 cm^3. The results have been good for a year or two. Many patients did not come regularly for follow-ups, and we do not know the final results.

We have observed a case of infection (abscess) in one breast, and a large oily cyst in another case. We seldom inject the retroglandular space now. Rather, we inject subcutaneously in the four quadrants of the breast, mainly the upper two. The technique is the same as that used in facial recontouring. When injecting the breast retroglandularly or for a body defect, we use a 60 cm^3 syringe and a 5 mm blunt cannula. The fat is washed in most cases, and general anaesthesia is used.

Hands

These give the most reliable results, with 12–15 cm^3 being injected subcutaneously in the dorsum of the hand. Long-lasting results are seen after four or five years. We believe that bones behave as a splint and prevent the retraction of the graft. The technique used for hands is the same as that used for the face.

SYRINGE FACIAL FAT TRANSFER

We shall now describe in detail the technique of syringe facial fat transfer – lipofilling – which is the most used.

Why facial recontouring?

Facial ptosis in the case of tissue involution is due to a loss of volume of the deep structures – particularly of the soft tissues of the lower two-thirds of the face. Therefore what concerns us is to restore the lost volume using the means at our disposal – prostheses made of silicone, bone, cartilage, dermis, adipose tissue blocks, or by fat injection – when the involution's location allows it.

Until recently, as far as rejuvenation surgery was concerned, the aesthetic surgeon was limited to practising surface surgery in all cases. The concept of volume restoration was never mentioned, whether for a rejuvenation problem or as an embellishment. Surface surgery was supposed to resolve all problems in all cases, the proposed treatment being above all a cutaneous one. According to the importance of the aesthetic anomaly or the age of the patient, different options were available: model lifting, prolonged model lifting, upper lifting, lower lifting or full lifting. A volume increase of the malar region was done only for the beauty it gave according to the patient's own request and never for rejuvenation purposes.

It was well known that the full lift had little or no effect on the T zone of the face, where the structure is bony and ages differently. The loss of volume of the V zone ('V' in shape as well as a symbol of vulnerability) was never mentioned, even though it was obvious that the support of this zone (Figure 50.4) – representing two-thirds of the medium and inferior laterals of the face – is above all adipose tissue, superficial as well as deep. This tissue's involution, its hypotrophy, produces a false ptosis in the lower half of the face (a true ptosis is when there is tissue proliferation).

A face lift improves only the cheeks; the term 'meloplasty' is more appropriate than the term 'face lift', since only the cheeks are helped and not the other areas of the face, particularly the T zone. Surface surgery for this area is an inappropriate technique; volume surgery is the only technique that should be used in such cases.

Facial analysis is of prime importance before any aesthetic surgery of the face and neck. In cases of tissue involution, there is too much cutaneous covering, which is no longer

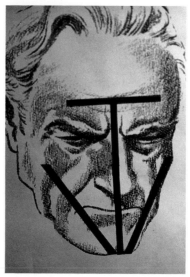

Figure 50.4 The T and V zones of the face in a case of tissue involution.

adapted to its content and which is at the same time its support, structure and framework. This cutaneous cover has been accused of being at the origin of aesthetic anomalies, whereas the true culprit is the hypotrophy of the superficial and deep structures of the V zone. A face lift – inappropriate treatment in such cases – will have consequences such as unnecessary scars, decrease of the side burn, a recession, and a stepping of the hair line in the postauricular zone.

The essential consequence of aging – tissue involution in the V zone, which has not been corrected – will continue, and a new false ptosis will occur, more or less rapidly. A volume surgery could avoid or delay this evolution by an aetiological treatment, which moreover has the advantage of simplicity. The skin's elasticity will once more be blamed – although it has nothing to do with the deep involution process. Lipofilling is not a panacea, and it is certain that some day we will have other techniques at our disposal.

Lipofilling does, however, have the advantage of being the only precise treatment that corrects, at least temporarily, the defect in question. Volume surgery also takes care of false ptosis; facial skin is only a cover for the deep structures, and should not be used as a means of traction or tension to give back the tonicity and firmness of the face when the framework is the source of the problem.

In other cases, patients do not come for rejuvenation purposes but rather to change an aspect of their appearance. These patients are candidates for one or more localized volume increases in the face because of insufficient development of the deep structures or a desire to modify a normal contour (e.g. cheekbones, hollow cheeks and chin). If a silicone prosthesis can be used, these patients can be treated by lipofilling as well.

Aesthetic facial rejuvenation and embellishment surgery were for a long time bidimensional surgery. It was often unjustified because aging was treated in an incomplete manner; the associated tissue involution was not corrected and the previous volume of the face was not restored.

The idea of volume surgery must therefore be added to the idea of surface surgery. The latter is in fact incomplete, and is justified only in cases of tissue proliferation; it is often performed at the same time as volume facial surgery when there is an associated deep soft tissue proliferation.

The use of adipose tissue or its derivatives is not the only option. Other means (prosthesis or other autologous tissue) leading to volume increase in the region to be treated can be used.

With the volume of the operated regions temporarily or permanently restored by a more logical implantation surgery, the consequences of aging – tissue hypotrophy – can be addressed. Lipofilling easily permits the surgeon to perform tridimensional surgery by acting on an element that has previously been ignored: volume.

Preoperative examination

The preoperative examination is very important. With the help of a mirror and the patient's cooperation, the surgeon should study the weak points of the face, where tissue involution begins, and the other zones of the face for which the patient is seeking to have an aspect modified.

If needed, a test can be done to temporarily show the effect obtained by the desired volume. A determined quantity (2, 4, 6 cm^3 or more) of lidocaine diluted to one-third is injected in the area or areas to be corrected. Thus the surgeon will have an idea of the quantity of adipose tissue needed for the correction.

The manoeuvre to find the false ptosis needs to be done systematically. The thumb is placed in the cheekbone area, and then an up-and-out traction movement is made. If there is a modification in the nasolabial or labiomental furrows or in the jowls, this manoeuvre shows hypotrophy in the region and the existence of false nasolabial or labiomental furrows and false jowls. The cheekbone region needs to be increased as well as the false nasolabial or labiomental furrows. The cheekbones, together with the chin, are the three pillars of the youth-and-beauty triangle.

In the case of wrinkles on the upper lip, its skin should be smoothed out with the help of both index fingers, each being placed on the external part of the white hemilip and performing an outward movement. If the wrinkles totally disappear, they are deep wrinkles caused by the involution of the underlying tissues; lipofilling is therefore indicated. If there is partial or total persistence of wrinkles then these are superficial wrinkles – true wrinkles caused by skin lesions. These lesions will be helped partially by lipofilling, but they will need additional treatment to be completely corrected (mechanical or chemical dermabrasion or collagen injection).

These facts should be carefully explained to

the patient. The examination should be done again when the patient has decided to have the operation. The conclusions should be written down, and a diagram of the face should be drawn.

When the operation date is set, generally after a second consultation to give the patient time to think it over, the surgeon will ask for the usual preoperative examination for surgery and give a routine preoperative treatment (vitamins C and K, phenobarbitone). Photographs should also be taken of the face at different angles, and a pre-estimation should be made of the amount of adipose tissue needed to do the filling (between 10, 30 and 40 cm^3 in general). Weak points should be isolated – symmetrical or multiple (small or large filling).

The total amount of local anaesthetic to use, the size of the extraction zone, the length of the operation, the postoperative reactions, and the return to normal of the region or regions treated depend heavily on this pre-estimation. These provisions should be explained to the patient as well as the fact that the treatment affects individuals differently.

Facial and harvesting zone markings

A good quality dermographic pen should be used for the drawings to assist in the preparation of the operation field. A green Pentel pen is recommended.

Face

The face is marked first. The marking should be done while the patient is standing and according to the results of the facial analysis.

The nasolabial, labiomental and glabellar furrows are marked with a line. The cheekbones, cheeks and extended surfaces should be marked with a circle or an oval. The lips are marked with a point. These drawings are symmetrical and identical on each side of the face. Sometimes one side of the face needs more correction than the opposite side, a very frequent aesthetic anomaly.

The quantity to inject in each area is evaluated, and the surface of the extraction zone will depend on the total volume necessary. In general, 4–6 cm^3 is injected in each malar zone, 2–4 cm^3 in each nasolabial furrow, 1–2 cm^3 in each labiomental furrow, 4–6 cm^3 in each cheek, 2–4 cm^3 in the glabellar region, 8–10 cm^3 in the total frontal area, 6 cm^3 in the temples, 2.5 cm^3 in each upper or lower lip, and 6, 8, 10 or 15 cm^3 in the chin. Once the marking of the face is finished, a photograph is taken and kept in the patient's file (slide or Polaroid).

Harvesting zones

The extraction zone surface will vary, depending on the quantity of adipose tissue to be extracted. Obviously, this extraction should not leave any surface irregularities.

The chosen zone should be marked while the patient is standing if this zone is located in the trochanteric region or the hip. It should be done lying down if it is in an exterior buttock or in the abdominal wall, since morphology is modified by the position.

The marking drawings should be either a circle, an oval, a square or a rectangle. The interior of the marked zone should be subdivided in small rectangles approximately 4 cm long and 3 cm wide. Their number should be approximately equal to the number of syringes necessary to do the filling. With one syringe, 5 cm^3 of adipose tissue can be extracted. A regular extraction can be performed easily and without leaving a residual deformation in the totality of the zone if only 5 cm^3 of adipose tissue is removed from each one of the rectangles, which thus serve as measuring units.

Operative zone disinfection

Rigorous asepsis is necessary. The tegument is usually disinfected with either 90% alcohol or any other product, according to the surgeon's preference. The surgeon will be gloved and masked. Draping of the operative zone should be done as for any other facial operation before the anaesthesia is given.

When using non-sterilized external refrigeration as anaesthesia or as a complement to local anaesthesia, disinfection should take place and the drape should be placed when this is finished.

Operative zone anaesthesia

Anaesthesia in the operative zone should be different than that used for reduction microlipoextraction. Recall that:

- in the case of microlipoextraction for reduction lipoplasty when a reinjection of tissues is not foreseen, 'the most important thing is not what one extracts, but what one leaves';
- in the case of microlipoextraction to reuse the tissues obtained during the extraction, 'the most important thing is not what is left, but what one extracts'.

In both cases, the tissues must be respected by the surgeon, but the tissues to be respected differ in each case.

The fraction that must live or relive is what matters, not the fraction that will be eliminated. A non-infiltrated 'dry' extraction is preferable to an infiltrated extraction, because of the hydraulic traumatism of the injection added to the chemical traumatism caused by the injection of adrenaline and lidocaine (Xylocaine). Therefore, in the case of microlipoextraction and reutilization of the extracted tissue, the utmost care should be taken by the surgeon for the tissue to be reinjected.

Anaesthesia of the harvesting zone

Anaesthesia of the donor zone should be performed first. The following should be done to extract the tissue to be reinjected.

Local anaesthesia

Even if local anaesthesia is not theoretically desirable for the above-mentioned reasons, it is often used. As in the case of a nerve block or regional anaesthesia, 1% lidocaine with 1/200 000 adrenaline is used. For anaesthesia through infiltration, the greater the surface to anaesthetize, the weaker the dilution. In general, a dilution to the fourth is used. The dilution is done using 2°C saline solution. A weaker dilution is perfectly possible (a fifth, an eighth or a tenth).

All the marked regions should be infiltrated at the same time; it will simply take longer for the anaesthesia's effect to be felt. The infiltration should be made in all the thickness of the layer of adipose tissue, but especially in depth. External refrigeration with ice bags should always be used for 20 minutes. The purpose is to obtain an extraction with as little bleeding as possible and to reinforce the anaesthesia.

We shall describe the Mazeas artifice, which is very valuable in certain cases of thick adipose tissue. When it is possible to create a thick fold with the left hand (on the abdomen, for example), one can use a long needle (spinal needle type, but finer), anaesthetize exclusively the depth of the adipose tissue in this fold, and obtain anaesthesia of the overlying tissues where an extraction can be easily obtained in a noninfiltrated zone.

Cryoanaesthesia

The best method is external cryoanaesthesia. However, we shall not describe this here, since it deserves an article of its own.

General anaesthesia

Sometimes patients want general anaesthesia rather than local. This is inconvenient, since the patient is kept in the clinic longer, but it is the ideal technique for large extractions. Twilight anaesthesia can also be used. Two or three zones can be refrigerated simultaneously, and the surgeon can perform the extractions satisfactorily. This anaesthesia is for ambulatory patients.

Anaesthesia of the facial zones

Anaesthesia of the receiving zone is performed second. Considering the fragility of the adipose tissue, Certain precautions should be taken.

- If the patient is under general or twilight anaesthesia, there is no problem.
- A nerve block is particularly convenient for the face: a block of the supraorbital nerves for the forehead and the glabella; a block of the infraorbital nerves for the upper lip, the nasolabial furrow and the cheeks; and a block of the mental nerves for the lower lip and the labiomental furrows.
- In certain cases, a wheal of lidocaine will be enough. It is the transcutaneous needle penetration that is painful; the subcutaneous injection is not really painful.
- We currently use external refrigeration, especially in the glabellar zone. The patient holds a block of ice between two pieces of cotton a few minutes before the injection. The skin should be anaesthesized as a priority because the deep tissues are a lot less sensitive. Small plastic bags filled with broken ice cubes are applied on the cheeks for about 10 minutes. Cryo-gel can also be useful, since it shapes itself to irregular surfaces. It needs special surveillance because it can burn the skin. Giorgio Fischer's artifice is recommended: instead of filling the bags with ice and water, he uses a mix made of two-thirds tap water and one-third antifreeze, after storing for a while in the freezer. The bags can thus be used several times.
- Local anaesthesia by infiltration of the zones to be increased is often used. There are no special recommendations. In general, a solution to the fourth is used. All infiltration on the face is preceded by the application of a plastic mask kept in the refrigerator. It is applied from the beginning of the anaesthesia of the donor zone. Facial infiltrations are therefore performed with no pain, with the help of an intradermic needle. Once finished, the mask is applied again until the adipose tissue is injected. This preparatory anaesthetic work, both time consuming and demanding a high level of skill can be carried out by the surgeon or an assistant.
- Premedication should be done from the beginning of the operation (0.25 mg of atropine sulphate by subcutaneous injection together with 10 cm^3 of phenobarbitone by intramuscular injection). An intravenous perfusion of saline solution can be made. If this is not done, a vein should be catheterized from the beginning of the operation.

Observations

External refrigeration of the areas to be operated on should be done before any kind of anaesthesia – general, twilight, block or local – as well as before any kind of extraction or injection of adipose tissue. It should be maintained for about 20 minutes.

Pure lipofilling technique

Instruments

The amount of equipment necessary for a face fill is very small:

- the 'classical' filling needle (2 mm outside diameter and 4 cm useful length); disposable ones now exist;
- 30- and 21-gauge needles for local anaesthesia;
- 10 cm^3 disposable plastic syringes;
- a 20 cm^3 saline solution ampule at room temperature or at 2°C, which will serve to dilute the local anaesthetic, to avoid all dead space in the syringe, to diminish the impact, facilitate the transportation, and to wash the adipose tissue;
- a 2 mm external diameter transfer needle;
- a wood or metal test tube holder.

We no longer use 2 cm^3 insulin syringes or 5 cm^3 syringes, which do not permit washing of the extracted adipose tissue. If the face fill is done at the same time as body liposculpturing, the adipose tissue extracted with the help of single-orifice cannulas of 3 or 4 mm outside diameter and 50 or 60 cm^3 syringes can be reused if it is transferred to 5 or 10 cm^3 syringes on which the usual 2 mm outside diameter filling needle has been mounted (14-gauge).

Extraction technique

The syringe allows the extraction, preparation and reinjection of adipose tissue in a closed space while respecting the integrity and sterility of the extraction. It also serves as a reservoir to conserve the extracted tissue in the freezer, if necessary.

Extraction of the adipose tissue

Using a 2 mm outside diameter filling needle mounted on a 10 cm^3 syringe, we first place 2 cm^3 of saline solution at room temperature or at 2°C in the syringe. The left hand makes a fold on one of the small rectangles marked on the extraction zone, and the needle is pushed through the skin in the middle of the adipose tissue. The left hand is then placed flat on the extraction zone and will stay that way throughout the operation. The right hand pulls out the syringe plunger completely, and the surgeon begins the extraction. During the whole extraction, the plunger will be kept in this same position.

Back-and-forth movements are made in a fan-shaped way almost the length of the needle. Four to five of these are made in one direction before going to the neighbouring region, without taking out the needle, which must remain under the skin. Between 30 and 50 seconds are needed to obtain 5 cm^3 of adipose tissue.

Once these 5 cm^3 have been obtained, the needle is removed, and 3 cm^3 of saline solution is drawn into the syringe. The latter is

placed vertically on a test tube holder, plunger up.

The needle that was used for this extraction is mounted on another syringe for use in another cylinder extraction. This takes place while the adipose tissue in the first syringe is going through a period of decantation, the first phase of washing.

Once 5 cm^3 of adipose tissue has been extracted with the second syringe in the same way, 3 cm^3 of saline solution should be added, and the syringe then placed vertically on the test tube holder. The predetermined amount of adipose tissue will be removed in each one of the rectangles marked on the extraction zone.

Washing

When the extraction is finished, the surgeon washes the adipose tissue with the saline solution. Once the 3 cm^3 of saline solution has been drawn into the syringe and it has been placed vertically on the test tube holder, one can see the mixture separate into two: the adipose tissue on top and the bloody saline solution on the bottom. This separation takes place after a few seconds.

This hydrohaematic fraction is emptied into a cup, and 5 cm^3 of saline solution is again drawn into the syringe. The syringe should once again be placed on the test tube holder in order to obtain the separation of the two fractions while performing the same manoeuvre on the other syringes.

There should be as many washings as necessary to obtain bloodless adipose tissue. In general, 2–4 washes are necessary – sometimes more if the sample is very bloody or if not enough time is allowed between each wash. A transfer needle will allow adipose tissue to pass from one syringe to another in order to get equal amounts for symmetrical regions. The reinjection can be done when all the syringes have been thus prepared.

Locally there should be an occlusive, slightly compressing dressing made of a few compresses kept in place by several

Elastoplast bands or a layer of Elastoplast. This dressing should be removed after 24 or 48 hours. It may have to be changed after a few hours if bleeding persists.

For a few years now, during the lipoextraction for lipofilling and for washing the fat, we have no longer been using normal saline (we use it only to dilute the local anaesthetic). Instead we use a 5% glucose solution.

Reinjection

Once the dressing is made, the injections should be done. The needle used for the reinjection should be of the same calibre as that of the extraction, namely 2 mm outside diameter. The needle will penetrate through the skin at the appropriate points of penetration for each region to inject. The vestibular approach is not recommended because of its potential for sepsis.

One must inject with caution and make sure of not being in a vessel. This manoeuvre can be performed if desired with the needle mounted on an empty syringe. Once this is done, the syringe full of adipose tissue is used and the injection begins. This is done in an intermittent fashion, 0.5 or 1 cm^3 every centimetre, always in a retrograde direction, while constantly verifying the evacuation of the syringe's content by its graduated scale (Figures 50.5 and 50.6).

The injection's track should be straight or curved, depending on whether the defect is linear or arched (lips or glabellar furrows). In the case of a larger defect (hollow cheeks or cheekbones), several retrograde injections should be made in a fan shape, starting from the cutaneous penetration orifice. If desired, a regular crossed increase can be performed by using another needle penetration point opposite the first.

The total content of a syringe should never be injected in the same place with or without the creation of a cavity. If necessary, the zone to be injected can be prepared with a full instrument (e.g. a tunneller) with a very fine point (e.g. a small awl). The preoperative grid

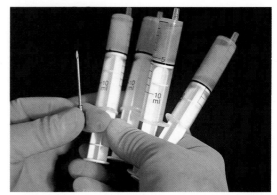

Figure 50.5 The 14-gauge needle should be used for extraction as well as for injection.

permits a more regular repartition of the ulterior injections, and will not overly traumatize the region as would a blunt cannula.

Remodelling of the injected region

After the injection, the operated regions should be remodelled carefully using the thumb and index finger, one of them being at the vestibule in the case of injections in the nasolabial furrows, the cheeks or the lips.

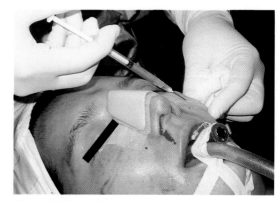

Figure 50.6 Injection of the malar region after a rhinoplasty.

Immobilizing the area with an Elastoplast band is not essential, but it cannot hurt. It is recommended for two or three days. It is nevertheless necessary after injection in the cheekbone area or chin. This is also true for implantation of prostheses in these areas (Steri-Strip and Elastoplast band).

The postoperative course is simple. Oedema varies from one patient to another. There are rarely ecchymoses, and patients do not mention any pain or discomfort. The patients have a normal appearance after 3–5 days.

The extraction zones take longer to return to normal. They have oedema and are indurated for several weeks. Sometimes patients should be warned that they will suffer more from the extraction zones than from the injection zones on the face.

When the filling is done on an ambulatory basis without general or twilight anaesthesia, the whole operation, including preparation, operation and patient rest, takes about 1.5–2 hours. Antibiotics are prescribed systematically. Vibramycin for 5 days is prescribed, more for medico-legal reasons than for risk of infection, which is minimal. Anti-inflammatories (Reparil) are, on the other hand, prescribed for 15 days. Analgesics are not necessary.

Delayed harvesting

Some years ago, we started to prepare the donor area as well as the receiving area to obtain better results and decrease the number of injections necessary for a long-lasting result. The aim is to create an inflammatory condition of the fat tissue and to graft a 'healing fat tissue' instead of a normal fat tissue. This possibility is explained to the patient, who will choose between 'fresh fat grafting' or 'prepared fat grafting'.

In this latter case, we give a conventional local anaesthesia and/or a cryoanaesthesia (external), and with a spinal needle or an ordinary 19-gauge needle give repeated strokes for one or two minutes in the whole thickness of the fat layer of the harvesting zone. No fat is extracted. A dressing is applied, and the patient returns home. The future receiving area may be prepared the same way. After 10 or 12 days, he or she will return, and a conventional fat harvesting will be performed and the first injection accomplished.

The remaining fat is kept in the freezer for future injections. Histological studies have shown that the specimen of fat obtained with this delayed harvesting has many new vessels, new collagen fibres and a great number of fibroblasts. Our clinical experience confirms that this 'prepared fat' decreases the number of injections necessary for a long-lasting result.

IMPLANT CONSERVATION

Conservation of implants in the freezer

Conservation of all types of implants coming from adipose tissue is easily possible through cold. The results do not differ from those with the fresh implants normally used. The purpose of this conservation is to save the excess implant extracted or to avoid a new extraction when repeated injections are foreseen. Many colleagues have followed this path and have confirmed the innocuousness and efficiency of this procedure (David Morrow of Palm Springs, California and Dimitra Dassiou of Volos, Greece, just to cite two).

Tissue conservation by refrigeration is a classic technique, as in the case of other cells (sperm), and the innocuousness and efficiency of the technique are also proven. All types of implants coming from adipose tissue have been kept in the freezer and reused, some after a whole year, for example:

- adipose tissue cylinder extracted with a 2 mm diameter needle (washed with saline solution);
- micro-implants extracted with a 12/10 mm (19-gauge) or an 8/10 mm (21-gauge) needle (washed with saline solution);

- implants extracted with 3–4 mm diameter cannulas and $60\,cm^3$ syringes that can be used with 5 or $10\,cm^3$ syringes and the classic 2 mm diameter fill needle (washed with saline solution);
- autologous collagen extracted with an $8/10$ cm or a $12/10$ cm diameter needle (washed with distilled water and kept in the freezer);
- this collagen can be used as a dermic implant (using an $8/10$ cm needle or dermojet) or as a subcutaneous implant.

Technique

After washing with either saline solution or distilled water to rid the implant of all traces of blood or haemoglobin, in every case the sterile cap of an injection needle is placed on the hub of the syringe. All extraction syringes are placed on a test tube rack, and are then placed in the freezer or refrigerator.

To reuse the implants thus kept, one need only take them out of the freezer compartment one hour before reutilization. This defrosting of the implant is done at room temperature ($22°C$) on a test tube holder. It is well-known that the freezing should be rapid whereas the defrosting should be slow.

A quicker freezing than that obtained using the freezer can be obtained with liquid nitrogen. The syringe is placed for a short time in a liquid nitrogen filled container before being placed in the freezer. A quicker defrosting than that obtained at room temperature can be obtained in warm water ($28°C$ or $30°C$). The syringe or syringes with the cap are placed in a container with faucet water warmed to this temperature.

Once again, the results obtained with the help of these conserved implants are no different than those obtained with fresh implants (on the face or hands). The repeated operations are more easily accepted by the patients.

COMPLICATIONS

Oedema is not a complication but rather a part of the operation. It varies from one patient to another: sometimes it is small, sometimes it deforms the area. The lips react the most readily. It is impossible to foresee to which category the patient belongs: that with a small reaction or that with a big one. The importance of this oedematous reaction is of course related to the amount of adipose tissue injected.

One can nevertheless tell the patient that in most cases after three days the deformation of the treated area is no longer visible to others – only to the patient. Less often, the treated regions can have abnormal oedema for about eight days.

Ecchymoses are rare because the adipose tissue is washed. There can, however, be small ones related to the anaesthesia or the adipose tissue injection. Sometimes they are delayed, and appear on the second or third day. They can be hidden with make-up.

Pain or discomfort are rare complications. The present author has never seen liquefaction of the graft or infection. Often a localized, sensible induration may be noticed in the treated areas, which is more palpable than visible, disappearing spontaneously in a few weeks, sometimes lasting more.

In order to avoid significant reactions, it is important not to hypercorrect in volume the region treated. One wants the patient to return to a normal appearance within a few days. Necessary hypercorrection can be done with repeated injections spread out over time. These are more easily accepted than a hypercorrection in volume that leaves the patient marked for a much longer time as a consequence of the operation. Moreover, small quantities take better than larger ones.

The only unfavourable evolution is the disappearance of the results obtained due to total reabsorption of the graft. This is noted in a certain number of cases. In fact, the reabsorption of the graft is due to the extreme diffusion of the implanted tissue in patients who have an important volume deficit in their sub-cutaneous structures. Most of these patients are older, and their facial adipose tissue capital has almost disappeared. It is rare for younger patients with individualized and limited weak points to be dissatisfied with their operations.

Of all the facial zones, the most difficult to treat are the lips.

RESULTS

The longest results that we have kept track of date as far back as 12 years, and we can affirm that the fraction that 'takes' (20–30%), takes definitely. We have never tried volume hyper-correction, and prefer to perform repeated injections throughout time upon our patients' request every 3–6 months or every year. Four or five are necessary to obtain a permanent or at least long-lasting result (Figures 50.7 and 50.8). Xerography after five years confirms the result (Figure 50.9).

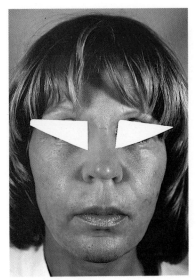

Figure 50.8 Result after five years.

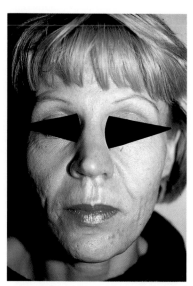

Figure 50.7 The patient had 20 cm³ of fat cylinders injected in the lower face twice, at a one year interval.

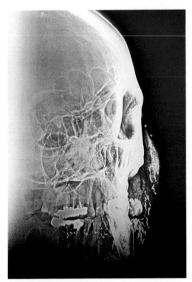

Figure 50.9 Xerography of the face after five years confirms the clinical result in a patient who has undergone malar augmentation.

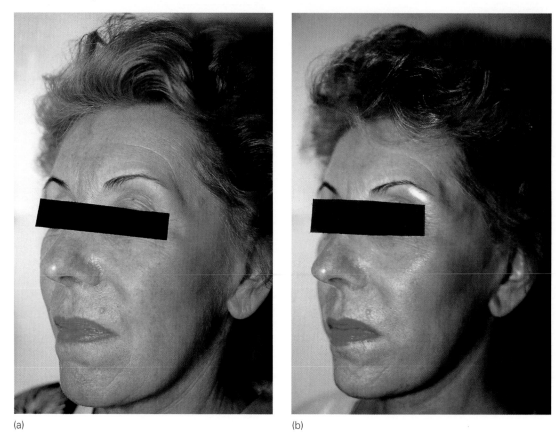

(a)　　　　　　　　　　　　　　　　　　(b)

Figure 50.10 Fat grafting of cheekbone area and nasolabial sulcus: four implantations of 5 cm³ at three-month intervals in the cheekbone area and 3 cm³ in the nasolabial sulcus. (a) Before. (b) After.

Grafting adipose tissue is not new, and the necessary hypercorrection is well known. The classic open complex technique with a scar and depression in the extraction area and a hypercorrection scar in the treated area used in reconstructive surgery has been replaced by an easy new closed technique with no scar or depression at the extraction area and no hypercorrection or scar at the treated area. The necessary hypercorrection is no longer performed all at once, but rather throughout time with repeated injections. The results of each injection adds to the result obtained by the preceding injection and so forth. Often, only one face fill is enough in case of a hollow face and moderate defect in a young and skinny patient.

In many cases, it has been noticed by Dr C Emelina (personal communication) that small volumes of injected fat (2 or 3 cm), when injected every six weeks in the same place, take better than larger volumes injected every three months. This better volume increase may be explained by the adjunction of the phenomenon of tissue expansion, which may also help in the final result (Figure 50.12).

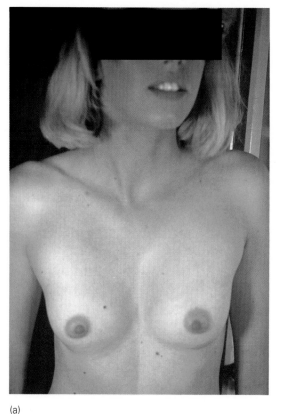

(a)

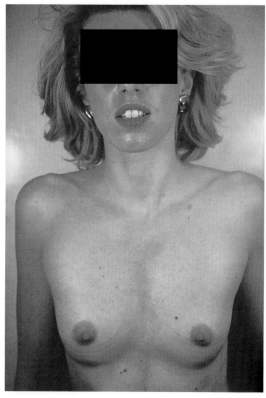

(b)

Figure 50.11 'Pes cavatum' fat grafting, delayed harvesting: good result after six years. (a) Before. (b) After.

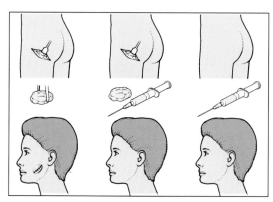

Figure 50.12 Evolution of fat grafting throughout time: open procedure; half-closed procedure; fully closed procedure.

SUMMARY

Fat grafting is an old technique. The old open procedure has been replaced by a completely closed procedure using a needle or cannula mounted on a syringe of variable size. The ease and safety of this procedure now allows the surgeon to perform as many injections as necessary to obtain a long-lasting result, without disfiguring the patient through hypercorrection in volume. Hypercorrection is one of the drawbacks of fat grafting, but at the same time it is an absolute necessity. Fortunately, it is no longer necessary to accomplish it in the space of one session, but rather it can be spread out in time over several sessions. The detailed technique for facial recontouring has been described here, as well as delayed harvesting.

Even though further research is necessary, the present procedure of syringe fat grafting is an important addition to soft tissue increase in aesthetic surgery.

REFERENCES

1. Fournier PF, *Body Sculpturing through Syringe Liposuction and Autologous Fat Re-injection*. Corona del Mar, CA: Samuel Rolf International, 1987.

2. Fournier PF, *Liposculpture: Ma Technique*. Paris: Arnette, 1989.

3. Fournier PF, *Liposculpturing: The Syringe Technique*. Paris: Arnette Blackwell, 1991.

RECOMMENDED READING

Fournier PF, *Liposculpture: Ma Technique.*, 2nd ed. Paris: Arnette Blackwell, 1996.

Gasparrotti M, Lewis CM, Toledo LS, *Superficial Liposculpturing: Manual of Technique*. Berlin: Springer Verlag, 1993.

51

Facial chemical peel

Randall K Roenigk

INTRODUCTION

Facial chemical peel is poorly defined, and includes a plethora of procedures. To some clinicians, it means treatment with a drug such as 5-fluorouracil, resorcinol or tretinoin cream. However, to most, it means the use of caustic agents like trichloroacetic acid (TCA) and phenol to produce an effective, long-lasting facial chemical peel (chemexfoliation). Some have referred to the facial chemical peel as 'chemabrasion', since the related and sometimes combined treatment modalities include dermabrasion, and laser resurfacing or 'laserabrasion'.[1] Chemical peels have been divided into superficial, medium and deep chemical peels, based on the depth of wounding caused by a particular agent.[2] Superficial peeling agents such as Jessner's solution, resorcin, 10–15% TCA, salicylic acid, solid carbon dioxide, tretinoin cream or 5-fluorouracil cause necrosis of the epidermis, and mildly stimulate collagen formation in the superficial papillary dermis. Medium-depth (unoccluded full-strength 88% phenol, 35–50% TCA) and deeper chemical peels (occluded or unoccluded Baker's phenol) produce more extensive dermal injury. The depth of wounding can extend to the upper reticular dermis with the medium-depth peels and to the mid-reticular dermis with deep chemical peels. Although there is no standard definition of facial chemical peel, we consider it to be a procedure that causes significant superficial dermal necrosis and produces long-lasting therapeutic or cosmetic benefits.

α-HYDROXY ACIDS: SUPERFICIAL CHEMEXFOLIATION

α-Hydroxy acids are derived from food sources such as sugar cane, sour milk and citrus fruits, and are carboxylic acids that have an alcoholic hydroxyl group in the alpha position. Acids that have a keto group at the alpha position (α-keto acids), such as pyruvic acid, have also been used to perform chemical peel. These chemicals work on the epidermis by reducing the thickness of hyperkeratosis in the stratum corneum by decreasing corneocyte adhesion.[3]

Glycolic acid is the most commonly used α-hydroxy acid, and is considered a versatile superficial peeling agent when used at 50–70% concentration. It may be used to treat many lesions that are predominantly in the epidermis or superficial dermis, including fine wrinkles, actinic keratoses, melasma, lentigines and seborrheic keratoses. To achieve consistently good results, a series of at least three to four repeated peels is necessary.[4] A double-blinded vehicle-controlled study of 34 patients with mildly photoaged skin revealed clinical improvement in those treated with 50% glycolic acid gel for five minutes once weekly for four weeks.[5] Glycolic acid at 50–70% concentration may cause dermal necrosis comparable to 30–50% TCA.[6] Full-thickness epidermal slough results in keratinocyte regeneration from appendages as well as new collagen formation in the papillary dermis. Glycolic acid has been shown to stimulate collagen production in human skin fibroblast culture in vitro and thus produce a new zone of collagen.[7]

Table 51.1 Some uses for TCA chemical peel	
Superficial peel (20% TCA)	
Acne	Photoaging skin
Aging skin	Rosacea
Alopecia areata	Sallow complexion
Blending (after deep peels)	Superficial acne scars
	Vitiligo
Freckles	Seborrheic dermatitis
Melasma	
Dilated pores	
Intermediate peel (35% TCA)	
Actinic keratosis	Lentigines (face, hands)
Actinic damage	Wrinkles (mild, moderate)
Aging skin	Blending (peel or dermabrasion)
Deep peel (50% or 60% TCA)	
Fine expression lines of face	Xanthelesma
Acne scars	Photoaging skin (severe)
Lentigines	Superficial epitheliomas
Perioral wrinkles	

TCA AND PHENOL: MEDIUM-DEPTH AND DEEP CHEMICAL PEELS

For the past several decades, Baker's formula with phenol has been used extensively to achieve effective facial chemical peeling.[8] McCollough et al[9] prefer a phenol-based formula combined with a moist dressing technique. The formula consists of 3 ml of phenol USP 88%, 3 drops of croton oil, 8 drops of septisol soap and 2 ml of distilled water. Since there is no tape placement or mask removal, there may be less risk of postoperative scarring. Although the cosmetic benefit obtained with phenol can be remarkable, this chemical is melanotoxic and may cause hypopigmentation ('china doll' or 'porcelain white' skin color). Also, phenol is known to cause systemic effects such as cardiac arrhythmia and renal toxicity.

For decades, TCA has been used to treat extensive actinic keratosis, solar elastosis and wrinkles.[10–12] Ayres[12] described its use for treating aging skin. Various application techniques have been used for TCA chemexfoliation, such as 20% TCA superficial peel, 35% TCA intermediate peel, 50% or 60% TCA deep peel; TCA peel with tape occlusion, chemical peels with TCA and tretinoin cream, 5-fluo-

rouracil, dermabrasion, phenol, solid carbon dioxide, Jessner's solution, α-hydroxy acids, resorcinol, pyruvic acid and salicylic acid.[13–15] Many cosmetic and therapeutic uses have been reported (Table 51.1).

TCA chemically destroys the epidermis and upper dermis, and causes the dead skin to slough within 5–7 days.[16,17] The sloughed epidermis is replaced within 7 days by new epidermis that migrates from the cutaneous adnexa. Regeneration of the dermis is evident in 2–3 weeks, but remodeling of the collagen usually continues for 6 months. The essentially permanent histologic changes in the skin are homogenization of superficial dermal collagen and an increase in the number of elastic fibers.[18] In addition, cytologically atypical keratinocytes are replaced by normal cells from the adnexae.

Premalignant lesions and actinic damage have been recognized as principal indications for facial chemical peeling.[19] TCA facial chemical peel compares favorably with 5-fluorouracil cream for treating extensive actinic damage. The severe reaction to 5-fluorouracil cream may last from 4 to 7 weeks (compared with 1 week for TCA), and retreatment is often necessary. In addition, TCA facial chemical peel removes some wrinkles from facial skin.

TCA facial chemical peeling is a versatile and elegant procedure that has several advantages: few medical contraindications, lack of systemic toxicity or allergic reactions, relatively less risk of scarring, and shorter wound-healing time than with 5-fluorouracil cream. The concentration of TCA is easily adjusted by the operator. Because the depth of dermal damage is based on the concentration of TCA, consistent results are obtained. We prefer to use standard concentrations of 20%, 35% or 50% TCA; however, 80% TCA causes unacceptable scarring of facial skin.

INDICATIONS

The patients best suited for TCA facial chemical peel have fair (type I or II), sun-damaged skin with actinic elastosis, fine facial wrinkles and extensive actinic keratosis (Figures 51.1

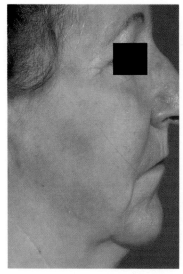

(b)

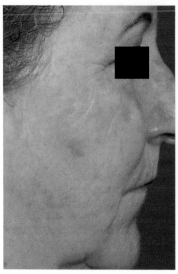

(c)

(a)

Figure 51.1 (a) Actinic keratosis and solar elastosis prior to facial chemical peel. (b) Note diffuse erythema at 6 weeks postoperatively. (c) At $4\frac{1}{2}$ months postoperatively, the erythema has resolved and the sun-damaged skin is much smoother.

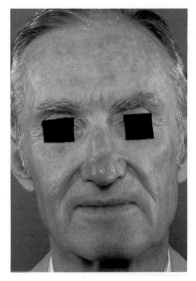

(a)

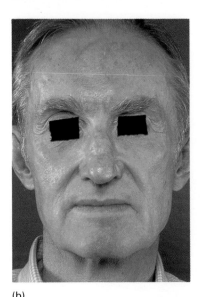

(b)

Figure 51.2 (a) Extensive sun damage in a fair-skinned person before 50% TCA facial chemical peel. (b) Appearance at 10 months postoperatively.

Indications for TCA facial chemical peel also include sun-related pigmentary disorders, especially lentigo simplex. Postinflammatory hyperpigmentation or melasma may respond to treatment with TCA. However, the results are not consistent, and the treatment may make the condition worse. For these conditions, it is suggested that, after detailed preoperative consultation, a patch of skin be tested (Figure 51.3). The treatment of vitiligo with TCA facial chemical peel depends on the chemical producing a diminution in the pigmentation of normal skin.

There are reports that superficial facial chemical peel with 20% TCA produces beneficial results in patients with acne vulgaris, rosacea, seborrheic dermatitis and radiation dermatitis.[20] Although mild-to-moderate superficial acne scarring has also been reported to be diminished with higher concentrations of

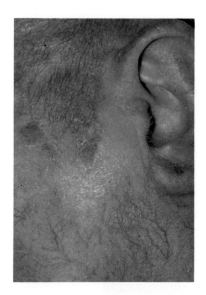

Figure 51.3 Application of 50% TCA to a test patch in the left preauricular area demonstrates that in this case a facial chemical peel will not only improve the sun damage but also remove some unsightly telangiectasias.

and 51.2). TCA is also used to treat fine cross-hatched facial wrinkles. TCA facial chemical peel may be effective for treating moderately deep wrinkles and perioral wrinkles, but not the deepest creases of facial expression.

TCA, in our experience TCA has not been very effective for treating this condition. Dermabrasion and CO_2 laser resurfacing may be considered in such instances. Although some dermatologists believe that facial chemical peel decreases the pore size of pilosebaceous units, our results are equivocal.

PROCEDURE FOR TCA CHEMICAL PEEL

Preoperative consultation may be more important than the procedure. The physician must not only determine the suitability of a patient for facial chemical peel, but also determine the patient's expectations and evaluate the patient psychologically. If the outcome is in doubt – as it is in the case of pigmentary disorders – a small patch of skin should be tested. Patients should understand that residual erythema can last from 2 to 3 months after chemical peel. The physician should emphasize the importance of avoiding sunlight for 6 months postoperatively.

Our patients are treated preoperatively with 0.05% tretinoin cream applied twice daily for 2 weeks. This treatment gently debrides the stratum corneum, including hypertrophic actinic keratoses, and degreases the skin by decreasing the secretory activity of facial sebaceous glands. Patients should be instructed not to use make-up, moisturizer, hair conditioner, styling mousse or hair spray for 24 hours preoperatively, because oils on the skin prevent transepidermal penetration of TCA.

On the day of the operation, the face is scrubbed with acetone for 10 minutes to remove the sebaceous oils. The skin will have the feel of fine sandpaper. The stratum corneum scale turns white as facial oils are removed. The eyes are protected with antibiotic ointment, gauze pads, and hypoallergenic tape or goggles. The patient may be sedated preoperatively with medication given orally or intramuscularly, but this is not always necessary. Local anesthesia is not used.

A cotton-tip applicator is moistened with

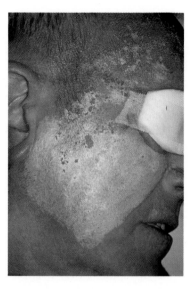

Figure 51.4 Frost (white area) produced by chemical coagulation of the epidermis with 50% TCA. The frost is beginning to fade from the forehead, which was treated first. Gauze patches protect the eyes.

TCA, and excess fluid is removed. The TCA is applied to an area approximately 2 cm by 3 cm by firmly rubbing the moistened applicator in a circular fashion.

The skin slowly turns whitish gray because of chemical coagulation of the epidermis. This color change is called a 'frost' (Figure 51.4). The greater the concentration of TCA, the more rapidly the skin frosts. However, if the skin was not adequately degreased, the frost may not occur. The greater the concentration of TCA, the greater the discomfort the patient may experience.

Some dermatologists perform facial chemical peel in a specific pattern by peeling anatomic units of the face in the same order in each patient. We treat the forehead first, and then, in order, the cheeks, nose, chin and lips, ears and eyelids. While the eyelids are being treated, particular care must be taken to avoid dripping TCA into the eye. Sterile water should be available to rinse the eyes in the event they are accidentally splashed with TCA. Ophthalmic antibiotic ointment is put on the eye before peeling the eyelids to protect the sclera and cornea from chemical burns.

Immediate postoperative care includes the application of a thin coat of antibiotic ointment (we prefer to use 2% erythromycin in petroleum) that is covered with a hydrogel dressing. The dressing provides immediate relief from the burning sensation because it decreases (neutralizes) the effective concentration of TCA and thus stops the chemical burn. A face mask fashioned from multiple layers of gauze is put over the wound, and left in place for 1 day. In some cases, a short-acting corticosteroid (betamethasone (Celestone), 1 ml) is given intramuscularly to minimize postoperative edema. The patient is instructed to sleep with the head elevated and to avoid excessive activity. Most patients go home and sleep or relax until the follow-up appointment the next day.

The dressing is changed twice daily. Re-epithelialization of the treated skin is usually complete in 1 week, after which time the wound is not dressed. However, lubrication of the skin and use of sunscreen is continued for as long as 6 months. Diffuse erythema lasts for 2–3 months, but after 1 week cosmetics may be used to cover the site.

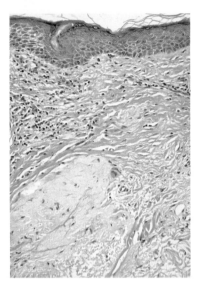

Figure 51.5 Biopsy specimen 3 months after 50% TCA facial chemical peel shows normal epidermis, fibroblasts with prominent nuclei in superficial dermis, and new collagen formation. The residual solar elastosis is now deeper in the dermis.

HISTOLOGIC EFFECTS OF TCA ON THE SKIN

The depth of the wound created by various concentrations and application techniques of TCA was evaluated by Stegman and by us in humans and hairless minipigs (Tables 51.2 and 51.3).[16–18] The therapeutic effects of TCA on the skin are due to the destruction of the epidermis and superficial dermis, and the subsequent re-epithelialization from epidermal adnexae and the stimulation of formation of new collagen (Figure 51.5). The depth of the peeling action correlates directly with the concentration of TCA, and dictates the therapeutic efficacy of the procedure.

Our studies have shown that the depth of tissue necrosis increased with increasing concentrations of TCA (Table 51.3).[18] Concentrations of TCA used to treat actinic keratosis should be at least 35–50%, because these are the concentrations necessary to remove the epidermis and superficial dermis completely to allow re-epithelialization by normal keratinocytes. Concentrations of TCA used for facial rejuvenation depend on the effect that is desired – whether partial exfoliation of the epidermis (20% TCA) or reduction of fine and medium wrinkles by inducing dermal necrosis (35–50% TCA).

Tape occlusion decreases the depth of dermal necrosis[18] because of interstitial humidifi-

Table 51.2 Depth of dermal necrosis produced by treatment with 50% TCA, 100% phenol or Baker's formula with and without tape occlusion[a]

	Wound thickness (mm)		Depth of scar at 60 days (mm)	
	Not occluded	Occluded	Not occluded	Occluded
Non-sun-damaged skin				
60% TCA	0.27	0.36	0.35	0.25
100% phenol	0.41	0.41	0.38	0.41
Baker's formula	0.5	0.65	0.41	0.40
Sun-damaged skin				
60% TCA	0.5	0.4	0.5	0.45
100% phenol	0.56	0.4	0.5	0.53
Baker's formula	0.63	0.85	0.57	0.9

[a]Modified from Stegman.[16]

cation and subsequent neutralization of TCA (decreased effective concentration of TCA). In contrast, tape occlusion increases the depth of penetration of other chemical peels such as phenol.

For a given concentration of TCA, the depth of dermal necrosis is inversely proportional to the thickness of the epidermis. Therefore thinning the epidermis by pretreatment with tretinoin and acetone causes a deeper dermal necrosis for a given concentration, and the result is a more effective and longer-lasting chemexfoliation.

Histological changes of TCA were studied in hairless minipigs.[21] Transient thinning and orthokeratosis of the stratum corneum were noted for 4 weeks postoperatively. From 24 hours to 4 weeks after TCA chemexfoliation, the zone of dermal necrosis was represented by collagen that had a distinct basophilic staining reaction. This change in collagen staining was still evident at 8 and 28 weeks. The collagen bundles were haphazardly organized, smaller and fragmented. The number of fibroblasts was increased in the superficial dermis at 4, 8 and 28 weeks in specimens of

Table 51.3 Depth of dermal necrosis produced by different concentrations of TCA with and without tape occlusion in the hairless minipig[a]

	Depth of necrosis (mm)		
TCA concentration (%)	Unoccluded	Occluded	Difference
20	0.044	0[b]	—
35	0.255	0.075	0.180
50	0.500	0.178	0.322
80	0.983	0.633	0.350

[a]From Brodland et al.[18]
[b]No measurable necrosis.
By permission of Elsevier Science Publishing Company.

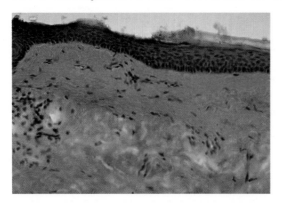

Figure 51.6 Biopsy specimen from scalp 1 year after 50% TCA facial chemical peel demonstrates normal epidermis and a zone of new, mature collagen overlying dense solar elastosis.

skin treated with 35%, 50% and 80% TCA. Greater concentrations of TCA induced a larger number of fibroblasts (Figure 51.6). Scarring and pigmentary alteration were clinically evident in some of the sites treated with 80% TCA, but not in those treated with 35% and 50% TCA. The elastic fibers were unchanged after treatment with 20% TCA. At 4 and 8 weeks, specimens treated with 35%, 50% and 80% TCA consistently exhibited a decrease in elastin. The amount of elastin at 28 weeks was greater than the baseline amount. Comparison of the long-term histologic effect of tape-occluded and unoccluded techniques showed that tape-occluded specimens exhibited significantly less long-term histologic alteration than occluded specimens.

COMPLICATIONS

When medium-depth or deep facial chemical peels are performed by experienced operators, complications are rare, and tend to be minor or easily corrected.[14,22] Superficial bacterial pustulation and eczematization are rare early complications, but, when they develop, they are managed with antibacterial therapy. Because latent herpes simplex virus may reactivate, patients with a history of herpes simplex should be treated with antiviral agents (e.g. acyclovir) administered orally 2–5 days prior until 5 days after the procedure. Milia frequently form soon after exfoliation, but are effectively treated with incision and drainage, with mild abrasive scrubbing, or resolve spontaneously.

Hyperpigmentation and hypopigmentation are common long-term problems. In general, the former occurs more frequently after superficial peels and the latter after deeper peels, especially in people with dark complexions. Hypertrophic scars may occur on the skin of the neck, dorsal aspects of the hands and arms, and on other areas not rich in cutaneous adnexa. Although hypertrophic scars may form on the face, especially on the upper lip and near the mandible, keloid formation is rare.

Other complications of chemical peel that may occur are accentuation of telangiectasias, enlargement of pilosebaceous pores, darkening of pigmented naevi, persistent erythema, and increased sensitivity to wind, sunlight and changes in temperature.

CO$_2$ LASER RESURFACING

The recent development of high-energy, short-pulse carbon dioxide lasers has introduced another method for facial rejuvenation and the treatment of photoaging and acne scarring. This instrument has also been used to treat actinic cheilitis, verruca vulgaris, seborrheic keratoses and lentigines.[23,24] The major advantages of pulsed-laser resurfacing include precise tissue ablation, minimization of residual thermal damage, and hemostasis.

The target chromophore of the CO$_2$ laser (10 600 nm wavelength) is intracellular water. Absorption of laser energy causes boiling, subsequent vaporization and cellular ablation. The disadvantage of the continuous CO_2 laser beam is that heat can accumulate in tissue after the water target is lost, causing thermal necrosis and scarring. However, if sufficient energy to vaporize tissue is delivered with a tissue dwell time less than or equal to the thermal relaxation time, there is little energy left for thermal conduction or thermal damage.[25] High-energy, short-pulse CO_2 lasers have been designed to deliver less than 1 ms pulses with energy fluences of 5–7 J/cm^2, which vaporize tissue to the 20–30 μm optical penetration depth of the laser and leave 40–120 μm of residual thermal damage. This thermal energy is helpful in sealing small vessels for hemostasis, yet is not enough to cause significant scarring.[26]

The high-energy, short-pulse CO_2 laser effectively removes the epidermis and part of the dermis. Shrinkage of the tissue is also noted during the procedure, which persists during the healing phase. Histologically, there appears to be new collagen formation in the dermis, and alterations in the density and distribution of elastic fibers. These findings are similar to those found in medium-depth peels.[27]

The early results have been impressive. Most studies have reported an average of 50% improvement in patients treated for photodamage. However, persistent erythema can be present for up to six months, which is significantly longer than originally described. Postinflammatory hyperpigmentation has been primarily reported in patients with Fitzpatrick skin type III or IV; the hyperpigmentation usually resolved after treatment with retinoic acid and hydroquinone creams. Contact dermatitis is uniquely more common after CO_2 laser resurfacing. Whether it is an irritant or allergic reaction has not been clearly delineated. However, common wound care agents such as Bacitracin and Polysporin are no longer commonly used, and have been replaced with bland ointments such as petrolatum. Other adverse effects and complications include edema, burning discomfort postoperatively, pruritus, tight sensation, excessive milia, contact dermatitis, hypopigmentation, bacterial infection and herpes simplex virus superinfection.[28] Isolated cases of hypertrophic scarring of the upper lip, induration of the vermilion border and focal atrophy of the cutaneous lip have been reported.[26] Full epithelialization takes place in 7–14 days. The use of hydrogen dressings and thick application of antibiotic ointment or petrolatum promotes wound healing. Crusting and drainage is reduced with wet dressing every 3 hours.

SUMMARY

Facial chemical peel encompasses a plethora of procedures and techniques. The development of high-energy, short-pulse CO_2 lasers has added yet another very useful tool for the treatment of photoaging and of acne scars, and for facial rejuvenation. Although there are many advantages of this procedure over the facial chemical peel or dermabrasion, more studies are needed to establish its long-term efficacy and safety. Facial chemical peel is a safe, effective and elegant method for treating common problems associated with photoaged fair skin. When standardized techniques are used, it is also possible to quantify the therapeutic effects and reliably predict the outcome.

REFERENCES

1. Fulton JJ, Dermabrasion, chemabrasion, and laserabrasion. Historical perspectives, modern dermabrasion techniques, and future trends. *Dermatol Surg* 1996; **22:** 619–28.
2. Brody HJ, In: *Chemical Peeling* (Brody HJ, ed.). St Louis, MO: Mosby Year Book, 1992:7–22.
3. Van Scott EJ, Yu RJ, Alpha hydroxy acids: procedures for use in clinical practice. *Cutis* 1989; **43:** 222–8.
4. Moy LS, Murad H, Moy RL, Glycolic acid peels for the treatment of wrinkles and photoaging. *J Dermatol Surg Oncol* 1993; **19:** 243–6.

5. Newman N, Newman A, Moy LS et al, Clinical improvement of photoaged skin with 50% glycolic acid. A double-blind vehicle-controlled study. *Dermatol Surg* 1996; **22:** 455–60.

6. Moy LS, Peace S, Moy RL, Comparison of the effect of various chemical peeling agents in a mini-pig model. *Dermatol Surg* 1996; **22:** 429–32.

7. Moy LS, Howe K, Moy RL, Glycolic acid modulation of collagen production in human skin fibroblast cultures in vitro. *Dermatol Surg* 1996; **22:** 439–41.

8. Baker TJ, The ablation of rhitides by chemical means: preliminary report. *J Florida Med Assoc* 1961; **48:** 451–4.

9. McCollough EG, Maloney BP, Langsdon PR, In: *Dermatologic Surgery: Principles and Practice*, 2nd edn (Roenigk RK, Roenigk HH Jr, eds). New York: Marcel Dekker, 1996:1147–60.

10. Roberts HL, The chloracetic acids: a biochemical study. *Br J Dermatol Syphilol* 1926; **38:** 323–34.

11. Monash S, The uses of diluted trichloractic acid in dermatology. *Urol Cutan Rev* 1945; **49:** 119–20.

12. Ayres SI, Superficial chemosurgery in treating aging skin. *Arch Dermatol* 1962; **85:** 385–93.

13. Brody HJ, Hailey CW, Medium-depth chemical peeling of the skin: a variation of superficial chemosurgery. *J Dermatol Surg Oncol* 1986; **12:** 1268–75.

14. Roenigk RK, Resnik SS, Dolezal JF, In: *Dermatologic Surgery: Principles and Practice*, 2nd edn (Roenigk RK, Roenigk HH Jr, eds). New York: Marcel Dekker, 1996:1121–36.

15. Coleman WPI, Brody HJ, In: *Dermatologic Surgery: Principles and Practice*, 2nd edn (Roenigk RK, Roenigk HH Jr, eds). New York: Marcel Dekker, 1996:1137–60.

16. Stegman SJ, A comparative histologic study of the effects of three peeling agents and dermabrasion on normal and sundamaged skin. *Aesth Plast Surg* 1982; **6:** 123–35.

17. Stegman SJ, A study of dermabrasion and chemical peels in an animal model. *J Dermatol Surg Oncol* 1980; **6:** 490–7.

18. Brodland DG, Cullimore KC, Roenigk RK, Gibson LE, Depths of chemexfoliation induced by various concentrations and application techniques of trichloroacetic acid in a porcine model. *J Dermatol Surg Oncol* 1989; **15:** 967–71.

19. Brodland DG, Roenigk RK, Trichloroacetic acid chemexfoliation (chemical peel) for extensive premalignant actinic damage of the face and scalp. *Mayo Clin Proc* 1988; **63:** 887–96.

20. Brody HJ, Update on chemical peels. *Adv Dermatol* 1992; **7:** 275–88.

21. Roenigk RK, Brodland DG, A primer of facial chemical peel. *Dermatol Clin* 1993; **11:** 349–59.

22. Resnik SS, Resnik BI, Complications of chemical peeling. *Dermatol Clin* 1995; **13:** 309–12.

23. Fitzpatrick RE, Goldman MP, Esparza RJ, Clinical advantage of the CO_2 laser superpulsed mode: treatment of verruca vulgaris, seborrheic keratoses lentigines and actinic cheilitis. *J Dermatol Surg Oncol* 1991; **20:** 449–56.

24. Fitzpatrick RE, Rutz-Esparza J, The superpulsed CO_2 laser. In: *Surgical Dermatology* (Roenigk R, Roenigk HH Jr, eds). London: Martin Dunitz, 1993:279–90.

25. Fitzpatrick RE, Goldman MP, Satur NM, Tope WD, Pulsed carbon dioxide laser resurfacing of photoaged facial skin. *Arch Dermatol* 1996; **132:** 395–402.

26. Hruza GJ, Dover JS, Laser skin resurfacing. *Arch Dermatol* 1996; **132:** 451–5.

27. Cotton J, Hood AF, Gonin R et al, Histologic evaluation of preauricular and postauricular human skin after high-energy, short-pulse carbon dioxide laser. *Arch Dermatol* 1996; **132:** 425–8.

28. Waldorf HA, Kauvar ANB, Geronemus RG, Skin resurfacing of fine to deep rhytides using char-free carbon dioxide laser in 47 patients. *Dermatol Surg* 1995; **21:** 940–6.

52

Dermabrasion for rejuvenation and scar revision

Henry H Roenigk Jr

INTRODUCTION

Dermabrasion is a method of correcting many cutaneous problems – from acne scars to removal of tattoos or tumors to the revision of scars.[1] The method has been modified over the past 40 years, from the sandpaper-type equipment to the fast and convenient motor-driven hand engines used today. The skill of the operator, judgment in selecting patients, and understanding of the cutaneous lesions are necessary to get good cosmetic results and to avoid serious complications that can result from dermabrasion.

EQUIPMENT

Although dermabrasion can be performed with manual units, almost all operators use an electric power source (Table 52.1).[2]

The older units are cable-driven, in which the motor rotates a cable approximately four feet long. The rotating cable turns the dermabrading end piece. The Robbins unit provides rotation speeds of 800–12 000 rev/min. In using cable-driven machines, the operator must be sure that the cable is kept straight or in no more than a very gentle curve. Sharp bends on the cable create excess friction, resulting in a broken cable. There is also more noise when using the cable.

Hand engines have been developed over the past 10 years, and are useful in dermabrasion because they are smaller, can be held in the hand, and are quiet. These electric engines with simple controls have a simple coiled cord that permits maximum flexibility. The torque is generally adequate for most dermabrasions. The combination of speed

Table 52.1 Instruments used in dermabrasion
Dermabraders
• Motor-driven
Bell International Hand Engine
Osada Hand Engine
Mill-Bilt Equipment Company
Robbins Instrument Company
Dremel Power Tool No. 370 (hand-held unit)
• Air-driven
Stryker Company
Dermatomes
• Laminar dermal reticulotomy
Davis, Davol or Brown dermatomes
• Schreuss (Derma III) machine
Schumann Precision Manufacturer
Brushes
• Diamond fraises
• Wire brush
• Small contoured fraises
Robbins Instrument Company

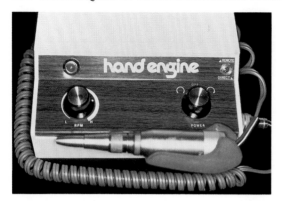

Figure 52.1 Bell hand engine, which is most often used for dermabrasion today

and torque of the machine and pressure applied by the operator provides the rapid cutting necessary. The Bell Hand Engine (Figure 52.1) has two models: Model 250 (speed crawl to 18 000 rev/min) and Model 28L (speed 2000–35 000 rev/min). These machines are primarily used today by most dermatologists doing dermabrasion.[3]

The end pieces or cutting tools for dermabrasion are diamond fraises, wire brushes and serrated wheels (Figure 52.2). Diamond

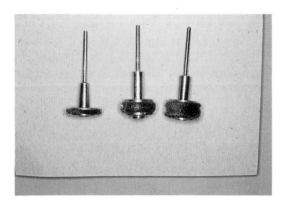

Figure 52.2 Wire brush fraises used at end piece as the cutting tools for dermabrasion

fraises are stainless-steel wheels to which are bonded diamond chips in two different grades of coarseness (regular or coarse). Most experienced dermabraders use the coarser of the two fraises. The wire brush is a stainless steel wheel with wires arranged at angles. The wires of the brush cut deeply and rapidly in frozen skin. Most experienced operators prefer the wire brush because it goes deep and thus gives better results, but for the novice or if only a superficial dermabrasion is necessary, diamond fraises work fine. The fraises are held by the mandrel on the chuck attached to the cable. A foot pedal rheostat to control speed is preferred.

LASER RESURFACING

The old CO_2 laser has been used to perform dermabrasion. It vaporizes tissue without bleeding and possibly with less pain than the standard dermabrasion. The healing time and postoperative care is similar. There is more delineation between normal and laserabrasioned skin (Figure 53.3) because it is more difficult to feather the edges as can be done with standard dermabrasion.

The CO_2 laser has been suggested as ideal treatment of multiple trichoepitheliomas, rhinophyma, epidermal nevi, syringoma, neurofibromas and tattoos. These problems have all been treated satisfactorily with standard dermabrasion. The CO_2 laser is probably the treatment of choice for rhinophyma (Figure 52.4) and actinic cheilits.

In 1993, Coherent Ultra-Pulse and Sharplan Silk touch systems developed a modification of the CO_2 laser with a continuous beam that could be used to ablate tissue in a controlled, bloodless, superficial way. With the use of computer-generated patterns, this has become one of the techniques of choice for treatment of wrinkles due to photoaging skin. The resurfacing lasers have also been used for acne scars, post-surgical scars and all the other indications for dermabrasion.[4]

Although the results have been excellent

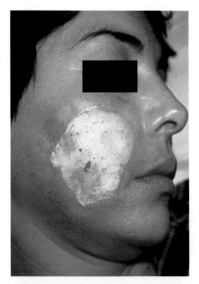

(a)

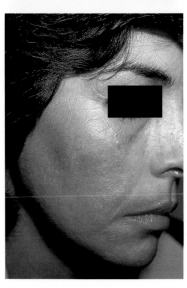

(b)

Figure 52.3 (a) Acne scars with white crust immediately after CO_2 laserabrasion. (b) Three months later, there is still delineation of the laserabrasion area.

for wrinkles, there still is debate about the long-term benefits, problems with wound healing, persistent erythema and other complications. Most clinicians still feel that dermabrasion works better for acne scars and the procedure will not be lost to the laser hysteria.

Newer lasers are being developed to deal with side-effects. The erbium YAG laser produces good results with less erythema, but requires 5–6 passes and has some bleeding just like dermabrasion. Collagen shrinkage, which is advantageous for lasers in photoaging skin, has no benefit in the treatment of acne scars. Certainly when more data have accumulated and good histologic studies have been completed and comparative studies between lasers and lasers versus dermabrasion versus chemical peel have been done, we shall learn which is the best technique for each condition. Increased experience with any new procedure produces more comfortable and ultimately better clinical results.[5]

PATIENT SELECTION AND PREOPERATIVE WORK-UP

The preoperative consultation is extremely important. The surgeon must tell the patient clearly what to expect from the procedure, as well as get a feel for the patient's expectations. The patient must understand the pitfalls and limitations of the procedure. Alternative procedures such as chemical peel, cryosurgery and collagen implants should be listed. The use of photographs to demonstrate the procedure, as well as before-and-after pictures (including those of complications), may be helpful in the consultation. This discussion should be documented in the chart.

Patients who seek cosmetic surgery to improve their appearance for a variety of personal reasons have unique personalities.

The surgeon must have a basic understanding of psychology and drive for perfection of the cosmetic surgery patient. Therapeutic dermabrasion may relieve some of the pressure to achieve perfect results. One should avoid promoting dermabrasion, and should list the other options available and the complications that can occur. There are adjunctive procedures that are often combined with dermabrasion, and these should be carefully covered in

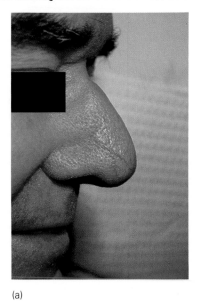

(a)

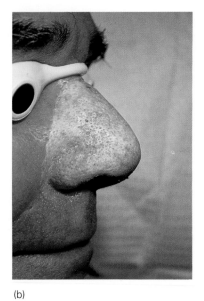

(b)

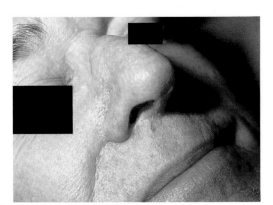

(c)

Figure 52.4 Rhinophyma: (a) before laserabrasion; (b) immediately after CO_2 laserabrasion; (c) improvement in texture and color of nose three months after CO_2 laserabrasion

the consultation. The physician must decide who is a good candidate and if a reasonable improvement can be expected. The patient who has a minimal scar and cannot tolerate what seems like a slight blemish should be avoided, as should patients critical of care given by previous physicians. The patient's criticism may be valid, but you too may be unable to live up to the patient's expectations.

Preoperative work-up includes a medical history – specifically other medication (especially aspirin) and diseases such as hepatitis, AIDS, venereal disease and recurrent herpes simplex.

Laboratory evaluations include complete blood count, serum chemistries and bleeding time. Other tests include evaluation for hepatitis B antigen and antibody and HIV III antibody titers after obtaining informed consent to perform the tests.

ANESTHESIA

Preoperative medicine should relax the patient and reduce the pain of dermabrasion, since most dermabrasions are done with local, not general anesthesia. Intramuscular meperidine (Demerol) and intravenous diazepam (Valium) (10–20 mg) give good preoperative sedation. Antihistamines or other sedatives may also be used. Motrin may help reduce edema and bleeding. Preoperative topical retinoic acid may reduce the incidence of milia postoperatively and improve wound healing. There should be constant monitoring of blood pressure, pulse and heart rate, and pulse oximeter when giving preoperative sedation. Keeping an intravenous line open during the procedure is helpful in giving more sedative medications during the procedure if necessary and for emergencies that might arise.

For small areas, such as tattoos, it is preferable to use local anesthetic with 1% or 0.5% lidocaine (Xylocaine) with or without epinephrine. Tumescent anesthesia to the entire face has also been used. Nerve blocks with lidocaine may be performed on the central face, with six points receiving 3 ml at each site.[6] The six points are bilateral

- supraorbital and supratrochlear
- infraorbital and
- mental nerves.

Prechilling of the skin with ice packs will enhance the local spray types of anesthesia usually used for dermabrasion. The spray anesthesia is performed by the assistant in a circular motion for 20–30 seconds until the skin becomes frigid and has a white frost on it. Care should be taken not to freeze too deeply, especially over the mandibular bone. Delineation of the area to be frozen usually is not greater than 2 or 3 cm. Towels will protect the adjacent skin.

The choice of spray anesthesia is important. Ethyl chloride is the oldest agent but is not used much because it is explosive and inflammable, has general anesthetic properties, and requires a blower for rapid evaporation. Frigiderm and Fluro-Ethyl are Freon 114 and Freon 114 plus ethyl chloride respectively. They generally freeze the skin surface to $-42°C$ in 25 seconds, according to work done by Hanke et al.[7] Other topical cryoanesthetic agents that contain pure Freon 111 and 112 can freeze to $-67°C$, and result in much more tissue necrosis. The risk of unpredictable hypertrophic scarring is greater with these sprays. The risk is greatest in areas overlying a bone, such as the mandibular ramus, zygomatic arch, malar eminence, and bossing of the chin and forehead. Frigiderm and Fluro-Ethyl are the preferred agents for cryoanesthesia.

General anesthesia is used more frequently by nondermatologic surgeons. Except for special circumstances, this only adds to the risk, cost and time in performing this procedure. The vast majority of dermabrasions are performed in office surgical suites.

TECHNIQUE

There are many variations on the technique. Dermabrasion requires at least one assistant to help with freezing and to hold the skin taut. Both operator and assistant should wear gowns, rubber gloves and plastic face shields. The assistant should wear cotton gloves over rubber gloves to protect the fingers. Cotton towels are preferred over gauze, which easily gets caught in the wire brush. The area to be abraded is painted with gentian violet (Figure 52.5). This not only serves as a guide, but gentian violet deep in the scars also indicates whether the abrasion has gone a sufficient depth to obliterate them. Vaseline and goggles are used to protect the patient's eyes, ears and nose. The patient lies supine on the table. Adequate ventilation and a cool ambi-

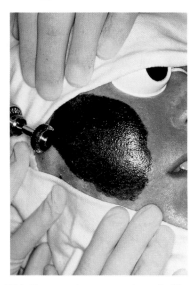

Figure 52.5 Preoperative preparation of skin prior to starting dermabrasion.

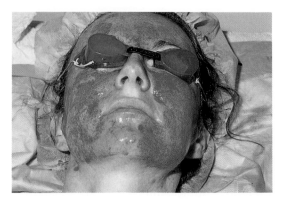

Figure 52.6 Immediate postoperative view of a full-face dermabrasion.

ent temperature of 17°C will help when freezing the skin.

Dermabrasion of the face is usually performed in sections: four on each cheek, two on the chin, two on the nose, two on the upper lip and three on the forehead. Spraying and abrading one area at a time, the surgeon starts at the outermost and dependent areas and moves towards the central and upper areas of the face. The operator moves the brush or fraise over the frozen skin with firm, steady, back-and-forth strokes and even pressure. In areas with deeper scars, more pressure may be applied. Dermabrasion is performed in anatomic units, so it is usually done to the natural folds of the face (nasolabial fold, hairline or submandibular) (Figure 52.6). This is to avoid obvious lines of demarcation that can occur with spot dermabrasion. Other portions of the body, such as the back, arms and legs, may also respond to dermabrasion for specific indications.

POSTOPERATIVE CARE AND DRESSING

The older method of dressing dermabrasion wounds was to apply an antibiotic ointment directly over the abraded area, covering this with nonadherent gauze and then an outer wrap of flexible surgical net.[8] This is removed the following day, and the wound allowed to form a crust. The crust will come off in 10–14 days, and antibiotic ointment can be applied to the slowly healing skin.

The new synthetic wound healing dressings have greatly improved the postoperative healing following dermabrasion. The healing time is reduced to 5–7 days, with virtually no pain and infrequent infections.

Op-site and Biobrane are new surgical dressings that provide some specific benefits. The biggest benefit is that the postoperative burning pain is reduced or completely eliminated. Op-site is a polyurethane material with an adhesive that will stick to stratum corneum but not to wet wounds. When using this, it is necessary to have a nonabraded section of skin around the hairline and in the preauricular area so that the Op-site can stick. On the other hand, Biobrane will stick to moist

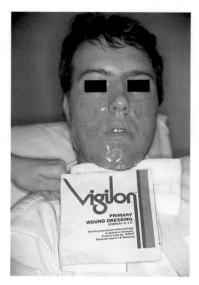

Figure 52.7 Patient immediately postoperative following dermabrasion, with Vigilon dressing applied.

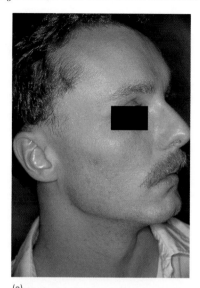

(a)

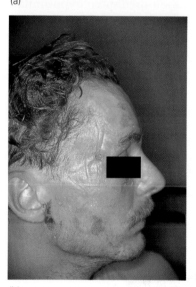

(b)

Figure 52.8 (a) Patient before dermabrasion, (b) The same patient after one month of Vigilon dressing.

wounds and can be placed over the completely dermabraded face.

Vigilon is another synthetic dressing that absorbs moisture and reduces postoperative pain. We find that the continuous use of Vigilon allows the skin to re-epithelialize in about seven days without going through the crusting phase, and it is our preferred dressing today (Figures 52.7 and 52.8). Prior to application, a polyethylene film is removed from one side of the dressing that will cover the wound. Vigilon, unlike other occlusive dressings, permits a moist environment while allowing for absorption of wound exudate. It is also nonadherent.

Pinski[9] evaluated these new dressings in a bilateral comparison study of patients undergoing full face dermabrasion. Occlusive dressings act by preventing dehydration to allow rapid epithelial migration. Vigilon may be the

best dressing to use following dermabrasion. It should be changed daily. Re-epithelialization will occur in 5–7 days without crusting compared with 10–12 days when crusts were allowed to form. Recent studies with Omni Derm by some investigators have shown this to be a desirable postoperative dressing for dermabrasion.

The patient is given written instruction for postoperative care. Pain medication such as acetaminophen (paracetamol) with codeine is helpful. Systemic antibiotics are usually used as well as a short course of systemic steroids to reduce postoperative edema. Acyclovir (Zovirax) to prevent herpes simplex should be used routinely.

The patient is seen in 24 hours for a dressing change. The Vigilon dressing is then changed on a daily basis at home. The patient should be evaluated regularly at 7, 14 and 30 days – more often if necessary. Avoidance of sun is important after dermabrasion. Exposure to the sun may easily burn the new skin, and will predispose to postinflammatory hyperpigmentation.

INDICATIONS

Dermabrasion was developed as a method of treating acne scars. It has been used to treat a variety of problems, including hypertrophic scars, traumatic scars, actinically damaged and wrinkled skin, and for correction of pigmentary abnormalities. The cosmetic indications for dermabrasion include

- acne scars (Figure 52.9)
- fine wrinkling (laser resurfacing may be better)
- scar revision
- melasma
- perioral pseudorhagades
- tattoo removal (Figure 52.10).

There are many other therapeutic reasons for selecting dermabrasion.[10,11]

- epidermal nevus (Figure 52.11)
- epithelioma adenoides cysticum (Figure 52.12)
- rhinophyma
- nevus angiomatosus
- syringoma
- adenoma sebaceum
- keloids

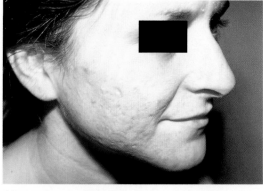

(a)

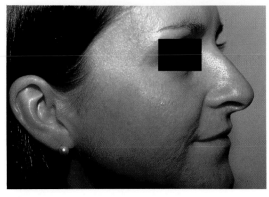

(b)

Figure 52.9 (a) Acne scars on right cheek. (b) Improved acne scars following a dermabrasion.

- discoid lupus erythematosus
- actinic keratosis and solar elastosis (Figure 52.13)
- seborrheic keratosis
- basal cell carcinoma
- Darier's disease

Hanke[12] provided a list of 50 conditions that have been treated with dermabrasion (Table 52.2).

The correction of old and new scars by dermabrasion is very effective. Superficial sharply demarcated scars can often be completely removed, while soft saucer-like depressions can be improved but not eliminated. It should be emphasized to the patient that improvement is expected, but there is no guarantee

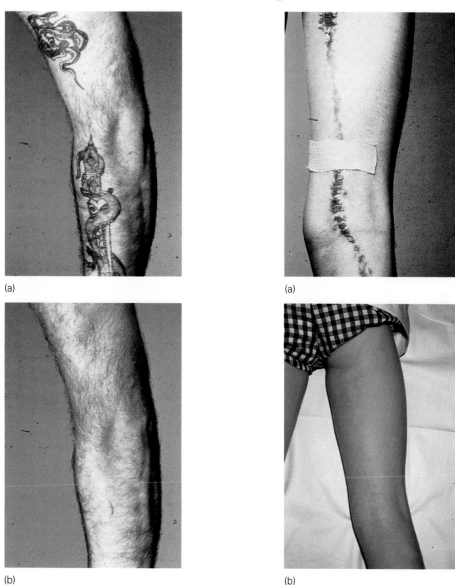

(a)

(b)

(a)

(b)

Figure 52.10 (a) Tattoo before dermabrasion. (b) Excellent cosmetic results of removal of tattoo by standard dermabrasion.

Figure 52.11 (a) Epidermal nevus prior to dermabrasion. (b) Removal of epidermal nevus by dermabrasion, with long-term results.

that all scars will be eliminated. Dermabrasion will soften sharp edges and improve the crater-like appearance of these scars caused by shadows in the depression. Deep ice-pick-type scars will require scar revision excision, punch elevation or punch grafting prior to dermabrasion. Dermabrasion can also be used for cysts or to marsupialize epithelialized sinuses when chronically infected. Scars from excisional surgery or trauma can be der-

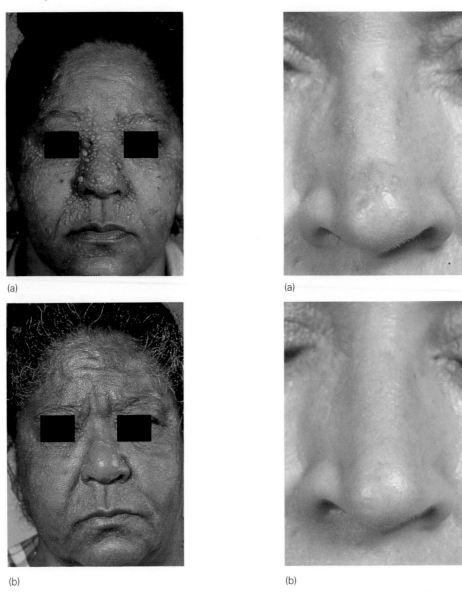

Figure 52.12 Epithelioma adenoides cysticum: (a) before dermabrasion; (b) five years after dermabrasion.

Figure 52.13 (a) Actinically damaged nose prior to treatment. (b) Postoperative view of dermabrasion of actinically damaged nose.

mabraded 6–8 weeks after sutures are removed, to camouflage these wounds by forming a more natural epidermal surface.

Older wounds do not respond as well unless they are re-excised, followed by dermabrasion.

Table 52.2 Various entities treated with dermabrasion	
Postacne scars	Adenoma sebaceum
Traumatic scars	Neurotic excoriations
Smallpox or chickenpox scars	Multiple trichoepitheliomas
Rinophyma	Darier's disease
Professionally applied tattoos	Fox-Fordyce disease
Amateur-type tattoos (indian ink)	Lichenified dermatoses
Blast tattoos (gunpowder)	Porokeratosis of Mibelli
Multiple seborrheic keratoses	Favre-Racouchot syndrome
Multiple pigmented nevi	Lichen amyloidosis
Actinically damaged skin	Verrucous nevus
Age- and sun-related wrinkle lines	Molluscum contagiosum
Active acne	Keratoacanthoma
Freckles	Xanthalasma
Pseudofolliculitis barbae	Hemangioma
Telangiectasia	Leg ulcer
Acne rosacea	Scleromyxedema
Chloasma	Striae distensae
Vitiligo	Early operative scars
Congenital pigmented nevi	Hair transplantation
Syringocystadenoma papilliferum	(elevated recipient sites)
Nevus flammeus	Linear epidermal nevus
Keloids	Syringoma
Dermatitis papilaris capilliti	Angiofibromas of tuberous
	sclerosis
Lupus erythematosus	Chronic radiation dermatitis
Basal-cell carcinoma	Xeroderma pigmentosum
(superficial type)	Lentigines

SCAR REVISION

The traditional approach for the revision of scars with dermabrasion has been to perform abrasion six months or longer after the original surgery or injury. The best esthetic results obtained were better when the scar was older. It was only 12 years ago that earlier intervention was first suggested. Burks[13] stated that 'pox scars, like other scars, may be dermabraded 6–8 weeks after their appearance.'

Collins and Farber[6] reported that, in selective cases, diamond fraise dermabrasion effectively enhanced the cosmetic outcome of nasal scars when treated 2–6 weeks after suture removal.

Yarborough[14] found that facial scars, when planed with a wire brush 4–8 weeks after injury, healed without evidence of residual scarring. These were compared with mature scars that were abraded 3 months to 13 years after injury, which were not eradicated.

The correction of scars by dermabrasion is very effective for both old and new scars. The more superficial ice-pick type of scars can often be completely removed, whereas deeper more saucer-like scars can be improved but not eliminated. Dermabrasion will remove sharp edges of acne scars and reduce their crater-like appearance. Occasionally, other procedures should be used to remove deep scars prior to dermabrasion. Fresh scars from excision surgery or traumatic accident repairs can be dermabraded about 6–8 weeks after sutures are removed, and the cosmetic appearance of these wounds can be greatly enhanced by the formation of a more natural epithelial surface over the healing wounds. Older wounds that have a white line are not usually improved much unless there is re-excision with scar revision followed by dermabrasion.

Larger, deep scars that do not respond well to dermabrasion alone should be treated by either

- punch excision of the wound (usually with a circular punch) and then suture closing of the wound;
- punch excision of the depressed scar and elevation of the plug to the flush surface of the surrounding skin (it can be held in place by a Steri-strip dressing); or
- punch excision with full-thickness graft replacement usually taken from the postauricular area.

Dermabrasion is usually then done about 6 weeks after these procedures have corrected the deeper scars, so there is a more uniform smoothing of all the skin surface.

Bovine collagen (Zyderm), Fibrel or fat transplants have been suggested as replacements for dermabrasion scars. My preference is to use these products if there are only a few isolated soft scars where dermabrasion seems unnecessary or as an adjunct to correct areas not completely repaired by dermabrasion.

The number of injections required to correct an individual scar depends on the degree of collagen response and depth of the defect. Dermabrasion can safely be performed after collagen injections into scars.

Examples of the results obtained with this technique are shown in the following examples:

- chicken pox scars – before, during and after punch elevation and dermabrasion (Figure 52.14);
- dermabrasion of traumatic wounds (Figure 52.15);
- dermabrasion of surgical scars (Figure 52.16).

Katz and Oca[15] have made a controlled study for which a split-scar paradigm was designed. Linear scars that were produced by full-thickness surgical excisions on the face, trunk and extremities were chosen randomly for abrasion 4, 6 or 8 weeks postsurgery. The results of spot dermabrasion of the left half of each scar were compared with the untreated right half of each scar. Ratings were performed by physicians, lay persons and the patients themselves after viewing color photographs of the scars taken at various time intervals. One operator performed all of the abrasions.

The summary of findings were as follows:

- dermabrasion significantly improved the appearance of surgical scars;
- the appearance of the scars was not worsened by dermabrasion;
- scars improved with dermabrasion at all time intervals, but was significantly improved ($p < 0.05$) at 8 weeks postsurgery, where 50% of the scars disappeared;
- the face, trunk and extremities showed comparable improvement with dermabrasion.

The authors coined the term 'Scarabrasion' for this procedure.

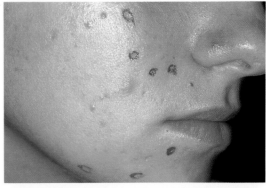

(a)

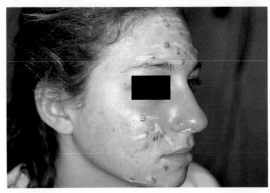

(b)

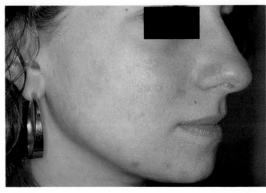

(c)

Figure 52.14 (a) Chicken pox scars on face outlined with gentian violet. (b) Immediately after a combination of punch excision and suturing, punch elevation and punch grafting. Full face dermabrasion was performed six weeks later. (c) Postoperative results at four weeks postdermabrasion.

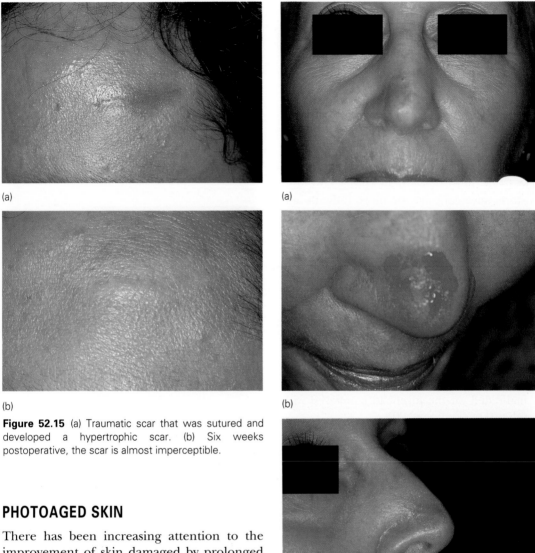

Figure 52.15 (a) Traumatic scar that was sutured and developed a hypertrophic scar. (b) Six weeks postoperative, the scar is almost imperceptible.

Figure 52.16 (a) Patient with basal cell carcinoma of tip of nose treated by Mohs surgery and full thickness skin graft. (b) Dermabrasion of the graft at two months postoperatively. (c) Five weeks postdermabrasion, with satisfactory cosmetic improvement of the graft.

PHOTOAGED SKIN

There has been increasing attention to the improvement of skin damaged by prolonged exposure to ultraviolet light. Many topical agents such as tretinoin (Retin A) and α-hydroxy acids will cause slow but gradual improvement in actinically damaged skin. Topical 5-fluorouracil has been advocated for patients with extensive actinic keratosis. These agents take a long time to show the improvement, and are sometimes very irritating to the skin.

An alternative approach to improving photoaged skin has been the use of chemical peels and dermabrasion, and more recently

CO_2 laser resurfacing with the new lasers. In his original book on dermabrasion, Burks[13] showed the significant improvement that could be obtained in an experiment he performed by dermabrasion on one half of the face of a patient with actinically damaged skin and observing the changes at one year. Superficial dermabrasion with a diamond fraise is an effective and rapid method of rejuvenating the skin of the face or scalp. The major problem that can occur is that aged skin heals more slowly than young skin, and postoperative care may be more difficult and prolonged.

The following are examples of cosmetic improvement of photoaged skin following dermabrasion:

- photoaged skin before and after dermabrasion (Figure 52.17);
- actinic keratosis of forehead before, during and after dermabrasion (Figure 52.18);
- perioral deep wrinkles before and after dermabrasion (Figure 52.19);
- actinic damage – note the area dermabraded on the forehead compared with other skin (Figure 52.20).

Certainly, similar results could be obtained today with full-face CO_2 resurfacing lasers.

COMPLICATIONS AND CONTRAINDICATIONS

Among the most common complications are

- hyperpigmentation
- keloids
- gouging of skin
- herpes simplex
- milia
- persistent erythema
- telangiectasia

Erythema is expected in the postoperative period, but it may sometimes persist for weeks or months along with some telangiectasia. Milia formation is very common, and can eas-

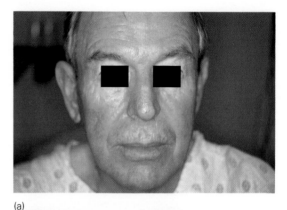

(a)

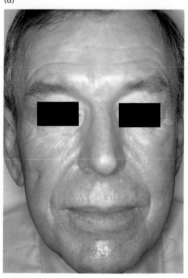

(b)

Figure 52.17 (a) Severe actinic damage with multiple actinic keratosis. (b) Six months after dermabrasion.

ily be corrected with abrasive soaps or simple extraction. Pinpoint electrodesiccation can also be used. The use of topical retinoic acid prior to dermabrasion may reduce the incidence of milia. Milia may be more common with the new occlusive wound dressings.

Hypertrophic scars or keloids may occur in a small number of patients. A personal or family history of keloid formation is a relative

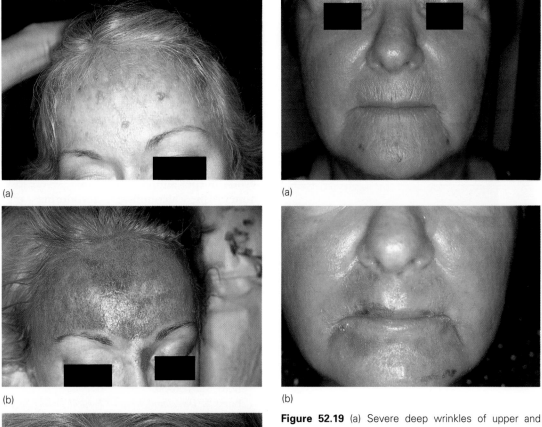

(a)

(b)

Figure 52.19 (a) Severe deep wrinkles of upper and lower lips. (b) One month after dermabrasion.

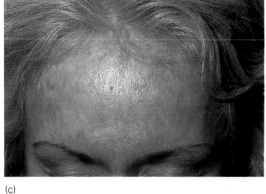

(c)

Figure 52.18 (a) Severe actinic damage and multiple actinic keratosis of forehead. (b) Immediately after dermabrasion. (c) Postoperative cosmetic improvement.

contraindication. Dark-skinned patients tend to form keloids more frequently. The use of refrigerants, especially on the mandible, may be partially responsible. Atypical keloids develop in atypical locations such as the buccal skin after dermabrasion of patients still on or having recently taken isotretinoin (Accutane) Keloids have also been seen in patients undergoing chemical peel and laser surgery after recent exposure to isotretinoin. Patients now wait one year after taking isotretinoin before the procedure. This has resulted in no atypical keloids in a follow-up study done by us. Treatment of these scars

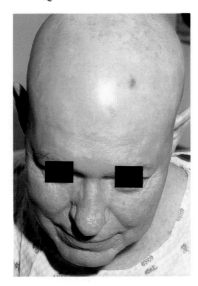

Figure 52.20 Severe actinic damage to entire face and scalp. Note the difference in color and texture of skin on forehead that has already been dermabraded.

with intralesional triamcinolone is helpful. Topical steroids may be used early for suspicious areas of hypertrophic scars.

Patients with a history of recurrent cold sores, possibly herpes simplex, should be approached with caution. The surgeon should avoid dermabrasion in the trigger areas of previous herpes simplex. Oral acyclovir (Zovirax), 200 mg five times a day for three days before and until the skin has re-epithelialized, should be given prophylactically. If disseminated herpes simplex develops, hospitalization and intravenous acyclovir are indicated.

Hypopigmentation and hyperpigmentation are common but usually temporary. Pigmentary problems are more common in dark-skinned patients (skin types IV–VI). They are most noticeable at the edges of the dermabrasion or in spot dermabrasion. Postinflammatory hyperpigmentation usually

fades in several months, and no treatment is necessary. Topical hydroquinone 4% and tretinoin cream 0.05% may cause fading.

Acne will occasionally recur after dermabrasion, although most patients with minimally active disease will actually improve. Infection with *Staphylococcus* and *Pseudomonas* occurs occasionally, and needs prompt topical and systemic therapy.

Dermabrasion is usually contraindicated in patients with chronic radiodermatitis, pyoderma, herpes simplex, psychosis, severe psychoneurosis, alcoholism, xeroderma pigmentosum, verrucae planae or burn scars.

REFERENCES

1. Roenigk HH Jr, Dermabrasion. In: *Dermatologic Surgery: Principles and Practice* (Roenigk RK, Roenigk HH Jr, eds). New York: Marcel Dekker, 1989:959–78.
2. Stegman SJ, Tromovitch TK, Dermabrasion equipment. In: *Cosmetic Dermatologic Surgery* (Tromovitch TK, Stegman SJ, eds). Chicago: Year Book, 1984:56–60.
3. Burks J, *Dermabrasion and Chemical Peeling in the Treatment of Certain Cosmetic Defects and Diseases of the Skin.* Springfield, IL: Charles C Thomas, 1979.
4. Roenigk HH Jr, Treatment of the aging face. *Dermatol Clin* 1995; **13**: 245–61.
5. Roenigk HH Jr, The place of laser resurfacing within the range of medical and surgical skin resurfacing techniques. *Semin Cutan Med Surg* 1996; **15**: 1–7.
6. Collins PS, Farber GA, Postsurgical dermabrasion of the nose. *J Dermatol Surg Oncol* 1984; **10**: 476–7.
7. Hanke CW, O'Brian JJ, Solow EB, Laboratory evaluation of skin refrigerants used in dermabrasion. *J Dermatol Surg Oncol* 1985; **11**: 45–9.
8. Schultz BC, Roenigk HH Jr, Debrisan as a postoperative dressing after dermabrasion. *J Dermatol Surg Oncol* 1979; **5**: 971–4.
9. Pinski JB, Dressings for dermabrasion: occlusive dressings and wound healing. *Cutis* 1986; **37**: 471–6.
10. Roenigk HH Jr, Dermabrasion for miscellaneous cutaneous lesions (exclusive of scarring from acne). *J Dermatol Surg Oncol* 1977; **3**: 322–8.

11. Roenigk HH Jr, Scar camouflage using dermabrasion. *Facial Plast Surg* 1984; **1**: 249–57.

12. Roenigk HH Jr, Dermabrasion: state of the art. *J Dermatol Surg Oncol* 1985; **11**: 306–14.

13. Burks JW, *Wire Brush Surgery.* Springfield, IL: Charles C Thomas, 1956.

14. Yarborough JM, Ablation of facial scars by programmed dermabrasion. *J Dermatol Surg Oncol* 1988; **14**: 292–4.

15. Katz BE, Oca AG, A controlled study of the effectiveness of spot dermabrasion ('scarabrasion') on the appearance of surgical scars. *J Am Acad Dermatol* 1991; **24**: 462–6.

53

Soft-tissue augmentation

C William Hanke, Jenette Michalak

INTRODUCTION

In recent years, scars and wrinkles and other soft-tissue defects have been treated successfully with injectable preparations. Collagen from bovine and porcine sources has achieved the most widespread use. Collagen from both sources received Food and Drug Administration (FDA) marketing approval in the United States during the 1980s.

ZYDERM/ZYPLAST

History and development

Following investigations by the Collagen Corporation in the late 1970s, Zyderm I was approved by the FDA in 1981. Zyderm II received FDA approval in 1983, and Zyplast followed in 1985. Samuel J Stegman, a dermatologist, served as the primary consultant to the Collagen Corporation, and became a leader in the development of new techniques and uses for Zyderm/Zyplast.

Zyderm is composed of purified bovine dermal collagen that has been pepsin-digested and suspended in phosphate-buffered saline. The antigenic telopeptide end-regions of the molecule are removed during digestion. The treatment syringe also contains 0.3% lido-caine to minimize discomfort during injection. Zyderm is 95% type I collagen and 1–5% type III collagen.

Zyplast is crosslinked with glutaraldehyde during processing. The concentration of collagen of Zyderm I and Zyplast is 35 mg/ml, and Zyderm II is 65 mg/ml (Figure 53.1). Zyderm I and Zyderm II lose a great deal of volume shortly after injection because of

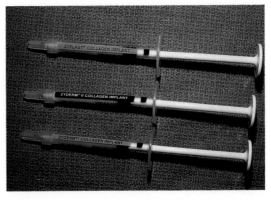

Figure 53.1 The three varieties of injectable bovine collagen are Zyderm I, Zyderm II and Zyplast. (Used with permission, C William Hanke, MD.)

saline absorption by tissue. Zyplast forms a more stable latticework in tissue, and saline absorption is less prominent.

Zyplast is colonized by connective tissue cells, which results in new collagen formation.

Contraindications and skin testing

Some patients are excluded from treatment with Zyderm/Zyplast. Patients with a history of hypersensitivity to lidocaine or other bovine products are excluded. Additionally, patients undergoing or planning to undergo desensitization to meat products should not be treated with Zyderm/Zyplast. People with multiple severe allergies should be treated with extreme caution. Zyderm/Zyplast is not to be used for implantation into breast, muscle, ligament, bone or tendon.

Two intradermal skin tests are recommended for most Zyderm/Zyplast patients.[1,2] There are several ways to perform double skin testing. Our current practice is to place the first skin test intradermally on the volar forearm. The patient returns in 48–72 hours for evaluation of the test. If there is no reaction four weeks later, a second skin test is placed on the opposite forearm. If both skin tests are negative at four weeks, treatment can begin. A positive skin test is characterized by local induration or redness that persists for more than six hours (Figure 51.2).

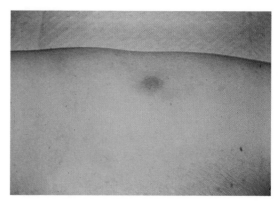

Figure 53.2 Erythema and swelling are indicative of a positive skin test to Zyderm. (Used with permission, C William Hanke, MD.)

placed in the thin eyelid skin (i.e. crow's feet) and is 'over-corrected'.

Cleansing of the skin with soap and water or alcohol pads before treatment should be performed. Most patients are treated in the sitting position, where side lighting can easily be utilized to identify subtle scars and wrinkle lines. Occasionally, ice will be applied to an area for 10 minutes before treatment, but most patients tolerate injections very well.

The physician and assistant should both wear gloves. The assistant should hold a gauze sponge to remove implant material that leaks

Indications and techniques

The most common indications for Zyderm/Zyplast are listed in Table 53.1, together with the products that are preferred by us for treatment. In general, Zyderm is used to treat superficial wrinkles and Zyplast is used to treat deeper wrinkles and furrows. Zyderm is placed in the papillary dermis and Zyplast is placed in the reticular dermis. If Zyplast is placed in the papillary dermis, 'beading' will occur and will last for several months. Beading will also occur if Zyderm is

Table 53.1 Indications for Zyderm (Zd) and Zyplast (Zp)	
Indication	**Recommended product**
Nasolabial furrows	Zp, Zd I or II
Glabellar frown lines	Zd I or II
Perioral lines	Zp, Zd I or II
Secondary cheek wrinkles	Zd I or II
Crow's feet	Zd I
Transverse forehead lines	Zd I or II
Marionette lines	Zp, Zd I or II
Vermilion–cutaneous junction	Zp, Zd I or II
Undulating scars	Zp, Zd I or II

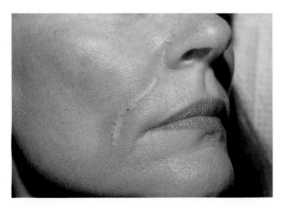

Figure 53.3 A white blanche is observed immediately following injection of Zyderm I. The white blanche indicates proper papillary dermal placement of Zyderm I. (Used with permission, C William Hanke, MD.)

Table 53.2 Duration of correction for Zyderm/Zyplast

Area treated	Duration of correction (months)
Nasolabial furrows	4–6
Glabellar frown lines	6–12
Perioral lines	6
Secondary cheek wrinkles	12–18
Crow's feet	6–12
Transverse forehead lines	6–12
Marionette lines	4–6
Vermilion–cutaneous junction	4–6
Undulating scars	6–18

onto the skin surface during treatment. A 30-gauge needle is ideal when bent at a 30°–45° angle with the bevel down. A serial puncture technique is used with Zyderm I and Zyderm II. An immediate white blanche is observed as the blood in the papillary dermal capillaries is temporarily compressed by the implant (Figure 53.3).

A linear threading technique is used when treating deeper wrinkles and furrows with Zyplast. The needle is inserted parallel to the skin surface at the level of the reticular dermis. In some patients with very deep wrinkles, a technique is used where Zyderm I is layered over Zyplast. Using the linear threading technique, Zyplast is placed in the reticular dermis. Zyderm I is then placed over the layer of Zyplast using the serial puncture technique.

When injecting sebaceous skin, a great deal of Zyderm or Zyplast may leak out onto the surface of the skin during treatment. The physician should attempt to advance the needle tip in the dermis until leakage is no longer observed.

Results

The approximate duration of correction following Zyderm/Zyplast for various soft-tissue defects is given in Table 53.2. The dynamic forces that are present in the perioral and lateral canthal areas reduce the duration of correction with Zyderm/Zyplast. Most patients with perioral rhytids, nasolabial furrows or crows' feet require re-treatment twice yearly to maintain correction (Figure 53.4). There is much less dynamic movement in the glabellar area and on the central cheek area. Consequently, the effects of Zyderm/Zyplast treatment may last as long as 12 months in these areas.

Human studies have shown that Zyderm and Zyplast are still present in the dermis nine months after treatment.[3] Zyplast, unlike Zyderm, is replaced by new host collagen. From a clinical standpoint, however, there is no difference in duration of correction for the two products. Zyderm/Zyplast does not persist following injection into the subcutaneous tissue, and correction is lost in a few weeks.

Adverse reactions

Adverse reactions to Zyderm/Zyplast can be divided into two categories: non-allergic and

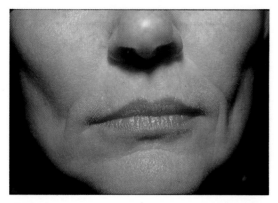

(a)

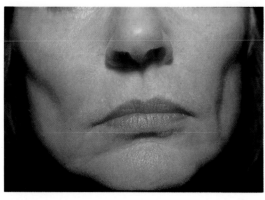

(b)

Figure 53.4 (a) Nasolabial lines are a common feature of aging of the lower one-third of the face. (b) The nasolabial lines have been obliterated following treatment with Zyderm I. (Used with permission, C William Hanke, MD.)

allergic. The non-allergic reactions will be discussed first, and include infection, bruising, local swelling/surface deformities, intermittent swelling and local necrosis.

The likeliness of infection (e.g. bacterial and herpes simplex) can easily be reduced through proper cleaning of the skin just before treatment.

Bruising of the skin is likely to occur in areas with thin skin such as the eyelids.

Bruising is also common in patients who are taking anticoagulant medications, and in patients who bruise easily on the legs.

A typical treatment site will exhibit mild localized swelling and redness for 1–24 hours following treatment. This may be covered with make-up. 'Beading' will occur if crow's feet are over-corrected with Zyderm I or if Zyplast is placed superficially in the dermis in any location. The surface deformity that results can last several weeks or months. 'Beading' is totally preventable with proper technique.

Intermittent swelling is an uncommon phenomenon that occurs in Zyderm/Zyplast-treated patients following beef or caffeine ingestion, menstruation, sun exposure, heat or exercise. It is our practice to perform repeat skin testing on these patients to be sure that allergic hypersensitivity has not developed.

Local necrosis is an uncommon occurrence that begins with blanching of the treatment site during injection, and may progress to superficial sloughing in subsequent days.[4] A wound may develop, and permanent scarring is possible. The physician may treat with systemic and topical antibiotics to cover the possibility of infection.

Allergic treatment site reactions occur in less than 1% of patients. These patients are then excluded from additional treatment with Zyderm/Zyplast. The typical patient with an allergic treatment site reaction develops red bumps or streaks at the treatment site following the first or second treatment (Figure 53.5). Allergic treatment sites have been treated with topical steroids, intralesional steroids, systemic steroids and systemic antibiotics with questionable efficacy. The best approach is observation at regular intervals until the reaction subsides.

Rarely, abscess/cystic allergic hypersensitivity reactions may occur. Nodules and draining abscesses develop, and they may cause pain. In order to relieve the pain, incision and drainage is necessary.

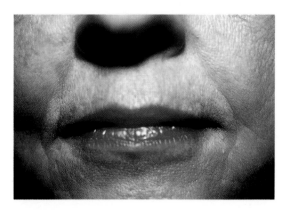

Figure 53.5 An allergic treatment site reaction is present in the nasolabial area several weeks following treatment with Zyderm I. (Used with permission, C William Hanke, MD.)

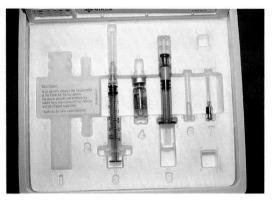

Figure 53.6 The Fibrel treatment kit contains ε-aminocaproic acid, absorbable gelatin powder and normal saline. (Used with permission, C William Hanke, MD.)

FIBREL

History and development

Fibrel was the second collagen-based injectable material to be approved by the FDA for the correction of soft-tissue defects. Fibrel evolved from the work of Spangler,[5] who mixed fibrin foam (Gelfoam) with human plasma and thrombin for injection into scars. Spangler's 1975 report[5] revealed excellent results in 89% of undulating scars. Gottleib[6] later modified Spangler's technique to the GAP repair technique, which involved gelatin foam (G), ε-aminocaproic acid (A) and human plasma (P). The gelatin foam served as a scaffold for the trapping of clotting factors and ultimately new collagen formation. ε-Aminocaproic acid inhibited fibrinolysis and allowed a solid clot to form. The clot later 'organized', and new collagen was laid down. The patient's plasma supplied supplemental fibrinogen. When the GAP mixture (Fibrel) is injected into a scar, the wounding process is duplicated and new collagen is synthesized. Fibrel was approved by the FDA for scars in 1988, and for age-related lines in 1990.

The Fibrel kit consists of 100 mg absorbable gelatin powder, 125 mg lyophilized ε-aminocaproic acid and a volume of normal saline (Figure 53.6). The gelatin powder is composed of porcine collagen (types II and III) that has been denatured.

Patients who are allergic to gelatin foam, ε-aminocaproic acid or benzyl alcohol are not candidates for Fibrel treatment. Fibrel is contraindicated in the following conditions: history of keloids, history of anaphylactoid reactions, previous hypersensitivity to Fibrel, or history of autoimmune disease. Implantation into breast, bone, tendon, ligament or muscle is also contraindicated.

A Fibrel skin test is required before treatment can be started. The dermis on the forearm is injected with 0.05 cm³ Fibrel (gelatin powder plus normal saline). A positive skin test is characterized by redness, swelling or inflammation that lasts more than five hours. The patient is seen for a final reading on the skin test at four weeks, unless a suspected positive test reaction occurs earlier. If the skin test is equivocal at four weeks, a second test is done on the opposite forearm. A positive test excludes the patient from Fibrel treatment. A negative test is not a guarantee that an aller-gic treatment-site reaction cannot develop during treatment. In the initial one-year clinical trial using Fibrel, 1.9% of patients had a positive skin test response and were excluded from the treatment.

Patients who are allergic to Zyderm/Zyplast may be skin-tested with Fibrel, and may be treated if indicated.

Indications and technique

When evaluating a scar for Fibrel treatment, a reliable clinical test is to stretch or pinch the scar with the thumb and index finger. If the scar disappears or improves on manual stretching, it will usually be improved by Fibrel (Figure 53.7).

Age-related lines such as nasolabial furrows and glabellar frown lines can be improved by Fibrel. However, superficial lines are difficult to treat because of the difficulty in placing Fibrel superficially in the dermis with a 27-gauge needle.

In our experience, Fibrel is very painful when injected without a local anesthetic. The face is cleansed with soap and water to remove make-up and dirt. The scars to be treated are then outlined with 1% gentian violet. Each scar is anesthetized with 1% lidocaine with 1:200 000 epinephrine (adrenaline) using a 30-gauge needle. After waiting 15 minutes, the scar is injected with Fibrel using a 27-gauge needle. An 'overcorrection' at 100–200% is desirable. If scars are atrophic or bound down, it is helpful to cut the vertical fibrotic bands with the 20-gauge custom undermining needle that is supplied in the Fibrel kit. The undermining needle 'releases' the scar and creates a pocket for the Fibrel implant.

Fibrel should be placed in the mid-to-deep dermis. Placement in the superficial dermis can result in prolonged surface irregularities. We generally use a serial puncture technique when treating scars. The number of needle entry points on the skin should be minimized

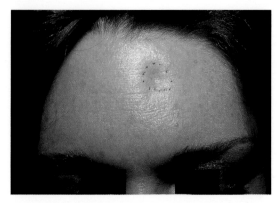

(a)

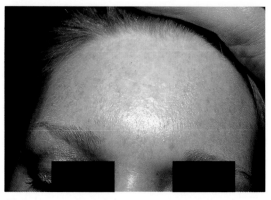

(b)

Figure 53.7 (a) A 37-year-old woman has an atrophic scar on the forehead. (b) The scar has been obliterated following one treatment with Fibrel. (Used with permission, C William Hanke, MD.)

so that Fibrel does not leak back out onto the skin surface through them. A linear threading technique is preferred for treating wrinkle lines. This technique limits the number of needle sticks, and postoperative bruising is minimized.

In our experience, 1 cm³ of Fibrel contains enough implant material to treat 10–20 scars in one sitting. Similarly, 1 cm³ of Fibrel is enough to treat nasolabial furrows in a single sitting.

A scar will usually require 1–4 treatments with Fibrel at 2–4 week intervals. Nasolabial furrows may also require treatments at 2–4 week intervals.

Results

Clinical trials with Fibrel began at 22 centers in 1984. A total of 840 scars in 300 patients were treated either once or twice with Fibrel following a negative skin test.[7] The results were evaluated using patient evaluation, physician evaluation and photogrammetric analysis.

Photogrammetric analysis involves computer measurement of scar volume as determined from scar molds. The results using the three techniques were similar; however, photogrammetric analysis demonstrated slightly higher improvement scores. In general, more than one-half of the scars showed more than 65% improvement at one-year follow-up.[7]

One-hundred and eleven patients with 302 scars were followed for two years, and showed 64.7% improvement.[8]

Eighty-seven patients were followed for five years. More than 50% of the scars maintained significant correction for five years.[9] The scars only lost an average of 35% of their original correction in five years.

Adverse reactions

Many patients treated with Fibrel will develop mild swelling at the treatment site lasting for 1–3 days (Figure 53.8). Minor adverse effects of this type occurred in 8% of the patients in the clinical trials. Occasionally, nodular swelling may occur, and can last 1–2 weeks before resolving. This occurs more commonly when the custom undermining needle has been used aggressively to release fibrotic scars and to create a 'pocket' for Fibrel. These patients, because of the increased needle trauma, will often show bruising for 5–7 days. Patients who are predisposed to bruising for other reasons (e.g. anticoagulant drugs) will also show bruising following Fibrel treatment.

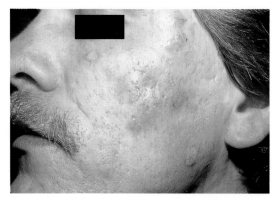

Figure 53.8 Considerable local swelling is observed following treatment of acne scars with Fibrel. The swelling usually resolves over several days. (Used with permission, C William Hanke, MD.)

As with Zyderm/Zyplast, local necrosis of the skin has occasionally been observed with Fibrel. Millikan et al,[8] reporting on the two-year clinical trial with Fibrel, described no allergic treatment site reactions. Similarly, Spangler reported no allergic treatment site reactions in 17 years, and Gottlieb observed none in 11 years. The gelatin powder has been shown to be a weak antigen, but antibodies to Fibrel developed at low levels in some patients.[10] The antibody levels, however, were lower or unchanged at five years post-treatment. These patients developed no allergic treatment site reactions or other serologic abnormalities, so the significance of the antibody level is unknown. In the five-year clinical trial, several patients were treated five or six times for unrelated scars.[9] The multiple exposures to Fibrel did not result in serologic abnormalities or increased antibody titers.

AUTOLOGOUS COLLAGEN

History and development

Autologous collagen involves the transplant of tissues from one part of the body to another.

The tissues most commonly used for the procedure are dermis and fat. In the 1980s the success of liposuction increased the interest in fat transplantation. Physicians utilized the fatty tissue through microlipoinjection to alter other areas of the patient's body. Fournier[11] researched and experimented with other procedures for fat transplantation. He harvested the intercellular fibrous septae from the discarded product of liposuction. He injected autologous collagen into soft-tissue defects and reported results comparable to those using Zyderm/Zyplast.

Autologous collagen can also be harvested from other sources, such as the excised dermis that is discarded during rhytidectomy. The dermis is minced and is suspended in saline for injection.

Contraindications and skin testing

The most important advantage of autologous fat collagen is there is no risk of allergic reaction or tissue rejection. This is beneficial for those who may have an allergic reaction to the foreign sources such as calf or pig collagen that are used in Zyderm and Fibrel. With autologous fat collagen, there is no need for skin testing. The second important advantage of autologous fat collagen is the theoretical unlimited supply at relatively low cost to the patient.

Indications and techniques

Autologous fat collagen has been most successful for treatment of large depressions in the nasolabial area and the chin, where it is necessary to use several cubic centimeters of filler. It is also useful for lip augmentation when injected at the vermillion and also intradermally in the body of the lips.

The primary disadvantage of using autologous fat collagen is that the material is so viscous that it generally requires a larger needle for injection than does Zyderm/Zyplast. The needle must be of at least 22 gauge.

Adverse reactions

The injection of autologous collagen results in much more bruising than with Zyderm collagen. This is due to the larger needle needed for the injection of autologous collagen. Injection with the 22-gauge needle also results in visible holes that may last for days or weeks at the treatment sites. The larger needle also requires local anesthesia to be used, which visibly alters the tissue, making correction more difficult. The larger-gauge needle also makes superficial dermal placement nearly impossible.

The risks carried with Zyderm/Zyplast should be considered when injecting autologous collagen. The physician must maintain caution when injecting all subcutaneous areas because of the risk of injecting into an artery.

AUTOLOGEN

Autologen is another process of autologous collagen preparation.[12] The procedure for obtaining collagen utilizes skin removed during abdominoplasty, breast reduction, excision, face lift or hair transplantation. Collagenesis Technologies, Inc (Boston, MA) processes the tissue specimen. The tissue must be frozen before it is sent to Collagenesis Technologies. The tissue is condensed to a powder, and the collagen is suspended in normal saline. The material is placed in a syringe and mailed back to the physician. Since the material is processed for use in the same patient, skin testing is not necessary. No allergic reactions have been reported. Corrections may last as long as 18 months.

ARTECOLL

History and development

Artecoll consists of fine poly(methyl methacrylate) (PMMA) microspheres suspended in a 3.5% collagen solution. It is injectable, and offers long-lasting correction of wrinkles and other dermal defects.[13]

Poly(methyl methacrylate) is commonly used for dentures, Plexiglas (Perspex), and bone cement in orthopedics. It was first synthesized by O Rohm, a German chemist, in 1928. Today, PMMA microspheres are synthesized by suspension–polymerization. The procedure involves the submerging of the microspheres in a heated 3.5% bovine spongiform encephalopathy (BSE)-free collagen solution. When the solution is cooled, it maintains a gel state.[13]

Artecoll is 75% collagen solution. At least one-half of the Artecoll collagen is replaced by fibroblasts and collagen fibers produced by the body. If the desired correction is not observed after the first treatment, Artecoll can be implanted again 1–3 months later.

Contraindications and skin testing

A skin test should be done on the left elbow of the patient 4–8 weeks before Artecoll is implanted. The patient may experience an allergic reaction from the bovine collagen, but the PMMA is chemically inert. Contraindications include allergic reaction to collagen, atrophic skin diseases, thin and flaccid skin, and susceptibility to keloids.[13] Artecoll should not be used to correct defects in the subcutaneous fat, since it will remain indefinitely as rubberlike nodules.

Indications and techniques

Artecoll has worked most successfully for the treatment of naturally occurring folds and wrinkles on the face, especially when the patient is between 40 and 50 years old.[13] Other successful treatments include the augmentation of the lips and philtrum. The lips are augmented relatively easily because of the 'natural pocket' between the skin and the muscle. Augmenting the lower orbital rim area improves the appearance of shadowed eyelids. Acne scars, deep glabellar frown lines, and horizontal chin folds may also be treated with Artecoll implants.[13]

Results

Clinical studies performed between 1989 and 1995 involved 118 patients with 200 folds implanted intradermally with Artecoll. The results of an anonymous questionnaire indicated that 89.5% of the patients were pleased with the result of the treatment.[13] Of the 118 patients, 62% received a single Artecoll treatment, 24% received two, and 14% received three or more.[13] Sixty-four percent of the patients reported obvious and lasting improvements in folds and wrinkles that had been treated with Artecoll. Moderate improvement was indicated by 25.5% of the patients.[13]

Adverse reactions

Common side-effects of the Artecoll implant are moderate discomfort, swelling, and redness of the treated areas, which usually subside after 2–3 days. Itching of the treated area usually subsides within a few weeks, but sometimes lasts for a few months. If the patient received lip augmentation treatment, common side-effects may be dry lips and possible discomfort when biting.

HYLAN GEL

Hylan Gel is an insoluble derivative of hyaluronic acid. Clinical trials began in 1991, and much interest in the product has transpired since then. A skin test is not necessary before treatment, because of the lack of hypersensitivity response. Therefore Hylan Gel has an advantage over Zyderm/Zyplast. In a clinical trial, when the subjects' age-related wrinkles were treated with Hylan Gel, only 60% of the wrinkles remained corrected at 18 months.[12] This short duration of correction will need to be lengthened for the product to be successful.

GORE-TEX

Gore-tex is a polytetrafluoroethylene filler substance for the correction of soft-tissue defects.[12] It is a thin suture-like thread that can be implanted under local anesthesia.

The material is threaded through a guiding needle and advanced into the deep dermis or subcutaneous tissue. The Gore-tex is then cut to the necessary length and the needle is removed. The physical effect of the procedure is seen instantaneously, and is also permanent. Fibrel, Zyderm or Zyplast may be layered over Gore-tex. The main indications for Gore-tex are deep nasolabial furrows and narrow lips.

Gore-tex does not promote allergic reactions. Occasionally, the Gore-tex thread will need to be removed from the patient.

INJECTABLE SILICONE

A number of medical specialties have utilized high-grade injectable silicone fluid for tissue augmentation. The experience of a number of physicians has extended beyond 20 years. Reports in the literature have indicated minimal adverse effects.[14] In 1991, the FDA announced that injectable silicone is an unapproved medical device and its use is illegal. Considering the FDA's position on injectable silicone, it would be improper to discuss it further in this chapter. The American Academy of Dermatology has instructed its members to follow the FDA guidelines.

REFERENCES

1. Elson ML, The role of skin testing in the use of collagen injectable materials. *Dermatol Surg Oncol* 1989; **15**: 301–3.
2. Klein AW, In favor of double skin testing. *J Dermatol Surg Oncol* 1989; **15**: 263.
3. Stegman SJ, Chu S, Bensch K et al, A light and electron microscope evaluation of Zyderm collagen and Zyplast implants in aging human facial skin. *Arch Dermatol* 1987; **123**: 1644–9.
4. Hanke CW, Higley HR, Jolivette DM et al, Abscess formation and local necrosis after treatment with Zyderm or Zyplast collagen implant. *J Am Acad Dermatol* 1991; **25**: 319–26.
5. Spangler AS, Treatment of depressed scars with fibrin foam – seventeen years of experience. *J Dermatol Surg Oncol* 1975; **1**: 65.
6. Gottleib S, GAP repair technique. Poster exhibit, American Academy of Dermatology Annual Meeting, Dallas, TX, December 1977.
7. Millikan LE, Rosen T, Monheit G et al, Treatment of depressed cutaneous scars with gelatin matrix implant: a multicenter study. *J Am Acad Dermatol* 1987; **16**: 1155–62.
8. Millikan LE, Alexander M, Baker W et al, Long-term safety and efficacy with Fibrel in the treatment of cutaneous scars – results of a multicenter study. *J Dermatol Surg Oncol* 1989; **15**: 837–42.
9. Millikan LE, Banks K, Parkail B et al, A 5-year safety and efficacy evaluation with Fibrel in the correction of cutaneous scars following one or two treatments. *J Dermatol Surg Oncol* 1991; **17**: 223–9.
10. Ring J, Messmer K, Incidence and severity of anaphylactoid reactions to colloid volume substitutes. *Lancet* 1977; **i**: 466–8.
11. Fournier P, Facial recontouring with fat grafting. *Dermatol Clin* 1990; **8**: 523–37.
12. Hanke CW, Coleman WP, Dermal filler substances. In: *Cosmetic Surgery of the Skin*, 2nd edn (Coleman WP, Hanke CW, Alt TH, Asken S, eds). St Louis, MO: Mosby Year-Book, 1997:217–30
13. Lemperle G, van Heimberg, Dippe B et al, PMMA microspheres (Artecoll) for skin and soft-tissue augmentation. Part II: Clinical investigations. *Plast Reconstr Surg* 1995; **96**: 627–34.
14. Clark DP, Hanke CW, Swanson NA, Dermal implants: safety of products injected for soft-tissue augmentation. *J Am Acad Dermatol* 1989; **21**: 992–8.

54

Gore-tex and facial rejuvenation

Claude Lassus

The author has been using Gore-tex for facial rejuvenation since 1986.[1-4]

GORE-TEX AND NASOLABIAL FOLDS

Ten years after the first use of this material to improve the deep nasolabial folds,[1,5] I should like to report my experiences.

All the anatomic assessments that have been made from the beginning of this century until now[6-8] have shown a close adhesion of the skin to the muscle all along the fold. With ageing, the cheek skin stretches and becomes ptotic, together with the underlying cheek fat pad, while there is no appreciable change in the muscle plane. The descent of skin and fat is stopped by the barrier due to the adhesion of the skin to the muscle plane all along the fold, accumulating over the fold and making it deeper and more acute in older subjects (Figure 54.1). This has been recently confirmed by Gosain, Amarante, Hyde and Yousif[8] from a dynamic analysis using magnetic resonance images.

Thus the surgical correction of nasolabial folds requires repositioning of the ptotic cheek fat pad as well as resection of the excess skin.[9-12] This can be achieved via a facelift

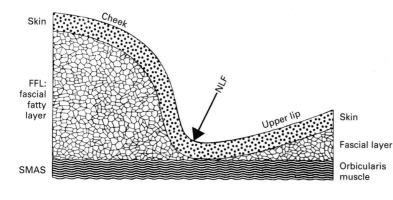

Figure 54.1 Diagrammatic representation of the deep nasolabial fold (NLF). SMAS, superficial aponevrotic muscular system.

(Hamra and Owsley) in older patients. But in younger patients (about 40 years old) who do not want to have a facelift, one must use another procedure that achieves long-lasting results.

That is why the use of Gore-tex in this indication seems to me, after 10 years, to be still valuable.

Moreover, with Gore-tex sheets of 4 mm thickness now available, the improvement of the deeper folds is more marked than it was with the 2 mm thickness sheets, although the technique remains the same.

Technique

Two incision lines are marked: one 4 mm long, in the alar crease, and one vertically at the inferior part of the nasolabial fold, 3 mm long. A tunnel is also marked along the fold, 3 or 4 mm medial to it. Lateral to the fold, the area to be suctioned is drawn; it must not communicate with the tunnel where the implant will lie (Figure 54.2).

Then, under local anaesthesia if the procedure is performed alone, or under general anaesthesia if a face lift is associated, the incisions are made with a No. II blade. Afterwards, with a special freer that enters through the inferior incision and emerges through the superior aperture, a tunnel is made just beneath the deep dermis and forward of the nasolabial fold (Figure 54.3).

The excess fat lateral to the fold is removed with a syringe or a machine, according to the surgeon, and with a 3 mm cannula (Figure 54.4).[13] A Gore-tex implant is shaped in a 4-mm-thick sheet. This implant is cut in a triangular shape (Figure 54.5). On moulding with the fingers, it becomes rounder. The inferior extremity of the implant is crushed with forceps (Figure 54.6).

A special needle is introduced through the inferior aperture and emerges through the superior one. The flat extremity of the implant enters the hole of the needle and is curved on itself (Figure 54.7). The needle is

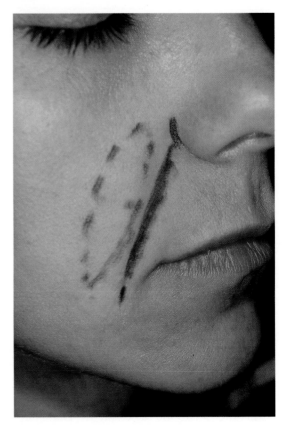

Figure 54.2 Preoperative markings.

then withdrawn, leaving the implant in the tunnel (Figure 54.8).

The extremities of the implant are cut and buried deeply beneath the skin. This is very important – it prevents the inflammatory reaction that can be seen when Gore-tex is too close to the surface.

A stitch closes each of the apertures (Figure 54.9); it is removed the next day. A compressive dressing is applied for 24 hours to minimize postoperative swelling and to maintain the implant in a good position (Figure 54.9). Thus the postoperative follow-up is generally very simple. It is very rare to see oedema or

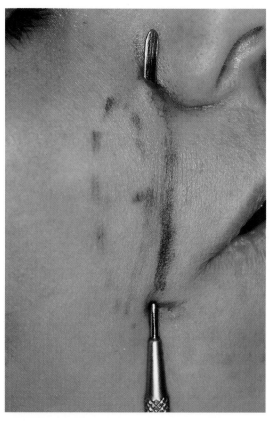

Figure 54.3 The tunnel is made forward of the nasolabial fold.

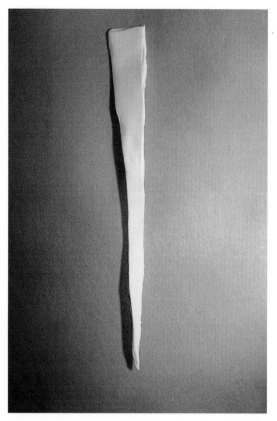

Figure 54.5 A triangular piece is cut from a Gore-tex sheet (2 or 4 mm thick).

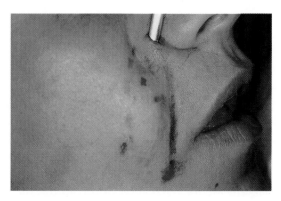

Figure 54.4 Liposuction of the excess fat above the fold using a 3 mm cannula.

ecchymosis, for example. However, of course, they may occur.

Improvement is seen very rapidly, but the patient must be warned that with this technique it is impossible to remove the deep nasolabial fold completely. Improvement is about 60%, and even more in certain circumstances. These results are long-lasting (Figures 54.10–54.12).

This procedure can be performed alone or during a face lift, which allows the removal of part of the excess stretched skin.

The treatment of nasolabial folds is only

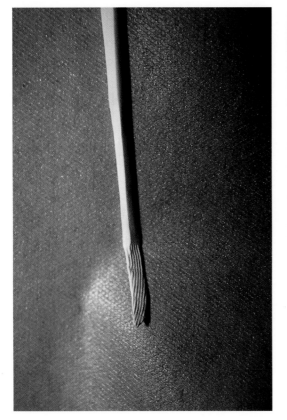

Figure 54.6 The lower extremity of the Gore-tex implant is crushed flat with forceps.

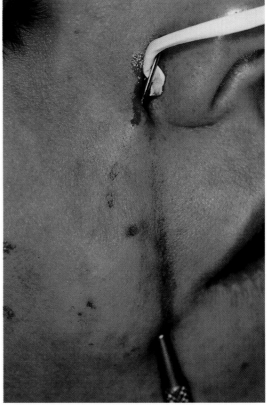

Figure 54.7 The flat extremity of the Gore-tex implant is passed into the hole of the pass and curved on itself.

slightly improved by superficial facial rhytidectomy,[10] and the problem is made worse by the manipulations on the SMAS.[14] Therefore other approaches to the treatment of deep nasolabial folds have to be considered, and the use of Gore-tex implants according to the technique described here achieves satisfactory and long-lasting results.

RESTORATION OF LIP ROLL WITH GORE-TEX

Prominent lips have been very much in demand for a few years now, because a youthful mouth is a full one. To enhance thin lips, fillers can be used,[11,15–17] as well as rearrangements of the local tissues.[18–23]

At present there is another demand: some patients ask for re-creation of the lip roll that could be palpated in their youth. Collagen injections achieve this, but unfortunately they

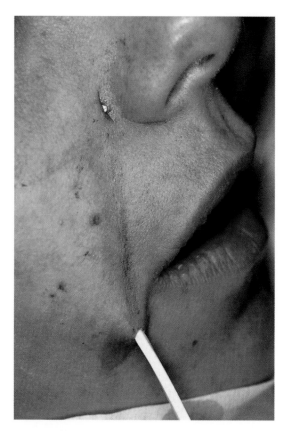

Figure 54.8 The implant is put into the tunnel.

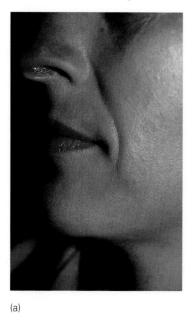

(a)

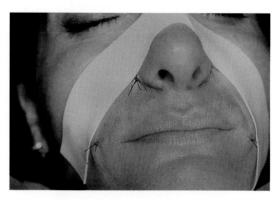

Figure 54.9 The apertures are closed with stitches, and a dressing is applied for 1 or 2 days.

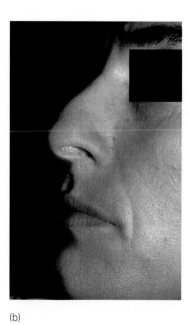

(b)

Figure 54.10 Improvement of deep nasolabial fold: (a) before; (b) after 5 years.

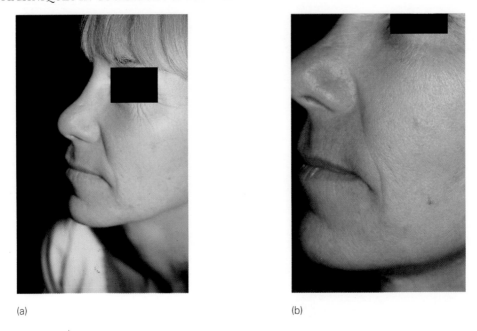

(a)   (b)

Figure 54.11 Improvement of deep nasolabial fold: (a) before; (b) after 8 years.

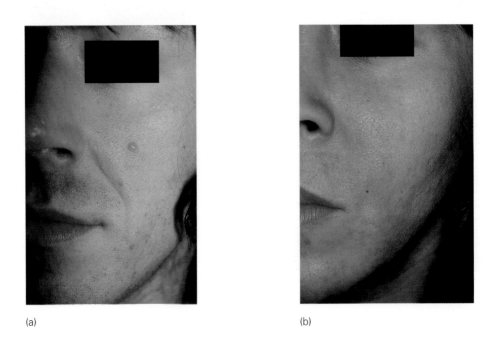

(a)   (b)

Figure 54.12 Improvement of deep nasolabial fold: (a) before; (b) after 9 years.

have to be repeated for the effect to be lasting.

For two years, I have been using Gore-tex to enhance the vermilion border of the lips:

- because there is a natural pocket between the skin and the orbicularis muscle all along the white roll where a Gore-tex implant can easily be placed;
- because the overlying skin here is thick, providing the necessary protection for the Gore-tex.

Technique

The tunnels into which the implants will be put are marked preoperatively (Figure 54.13). Then, under local or general anaesthesia according to the wish of the patient, two incisions are made at each extremity of the lip, at the junction of skin and mucosa. Then, with the same freer as is used for deep nasolabial folds, a pocket is easily created between the skin of the Cupid's bow and the underlying orbicularis muscle at the upper lip (Figure 54.14).

The same is done at the lower lip.

A sling of Gore-tex is cut into a 2-mm-thick sheet. It is then moulded with the fingers to make it rounder. One extremity is crushed with forceps (Figure 54.15). The Gore-tex

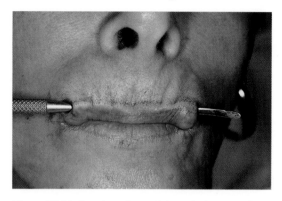

Figure 54.14 Creation of tunnel through the upper lip.

pass is introduced through one aperture, and then emerges through the other (Figure 54.16).

The flat implant extremity is introduced into the hole of the pass; then it is curved on itself (Figure 54.17), and the needle is withdrawn, pulling the implant through the pocket (Figure 54.18).

The extremities are cut, and buried well beneath the skin surface, and a stitch closes each of the openings.

The postoperative follow-up is very simple: some swelling may be seen for four or five

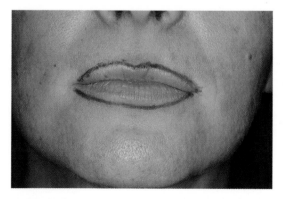

Figure 54.13 Drawing of tunnels into which implants will be placed.

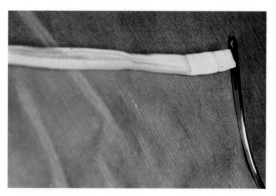

Figure 54.15 An extremity of the Gore-tex implant is crushed flat with forceps so that it can enter the hole of the pass.

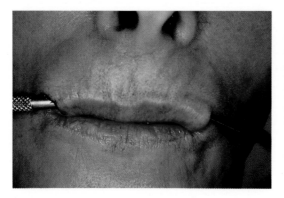

Figure 54.16 The Gore-tex pass in place.

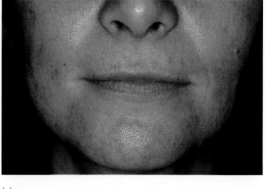

(a)

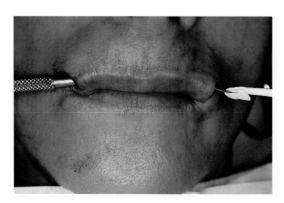

Figure 54.17 The flat extremity of the implant is introduced into the hole of the pass and curved on itself.

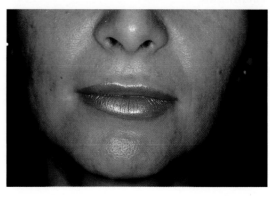

(b)

Figure 54.19 Restoration of lip roll: (a) before; (b) after.

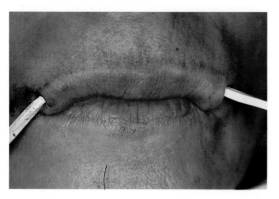

Figure 54.18 The implant in position.

days, and that is all. The stitches are removed two days postoperatively.

The results of this technique are shown in Figures 54.19–54.21.

Complications

So far, only one complication has been seen: on the left side of an upper lip, in the immediate postoperative course, the implant moved upwards for an unknown reason. A month and half later the implant was easily removed through the same openings. A new pocket was created at the right place, and a

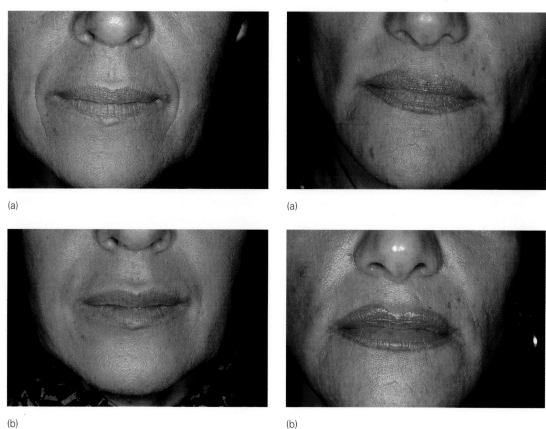

(a)

(b)

Figure 54.20 Restoration of lip roll: (a) before; (b) after.

(a)

(b)

Figure 54.21 Restoration of lip roll: (a) before; (b) after.

new implant was inserted, finally achieving a satisfactory result.

This shows the advantage of using Gore-tex: in the rare case of any problem, the implant can easily be removed without any damage, and this is the main reason why I use this material. No other complications have occurred.

REFERENCES

1. Lassus C, Utilisation d'un matériau de renforcement dans le traitement des ridules et des rides du visage. Présenté au 14 ème Congrés National de Médecine Esthétique et de Chirurgie Dermatologique, Paris 25–27 Septembre 1987.

2. Lassus C, Utilisation d'un tissu de renforcement pour le traitement des rides faciales. *J Soc Chir Esth* 1989; **14**(54): 29.

3. Lassus C, Expended PTFE in the treatment of facial wrinkles. *Aesth Plast Surg* 1991; **15**: 167.

4. Lassus C, Treatment of the deep nasolabial folds with Gore-tex implants. Presented at the 61st Annual Scientific Meeting of the American Society of Plastic and Reconstructive Surgeons, Washington, DC, September 20–24, 1992.

5. Horibe EK, Horibe K, Yamaguchi CT, Pronounced nasolabial fold: a surgical correction. *Aesth Plast Surg* 1989; **13**: 99.

6. Millard DR Jr, Yuan RTW, Devine JW Jr, A chal-

lenge to the undefeated nasolabial folds. *Plast Reconstr Surg* 1987; **80:** 37.

7. Yousif NJ, Gosain A, Matloub HS et al, The nasolabial fold: an anatomic and histologic reappraisal. *Plast Reconstr Surg* 1994; **93:** 60.

8. Gosain AK, Amarante MTJ, Hyde JS, Yousif NJ, A dynamic analysis of changes in the nasolabial fold using magnetic resonance imaging: implications for facial rejuvenation and facial animation surgery. *Plast Reconstr Surg* 1996; **98:** 622–36.

9. Pensler JM, Lewis SR, Parry SW, Restoration of the upper lip and nasolabial area by the means of an intraoral approach. *Plast Reconstr Surg* 1986; **78:** 449.

10. Riefkohl R, The nasolabial fold lift. *Ann Plast Surg* 1985; **15:** 1.

11. Jost G, Levet Y, Parotid fascia and face lifting: a critical evaluation of the SMAS concept. *Plast Reconstr Surg* 1984; **74:** 42.

12. Barton FE Jr, The aging face: rhytidectomy and adjunctive procedures. In: *Selected Readings in Plastic Surgery*. Dallas: University of Texas Southwestern Medical Center, 1989.

13. McKinney P, Cook JQ, Liposuction and the treatment of nasolabial folds. *Aesth Plast Surg* 1989; **13:** 167.

14. Guyuron B, Michelow B, The nasolabial fold: a challenge, a solution. *Plast Reconstr Surg* 1994; **93:** 552.

15. Meyer R, Kesserling UK, Aesthetic surgery in the perioral region. *Aesth Plast Surg* 1976; **1:** 61.

16. Knapp TR, Kaplan EN, Daniels JR, Injectable collagen for soft-tissue augmentation. *Plast Reconstr Surg* 1977; **60:** 398.

17. Kesserling U, Rejuvenation of the lips. *Ann Plast Surg* 1986; **16:** 167–74.

18. Austin H, Weston G, Rejuvenation of the aging mouth. *Clinics Plast Surg* 1992; **19:** 2.

19. Delerm A, Elbaz JS, Cheiloplastie des lèvres minces. Proposition d'une technique. *Ann Chir Plast* 1975; **20:** 243.

20. Lassus C, Thickening the thin lips. *Plast Reconstr Surg* 1981; **68:** 959.

21. Lassus C, Surgical vermilion augmentation: different possibilities. *Aesth Plast Surg* 1992; **16:** 123–7.

22. Robinson DW, Ketchum LD, Masters FW, Double V-Y procedure for whistling deformity in repaired cleft lip. *Plast Reconstr Surg* 1970; **46:** 241.

23. Wilkinson T, Lip enhancement. *Technical Forum* 1990; **13:** 4.

55

Hair loss: Surgical treatments

Henry H Roenigk Jr

INTRODUCTION

The loss of hair by men and women, although generally not a serious health problem, can create psychological and self-esteem problems. The desire for a youthful and athletic image (especially in men) is not necessarily associated with a bald scalp. The media and advertising of all items is youth- and beauty-oriented, and the maintaining of a youthful appearance may be important in obtaining and keeping a job, spouse or girlfriend in today's society.

The most frequent indication for surgical repair of hair loss is male pattern alopecia (androgenetic alopecia). Androgenetic alopecia is also common in women even at an early age; however, they can frequently cover it up because they maintain a partial hairline and can style their hair to hide the thinning more easily than can men, who have shorter hair styles and more frontal balding. Other diseases of the scalp that result in permanent hair loss can also be corrected by surgical procedures.

Hair loss: options for treatment

Loss of hair – whether as a result of androgenetic alopecia, illness, burns, accidents, operations, radiation or other causes – can often detract from one's appearance. But in recent years, more and more people affected by hair loss have been able to improve their appearance through cosmetic surgery and other options.

Among the possible solutions to the problem of hair loss are hairpieces, drug treatment (minoxidil) and hair replacement.

The advantage of toupees, wigs and other hairpieces is that they can provide a full head of hair immediately. The disadvantages are that the hair is false, it will fall off, and it usually must be removed at night.

Most tonics and vitamins are worthless in treating baldness. A topical medication called minoxidil (Rogaine), however, has been found to be effective for some types of hair loss, and may be a reasonable option. Minoxidil is somewhat costly, and must be used continuously to maintain results. Furthermore, it does not work for everyone. Minoxidil 2% (Rogaine) is currently an over-the-counter product. Other new topical agents and oral agents such as fenestride (Phoscar®) 1mg are soon to be approved for other medical options.

Surgical options available, include the following:[1]

- hair transplantation
- micro- and mini-hair transplants
- strip grafting
- scalp reduction
- tissue expanders and flaps
- combination procedures
- rotational flap techniques.

HAIR TRANSPLANTATION TECHNIQUE

Patient preparation for punch-graft hair transplantation is minimal.[23] The patient is instructed to maintain maximum hair length at the donor and recipient sites. An antiseptic shampoo (Hibiclens or pHisoHex) is used daily for three days before surgery, and any underlying scalp disorder is treated appropriately. A light meal two hours before surgery is recommended to avoid syncope associated with fasting.

Premedication is often used to relax the patient. Diazepam (Valium), given in small dosages intravenously or sublingually, provides safe, rapid, light sedation, with the benefits of easy arousability and postsurgical amnesia.

The donor site is prepared by trimming the hair to a length of 1–2 mm. The donor and recipient sites are then scrubbed with antiseptic soap. The occipital donor site should be a narrow (less than 2.5 cm) transverse band, to allow good postsurgical camouflage by the longer surrounding hair. The patient is maintained in the prone or supine position during administration of local anesthesia (1% lidocaine with 1:100 000 epinephrine (adrenaline)) or tumescent anesthesia and cutting of donor grafts and recipient holes. Normal saline is injected into the donor area, and a power punch is routinely used to produce better donor transplants.[7]

Caution should be maintained in orienting the punch angle of the donor grafts to correspond with the angle of the hair emerging from the skin. Following punchcutting to the subcutaneous level, the donor transplants are removed at the lowest depth with curved iris

scissors and stored in a sterile, saline-filled petri dish. Next, any fat is trimmed from the donor transplants, and they are grouped according to density while the recipient sites are cut. Any arteriolar or brisk venous bleeding should be sutured before pressure is applied to the donor graft holes.

The recipient area hairline should be carefully planned to maintain a gentle widow's peak (Figure 55.1). Frontal rows are often

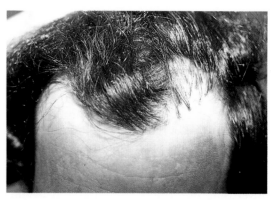

(a)

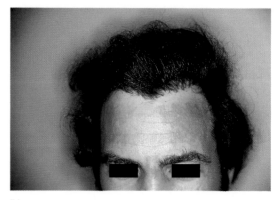

(b)

Figure 55.1 (a) Male pattern baldness with bilateral temporal loss. The planned hair transplants will allow a natural appearance with aging. (b) One year after multiple 4.0 mm hair transplants into the frontal hair line.

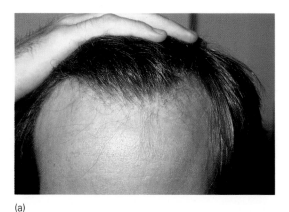

(a)

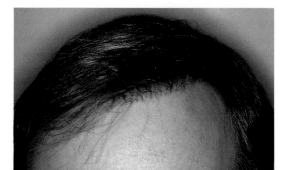

(b)

Figure 55.2 (a) Early thinning of the frontal hairline. (b) Mini-transplants used alone for the frontal hairline.

plants will fit like keys in locks because they were cut at a forward angle corresponding to surrounding frontal area hair growth, and because the donor transplants are 0.5 mm larger than the recipient sites. Any misplacement of these grafts will change the direction of growth and result in an abnormal frontal appearance. All transplants are carefully placed to full depth, giving a smooth skin surface.

After surgery, the transplanted hairs usually enter a resting phase, and are shed. This leaves the grafts bare for as long as three or four months. Often, several subsequent sessions are required to fill in these areas; these should be performed no more frequently than every three weeks. Usually no more than 50–75 regular transplants are done at one session, although 300–3000 mini-transplants can be done at one session. The end result takes many months to look natural (Figures 55.3–55.7).

MINI-TRANSPLANTS

The standard size grafts can frequently leave a 'row of corn' appearance, especially in the frontal hair line. Mini-grafts and micro-grafts can help correct that problem. Mini-grafting is a relatively new procedure, which is often

spaced 2–3 mm apart, but subsequent rows are 4–5 mm apart. Donor grafts are generally 4 mm or less in diameter and recipient sites are 3.5 mm or less. Mini-transplants (1.0–1.5 mm donor transplants with two or three hairs per transplant) are preferred for the frontal hairline (Figure 55.2) or to fill in between larger donor transplants. The tissue is cut at a corresponding angle to the donor grafts, pointing in the direction of natural hair growth.

The placement of grafts is a crucial step for success in orienting hair growth. The trans-

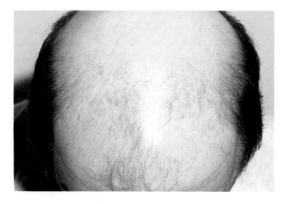

Figure 55.3 Extensive male pattern baldness.

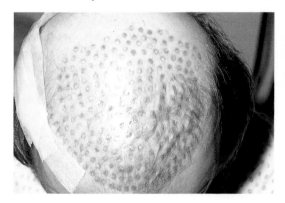

Figure 55.4 Early hair transplants, with some having lost hair after transplantation and others showing early growth at 3–4 months.

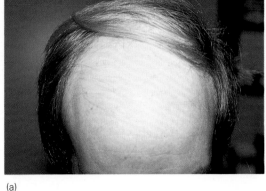

(a)

performed after hair transplantation to soften the hairline and fill in between the larger grafts. Mini-grafts can be used alone to provide a soft natural hairline (Figure 55.2). The procedure is similar to hair transplantation, except that the hair grafts are much smaller. Mini-grafts help to blend grafted hair with normal hair, and eliminate the 'cornstalk' appearance that can sometimes result from transplantation.

(b)

Figure 55.6 (a) Male pattern baldness. (b) The same patient after one year and several hundred hair transplants.

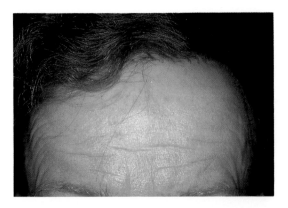

Figure 55.5 Full growth of hair after over 500 hair transplants.

The harvesting technique is similar to standard hair transplants although I prefer a rectangular strip of donor hair to be harvested and then 1 mm slits cut off the strip. A slit is made in the recipient frontal area, and the 1.0–1.5 mm slit is teased into place after stretching the slit with a dilator and jeweler's forceps. Another technique is to take individual hairs off a graft and then put them in recipient holes created with an 18-gauge needle and stretched with special expanders. Another technique is to use the CO_2 laser to create the recipient holes.

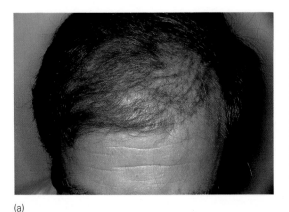

(a)

(b)

Figure 55.7 (a) Diffuse frontal thinning soon after hair transplants to frontal area. (b) Six months later, with thick transplant giving an excellent cosmetic result.

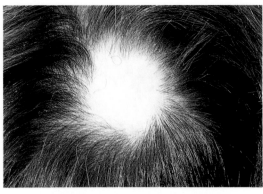

(a)

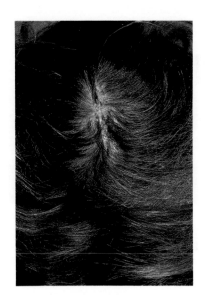

(b)

Figure 55.8 (a) Vertex baldness, with other areas having good hair growth. (b) After one scalp reduction.

Some surgeons have treated entire frontal scalps by micro- or mini-transplants with excellent results. My preference is to combine these with the standard size hair transplant.

SCALP REDUCTION TECHNIQUE

The preoperative preparation is the same as the hair transplantation.[4–7]

The technique, when used alone, is most applicable to patients who have vertex balding with an intact frontal hairline (Figure 55.8). Flexibility of the scalp (a compressible motion of 2 cm is optimal) is the most important determinant of appropriate patients.

An ellipse, the length of the bald area and between 2.0 and 4.0 cm wide, is drawn. It should not extend further anteriorly than the proposed transplanted frontal hairline.

The length of the excision will vary, but is often 12–15 cm. Several different patterns are

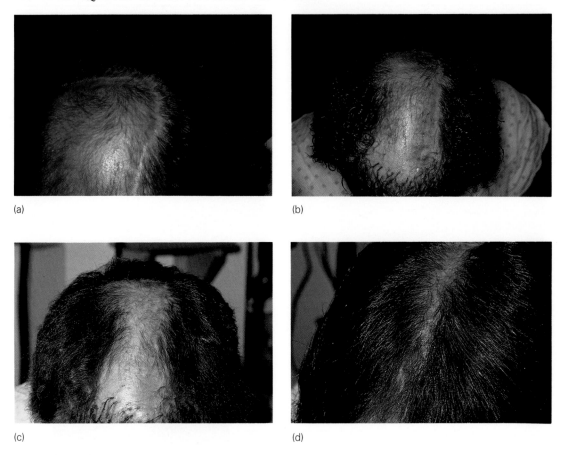

(a)

(b)

(c)

(d)

Figure 55.9 (a) Extensive baldness after first paramedian scalp reduction. (b) Further scalp reduction. (c) Yet further scalp reduction. (d) Complete elimination of bald scalp by scalp reduction.

used, including the midline sagittal excision (which is the most common), or the J-shaped or S-shaped paramedian incision (Figure 55.9). The crown area can be incised with an M-plasty, butterfly-shaped reduction, or other modification such as a T-shaped or C-shaped excision.

The scalp is cleansed, and local anesthesia with either 1% or 0.5% lidocaine with epinephrine (adrenaline) 1:100 000 is injected circumferentially along the edges of the planned excision lines and then extended to

the maximal distal area of undermining in the hair-bearing skin. The lower concentration of anesthesia (tumescent technique without sodium bicarbonate) is preferable, because higher quantities of anesthesia (up to 100 cm^3) are needed for scalp reductions than for hair transplantation.

One side of the ellipse is incised through the galea. Hemostasis is obtained with electrocautery. It is helpful to have one or two assistants and to have suction available. The edges of the scalp are everted, which allows the surgeon to desiccate those few large vessels quickly and easily. The bleeders are at the level of the galea and the deep dermal plexus.

After hemostasis has been achieved, extensive undermining in the galeal–periosteal plant is accomplished with minimal bleeding by spreading blunt-edged extra long Metzenbaum scissors or the index and third fingers. Undermining can also be done with the Iconoclast, which is used for undermining in face lifts.

When the undermining is completed, the surgeon and assistant push or pull the scalp toward the midline so that the sides of the incised scalp overlap. Using this maneuver – which can be accomplished with the fingers, skin hooks, forceps or towel clips – it is easy to estimate the amount of bald skin that can be excised. If this amount seems inadequate, further undermining can be performed. If more or less skin than initially was planned can be excised, adjustment is made in the location of the second incision before proceeding with incision of the other side of the ellipse. Various devices have been used to get more reduction and less stretch back. These include interoperative tissue expanders and Fetchet expanders.

Lateral undermining usually extends anteroposteriorly, and should stop at the insertions of the frontalis and occipitalis muscle to avoid bleeding. When the wound width is 4 cm or larger, easier closure is facilitated by galeotomy. This involves incisions upward through the galea running parallel to lengthwise at 3 mm intervals, which thereby relax the galea aponeurotica. The wound is then brought together with towel clips. If there is a problem in getting the wound edges together, one should go back and do more undermining. The clips are removed one by one as suturing is done.

Layered closure is carried out with galea and subcutaneous tissue closure with 1-0 or 2-0 Vicryl, 2-0 surgical gut or Dexon. The skin is closed with staples.

There is usually no need for a dressing, although a bulky dressing similar to that used in hair transplants can be used. Prophylactic systemic steroids and antibiotics are frequently used to prevent edema and infection. There is frequently severe postoperative pain, and adequate narcotic analgesics are necessary. The staples are removed in three weeks. The patient should massage the skin to keep it loose in preparation for the next scalp reduction, 6–10 weeks after the original one.

STRIP GRAFTING

The development of strip grafts by Vallis in 1969 was an attempt to avoid the problem with hairlines and to give a more even full hairline.[8] Hair-bearing donor strips are taken from the occipital or occipitoparietal area of the scalp. They may be excised horizontally or vertically, depending on the hair direction required along the hairline. The strips may be placed bilaterally for the entire hairline or unilaterally for just the part side.[9]

Hairline strip grafts may be backed by placing either strips or plug grafts posteriorly. Apposing the second strip graft immediately behind the frontal graft usually leaves an obvious linear defect between the two strips. For this reason, it is usually more acceptable to place transplants behind the hairline strip graft.

Special instruments have been developed for this procedure. Vallis developed a parallel double blade holder that enables one to cut accurate incisions 5–6 mm apart. The strip itself should not exceed 6 mm in width. Vallis also developed a running W knife to give the irregularity necessary for a natural-appearing hairline. The final length may vary, but 8 cm is usually the maximum.

There has been a high incidence of unsatisfactory technical problems with this technique, and thus a high failure rate of these larger strip grafts. The procedure is not used much today among dermatologists performing hair replacement surgery.

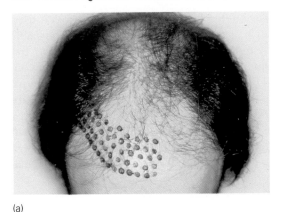

(a)

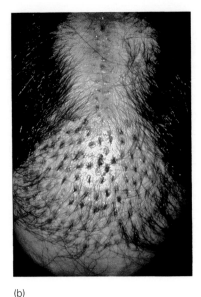

(b)

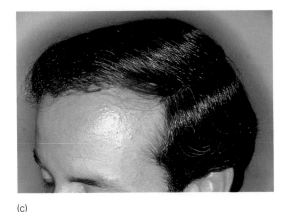

(c)

Figure 55.10 (a) Male pattern alopecia that will be connected by a combination of hair transplant to the frontal hairline and then scalp reduction behind the transplant. (b) Hair transplants and scalp reduction completed. (c) End result one year later.

COMBINATION PUNCH AUTOGRAFT AND SCALP REDUCTION

Patients with male pattern alopecia of Type IV or greater often have such extensive balding that conventional punch autografting alone is not sufficient. The donor area will not yield enough grafts to cover the bald area in an acceptable density. The use of a combination of scalp reduction and hair transplants can correct that problem (Figure 55.10).[10] Scalp reductions behind the hair transplant area are performed in serial sessions at 8–12-week intervals. The final punch autograft sessions for filling in come either after all bald tissue is reduced or when scalp laxity is too small for further reduction. Hair transplantation can be used to cover up the scar of scalp reduction.

ROTATIONAL FLAPS OF SCALP

The hair-bearing temporoparietal flap pioneered by José Juri has become an important adjunct to the previously described procedures. The desired result is to immediately establish more natural-appearing hair in the frontal region than is possible with the punch autograft method.

The most esthetic result for extensive baldness may be obtained by the Juri temporoparieto-occipito-parietal flap. This procedure allows a complete frontal hairline with hair orientation forward.

The flap is designed with a single temporal pedicle running continuously around the parietal and occipital areas to the opposite parietal side. The flap, usually 35 cm long, is transposed back upon itself to the homolateral frontal area.

Two weeks later, the flap is severed at the opposite frontal side and sutured in place as the natural-appearing frontal hairline. The vascularization is provided by the frontal scalp.

The methods of rotating bilateral temporoparietal pedicle flaps have been described as practical office procedures. The technique of de-epithelializing the anterior portion of the new hairline flap, so that hair follicles are buried and will camouflage the scar, allows for a more natural hairline. This allows upward growth of the grafted hairline, which is virtually natural in appearance.

The more extensive Juri procedure should be performed under general anesthesia by surgeons experienced in this procedure. Tip necrosis of a flap can result in a disastrous cosmetic result.

COMPLICATIONS

The complications of hair transplantation are well known, and are mostly a result of poor technique and judgement in planning a proper hairline. Good transplants are obtained with sharp power punches and use of saline to harden the donor tissue. Proper placement of transplants and attention to detail are important.

Complications from scalp reduction can be preoperative, in the improper selection of patient, or operative, due to bleeding and problems with closure of the wound.

More anesthesia and deeper undermining all the way to the level of the ear may be needed. Bilateral galeotomies will help. Occasionally, a relaxing incision either parallel to the wound or just above the ears will be necessary. If the wound will still not close then it should be allowed to scar by secondary healing and the scar should be revised later with another mini scalp reduction.

Other operative problems include poor choice of excision patterns that create closure problems or cosmetic scars that are too noticeable. The use of scar camouflage by the flap angle and de-epithelialization, which will allow hair to grow through the scar, will give a better cosmetic result.

Postoperative problems include edema of the entire scalp, which can be partially controlled with systemic steroids. There is usually much more pain and tension in the scalp area than are experienced with hair transplants, and strong narcotic analgesics are necessary. Systemic antibiotics are used routinely to prevent wound infection. Systemic steroids will help reduce tissue edema. Hematomas occur most frequently in the occipital area below the tip of the wound. Unless they are large, aspiration or evacuation is not carried out, and they should resolve spontaneously. There can be necrosis of the wound edges, especially if there is too much tension on the wound, and hypertrophic, keloid or stretched scars. One of the problems that creates the most anxiety on the part of the patient and surgeon is the postoperative hair loss a few weeks after surgery. This is due to the trauma of scalp reduction; the hair will regrow in several months. One should not rush into a second scalp reduction until adequate time has elapsed to allow determination of whether regrowth will occur along the lines of excision.

REFERENCES

1. Roenigk RK, Roenigk HH Jr (eds), *Dermatologic Surgery: Principles and Practice.* New York: Marcel Dekker, 1989:Chaps 55–9.
2. Orentreich N, Hair transplantation. *NY State J Med* 1978; **72:** 578.
3. Unger WP, *Hair Transplantation.* New York: Marcel Dekker, 1988.

4. Alt TH, Scalp reduction as an adjunct to hair transplantation. *J Dermatol Surg Oncol* 1980; **6:** 1011.

5. McCray MK, Roenigk HH Jr, Cosmetic correction of alopecia. *Am Fam Pract* 1983; **28:** 207.

6. Schultz BC, Roenigk HH Jr, Scalp reduction for alopecia. *J Dermatol Surg Oncol* 1979; **5:** 808.

7. Tromovitch T, Stegman S, Scalp reduction for alopecia. In: *Cosmetic Dermatologic Surgery* (Tromovitch T, Stegman S, eds). Chicago: Year Book, 1983:25–9.

8. Vallis CP, Surgical treatment of the receding hairline. *Plast Reconstr Surg* 1969; **44:** 271.

9. Vallis CP, The strip graft. *Facial Plast Surg* 1985; **2:** 245–52.

10. Roenigk HH Jr, Combined surgical treatment of male pattern alopecia. *Cutis* 1985; **35:** 570–7.

56

Electrical stimulation of skin (ESS) in skin aging and scars: 13 years' experience with electrorhytidopuncture[†]

Liliane Schnitzler, Philippe Simonin

INTRODUCTION

Of all the ways of fighting skin aging, electric stimulation of skin (ESS) appears to be a therapy of choice. As long ago as the last century, galvanotherapy was proposed not only for the skin but also for bones, and Lefort advocated gold-needle electrolysis on fracture sites in 1870.

The principle of this method (electrorhytidopuncture, ERP – Top Derm) lies in two techniques: either

- a transepidermal introduction of electrodes in the dermis and hypodermis on a route parallel to the epidermis, or
- an electric stimulation of the skin surface,

in both cases with the development of efficient, appropriate and non-traumatizing currents.

Since 1983, we have been applying this treatment to slack skin on the face and neck, to age-related, average (and even deep) wrinkles, and to scars, whatever their aetiology. In addition, new hopes have arisen regarding the treatment of hair loss.

† Note that 'Electroridopuncture', 'Electroridolyse' and 'Top Derm' are official trademarks,[1,2] and there are patents on both the process[3] and the device (the multineedle holder with seven electrodes, and simple electrodes, sledge, roller, triangle).[4]

SIMONIN'S APPARATUS

The functioning of this apparatus[†] is relatively simple. There are two functions: ERP and Top Derm.

ERP

This delivers a soft, rectangular, galvanic current of 0.3 mA intensity correlated with a 0–12 V potential. The stainless-steel needles are of 0.2 mm diameter, with 50 µm points. Other characteristics include the following:

ERP Mono
- Frequency: 330 Hz
- Length of treatment: 8 s
- Fixed impulse: 1.4 ms
- Fixed period: 3 ms

The current supply is connected to a single needle introduced in a single holder and used for selective improvement of wrinkles and scars. The practitioner uses the positive terminal. The impulse can be repeated several times at different insertion sites, in a scar or following each wrinkle (e.g. crow's feet, nose wrinkles, upper and lower eyelid areas, lips, forehead, and throat).

ERP Multi

- Frequency: 253 Hz
- Length of treatment: 8 min
- Fixed impulse: 1 ms
- Fixed period: 2.95 ms

Two multineedle holders, each connected to seven electrodes, are used with alternate polarity on areas of slack skin (lower face and neck).

Top Derm

- Peak-to-peak voltage: 200–1200 V
  Roller: 200–500 V peak to peak
  Sledge: 400–800 V peak to peak
  Triangle: 600–1200 V peak to peak
- Period t: 1 µs
- Width of one impulse: 0.5 µs
- Frequency: 1 MHz

A block diagram is shown in Figure 56.1.

The different electrodes are all applied *on* the skin – *not under*.

- the roll is preferably used to treat the wrinkles of the neck;
- the slide is used for the lines of the forehead, eyes and upper lips;
- the triangle is applied back and forth on the entire surface of the face and the neck.

A comparative study of ERP and Top Derm

The resistance on the skin is much greater than that under the skin:

- 500 kΩ on the skin
- 5 kΩ under the skin.

It must be noted that the resistance on the skin varies depending of the person, the area treated, the type of skin, and the size and form of the electrode, necessitating adjustment of the voltage in each case.

An explanation of the three principles used on ERP and Top Derm is given in Figure 56.2.

We must create a limited trauma to make the dermis react and compel the fibroblasts to produce elastin and collagen.

With ERP, the penetration of the needle in the skin limits the current to a low voltage and a very weak intensity of the order of 1mA.

With Top Derm, the application on the skin of a gold or gold-plated electrode (non-corrodible material) requires a high-voltage current with a much weaker intensity than the ERP, of the order of 1µA instead of 1mA.

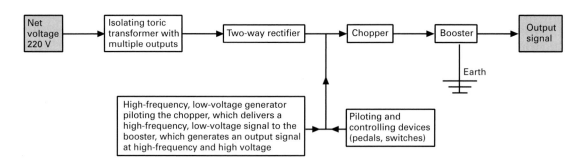

Figure 56.1 Block diagram of Top Derm.

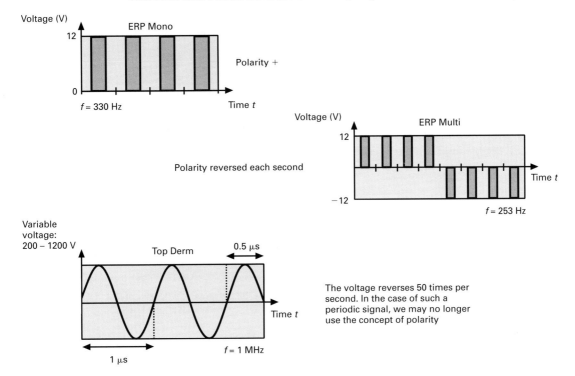

Figure 56.2 The three principles used in ERP and Top Derm.

SELECTION OF PATIENTS

Skin aging

The treatment is most strongly indicated for *loss of elasticity* and *decrease of collagen* generated by photoaging.

For practical reasons, developments have been limited to the face, neck and low neck, but there is no reason to avoid using the treatment on other zones of the skin, such as the upper sides of the hands, which easily reveal the age of the patient.

The loss of elasticity responsible for ptosis and wrinkles occurs unevenly – sometimes at a relatively young age, sometimes after 50. This irregularity is due to numerous factors: genetic, hormonal and environmental (mainly sun and tobacco, but also malnutri-tion, worry and stress). Patient age varies from 25 to over 80. Most patients are women, but not exclusively: the typical patient is an active post-menopausal woman on a hormone-sub-stitution treatment who wishes to delay the visible effects of age.

Scars

All scars can be electrically stimulated:

- recent or old, depressed or indurated scars;
- post-traumatic or excisional scars;
- fibrous scars resulting from acne, varicella zoster viral infections or burns;
- soft distensible scars with smooth margins, or 'icepick' lesions with sharp borders, as in acne or Winer's pores.

THERAPEUTIC PROCEDURE

Skin aging

Each session includes the treatment of the entire face and neck, and sometimes the décolleté (ERP Mono, ERP Multi, Top Derm). The initial treatment comprises 10 sessions of 30 minutes over 2–4 months, beneficial effects being perceptible after the sixth session.

Scars

These are treated in 4–6 sessions of roughly 15 minutes:

- ERP Mono for the deep scars;
- Top Derm for the fibrous scars.

RESULTS

Aging

Modes of appreciation
Subjective (by patients)
Some patients notice unhoped-for results, and talk of 'surprising' or 'fabulous' effects, or a 'wonder solution'. For most, however, effects are more soberly evaluated as favourable – mainly on tone but also on certain wrinkle zones, periorbital, perioral or frontal. Other patients find no amelioration. All agree on the *absence of any medium- or long-term side-effects.*

Objective (medical)
Before and about one month after a series of 10 sessions, a strictly comparative iconography is carried out on each patient, and negative imprints are taken with synthetic resin on a duly marked zone (Figures 56.3 and 56.4). The imprints are read either with the naked eye or with a binocular magnifying glass. This comparison – to which is added the subjective opinion of the practitioner – allows the most objective conclusions to be drawn. Of course, one must be aware of the limits of evaluation on these sole clinical criteria.

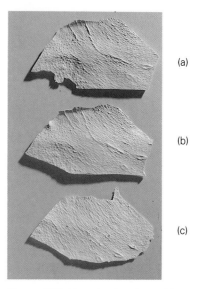

Figure 56.3 Negative imprints of lower lip: (a) before; (b) after 7 sessions; (c) after 11 sessions.

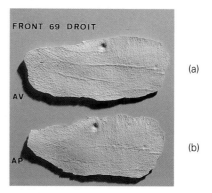

Figure 56.4 Negative imprints of forehead: (a) before; (b) after 10 sessions.

Global results
We have made a single-centre study of about 700 cases: they confirm Simonin's results on over 2500 studied by him in Geneva, Paris, Baden-Baden and Munich.

Two-thirds of patients show a positive response to electrical stimulation after 10 sessions, and even more after regular long-term treatment:

- 40% very good results
- 22% good results
- 13% average results.

On the whole, the face appears younger (Figure 56.5).

- The effect on tone, evaluated by traction and palpation, is often clear: the oval of the face is outlined again, the neck is firmer, and the hollow of the cheeks is filled in.

- The effect on wrinkles is visible at rest: deep wrinkles are attenuated, medium wrinkles are sometimes reduced, and small wrinkles have disappeared; mimic expression wrinkles persist, but are attenuated.

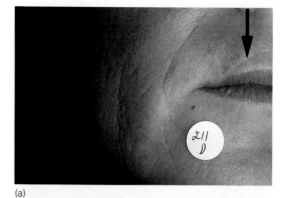

(a)

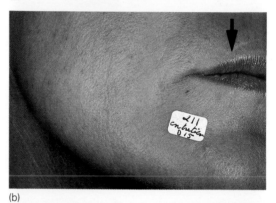

(b)

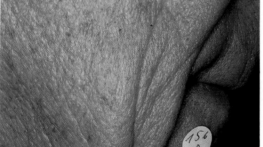

(a)

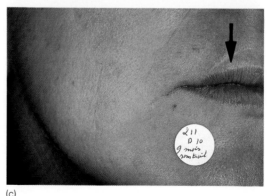

(c)

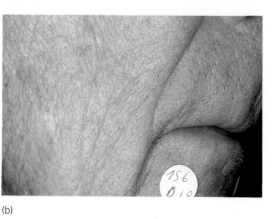

(b)

Figure 56.5 A 72-year-old man who did not want a face lift. Very good results on tonicity were obtained after 10 sessions: (a) before; (b) after.

Figure 56.6 A 42-year-old female patient: (a) before treatment; (b) after 15 sessions; (c) persistent improvement after nine months without ESS. Note that the untreated scar on the upper lip remains unchanged.

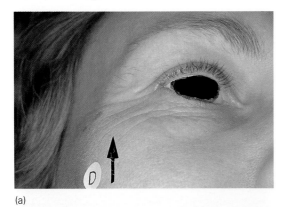

(a)

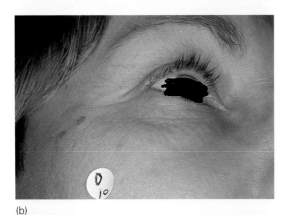

(b)

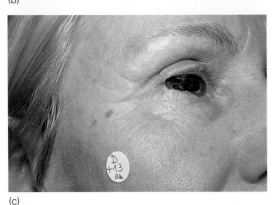

(c)

Figure 56.7 Long-term beneficial effects on a 45-year-old patient: (a) before treatment; (b) after 2 months (10 sessions); (c) 13 years later (8 sessions per annum, 1983–1996).

A certain unevenness of results is also noticeable, some areas on the same face being greatly improved and others less so. Disparity also appears with time: while positive effects are sometimes noticed as soon as the sixth or seventh session, they can be delayed, becoming visible only a few months after the tenth session, when treatment has been discontinued. In some cases one must increase the number of sessions to about 15 to obtain a visible and palpable amelioration. Finally, 20% of patients remain unresponsive and present no visible amelioration.

To conclude, we should stress the *long-term persistence of the results,* with amelioration

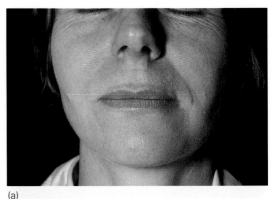

(a)

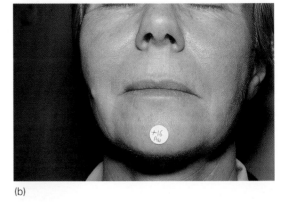

(b)

Figure 56.8 ESS between 1983 and 1996 (15 sessions first, followed by 8 sessions per annum): (a) a 42-year-old female in 1980; (b) the same patient – now 58 years old – in 1996 (no other treatment was given).

continuing for several weeks or months after discontinuation of treatment, as shown by the imprints and photographs (Figure 56.6).

However, although ESS induces new collagen and elastin formation, it does not, of course, stop the degradation process. Therefore, when satisfactory results have been obtained, *a monthly maintenance session is advised*. We presently have a follow-up of several years – 13 years even for certain patients. Studies of these show stabilization in aging or even a rejuvenation over several years, without the need for other forms of treatment (Figures 56.7 and 56.8).

Scars

More than 60% are improved in just five or six sessions. The best results are observed with old fibrous and depressed scars, which become more supple, with the depression filling in (sometimes completely). Such results have been achieved even when no other complementary therapy was used (Figures 56.9–56.12). When obtained, the beneficial effect seems permanent (Figure 56.13). We have not obtained any results for cheloids.

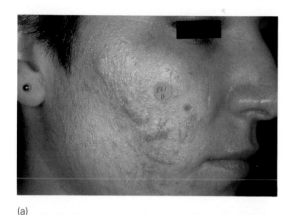

(a)

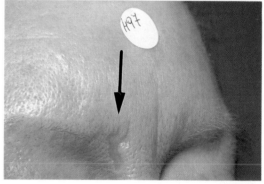

(a)

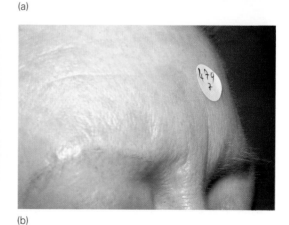

(b)

(b)

Figure 56.9 Three-year-old persistent acne scars, with good results obtained after 6 sessions: (a) before; (b) after.

Figure 56.10 Depressed and atrophic scar following necrotizing zona, with complete improvement after 7 sessions: (a) before; (b) after.

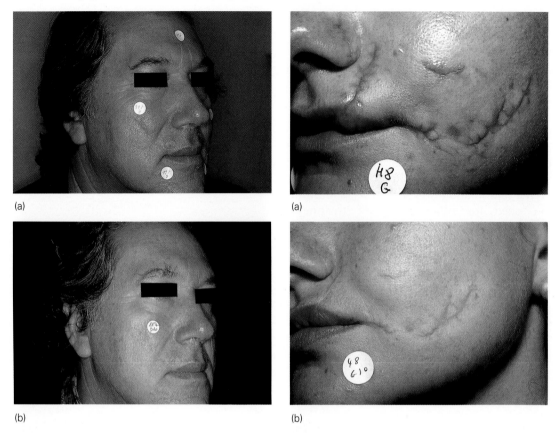

(a)

(b)

(a)

(b)

Figure 56.11 ESS on the face and on an old fibrous cheek scar: (a) before; (b) after. The amelioration seems evident on both scar and facial appearance (wrinkles on crow's feet, nasolabial fold and glabella frown lines).

Figure 56.12 Recent windscreen scars: (a) before; (b) after 10 sessions.

Side-effects

In the short term, the following may be observed.

- With ERP, there can be low-intensity pain on implantation of needles, receding in a few seconds; this is greatly reduced by the prior application of a lidocaine- and prilocaine-based cream (EMLA). Exceptionally, some temporary papulous lesions can arise at the needle implantation sites due to allergy to the metal of the needle, necessitating interruption of the treatment.

- With Top Derm, there is a sensation of great heat to the point of a burning sensation felt by the patient; this lasts about one hour, but *no sign of burn* is visible on the skin. After two days, the epidermis seems to be slightly dehydrated and to have gone through a light micropeeling, although this is invisible.

However, in the *medium and long term, no side-effects whatsoever* are noticed – which is quite remarkable: there is neither sclerosis nor any trace of pigmentation or scarring at the needle insertion site, or after sweeping of the Top Derm electrode over the epidermis, independently of the patient's complexion and even during sunny times of the year.

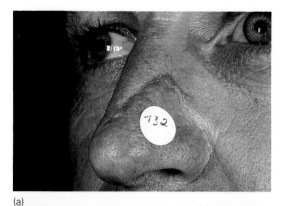

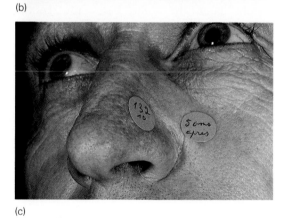

(a)

(b)

(c)

Figure 56.13 A recent postsurgical scar: (a) before; (b) after 4 sessions; (c) after 5 years.

DISCUSSION

The mode of action of electrical stimulation of skin is probably a complex and multifactorial one, and requires fundamental studies.

Clinical applications conducted by ourselves[5,6]

After unilateral treatment

In 1984 and 1985 five patients (two doctors, one journalist and two elderly patients) accepted electrical stimulation on one half of the face in order to compare the results with the untreated side. In all cases the difference was significant, visible, and apparent on photographs; on the treated side wrinkles were clearly diminished and tone was improved, in less than three months (Figures 56.14 and 56.15).

In 1987 ten other cases were the subjects of a detailed comparative study on crow's feet:

- *left*: introduction of a needle without electrical stimulation;
- *right*: electrical stimulation by low frequency alone.

In most cases, after 10 sessions, and particularly three months after discontinuation of treatment, a significant difference in the comparative imprints was observed by binocular magnifying lens, the residual amelioration on the right-hand side contrasting with the unchanged, or even worsened, aspect of the left-hand side.

R   L

Figure 56.14 A 78-year-old female patient: right-hand side treated (12 sessions); left-hand side untreated.

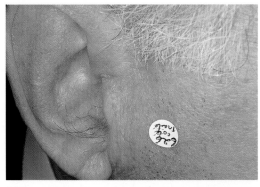

(a)

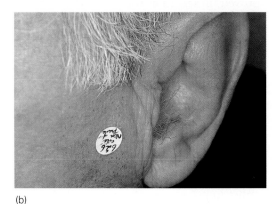

(b)

Figure 56.15 A 65-year-old physician: treatment was applied in the pretragal area on the right-hand side only (a); the left-hand side was untreated (b).

After treatment of the whole face

In 1986, in four cases treated in Geneva, *quantitative histochemical studies* were performed by the INSERM Conjunctive Tissue Biochemical Laboratory (L Robert, Paris), including a study of the three-dimensional skin microrelief and of semifine and ultrastructural sections, the results of which have been reported by Simon.[7]

These studies all led us to suspect the involvement of numerous factors causing reorganization of the dermo–epidermal structures similar to the tissue healing process. They showed, correlatively, the following:

- the development of an additional dermo–epidermal zone giving the impression of an abnormally thickened basal membrane, equivalent to the precollagenic network observed at the second month of embryonic development;
- intensification of specific collagen stainings, reduced fragmentation of the bundles, which were more structured and compact, and a probable increase in type III collagen;
- reorganization of elastic tissue, with reappearance of the oxytalan fibres and a reconnection of the elaunin fibres;
- reorganization of fibronectin into a diffuse dermal network;
- reconstruction of cutaneous microrelief, with dense and multidirectional folds and particularly a reduction of the development surface – these two results characterizing a skin with a younger texture.

In 1987, *cutaneous elasticity* was measured (with a twistometer) in 10 cases at neck level before treatment, after 10 sessions and three months later. In some cases the results demonstrated an indisputable durable residual amelioration.

In 1994, a *profilometric analysis* (using an image analyser) was reconducted on skin replicas recorded during 1985–1986 from 33 patients – many of whom had actually been out of touch for a long time (Laquieze–Thérapharm Research). The results confirmed what could already be seen with the naked eye, namely an objective improvement in more than 70% of the cases after 10 sessions.

The *habitual retained parameters* are

- RA: ruggedness
- RZ: average amplitude of the micro-ruggedness
- Number of wrinkles per field (treated surface unit)
- PF: average depth.

Within the 33 treated and analysed sites,

the study reveals an *average significant diminution of the following parameters:*

- ruggedness: -18%
- amplitude: -7%
- depth: -19.3%

In terms of *the number of improved cases*, the following results were obtained for the parameters examined:

- ruggedness: 82%
- amplitude: 64%
- depth: 61%

We observed an average global improvement of more than 15% of the skin relief in 70% of the cases, regarding the best results as a 50% improvement of the ruggedness and depth of the wrinkles and a 25% improvement of the micro-relief.

After treatment of scars

Our personal results are beneficial even for sclerous old scars that had resisted other therapy. It appears that ESS induces fibroblasts to increase normal new collagen production and modifies glycosaminoglycans in the intercellular substance.

ESS: other publications about experimentation or fundamental research on human and animal cicatrization

The benefits obtained by electrical stimulation were reported in the last century, but it is only recently that this therapeutic technique has been used again on bone, on the nervous system, and even more recently on skin and subcutaneous fat. The relationship between the biological effects of pulsed electrical fields and the growth of mammalian tissue is presently a subject of great interest.[8–10]

We should mention here some North American studies, notably those by Alvarez et al[11] on the effects of superficial electrical stimulation on skin wounds, those of Smith, Brown et al[12,13] in rabbits and mice, and those of Davis et al[14] on the effects of a polarity change during pulsed electrical current in experimental pathology. Bourguignon and Bourguignon[15] investigated the effects of electrical stimulation by high-voltage pulsed galvanic currents on human fibroblast cell cultures, demonstrating, reproducibly, that, between 50 and 75 V at 1 MHz frequency, *ESS increases protein synthesis of fibroblasts as well as nucleoplasmic activity*. In their conclusions, they noted this technique's advantage for accelerating cutaneous healing. It does seem that ESS triggers multiplication of dermal fibroblasts and an increase in their activity, *with production of both collagen and elastic fibres*, which would explain the beneficial effects of ERP observed with Simonin's method.

The work of Wood et al[16] should be noted. They evaluated the efficiency of a pulsed low-intensity direct current (300–600 µA, 12 V, 0.8 Hz) used in a double-blind placebo multicentre study in the treatment of chronic stage II and stage III decubitus ulcers. In the treated group, 58% of ulcers healed in 8 weeks, whereas in the placebo group only 3% healed and most increased in size, showing that low-intensity direct current had a significant influence on the healing rates for these ulcers.

Animal studies (guinea-pigs, $n = 10$) have demonstrated that mean specific activities for membrane-associated thioredoxine reductase revealed a 62% increase in thioredoxine activity over control subjects, indicating that enzyme activation is most likely caused by a calcium flux in the epidermis due to direct current; ESS provoked an increase in the expression of the TGF-β receptors, which improved the cicatrization. These authors (Wood et al) believe that the growth of fibroblasts and keratinous may be enhanced by pulsed low-intensity direct current owing to changes in calcium homeostasis.

ESS in the medical treatment of aging

In our opinion, this procedure is one of the best medical treatments for aging of the face,

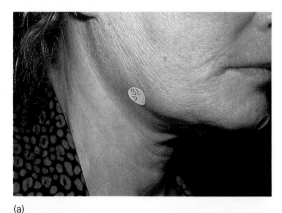
(a)

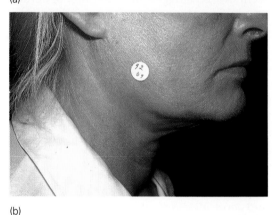
(b)

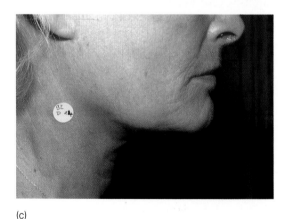
(c)

Figure 56.16 (a) A 63-year-old patient 2 years after a face lift. Good results are obtained after 9 sessions (b), and even better ones after 14 sessions (c).

either in isolation or associated with other therapies, but in particular in two circumstances:

After a face lift

If redundant tissue has been well excised, the quality of the skin is only slightly improved: action on collagen and elastic tissue remains desirable after surgery (Figure 56.16).

In association with other medical methods

Application of topical products (e.g. tretinoin, retinaldehyde or α-hydroxy acids such as glycolic acid)

Studies, some very important and double-blind controlled, especially North American ones, prove that the use of such products increases the thickness of the epidermis as well as new collagen formation in the papillary dermis, but it does not appear to have any action on elastic tissue. The complementary use of ESS is profitable.

Collagen implants

These are not indicated when elastosis is important, the wrinkles' origin being double: expression, of course, but also flabbiness. Preliminary ESS sessions improve the tone and therefore the efficiency of collagen implants.

Chemical peels

Soft peels do not seem to provoke any resurgence of elastic fibres, in contrast to TCA or phenol peels. ESS could be a good substitute.

Dermabrasion and microdermabrasion

When these treatments are combined with ESS, we can detect an improvement of the already good results.

Laser resurfacing

This promising new technique is applied to multiple superficial wrinkles, and may supersede phenol peels or dermabrasion. ESS appears to be the ideal complement, principally Top Derm, which achieves a 'soft, real electric resurfacing'.

CONCLUSIONS

Clinicians and research workers are aware of the beneficial effects of electrical stimulation on the body and know most of its modes of action, but are uncertain about its exact mechanism. While the great majority of North American studies have concerned fundamental research or animal experimentation, the process is beginning to be studied in vivo in man: thus the same process can help join a bone fracture, tone a neurological bladder, heal a wound, soften a scar or rejuvenate a face. The scope of this action is probably even vaster than it seems, and it is likely that in the years to come this treatment, originally geared towards cosmetology, will become a therapy in its own right. Much is expected from the pursuit of fundamental studies allowing a better understanding of the processes triggered by pulsed electrical currents on living cells, but hope also lies with clinical research, with physicians using Simonin's method (essentially in Europe – mainly Switzerland and France) becoming every day more numerous and, it is hoped, desirous of sharing the results of their own practice.

REFERENCES

1. Electroridopuncture. *Official Trademark* 808682.
2. Electroridolyse. *Official Trademark* 846842.
3. *French Patent* 8205796; *European Patent* 0091853; *Canadian Patent* 121365; *US Patent* 452210.
4. *French Patent* 2567762; *Swiss Patent* 6637719; *Luxembourg Patent* 86009; *Belgian Patent* 902903; *Spanish Patent* 288234; *British Patent* 2163355.
5. Schnitzler L, Stimulation électrique cutanée (vieillissement et cicatrices). Electroridopuncture suuivant le procédé de Ph. Simonin. *Rev Eur Dermatol MST* 1989; **1**: 495–504.
6. Schnitzler L, Simonin Ph, Le traitement des rides par électroridopunctures. *Bull Esth Dermatol Cosmetol* 1986; **15**: 46–50.
7. Simon V, Electroridopuncture: méthode, technique d'analyse, résultats. Mémoire pour Diplôme d'études Approfondies de Biologie Cutanée et Cosmétologie, Faculté de Pharmacie de Chatenay–Malabry, 1986: 1–177.
8. Haines E, Shocking therapy: uses of transcutaneous electric nerve stimulation in dermatology. *Dermatol Clin* 1991; **9**: 189–97.
9. Reich JD, Cazzaniga AL, Mertz PM et al, The effect of electrical stimulation on the number of mast cells in healing wounds. *J Am Acad Dermatol* 1991; **25**: 40–6.
10. Reich JD, Tarjan PP, Electrical stimulation of skin. *Int J Dermatol* 1990; **29**: 395–400.
11. Alvarez OM, Mertz PM, Smerbeck RV et al, The healing of superficial skin wounds is stimulated by external electrical current. *J Invest Dermatol* 1983; **81**: 144–8.
12. Smith J, Romansky N, Vomero J et al, The effect of electrical stimulation on wound healing in diabetic mice. *J Am Podiatry Assoc* 1984; **74**: 71–5.
13. Brown M, McDonnel MK, Menton DN, Polarity effects on wound healing using electric stimulation in rabbits. *Arch Phys Med Rehab* 1989; **70**: 624–7.
14. Davis SC, Cazzinaga A, Reich JD et al, Pulsed electrical stimulation: the effect of varying polarity. *J Invest Dermatol* 1989; **92**: 418.
15. Bourguignon GJ, Bourguignon YW, Electric stimulation of protein and DNA synthesis in human fibroblasts. *FASEB J* 1987; **1**: 398–402.
16. Wood J, Evans PE, Schallreuter KV et al, A multicenter study on the use of pulsed low-intensity direct current for healing chronic stage II and stage III decubitus ulcers. *Arch Dermatol* 1993; **129**: 999–1009.

Cosmetic cutaneous laser surgery

Timothy J Rosio

INTRODUCTION

Defining, understanding and learning cosmetic laser surgery

What is 'cosmetic laser surgery'? It implies that a desirable change in appearance is accomplished by laser alteration of macroscopic or microscopic structures of the skin. Ideally, a laser is chosen to exploit special tissue interaction benefits unavailable from other surgical instruments via immense quantities of monochromatic photons delivered with great spatial and temporal precision.

A distinction between cosmetic and reconstructive surgery may be easy at times and difficult at others. A commonly accepted definition states that 'reconstructive' surgery seeks to restore a more normal appearance relative to one's societal peer group, while 'cosmetic' surgery strives for an appearance better than one's normative group. Wide latitude in interpretation of 'normal' exists, and much reconstructive surgery improves appearance simultaneously with function. A broad interpretation of cosmetic laser surgery will be used here, including some overlapping conditions and procedures. Greater emphasis will be placed on conditions traditionally recognized as primarily cosmetic. Table 57.1 outlines the subjects considered here.

Table 57.1 Outline of considerations in cosmetic laser surgery

Potential advantages/benefits versus potential disadvantages

Laser categories (accessories available e.g. scanning/pulsing attachments)
- CO_2, excimer, Er-YAG
- Green- and yellow-light CW lasers: argon, KTP, copper-vapor, CW tunable dye
- FEDL
- Q-switched: ruby, alexandrite, YAG; normal ruby

Techniques
- Organ-level cutaneous surgery:
    Resurfacing (superficial)
    Recontouring (dermis)
    Incisional: hemostatic scalpel
- Tissue-level:
    Vascular photothermolysis
- Cellular-level selective photothermolysis:
    Melanocytes
    Tattoos (decorative; traumatic: gunpowder, asphalt)
    Hair (melanocytes or exogenous chromophore)

Disorders
- Vascular:
    Malformation
    Hyperproliferation
- Dyschromias:
    Melanocytic
    Tattoos
- Tissue hypertrophy or proliferation or dysmorphogenesis (scars, tumors, etc.):
    Actinic cheilitis
    Adnexal tumors, angiofibromas, syringomas, neurofibromas, trichoepithelioma keloid or thickened scar
    Xanthelasma
    Rhinophyma
- Hirsutism

CO_2, carbon dioxide; CW, continuous-wave; KTP, potassium titanyl phosphate; FEDL, flashlamp-excited dye laser; Er-YAG, erbium-YAG (erbium-doped YAG crystal).

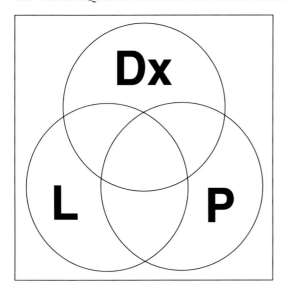

Figure 57.1 Integration of perspectives: consideration of available laser hardware (L), procedural options (laser and non-laser) (P), and diagnoses associated with specific laser treatment results (Dx).

The main goal of this chapter is understanding how to logically approach the selection of lasers in cosmetic surgery, promoted by simultaneously considering three perspectives (Figure 57.1):

• What are the currently available cutaneous lasers and how are they functionally grouped?
• How do cosmetic laser procedures compare with traditional procedures?
• What diagnoses are frequently treated successfully with particular laser approaches?

Integration of these complementary perspectives with clinical judgment helps the surgeon to weigh which, if any, cosmetic surgical approach (laser or non-laser) is indicated for a particular patient. This follows what thoughtful experienced surgeons do when they ask what procedures are available to treat a problem, what hardware is accessible and how they can use it procedurally to get the best cosmetic results, and (for a given diagno-

sis) the degree to which a particular cosmetic laser approach is indicated.

Relative indications

Some cosmetic procedures discussed in this chapter are now considered 'strongly indicated' to be performed by a particular laser and technique (Table 57.2). *Strongly indicated* implies that results achieved with the laser technique are superior, or safety benefits or both results and procedure safety occur reliably enough to warrant this choice over all other approaches if available. Other procedures deserve a *selective indication*. 'Selective' suggests superior results or that safety benefits may be attributed to a specific laser technique versus a conventional surgical approach under specific conditions. In the absence of such specific conditions, conventional surgery may offer equal or superior benefits in results, safety, cost or other aspects. *No indication* implies a lack of benefits sufficient to recommend its use under most circumstances, or the potential for worse than usual results.

Laser training

Even with a strong indication, proper training in each laser technique is vital, whether or not the surgeon has prior cosmetic surgery experience for comparable problems with non-laser techniques. Specific courses are now available, offering 'hands-on live-tissue exercises' simulating disorders that surgeons treat with lasers. These live-tissue workshops help develop the necessary hand–eye coordination and judgment required in each technique.

Basic descriptions of various cosmetic cutaneous laser surgery procedures will be given after an overview of the increasingly diverse lasers available. Laser procedures will be mentioned both from the perspective of the type of surgical process or procedure employed (e.g. resurfacing tissue) and additionally organized by diagnosis.

Table 57.2 Relative indications for cosmetic laser treatment

Disorder	Laser type(s)	Degree of indication[a]
PWS (infants)	FEDL	+++
PWS (adults)	CW[b] yellow/green or FEDL	+++
Hemangioma ≤9 months	FEDL	+++
Poikiloderma of Civatte	FEDL	+++
Spider angioma	CW[b] yellow or green	+++
Large linear telangiectasia (face)	CW yellow or green systems	+++
Small linear telangiectasia (face)	FEDL or CW yellow or green	+++
Small leg veins	FEDL or CW[b]	++
Matte telangiectasia	FEDL or CW[b] yellow or green systems with scanner	+++
Rosacea erythema	FEDL or CW[b] yellow or green	+++
Scar or striae remodeling/ fading	FEDL or CW[b]	+++
Tattoos	Q-switched (ruby, YAG, alexandrite)	+++
Ephelid, lentigo	Q-switched or PLDL	+++
Café-au-lait	Q-switched	+++
Chloasma	Q-switched (ruby, alexandrite)	++
Nevus of Ota	Q-switched (ruby, YAG, alexandrite)	+++
Hirsutism/hair removal	Normal-mode ruby, or Q-YAG with exogenous chromophore	
Adnexal tumors	CO_2 or CW[b] yellow or green systems	+++
Blepharoplasty	CO_2	++
Neurofibromas	CO_2	++
Keloids	CO_2	++
Graft, flaps	CO_2	+++
Incisional lines, scar resurfacing/recontouring	CO_2	+++
Xanthelasma	CO_2 or FEDL	++
Wrinkle resurfacing	CO_2	+++
Face lift	CO_2	+
Full face laserbrasion	CO_2	+++
Actinic cheilitis	CO_2	+++
Rhinophyma	CO_2	+++

[a] +++, strong indication; ++, selective indication; +, no indication.
[b] High-power CW (e.g. KTP) system preferable to limit exposure time.

LASERS IN COSMETIC CUTANEOUS SURGERY (Figure 57.2)

Practical approach to lasers in cosmetic surgery

Practical understanding and appropriate selection of lasers for cutaneous cosmetic surgery requires knowing the wavelength of the laser, the relative absorption efficiencies and arrangement of the chromophores in the skin for the wavelength in question, and the temporal–spatial distribution of a quantified beam. The relative chromophore absorption efficiencies along with the beam intensity and fluence determine the type of reaction at the target and the effects on surrounding cells. In other words, will the target be *warmed, coagulated, vaporized* or *photomechanically fragmented,* and how confined will the damage be?

Cosmetic surgery techniques operate by either photothermal or photomechanical reactions. Photothermal reactions are of three different types, depending upon the tissue

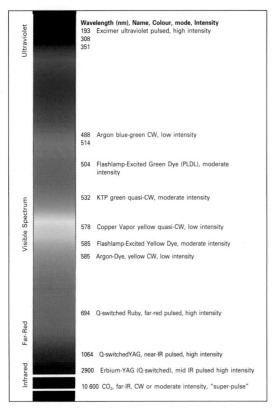

Figure 57.2 Lasers with potential use in cosmetic surgery. Most of these lasers have demonstrated use in cosmetic surgery. Both the erbium–YAG and excimer lasers may have future applications in superficial resurfacing. The excimer laser's putative UV carcinogenesis may preclude its application in cutaneous surgery.

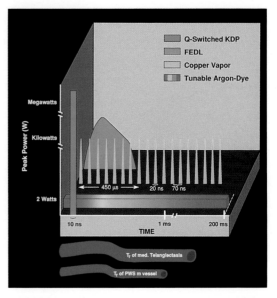

Figure 57.3 Thermal relaxation time related to laser power and exposure times of selected cutaneous lasers. Microvessels are characterized by thermal relaxation times of approximating 100–1000 μs. Shorter (nanosecond) high-energy exposures completely destroy the vessel; lower fluences with much longer exposures cause coagulation, but also allow sufficient heat to diffuse to surrounding tissue, resulting in nonspecific epidermal and dermal damage (and possible visible scarring). Very brief (nanosecond) lower-power pulses closely spaced (e.g. 2–5 kHz) are 'quasicontinuous' (e.g. with copper-vapor and non-Q-switched KTP lasers). The total energy contained in an individual pulse is low despite a moderate peak power due to the brief duration.

temperature achieved: temperatures less than 50°C for brief periods may cause reversible thermal injury. Temperatures of 50–70°C cause irreversible thermal injury and coagulation; cells reaching 100°C vaporize when their tissue water boils.

The time course of elevated temperature is important too (Figure 57.3). Slow heat delivery achieves lower peak temperatures, and conducts the heat injury to a broader area. Rapid delivery of energy causes much higher temperatures for shorter periods of time, and confines thermal injury closer to the target. Extremely high-intensity very short pulses (e.g. nanoseconds) produce photomechanical (i.e. non-thermal) effects, resulting in disintegration of the target and minimal damage to surrounding tissues. An example is the photodisruption of tattoo pigment particles or melanocytes by the ruby laser.

Three functional categories of cosmetic surgical lasers

The lasers for cosmetic applications under discussion may be placed in three functional categories: whole-tissue surgical lasers, superficial-pigment lasers and deep-pigment lasers.

Whole-tissue surgical lasers

These include the carbon dioxide (CO_2) laser, the erbium–YAG laser and (still experimental) the excimer laser. Incising, planing and sculpting tissues is the forte of lasers in this category. The CO_2 laser and erbium–YAG laser wavelengths are absorbed with extremely high efficiency by tissue water. The excimer laser is highly absorbed by tissue proteins. Since tissue water and proteins are ubiquitous in all cells, very little scattering occurs, and intense photothermal transformation coagulates or vaporizes tissue very efficiently. High-intensity brief tissue exposures lead to extremely sharp scalpel or ablational effects with high precision, where no hemostasis is achieved. Lower intensities and longer exposures allow adjacent thermal injury, which coagulates small blood vessels, leading to a bloodless field. The surgeon therefore may choose which properties are most attractive in a given situation – for example vaporizing a few cell layers at a time in very small areas or achieving varying degrees of hemostasis to improve observations in the surgical field.

Superficial-pigment lasers

These include all the green- and yellow-light laser systems: the argon, KTP, krypton, copper-vapor and continuous-wave (CW) argon pumped dye lasers as well as the flashlamp-excited green dye or pigmented lesion dye laser (PLDL), the flashlamp-excited yellow dye laser (FEDL) and the Q-switched KTP/YAG (532 nm) laser. These laser wavelengths transmit through water but penetrate the skin poorly; they are absorbed in less than 0.1 mm by melanin, or in 0.5 mm by blood and to a lesser degree other tissue constituents.

Long temporal exposures to the wavelengths from any of these lasers coagulates tissue widely. Short intense exposures of the order of hundreds of microseconds up to milliseconds allow thermal spatial confinement to superficial melanin and hemoglobin targets. This category of lasers is therefore ideal for treating superficial vascular lesions and superficial melanocytic pigmentary disorders.

Deep-pigment lasers of extremely high intensity and short duration ('high fluence')

These are all Q-switched lasers, including the ruby, Q-switched YAG and alexandrite lasers. Q-switching (pulsing) results in such high-intensity photon delivery to tissue targets that photomechanical effects (fragmentation) are seen. Surrounding tissues are protected from thermal injury. This occurs because delivery of the photons takes place over a period shorter than the thermal relaxation time of the target, i.e. before significant heat dissipation can occur.

Selective photothermolysis can occur in any chromophores that absorb these wavelengths efficiently enough. This is true for most tattoo pigments over a broad range. The far-red and near-infrared wavelengths of these lasers are capable of penetrating several millimeters through the skin because of long-wavelength transmission and poor absorption by other chromophores. The Q-switched YAG infrared wavelength is less efficiently absorbed by melanin than exogenous pigments, compared with ruby and alexandrite wavelengths.

PROCEDURES

Cosmetic laser surgical procedures range from those similar to standard surgical techniques to those taking place at progressively more specific levels: the whole-skin organ level exemplified by procedures such as resurfacing, recontouring and incisional surgery; the tissue level (e.g. vascular); and finally selectivity at the cellular or subcellular level.

ORGAN-LEVEL CUTANEOUS SURGERY: SPLIT-THICKNESS OR FULL-THICKNESS REMOVAL

Resurfacing

Resurfacing is superficial removal of the skin similar to a chemical peel or mechanical abrasion. The laser in widest use is the CO_2 laser, but exciting potential also exists for the erbium–YAG laser because both have high absorption efficiencies in water and the ability to achieve efficient vaporization with even shorter tissue exposure times. This absorption efficiency, high fluences and proper technique confines thermal injury to a very narrow zone and reduces the risk of scarring.

Resurfacing techniques have been applied to actinically damaged skin to improve hyper- and hypopigmentation, telangiectasia, elastosis and precancerous changes including actinic keratoses and actinic cheilitis, and also for superficial wrinkles.[1–4]

Perioral resurfacing may include treatment of actinic cheilitis i.e., vermilionectomy, perioral wrinkle removal, or both.

Actinic cheilitis presents as a scaling, mottled, faded, sometimes wrinkled lip, occasionally with hyperpigmentation. Laser resurfacing replaces these changes with a more uniform, pink vermilion and a smooth-appearing labial surface that appears many years younger. Laser rhytid removal offers greater precision control over localized deeper wrinkles (see Figure 57.5 below).

The method is superficial destruction of the skin into the papillary dermis level with photocoagulation or vaporization. Depth precision and uniformity of tissue removal are the primary goals of the surgeon. The laser is a non-touch technique, and therefore provides no tactile feedback. Secondly, the margin for error is extremely slim. That is, the difference between delivering too little laser energy (inadequate therapeutic response) and excess laser energy (scarring and other undesirable effects) may arise in fractions of a second.

Therefore it is imperative for the surgeon to anticipate how much energy is needed and how to control the temporal and spatial delivery of that energy. The surgeon orchestrates power settings, beam profiles via lens selection and distance from handpiece to tissue, rate of hand movement as well as the optional use of electromechanical shuttering, pulsing or scanning of the laser beam. *The goal is tissue*

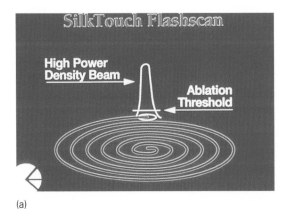

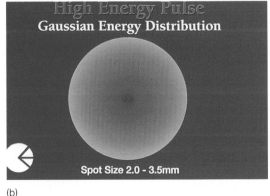

(a)

(b)

Figure 57.4 Resurfacing technologies. Scanned continuous wave (a) and 'pulsed' laser beam (b) delivery patterns used in skin resurfacing. These technological methods help to control temporal and spatial energy delivery for safer, reproducible resurfacing.

vaporization within the thermal relaxation time of skin (≤1 ms), requiring a fluence of 5 J/cm³. Figure 57.4 displays scanned samplings of continuous-wave and pulsed high-energy beam delivery techniques and patterns used in skin resurfacing. The energy density may be modified to vary the penetration depth. The pulsed beam may also be delivered in an array of varying densities by a pattern generator similar to those used in some vascular lasers (see Figure 57.15 below).

Technique tips

Local, nerve-block or tumescent anesthesia may be used. If nerve blocks are employed, or occasionally general anesthesia, local anesthesia may be of use in distending superficial wrinkles and theoretically adding a small margin of additional safety from subjacent thermal damage. Facial zones, cosmetic junctions and subunits may be delimited with a surgical marker as for dermabrasion or chemical peeling. Nerve blocks frequently utilized include supraorbital, supratrochlear, dorsal external nasal, infraorbital and mental. It is important to place a moistened gauze over the teeth, the eyes, and possibly just within the nares prior to resurfacing the adjacent areas.

The clinical endpoint for superficial tissue resurfacing (e.g. of wrinkles) is epidermal removal with dusky color change in the tissue, i.e. a light pink-gray or chamois color.[2,5] Limiting vaporization to the superficial dermis reduces risk of deeper dermal injury and scarring. This is especially true when resurfacing scar-prone areas of the body such as the upper lip or eyelids, where a poor cosmetic result from hypertrophic scarring may be catastrophic.

Labial resurfacing – After bilateral mental nerve blocks with 1% lidocaine (Xylocaine), locally infiltrate the vermilion from the vermilion glabrous junction to the line of occlusion, and include the corners of the mouth (not anesthetized by the mental nerve block). Place moistened gauze sponges in the labial gingival sulcus to both protect the teeth and

induce a more convenient protrusion of the lower lip. Make one pass. Ensure that uniform superficial coagulation has been achieved. A gentle wiping or peeling of the coagulum is performed. Any thickened and granular surface tissue previously undetected should be inspected closely and palpated. If sufficiently suspicious, a biopsy should be taken. If the tissue only appears slightly thicker or more tenacious then a second pass over this focus may be warranted. The higher-power pulse technique is preferred if a second pass is required over such foci. This reduces the chance of a bead scar or localized discoloration. Occlusive ointment wound healing is routinely employed as with other resurfacing surgeries. Unguent is applied, followed by petrolatum-impregnated gauze; then non-adhering gauze is secured with tape.

Glabrous skin resurfacing – Careful technique includes limiting the number of passes, pattern overlap, careful debridement between passes, patient selection, and pre- and postoperative management. Herpes simplex virus prophylaxis is recommended from the time of the surgery until reepithelialization is complete, or for a period of 7–10 days. Bacterial or candidal infections occur in less than 5% of cases, and are treatable with standard oral antibiotics effective against *Staphylococcus* and *Streptococcus*, or a topical anticandidal agent. Moist wound healing is routinely employed in all resurfacing surgeries. Emollients and emollient-impregnated gauze, hydrogels and polyurethane dressings as well as special semipermeable knits that do not adhere to the wound are all valid approaches used alone or in combinations.

Simple moisturization and avoidance of irritants are indicated for the first couple of weeks after resurfacing. Makeup may be carefully reinstituted after reepithelialization. Two to three weeks post epithelialization, some patients are ready to shift from sunblocks to sunscreens, and may be ready to institute or resume melanin inhibitors. Inflammation during this stage may be helped by low-

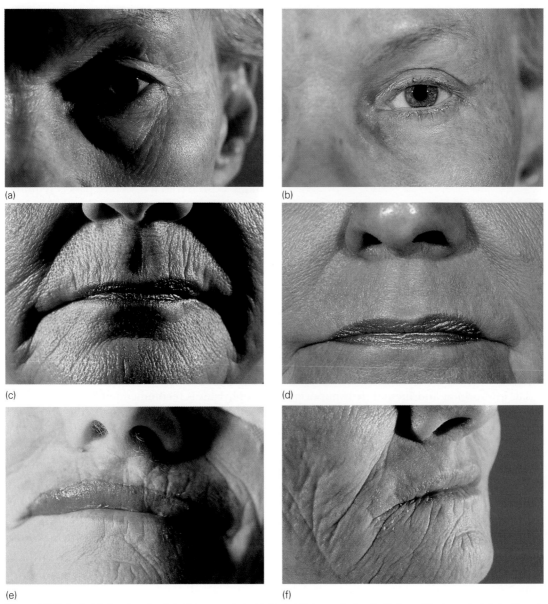

Figure 57.5 Periorbital and perioral rhytid removal. (a, b) Periorbital resurfacing (with laser blepharoplasty); (c–f) perioral resurfacing in two patients shown before (c, e) and 8–10 weeks after (d, f) laser surgery. Note the improvement in the superficial rhytids, tissue color and texture.

potency steroid creams. Generally, another two to three weeks is required before the patient is able to resume α-hydroxy or retinoic acids. At the earliest sign of focally prolonged erythema or increasing localized induration, dilute steroids (e.g. triamcinolone 2.5–5 mg/cm^3) should be injected at one to two week intervals to the mid to deep dermis with low volumes, or else a blister may be formed.

As illustrated in Figure 57.5, a full-thickness epithelial coagulation and resurfacing technique is used to de-epithelize transitional or mucosal surfaces – for example vermilion with actinic cheilitis (laser vermilionectomy). The pictures show that both the lower-power 3–5 W continuous-wave 'airbrush' or 'painting' technique with 2–5 mm spot size and the higher-power shuttered technique at 20 W with 0.05 s tissue exposure and 3–5 mm spot size give clinically equivalent results when performed meticulously. Scaling, mottled, faded lip, occasionally with hyperpigmentation, is replaced by a more uniform pink smooth appearing labial surface that appears many years younger.[4,6,7]

Advantages over the lip shave are greater uniformity, natural cosmetic texture and color, and avoidance of the band and bead scars not uncommonly seen with shaves. Advantages over the mucosal advancement flap are ease of performance (when removal of deeper tissue is not required), and superior cosmesis and function. The narrowed and thin-lipped appearance so common after mucosal advancement is avoided. In other words, the anterior–posterior lip diameter and the cephalocaudal lip thickness are both normally maintained with laser

vermilionectomy. Upper-lip discomfort from recurring pricking by redirected lower-lip whiskers, frequently encountered after mucosal advancement, is also avoided by laser vermilionectomy.

Cosmetic laser recontouring of the dermis: mid- or deep-thickness tissue removal

Recontouring implies a deeper wounding and removal of skin past the papillary dermis. This is analogous to mid to deep chemical peels, dermabrasions or split-thickness planing. Focally, even full-thickness tissue may be removed. Examples include the treatment of rhinophyma, removal of adnexal tumors, treatment of xanthelasma, pitted acne scarring, scar revision via improving incision lines and reducing differences in tissue contours, removal of deeper wrinkles, and tattoo removal techniques with the CO_2 laser.

Scar revision and pitted acne scars (Figure 57.6)

High tissue fluence producing instant vaporization is required for cosmetic laser recon-

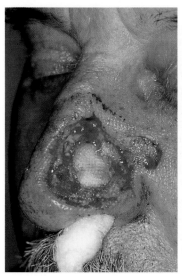
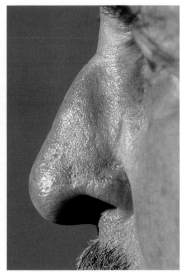

Figure 57.6 Nasal flap and scar revision through laser recontouring treatment. (a) Initial nasal side wall skin cancer defect. A hinge flap (not shown) restored the mucosal lining; the resultant defect, 200% larger than shown here, was covered with a forehead flap. Laser recontouring of the flap and incisional scars yielded the final cosmetic result (b).

(a)   (b)

touring surgery. High fluences briefly applied narrow the zone of thermal injury that can result in unintended scarring. Methods for revision of scar lines and pitted acne scars[8] employ split-thickness dermis removal and feathering techniques; so do xanthelasma, rhinophyma, adnexal tumors and genodermatoses. Therefore they are considered together.

Technique

Routine surgical preparation of the skin is followed by local anesthesia with or without nerve blocks. General anesthesia may be employed instead. When local anesthesia is used for the treatment of incision lines and pitted acne scars, care must be taken not to distort the scar-tissue contours, since these are used to ascertain the clinical endpoint with the laser.

One to several resurfacing passes are made in 'steps' over the peripheral contours of sharp-edged deep wrinkles or a prominent depressed or step-off scar line. This graduates the difference between the adjacent tissue height of the peripheral tissue and the base of the scar.

After this has been accomplished, the base of the scar is barely de-epithelialized using the superficial resurfacing technique described above. Localized feathering is performed to avoid abrupt transitions. This technique works extremely well in combination with the punch graft transplantation method of correcting ice pick or pitted scars.[9]

Between passes, a moistened Q-Tip or gauze should be employed to remove carbonized tissue. Higher power densities are required to vaporize scar tissue than unscarred epithelium. Extra caution is required in scar-prone areas such as the upper lip, eyelids and angle of the jaw, as with other resurfacing techniques. On thicker scarred areas, making too many passes in an attempt to completely smooth scar contours is likely to result in excessive formation of new scar tissue. Close follow-up in the postopera-

tive period at 3, 6 and 8–10 weeks is important so that early intervention with intralesional steroids and/or silicone gel can inhibit undesired scar tissue formation.

Xanthelasma

Small xanthomatous plaques are often easily removed by scalpel incision. Large plaques or those in unfavorable locations on the lids may lead to unfavorable scars or ectropion. The CO_2 laser may be used with selective indication in large xanthomatous plaques or smaller ones in sensitive or scar-prone locations.[10] The laser treatment method for xanthelasma employs repeated superficial vaporizations with either the continuous-wave technique or (preferably) the electromagnetically shuttered technique until the majority (but not necessarily all) of the yellowish adherent xanthomatous plaque is removed. Vigorous cleansing with moistened Q-Tips or wet gauze is employed between passes. Plaques may be treated with one to several passes to a split-thickness level, but without penetration to the orbicularis muscle. Fastidious technique is required throughout to obtain immediate vaporization and a smooth plane. Occlusive antibiotic ointment dressings are maintained until re-epithelialization. A recent case report using a series of five FEDL treatments in one patient at an average fluence of 7 J effectively eliminated xanthelasma plaques.[11]

Rhinophyma (Figure 57.7)

Rhinophyma treatment with the CO_2 laser is 'strongly indicated' because of the precise control it offers for nasal tissue sculpting. Esthetic judgment is invaluable in assessing how much tissue to remove and obtaining a symmetrical and pleasing end result. Photographs from 10–30 years prior or more may be helpful in estimating the patient's underlying soft-tissue structure prior to rhinophymatous hypertrophy.

The clinical endpoint for treatment of rhinophyma requires an acceptable contour while maintaining some reticular dermis and

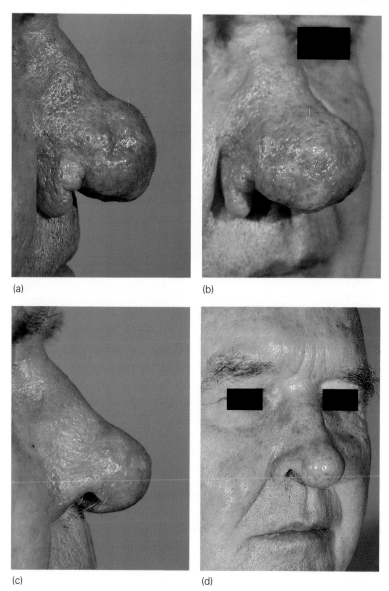

(a)

(b)

(c)

(d)

Figure 57.7 (a–d) Rhinophyma excisions by laser.

associated deeper sebaceous glands. Superficial technique is required in peripheral and less hypertrophic areas, and particularly along the lateral alar groove, which lacks cartilaginous support. Excessive depth in these locations will result in undesirable texture change (scarring) and alar retraction.

Sequential laser passes result in progressive visualization of more numerous sebaceous glands, which appear to become larger in diameter with each layer. After a mid-dermal depth is passed, the size of sebaceous glands may still increase slightly, but their number begins to decrease.

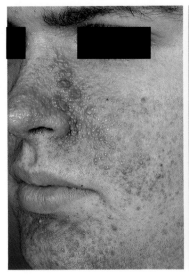
(a)

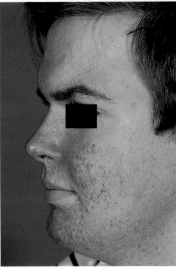
(b)

Figure 57.8 (a, b) Tuberous sclerosis: CO_2 laser vaporization of angiofibromas is achieved even in the delicate areas of the eyelids and periorbital skin.

Anesthesia is achieved using a dorsal external nasal block and also infiltration of the columella initially with 1% lidocaine without epinephrine (adrenaline) followed by 0.25% bupivacaine (Marcaine) with 1 : 200 000 epinephrine. Once these nerve blocks are placed at the nasal root and the nasal tip, lines of anesthesia are infiltrated along the meilonasal junctions and also locally into the base of the ala nasi. To make this process even more comfortable for the patient, I commonly employ two infraorbital nerve blocks with 2% lidocaine without epinephrine a few minutes before the local infiltration.

If large rhinophymatous nodules are present, focused-beam excisions may be accomplished with 10–20 W and 0.1–0.2 mm spot size in continuous mode.

After removal of more gross amounts of rhiniphymatous tissue, or in milder cases even initially repeated overlapping passes are performed with careful removal of charred tissue between passes.

A 1–2 mm beam size may be employed to recreate an alar sulcus if this has been obliterated by hypertrophic tissue. Under-treatment is preferable to an overly aggressive approach. Repeat surgery may be performed if inadequate tissue removal is judged after healing.

The surgeon should expect (and the patient informed prior to surgery) that dilatation of some pores will be evident after healing. This should be discussed with the patient as an anticipated side-effect rather than a complication of this procedure.

Non-rhinophymatous areas of the nose should be superficially resurfaced to feather the surgical area of the nose into adjacent cosmetic units. A strong benefit of the CO_2 laser technique is that smoother blending at cosmetic unit junctions can be easily performed compared with electrosurgical or blade techniques. Proper technique with the laser also achieves better visualization of the surgical endpoint of the mid- to deep-level glands than is achievable with the scalpel technique. Additionally, precisely limiting subjacent tissue injury is a hallmark of the laser technique in contrast to electrosurgery, which damages the tissue to a greater depth.

The patient should be seen minimally at four, six and eight weeks after the surgery to observe for any excessive scar tissue formation, which should be managed early on with steroids. Very small volumes of 2.5–10 mg/cm^3 triamcinolone is efficacious when administered intralesionally to focal early scar tissue formation.

The distinct advantages of laser treatment of rhinophyma have resulted in numerous papers since 1980.[12,13]

Thickened scars or keloids

Treatment of either hypertrophic or keloidal scars remains a controversial topic concerning a difficult-to-predict condition. In general, the anatomic area and the individual patient's scar-tissue-forming tendencies are decisive variables. Suffice it to say that no technique can be routinely advised. There is a lack of controlled studies comparing laser treatment techniques of scars with other conventional surgical methods. However, I and other investigators have found the focused incisional CO_2 laser technique to be valuable in treating keloids of the head and neck region. Notably, earlobe keloids respond very well to the incisional technique, and often 'shell out' from surrounding tissue.

A continuous focused beam at 10–15 W cuts the firm keloid from surrounding tissue. The keloid is grasped by a towel clamp with strong traction, while the third digit of the nondominant hand palpates the anterior surface of the lobule (usually non-involved). Second-intention healing is favored to minimize foreign-body reaction.

Laser removal is combined with intralesional steroids at the time of operation and for one to several visits afterwards as indicated by the patient's progress monthly. The patient should be followed for at least one year, and intralesional steroid progressively withdrawn. Injections are reinstituted at the first palpable or visible sign of recurrence.

Scar and striae fading and remodeling

A few investigators have found that persistent hypertrophic scars on the face, sternum, presternal area and other locations may be induced to atrophy or remodel through either CO_2 or argon laser focused impulses ('drilling').[14,15] After local anesthesia, 0.1–0.2 mm spot sizes are used with 0.1 s tissue exposure time (or 0.5–1.0 s exposure time for the argon laser) in a grid of impulses perpendicularly applied to the scar tissue with impulses separated by 3–4 mm. After laser treatment, the area may be intralesionally injected with 20–40 mg/cm^3 triamcinolone. It must be acknowledged that the potential for exacerbation of hypertrophic scar tissue exists with either of these techniques. I regard this technique as non-indicated routinely, but deserving wider investigation.

Hypertrophic or atrophic scars and some striae may be lightened (if erythematous or violaceous) or possibly remodeled by FEDL treatments. A few investigators have reported success with minimally purpuric doses. A series of 3 or 4 treatments over 6–12 months may soften and partially improve contours by 25–60%. Further work needs to be done to confirm and refine these observations.

Scalp reduction

Standard scalp-reduction procedures may be performed with the CO_2 laser in order to obtain hemostatic benefits. The method involves focused incisions with the CO_2 laser using it as a 'light scalpel'. If the patient has a bleeding tendency or is on blood thinners or antiplatelet medications, the use of a laser would be a 'selective indication'. Advantages besides less bleeding and better visualization include increased speed of the procedure, since less time has to be devoted to electrosurgical coagulation of blood vessels. No other long-term advantage is attributed to the laser approach. The surgeon must also have electrosurgical equipment to properly electrocoagulate vessels greater than 0.5–1.00 mm diameter.

The patient is prepared in the usual fashion, preferably with ring block anesthesia. The scalp is placed under moderate tension perpendicular to the long axis of the incision.

A high-power continuous mode employing 15–30 W and 0.1–0.2 mm spot size is selected. A smooth even movement of the handpiece along the intended incision path is performed, keeping the beam perpendicular to the skin surface. The speed is adjusted to maintain the proper depth. The depth is ordinarily truncated at the adipose layer, and an additional pass or two may be required to incise through the galea.

A supplementary technique is favored by some, with an initial full-thickness penetration at one pole of the incision, through which either a back stop of moistened gauze or a long metallic back stop is introduced underneath the tissue to be incised.

Potential disadvantages cited for this approach are primarily the presence of additional equipment and an assistant to handle the smoke evacuation system. Otherwise the technique is rapid, safe and efficient. An important technique tip is to remember that, as with all incisional laser surgery, maintaining the skin under greater lateral tension than is ordinarily required with scalpel surgery greatly facilitates an even incision line.

Adnexal tumors and genodermatoses (Figure 57.8)

Vaporization planing of adnexal tumors and tumors, e.g. sebaceous adenomas, associated with genodermatoses such as angiofibromas or tuberous sclerosis and neurofibromas is 'strongly indicated' and readily achieved with the CO_2 laser.[16–19] Patient preparation and anesthesia are similar to those described in preceding sections, with local anesthesia or nerve blocks. The clinical endpoint for angiofibromas and small adnexal tumors is vaporization to upper- or mid-dermal level or until the growth is grossly removed – whichever is obtained first.

A minimal spot size for small papules or a larger pattern for plaques and tumors is used for ablation. Resurfacing and pulsed drilling techniques works well for large plaques and small papules respectively.

Moderate and larger lesions of neurofibromatosis often benefit from thumb and forefinger pressure on the lateral aspects of the lesion, causing it to protrude slightly after superficial vaporization has been performed. Further partial vaporization of the prominently protruding portion is usually sufficient; if the tumor is quite large and the resulting defect is quite deep then suturing may be of benefit.

An alternative to the CO_2 laser technique is the use of the argon or KTP system with 1–20 W shuttered continuous-wave photocoagulation of angiofibromas. The clinical endpoint, while less precise than with the CO_2 laser, involves a whitish coagulation and shrinkage of the superficial portion of the lesion.

Another example of the laser's advantage over other resurfacing methods is the precision achievable for small individual syringomas. Precise vaporization is achieved even in the mobile delicate areas of the eyelids and periorbital skin. Use of dermabrasion or electrosurgical techniques this close to the eye is not feasible or is contraindicated. Repeat treatments over time are easily administered if new tumors develop or recur. Commonly a 0.2–0.4 mm spot size is employed for ablation.

Patient preparation includes protection of the eyes with moist occlusive dressings or corneal eye shields for lesions close to the eyelids.

CO_2 laser tattoo removal (Figure 57.9)

CO_2 laser tattoo removal in my practice is reserved for patients who refuse or are unresponsive to Q-switched pigment lasers. The technique employs a combination of recontouring and microspot incisional techniques in an advanced method that I refer to as the 'Swiss cheese technique'[20] (Figure 57.10). A superficial ablation technique is used to remove gross amounts of tattoo pigment at a superficial to mid-dermal level.[21,22] Subsequently, pinpoint vaporization of scattered residual pigment depots is accomplished

- Of major importance is thorough knowledge of blepharoplasty procedures and complete familiarity with the use of the surgical instrument, be it scalpel or laser, being utilized.
- No major permanent advantage of either the laser or the scalpel exists when one is compared with the other.
- Significant short-term advantages are possible with the all-laser technique (used throughout the procedure), including less swelling, less ecchymosis, and significant potential speed advantages after much practice with the technique.

Potential disadvantages cited include

- the learning curve required with the laser technique;
- the extra assistant needed for smoke evacuation;
- the utilization of additional equipment.

With proper techniques, there does not appear to be any greater risk for the experienced laser surgeon than exists in the use of the scalpel technique. In fact, surgeons familiar with both techniques note that the routine employment of corneal shields for the patient undergoing the laser procedure places the patient at greater safety than the unprotected patient undergoing the scalpel surgical technique, for which there have been documented cases of injury to the globe.

Technique

As described by David,[25] the patient is prepared and draped using sterile saline soaked sponges, and standard lines of incision are drawn using a conventional marking pen. Topical ophthalmic anesthesia is used, with 2% tetracaine. The conjunctivae of the lower eyelids are infiltrated with 1% lidocaine and epinephrine 1 : 100 000. Infiltration is extended into the lower lid fat compartments transconjunctivally using an additional 2 cm³ of local anesthetic. The skin of the upper eyelids may be injected by either the usual transcutaneous method or transconjunctivally if preferred.

Lower-lid technique – The lower lid is retracted while a protective lid plate (e.g. Jaeger) is placed over the globe and into the fornix. Light pressure from the protective plate directly superiorly and posteriorly on the globe induces fat bulging and some protrusion of the conjunctiva.

A CO_2 laser is used, with a focused 0.1–0.2 mm spot size and power setting of 7 W, and is moved at approximately 1–1.5 cm/s to make an incision through the conjunctiva. Incision placement is approximately 5 mm inferior to the lower dorsal border overlying the subconjunctival fat protrusion. The incision may extend from the punctum laterally to the end of the tarsus parallel to the contour of the globe.

The incision is deepened into fat compartments. Fat elevation over a back stop is performed and then excised.

Upper lid technique – The protective Jaeger plate is once again positioned to protect the cornea and globe. A focused incisional laser at similar settings as before is employed to excise skin and muscle in a fashion similar to scalpel surgery. Skin and muscle are undermined and removed from the underlying septum. Lateral traction is applied as the incision is made. Non-laser surgical instrumentation may be used to incise or dissect tissue as judged desirable or necessary; however, all such maneuvers increase bleeding, bruising and swelling, and counter the potential advantages of the laser technique. Closure of upper-eyelid incisions is with standard 6-0 nonabsorbable suture; no closure is required for the lower lids. Cold compresses are applied immediately after the surgery and continued for 24 hours. Upper-lid sutures may be removed in 5–6 days, or will separate after a few days if mild chronic or plain gut has been used.

Morrow and Morrow[24] demonstrated that

chemical peeling of eyelids can be safely performed during laser blepharoplasty, yielding more impressive results and a single recuperation.

TISSUE-LEVEL CUTANEOUS SURGERY

Vascular photothermolysis

The treatment of unwanted superficial blood vessels is one of the most commonly requested and performed cosmetic cutaneous laser procedures. The vessels may be one or a few in number but abnormally dilated; conversely, vessels may be normal in size or slightly dilated but increased in number and density. Examples of 'dilated' vessels are single enlarged nasal blood vessels or a spider angioma. In contrast, the density of minimally dilated vessels is greatly increased in erythema in rosacea, actinic erythema or postsurgical telangiectasia.

The goal of vascular photothermolysis is to raise the temperature of the vessel to between 50°C and 70°C for long enough to achieve complete vessel-wall coagulation but short enough to prevent unwanted heat dissipation and damage of surrounding tissues with subsequent fibrosis and clinical scarring. The success of cosmetic laser treatment of unwanted vessels and excellent results earns a 'strong indication' for this application of lasers. The crucial questions become: which laser and laser wavelength, which settings and which diagnoses? These issues will also be discussed under the approach to vascular disorders in the 'disorder category' section in two groups: vascular malformations and hyperproliferations.

To help understand preferences of lasers for vascular problems, I have composed a 'visual conceptual blueprint' for selection of superficial vascular lasers (Figure 57.12).[26] In this algorithm the current choices of flash-lamp-excited dye lasers, continuous-wave lasers operated with scanners and continuous-wave lasers in freehand mode are selected by a series of clinical criteria. These criteria prominently include the *size of vessels* (ranging from microvessels to large telangiectasias), the *age* of the patient (from infant to mature), the *vascular pattern* from confluent or matte to prominent linear or solitary vessels, and the *flow pattern* and *type* of vessel (e.g. from a low-flow-rate capillary up to a high-flow-rate arteriole). Laser preference in the algorithm figure is strong (and functional overlap is least) where one gradient bar is the darkest; lighter shades of gray signify less efficacy, safety or efficiency – therefore consideration of the alternate laser type is warranted.

The first criterion is vessel size. The smallest blood vessel in young patients responds readily to all systems due to the low energy required and the short '*thermal relaxation time*'. The safest system then is one that delivers light energy in a pulse most closely matching this vessel-volume-related time value. As the size of the vessel increases, the amount of energy and time required to achieve coagulation increases beyond the current 450 μs FEDL systems, to the point where tissue injury is only partially selective.[27] It is on larger vessels, which are generally linear and solitary to a few in number, that freehand continuous-wave shutter techniques are relatively more effective and easier to apply. Scanners facilitate treatment of larger areas, more safely and consistently than freehand methods, and with less surgeon fatigue.

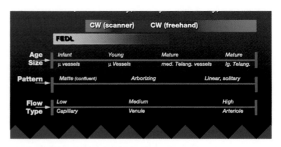

Figure 57.12 Blueprint for selection of lasers for treating superficial vascular problems.

More recently, higher-fluence vascular laser systems have improved the results of small leg telangiectasia treatment. In addition, an incoherent broadband light source originally developed to burn off military aircraft paint has been drafted to treat vascular lesions.

All these new leg vein systems have in common the capability to deliver 20 J/cm^2 or more within a few milliseconds.

Techniques

Pain relief for vascular photothermolysis treatments

I use nerve blocks routinely for comfort, local anesthesia occasionally in very sensitive areas, non-nerve-block regions, such as the eyelids, and 30% lidocaine or EMLA cream for neck areas, or i.v. sedation analgesia for very young patients or patients with large sensitive areas. Empathy and responsiveness to the individual patient's perception of pain is more important than rigid protocols. For young children, I believe sedation-induced amnesia is more important than analgesia, since fear is compounded with multiple treatments even when analgesia is near-complete.

Test spots and treatment administration

We begin FEDL treatments for microvessels with sketches of the patient's anatomic area in, for example, a portwine stain. Three barely overlapping test impulses are placed in each selected representative cosmetic unit (e.g. neck, cheek or forehead). Energy settings are begun at 1–1.5 times the minimum energy to elicit purpura, and several are done at 0.5 J increments. The response is judged for noticeable lightening and degree of epidermal tissue reaction graded by the patient at home with their 'report card'. Slight flaking or no change suggests that energy levels may be increased to achieve or maintain lightening; focal crusting for up to 3–5 days commonly accompanies a very effective dose for initial portwine stain treatments; crusting beyond 5–7 days or a dense scab argues for energy reduction in the early stages of treatment.

Common FEDL test spot energy settings begin at 4–5 J in younger patients and neck areas, while 5.5–6.0 J is used initially in other areas and older patients. Antibiotic ointment and a protective dressing are optional except with prominent crusting, or in young children who may traumatize test spots. Makeup may be applied and removed carefully after 3–5 days in areas without thick crusting. Repeat treatments may be performed at 6-week intervals.

Figure 57.13 shows the results of FEDL treatment of a portwine stain.

Continuous wave

The basic approach is selection of the highest power but briefest shutter duration for all the continuous-wave (CW) systems and titration to the shortest tissue exposure giving adequate coagulation of the vessel. The immediate blanching endpoint in CW laser treatments is much less noticeable than the FEDL purpura. However, the high energies and exposure times required in some CW treatments may elicit greater delayed crusting or scabbing, for up to 10–14 days. Assessment and retreatment intervals are best delayed for 6–12 weeks.

Continuous-wave KTP, dye, copper-vapor or argon lasers are more safely used with electromechanical shuttering. Commonly I choose a 100 μm spot size for the smallest facial telangiectasias and a 1–2 mm spot size for larger facial or leg vein treatments. Initial time settings of 2–3 ms for small facial vessels, beginning with 10 ms, ultimately delivering a range of 10–25 J/cm^2 to the vascular target. Lower settings are common for tracing small, fine superficial vessels, especially in children.

Figure 57.14 shows the results of CW laser treatment of a large nasal telangiectasia.

When tracing is impractical, the freehand grid approach employs small (1–2 mm) spots applied in a uniform array of contiguous impulses over the vascular lesions. Freehand continuous 'airbrushing,' while successful in some hands, varies energy delivery by

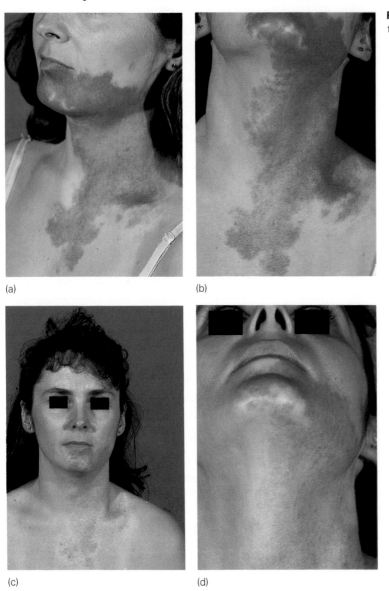

(a)

(b)

(c)

(d)

Figure 57.13 (a–d) FEDL treatment of a portwine stain.

100–1000-fold to adjacent areas, with accompanying under/overtreatment potential.

Scanners

Scanners are electromechanical and software light-delivery devices that provide CW lasers with more predictable and precise spatial and temporal distribution for treating confluent surface areas.[28] Treatments are accomplished with less surgeon fatigue than by tracing.[29] Scanners conduct preset impulses (e.g. 127×1 mm spots) to a predetermined 13 mm hexagonal area. The hexagon is covered by confluent pulses, which are delivered in a discontiguous sequence to allow cooling between adjacent tissue pulses. A feature of the hexagonal shape is *tessellation*, fitting multiple polygon edges together like a mosaic,

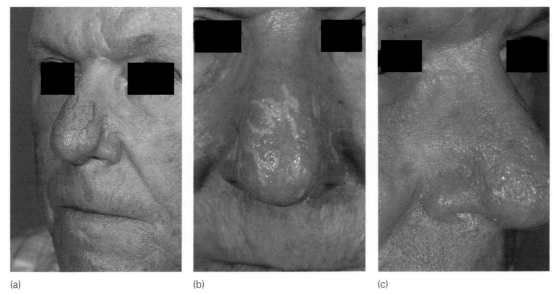

(a) (b) (c)

Figure 57.14 (a–c) Shuttered CW laser treatment of telangiectasia.

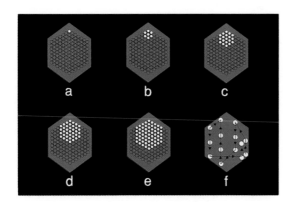

Figure 57.15 (a–f) Scanner impulse delivery and pattern: variable-size hexagons may be selected for treatment. Part (f) shows the discontiguous delivery of overlapping laser impulses, allowing tissue cooling between adjacent sites.

completely covering the combined surface area. See Figure 57.15.

The CW scanner is attached to CW lasers for small- to medium-sized vessels, particularly those that are more confluent over a large

area and those with lower flow rates. Scanner settings may be performed to specify either time or joules. Setting the laser at maximum power input to the scanner provides the required joules with minimal temporal tissue exposure. The highest-power lasers need special scanners designed to work with them. These allow treatment in the 1–30 ms exposure range. Other scanners can only use low power and longer exposure times. Total joules, 25–150% greater than standard FEDL systems, may be delivered. Test spots are applied in cosmetic units. Minimal or no purpura to mild blanching of the skin is the initial clinical endpoint. Total energy is then modified by adjusting the *exposure time* as indicated to achieve lesion lightening, or decreasing excessive tissue reaction. Readiness for retreatment is judged at 8–12 week intervals. Antibiotic ointment is used for any crusting.

Shuttered vascular drilling and tracing

Arteriovenous malformations (spider angiomas) of small size may be treated with either FEDL or CW lasers. However, medium to large 'feeding' vessels are approached with CW (freehand) in a particular fashion. Treatment of spider angiomas requires special techniques because of the depth of the feeding vessel and its frequently high flow rate; therefore the central vessel technique will be discussed first.

Lidocaine 2% is sparingly injected beneath the spider angioma central vessel (or a nerve block) to make the vascular drilling and coagulation procedure painless. One should take care not to blanch or inject the malformation. A CW visible-light vascular laser at 1–20 W may be shuttered at 10–100 ms with a spot size of 0.1–1 mm in superimposed impulses over the vessel. The beam is maintained in exactly the same axis. Fluences of 100–300 J/cm^2 are used to achieve vaporization for drilling. Diascopy may facilitate locating one or more feeding vessels. Deeper or more resistant vessels may require preliminary ink markings with a fine-tipped liquid-ink pen. This causes pinpoint vaporization of the overlying epidermis, facilitating high-intensity beam penetration to deeper, high-flow and slightly larger-diameter feeding vessels.[30]

A repeat shuttered tracing technique applied to dilated radiating runoff vessels from the central spot may be used with a power setting of 1–20 W, a pulse duration of 6–100 ms and a spot size of 0.1–2 mm. In general, the highest peak power and shortest tissue duration minimizes thermal spread and maximizes patient comfort. Fluences achieved are generally in the range 10–20 J/cm^2. Tissue exposures for draining vessels are not superimposed. Instead, individual spots are separated by 1–2 mm along the length of the vessel, while disappearance of the blood within the vessel or extremely faint blanching is the clinical endpoint as one traces toward the origin. Alternatively, for very fine, numerous, perhaps confluent draining vessels, a scanning attachment to the continuous wave system or incorporation of an FEDL system in the treatment for the small vessels is desirable.

Photothermolysis of spider angiomas is highly successful, and yields excellent cosmetic results consistently, and therefore is highly indicated. This is in contrast to treatment of medium- and larger-sized spider angiomas with electrodesiccation and epilating needle techniques, where more frequent failures and depressed hypopigmented scars are more commonly encountered than when applied to small superficial vessels.

Tracing of leg veins in skin types I and II is generally performed with spot sizes of 1–5 mm. The larger spots are restricted to the FEDL systems, some of which offer an elliptical spot. Fluences of 12–25 J are often required. As with sclerotherapy, treatment failures, recurrences and prolonged hyperpigmentation must be anticipated. Proper vessel selection enhances chances of patient and physician satisfaction. The advantages of this method include treatment of superficial vessels that are difficult or too small or fragile to inject. Currently several of these systems are under study to evaluate their efficacy and best treatment parameters. As with facial vessels, there appears to be a strong niche for both FEDL systems and the non-purpura-producing vascular lasers.

Photocoagulation of larger volume lesions

Another photocoagulation technique used for lesions several millimeters and larger employs a moderate spot size, approximately 2 mm in diameter. This is used in the treatment of lesions such as venous lakes[31] and cherry angiomas with a continuous wave. Visible vascular lasers are employed, such as the KTP, tunable dye and copper-vapor lasers. High power settings from 3 to 10 W, CW mode, in an airbrush or painting fashion are used.

For raised or thickened lesions, a clear glass slide is used to partially compress the lesion, reducing its volume and the distance from the anterior to the posterior wall (Figure 57.16).[32] A thin layer of blood should remain within the lesion to provide the chromophore. A smooth continuous motion is employed that is just sufficient to lightly blanch the tissue. This should be carefully carried to the peripheral border of the lesion, or recurrence is likely. This approach is highly indicated because of its ease of application for both cosmetic surgeon and patient and also the consistency of excellent results. The color and texture are most often excellent, and indistinguishable from adjacent untreated tissue after healing is accomplished. This is in contrast to other techniques, which frequently leave a small bead scar or at least prominent discoloration of a focal area.

CELLULAR-LEVEL SELECTIVE PHOTOTHERMOLYSIS

Cellular-level selective photothermolysis is currently used to treat dyschromias caused by either excess melanocytes or pigment in deco-

rative or traumatic tattoos. Also under investigation are hair-removal lasers that depend on melanin content or an exogenously applied chromophore that penetrates close to germinative cells. Tissue-level cosmetic laser surgery is exemplified by the use of *moderately high fluences* of vascular selective wavelengths to photocoagulate the desired blood vessels. In contrast, cellular or subcellular photothermolysis employs *extremely high fluences*, and wavelengths that photomechanically disrupt individual cells or pigment particles found intracellularly or extracellularly. Mechanical disruption of pigment is 'highly indicated' compared with other approaches because of spatial confinement of injury. Photofragmentation of selected chromophores is accomplished while leaving adjacent nontarget cells and tissues unharmed. Excellent cosmetic results are accomplished more reliably

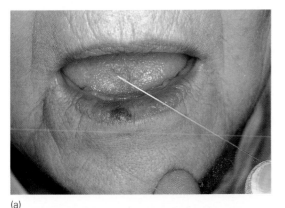

(a)

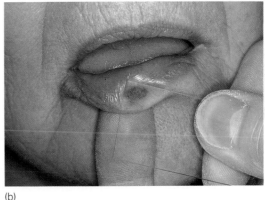

(b)

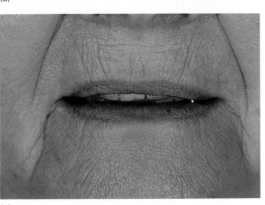

(c)

Figure 57.16 (a–c) Coagulation of labial venous lake with a CW laser.

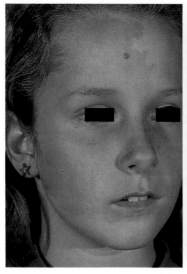 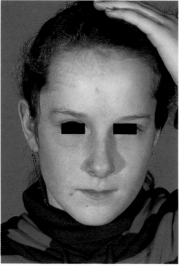

(a)   (b)

Figure 57.17 (a, b) Café-au-lait removal by ruby laser. An extensive right-hemiface congenital café-au-lait has normal pigmentation restored without scarring.

and frequently than with previous methods.[33] Figure 57.17 shows the result of ruby-laser treatment of café-au-lait hyperpigmentation.

Advantages of cellular-level photothermolysis include great precision and minimal trauma to adjacent tissue, frequently no need for anesthesia, greater safety, and reduced risk of infection since the skin surface remains wholly or largely intact. Ultimately, a better immediate and long-term appearance relative to other surgical approaches is likely. Disadvantages include the use of sizeable and expensive equipment and multiple treatments, and some pigments are resistant. Surgical excision and dermabrasion may have undesired and less predictable cosmetic results, but they are frequently accomplished in a single session.

Laser hardware

The Q-switched ruby laser, the Q-switched YAG/KTP laser, the flashlamp-excited green dye laser (pigmented lesion dye laser or PLDL) and the alexandrite laser are the preeminent systems available today for selective photothermolysis of melanin and tattoos. While the argon and CO_2 lasers remain valuable and may be used for superficial resurfacing and removal of extremely superficial melanocytic lesions, precise technique is crucial and the cosmetic results are far less predictable compared with selective photothermolysis. The argon and CO_2 lasers use a photocoagulative mechanism, which injures adjacent and subjacent tissue to a variable degree and can result in undesired pigmentary and textural changes. This earns the CO_2 and argon lasers the more limited indication ('selective indication') for superficial pigmentary disorders or for the treatment of tattoos.

Not all of these high-fluence lasers are equally applicable to various dyschromias. Their particular suitability is best understood by analyzing the wavelength absorption in the various pigments, as well as the wavelengths'

Table 57.3 Comparison of lasers for treating pigmented lesions

Laser	Melanin		Tattoo		
	Superficial	Deep	Black-blue/black	Red	Green
PLDL	++	0	0	+	0
Q-KTP	++	0	+	++	0
Q-Ruby	+++	++	+++	+	++
Alexandrite	+++	+	+++	+	++
Q-YAG	+	+	++/+++	0	0

relative transmission through the dermis to reach deeper pigment. Table 57.3 shows a comparison of various types.

The short wavelength of the green flash-lamp-excited dye laser (PLDL) and the moderately high melanin absorption efficiency make it well suited for extremely superficial melanocytic lesions. The poor penetration of the short wavelength actually protects deeper chromophores and tissue (e.g. vascular) that could non-selectively absorb the laser energy. The Q-switched ruby and alexandrite lasers (694 and 755 nm respectively) are poorly absorbed by any chromophores in the dermis except for melanin or tattoo pigment. Many red tattoo pigments are removed partially or completely by these lasers; however, a few are resistant. The Q-switched YAG/KTP offers two

wavelengths: 1064 nm (YAG) and 532 nm (KTP). The 1064 nm wavelength is used for tattoo removal like the Q-switched ruby and alexandrite lasers; however, it is not effective for the removal of green pigments. At least one research study has shown the Q-switched YAG/KTP at 532 nm to remove red tattoo pigments faster and significantly better than the ruby and alexandrite lasers. Q-YAG-induced 'epidermabrasion' likely explains a significant amount of its red advantage. Figure 57.18 shows the results of tattoo removal by a ruby laser.

Another notable clinical difference between Q-ruby and Q-YAG laser treatment of tattoos is the immediate tissue effect. Q-YAG laser total energy outputs per pulse are significantly lower than those of ruby and alexan-

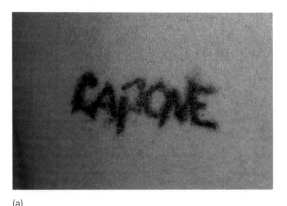

(a)

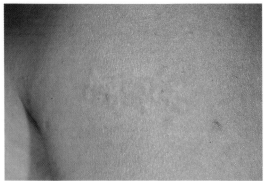

(b)

Figure 57.18 (a, b) Tattoo removal with the ruby laser.

drite lasers, but Q-YAG lasers can fire repeated pulses more rapidly. The net result is that the Q-YAG laser fires smaller, briefer, more rapid impulses to achieve comparable tattoo removal efficacy. The immediate clinical difference is purpura, and more epidermal disruption and bleeding from Q-YAG treatments (seldom seen with the ruby or alexandrite). Approximately 80% of tattoo patients experiencing both Q-YAG and Q-ruby treatments would prefer to avoid the skin disruption. However, many found Q-YAG discomfort preferable to Q-ruby.

The Q-switched YAG infrared wavelength (1060 nm) is poorly absorbed by melanin compared with tattoo pigments, with only 10% efficiency compared with the ruby laser's melanin absorption efficiency. Q-switched YAG is generally not efficacious for deep melanin (except nevus of Ota). A benefit for darker skin types treated with the Q-YAG laser may be less hypopigmentation – for example, especially in the first 6 months after treatment.

Techniques

Usually topical anesthesia cream (e.g. EMLA) is used; however, nerve-block anesthesia or occasionally local anesthesia may be used for more sensitive and larger areas of the face (e.g. moderate to large café-au-lait or large lentigos) and also for particularly sensitive areas over the anterior chest, breast, finger and ankle. Average initial settings are 2–5 J, depending on laser, pigment, etc., derived from individual patient test spots and experience.

Ruby or alexandrite lasers often cause a prominent temporary whitening of the impact site, which usually fades within minutes. This whitening is not photocoagulation as observed in low- to moderate-fluence laser treatments. Instead, it represents tissue-water cavitation bubbles. Initial settings for decorative and traumatic carbon-based tattoos are 2-5 J. Melanocytic lesions, depending on

wavelength, may require settings of 2–10 J. Superficial dark lesions generally require lower energies, while deeper, lighter colored lesions require higher energies. Energies are increased as required to achieve immediate tissue reaction or maintain clinical fading progress.

While punctate bleeding occasionally occurs with the ruby laser, it is extremely common and more pronounced with the Q-YAG/KTP laser because of the shorter pulse width. Q-switched lasers and PLDL frequently ablate superficial melanocytic lesions. Antibiotic ointment and bandage dressing are frequently used to protect the site for 3–5 days.

Treatment impulses generally should not be superimposed. This is seldom helpful in destroying pigment, but may damage tissue. The number of treatments is determined by a combination of pigment type(s), quantity and depth. Energy settings are increased as needed to see immediate tissue reaction or clinical progress, without scarring. Some tattoos may be removed in as few as one or two treatments, as is seen for some lentigos and ephelides. Responsive café-au-lait patches may require three or five treatments, while an average number for denser tattoos is five to eight treatments. Treatment interval recommendations range from three to six weeks. There should be no prominent inflammation prior to repeat treatments.

DISORDER CATEGORIES

An overview of disorders readily treated with lasers will be listed by disorder categories: *vascular problems* are divided into malformations and hyperproliferations; *dyschromias* will be discussed as melanocytic and exogenous pigments; and a third category of *tissue hypertrophy* or *proliferation* or *dysmorphogenesis* will be included. Practical points and comparisons of various approaches will be mentioned. More thorough technique descriptions are listed in the preceding section.

Vascular problems: malformations and hyperproliferations

There is a series of important decisions to make in the selection of lasers for cutaneous vascular lesions. The first and most important one is whether the vascular anomaly is a malformation or a hyperproliferation. A *malformation* is an expansion or dilatation of vascular elements, which may be caused by a variety of factors, including anomalous connections, genetic constitution of the vascular wall, acquired damage (as seen in poikiloderma of Civatte and post-rhinoplasty erythema) and hormonally induced effects. *Hyperproliferation* implies an actual increase in the number of blood vessels (which may or may not be normal), as is commonly seen in proliferative hemangiomas of infancy and pyogenic granuloma and neovascularization, which may occur after surgery, trauma or spontaneously. We shall discuss malformations first.

My basic approach to preferences of lasers and techniques employed in the treatment of malformations is best viewed in the 'visual conceptual blueprint for laser preferences and vascular criteria' (based on safety, efficacy and efficiency) (see Figure 57.12). In this context, consider the treatment of an infant with non-distinguishable individual microvessels, or a patient with matte telangiectasia nearly confluent on the face, or a patient with a dark ruddy skin from rosacea or a bright confluent blush from a rhinoplasty or other similar surgery. These patients' extensive conditions would be considered to be preferentially treated with highly reproducible, precisely quantified laser exposures administered most efficiently. Preferences lie with either the flashlamp-excited dye laser[34,35] or a scanner attachment to the highest-power CW visible laser system that will allow a minimum tissue exposure time (e.g. a KTP) or high-powered argon, dye or copper-vapor system.[26]

Poikiloderma of Civatte

This condition on delicate mobile areas of neck skin is very well suited to the FEDL approach, particularly when the surface area is large and the pattern is discontinuous. Relatively low fluences (3–5 J) are safest initially. One should reduce fluences toward the treatment periphery (by laser settings or by further defocusing the handpiece to obtain a larger spot) to feather the laser-treated area for better cosmesis. In some cases melanocytic pigmentation may be treated with the Q-switched ruby or other lasers recommended for superficial melanin pigment. Variable amounts of brown pigment remaining are likely hemosiderin or postinflammatory hyperpigmentation. This often responds poorly to further treatment, and a test spot is advisable prior to extensive pigment laser treatment. In some cases clearance may be best left to time with assistance from fading creams and sunblock.

Telangiectasias

Larger, higher-flow, arborizing or linear telangiectasias possess a greater volume of blood. I often prefer to treat with CW or quasi-CW visible-light laser vascular systems in a freehand shuttered fashion.[36] This larger type of vessel is seen frequently in rosacea, essential telangiectasia, actinic damage, radiation damage and spider angiomata.

Advantages of the electromechanically shuttered CW laser approach for telangiectatic malformations include the high success rate in a single treatment, excellent cosmetic results, minor patient discomfort, low risk of any noticeable scar, and the absence of purpura associated with FEDL treatment. The use of black liquid, fine-point pen ink applied in a pinpoint dot over the center of the feeding vessel allows vaporization of a very narrow channel down to the feeding vessel with enhanced success and cosmetic results.[30] Surgeons and patients should be aware of the high rate of recurrence of vessels located close to the floor of the naris. FEDL treatments may be slightly more efficacious and minimize risk of texture change.

Treatment of leg telangiectasias benefits from some knowledge of phlebology. Carefully selected linear or arborizing telangiectasias on the lower legs can respond well to laser treatment. Recall that with lasers and sclerotherapy, prolonged hyperpigmentation, recurrence and/or scarring may be encountered increasingly as one progresses from proximal to distal.[37,38] The best responding telangiectasias are small (0.1–0.5 mm), bright red to violet in color, very superficial, blanche on mild pressure and gradually refill after blanching. It is my impression that their superficial location, relatively low flow and thin wall account for their response to moderate laser fluences compared with other leg veins.

Neovascularization after surgery, trauma and sometimes sclerotherapy is sometimes listed as a hyperproliferation; but generally I regard it and treat it as a telangiectatic malformation; combining laser therapy with sclerotherapy for various sizes and types of vessels helps optimize results.

Hyperproliferation

Hemangiomas and pyogenic granulomas are caused by proliferation of vascular elements. A treatment decision requires the location and thickness of the hemangioma, the age of the patient and the growth pattern that the hemangioma has been exhibiting. A thorough discussion of this subject is beyond the scope of this chapter. However, cosmetic laser treatment of hemangiomas also has an important medical and functional basis, and therefore earns this application a high indication.

Macular hemangiomas appearing at birth or shortly thereafter in important cosmetic or functionally important locations may be treated early with laser therapy to retard growth, to stabilize the lesion or even in some cases to achieve a major regression or complete disappearance.[39] These proliferating vessels are individually very small and densely confluent – locating these characteristics on my conceptual blueprint of laser preferences and vascular criteria indicates treatment with the FEDL or CW sources with very short electromechanically shuttered tissue exposures. In infants with small- to moderate-size hemangiomas no anesthesia is used. In larger lesions nerve-block (preferably) or possibly local anesthesia is considered. FEDL treatment is normally administered at 6–7 J, and a repeat evaluation and possible treatment is scheduled usually 4 weeks later. Initial treatments of proliferative hemangiomas with CW scanner or shuttered freehand approaches should strive for very slight superficial blanching. Stabilization and regression of hemangiomas can frequently be achieved with considerably milder photocoagulation endpoints than required for vascular malformations. If a nearly macular hemangioma continues to increase in size despite a first or second treatment as described, or is already thicker than 2–3 mm, then steroid therapy needs to be considered in the therapeutic program.

Once a hemangioma has been stable for months or has even shown some regression on its own (most likely after the age of 9 months), I find it the best course to allow natural regression to take place if at all possible to a maximum point most often reached by age 5 or 6 years. Subsequently surgical incision of remaining hemangioma or redundant skin and fibrofatty degeneration can be accomplished. It is during the first 9-month period of growth that proliferative hemangiomas are most laser- and steroid-responsive. However, after the age of maximum spontaneous improvement, laser therapy again has a considerable role in cosmesis for treating telangiectasias or small residual amounts of hemangioma. I believe the early application of laser therapy to selected superficial hemangiomas does significantly improve long-term cosmesis. It is uncertain whether laser therapy can play a significant helpful role in subcutaneous hemangiomas or the deep component of transcutaneous hemangiomas.

Pyogenic granuloma

Pyogenic granulomas may be treated by excision with a CO_2 laser in incisional mode alternating with spot coagulation as required or direct vaporization. More recently, treatment with visible light lasers has been found to be successful in a limited number of cases.[40,41]

Dyschromias: melanocytic and exogenous pigments

Dyschromias will be divided into melanocytic and exogenous pigment dyschromias.

Melanocytic dyschromias

These include freckles, lentigos, chloasma, café-au-lait, benign nevi and postinflammatory hyperpigmentation (particularly that of long standing, such as is associated with burns). The treatment of melanocytic dyschromias is best divided into two categories: superficial dyschromias and deep dyschromias.

Superficial dyschromias

Numerous options in cosmetic cutaneous laser surgery treatments exist for freckles, lentigos and some junctional nevi. Certainly liquid nitrogen, argon-laser coagulation and CO_2-laser resurfacing are capable of removing many superficial melanocytic dyschromias with good to excellent results. However, occasional and unpredictable postinflammatory hyperpigmentation, permanent hypopigmentation and, rarely, undesirable texture changes do occur. The availability and low cost of 'low-tech' approaches argues for their early consideration in superficial melanocyte dyschromias.

The high degree of patient satisfaction with the results of high-fluence lasers such as the Q-switched ruby and alexandrite lasers and the PLDL, the lack of need for injectable anesthesia and the good cosmetic results, earn at least a selective indication for the high-fluence laser results.

Moderate- or high-fluence lasers offer insurance against undesired hypo- or hyperpigmentation and textural change, as well as avoidance of the need for anesthesia. The Q-switched ruby laser, green FEDL (PLDL), alexandrite laser and Q-switched YAG/KTP laser may all be used to safely eliminate such superficial melanocytes.

The CO_2- or argon-laser technique depends a great deal on the speed of hand movement.[5,42]

Deep dyschromias

For deeper melanocytic lesions such as chloasma, café-au-lait, compound melanocytic nevi and postinflammatory hyperpigmentation, only the Q-switched ruby laser has been proven effective. The alexandrite laser has potential to be shown likewise effective, since its wavelength is closer to that of the ruby than to that of the infrared YAG laser (1060 nm). The patient ordinarily needs no anesthesia, and discomfort is approximately that of a rubber band snap against the skin. Several to many weeks may be required before fading is appreciated. Repeat evaluation and potential repeat treatment are conducted at 6–8 weeks. Commonly 10–12 weeks are recommended for conditions such as chloasma that may develop temporary postinflammatory hyperpigmentation, which we allow to subside before judging the effects of treatment. Nevus of Ota patients may require several treatments, and delays of 3–6 months are not uncommon before fading is noted. These patients frequently require a treatment course of two years or more to accomplish maximal lightening. Frequently, elevated compound nevi are treated with split-thickness removal of the nevus primarily, and a Q-switched ruby laser is secondarily utilized to remove any residual pigmentation. This accomplishes a nearly scarless texture of the skin while obtaining removal of color without incision lines.

Tattoos

Exogenous tattoos include decorative tattoos as well as traumatic tattoos obtained from gunpowder blasts or asphalt and similar road substances. Photothermal means of treating tattoos have included the argon and CO_2 lasers. Argon-laser treatments produce accentuated scar tissue in the vicinity of the pigment because of enhanced laser absorption. While most pigment is not removed with this approach, scar tissue partially obscures pigment by light scattering and absorption, resulting in apparent lightening of the tattoo. Unfortunately, incomplete blocking of the tattoo color and undesirable texture change are most common with this technique.

The CO_2 laser technique has been successful at removing tattoo pigments. However, early attempts were frequently criticized because of scar tissue being sharply demarcated in the shape of the original tattoo and because of hypertrophic scarring. Improvements in the methodology combined in what I have dubbed the 'Swiss cheese technique' are described in detail in the technique section of this chapter. The combination of uniform laser beam exposure and high fluences is used to vaporize the most superficial layers of skin and remove gross amounts of tattoo pigment. The outline of the tattoo shape is feathered into adjoining tissue such that a graduated transition blends texture, color and shape much more harmoniously.

The second major component of the technique is the employment of very small spot sizes and electromechanically shuttered or pulsed tissue exposures directed to very small pigment depots at mid and deeper levels of the dermis. The Swiss cheese technique accomplishes goals of more complete pigment removal with better wound healing than either dermabrasion or salabrasion can. This approach is selectively indicated for tattoos that have proven partially or largely resistant to Q-switched laser removal or where multiple visits are not an alternative or the newer technology is not available.

The best cosmetic results in decorative or traumatic tattoo removal are accomplished with Q-switched ruby, Q-switched YAG or alexandrite lasers.[33,43] The relative advantage of the ruby and probably the alexandrite laser is the removal of green pigments, for which the Q-switched YAG is less effective. The YAG laser has been shown to be somewhat more effective in the removal of certain types of red tattoo pigments. The clear superiority of results and even complete clearing of tattoos in 75% of cases earns the Q-switched-laser approach a strong indication for treatment of decorative and traumatic tattoos.

Tissue hypertrophy, proliferation or dysplasia

This category combines very disparate disorders that have in common undesirable thickening or elevation of tissue. This includes tissue hypertrophy, proliferation or dysmorphogenesis conditions amenable to cosmetic cutaneous laser surgery. This category comprises four groups:

- chronic solar injury, including actinic cheilitis and solar photoaging (elastosis, hyperpigmentation and wrinkling);
- genetic and congenital conditions, including localized adnexal tumors, angiofibromas, syringomas and nuerofibromas;
- excessive or undesirable wound healing with thickened and hypertrophic scars and keloids;
- xanthelasma and rhinophyma, whose cause is currently unknown – although xanthelasma is associated in a minority of cases with hypercholesterolemia, and rhinophyma's association with rosacea is well known.

Actinic cheilitis and photoaging

Treatment of actinic cheilitis with the CO_2 laser is strongly indicated. Results have been documented in numerous studies to be superior to lip shaves and vermilionectomy followed by mucosal advancement flap. Treatment of actinic cheilitis and photoaging is discussed on pages 665–668. Local and nerve-block anesthesia allow painless and rapid treatment with excellent cosmetic and functional results. Laser resurfacing has caused a major paradigm shift in the treatment of lower-eyelid blepharoplasty: in combination with transconjunctival laser fat removal, *both* better removal of fine periorbital wrinkling *and* lower complication rates have occurred. Additionally, the precision of laser resurfacing has greatly expanded the number of people willing to seek textural improvement of their skin.

Adnexal tumors, genetic syndromes

Localized sporadic adnexal tumors as well as genetic syndromes may frequently result in scattered elevated lesions of great cosmetic concern. Laser treatment allows rapid treatment of many or few lesions, is repeatable over time (many new lesions are likely to appear in certain genetic disorders), and allows treatment in highly mobile areas with difficult access to other instruments (e.g. the periorbital zone, lip and nares). Therefore in properly selected cases the use of cutaneous laser treatment for cosmesis is highly indicated. The technique is accomplished under local anesthesia, and is described in detail on page 672.

Scar tissue

The treatment of keloids and thickened scars and hypertrophic scars with lasers is controversial. The CO_2 laser has been used successfully by numerous investigators to excise keloids, followed by steroid treatment intralesionally, or to superficially plane thickened scar tissue. Hypertrophic scars have been treated with the CO_2 and/or argon lasers with a small focused drilling technique and very brief tissue exposures to induce scar atrophy, with or without a supplementary intralesional steroid (see page 671).

Rhinophyma

CO_2-laser treatment of rhinophyma is strongly indicated for its superior precision and results compared with other modalities for recontouring and for the superior blending into adjacent cosmetic units. Superior visualization of tissue level is accomplished in both rhinophyma and xanthelasma. An ablational technique is used, and a bloodless field and lack of aerosol enhance the surgeon's precision and safety. Recent reports of FEDL treatment for xanthelasma suggest that greater safety may be available as a trade-off for numerous treatments.

HIRSUTISM

Hirsutism, or simply unwanted hair, is now removable with lasers. Although the procedure is still experimental, there is no question that hair can be removed with several laser systems, including the normal-mode ruby and the Q-switched YAG (which may be used with a topically applied chromophore), and photodynamic therapy using photosensitizers such as δ-aminolevulinic acid. The main questions are what is the long-term efficacy of the various approaches and what are the relative side-effects? Side-effects can include hyperpigmentation, prolonged follicular or diffuse erythema, hypopigmentation, and scarring. Without a chromophore or a photosensitizer, primarily pigmented terminal hairs respond, with their melanin acting as the target. Fluences much higher than that required for tattoo removal are employed. An externally applied chromophore that penetrates down the follicular orifice allows pale hair to be treated, as well as the use of lower fluences.

To date, multiple treatments are required for all systems, and some regrowth is inevitable. Early results suggest that ruby-laser treatment efficacy is probably better with the ruby laser on terminal hairs, but hyperpigmentation may be slightly higher as well. Q-YAG with chromophore offers some chance of improvement to the otherwise nonresponding, nonpigmented hairs. Therefore it is likely that several wavelengths and devices will be used, giving physicians flexibility for various skin types and hair colors as well as for patients with varying tolerances to side-effects.

SUMMARY

A broad definition of cosmetic cutaneous laser surgery has been used here to introduce three perspectives that cosmetic laser surgeons subconsciously employ in contemplating a laser-therapeutic approach. These three perspectives serve as a framework to support a decision-making process that weighs the available lasers, their functions, surgical techniques achieved with or without lasers, their relative benefits, and finally the perspective of individual diagnoses.

Specific techniques have been described and referenced and conceptual approaches described in novel ways so that new or experienced cosmetic laser surgeons will be better able to integrate new information on laser wavelengths, types, settings and 'recipes' offered in textbooks and at conferences. The cosmetic surgeon is encouraged to apply the three-perspective approach, incorporating laser hardware, procedures and diagnoses, in cosmetic laser surgery to help solve real-world cosmetic surgical problems.

REFERENCES

1. Abergel RPF, David LM, Aging hands: a technique of hand rejuvenation by laser resurfacing and autologous fat transfer. *J Dermatol Surg Oncol* 1989; **15:** 725–8.

2. David LM, Lask GP, Glassberg E et al, Laser abrasion for cosmetic and medical treatment of facial actinic damage. *Cutis* 1989; **43:** 583–7.

3. Spadoni D, Cain CL, Facial resurfacing. Using the carbon dioxide laser. *Aorn J* 1989; **50:** 1009–13.

4. Rosio TJ, Actinic cheilitis and in-situ squamous cell carcinoma. In: *Atlas of Cutaneous Laser Surgery* (Apfelberg DB, ed.). New York: Raven Press, 1992:39–41.

5. Dover JS, Smoller BR, Stern RS et al, Low-fluence carbon dioxide laser irradiation of lentigines. *Arch Dermatol* 1988; **124:** 1219–24.

6. David LM, Laser vermilion ablation for actinic cheilitis. *J Dermatol Surg Oncol* 1985; **11:** 605–8.

7. Zelickson BD, Roenigk RK, Actinic cheilitis. Treatment with the carbon dioxide laser. *Cancer* 1990; **65:** 1307–11.

8. Garrett AB, Defresne RJ, Ratz JL et al, Carbon dioxide laser treatment of pitted acne scarring. *J Dermatol Surg Oncol* 1990; **16:** 737–40.

9. Solotoff SA, Treatment for pitted acne scarring – postauricular punch grafts followed by dermabrasion. *J Dermatol Surg Oncol* 1986; **12:** 1079–84.

10. Apfelberg DB, Master MR, Lash H et al, Treatment of xanthelasma palpebrarum with the carbon dioxide laser. *J Dermatol Surg Oncol* 1987; **13:** 149–51.

11. Schonermark MP, Raulin C, Treatment of xanthelasma palpebrarum with the pulsed dye laser. *Lasers Surg Med* 1996; **19:** 336–9.

12. Shapshay SM, Strong MS, Anastasi GW et al, Removal of rhinophyma with the carbon dioxide laser: a preliminary report. *Arch Otolaryngol* 1980; **106:** 257–9.

13. Wheeland RG, Bailin PL, Ratz J et al, Combined carbon dioxide laser excision and vaporization in the treatment of rhinophyma. *J Dermatol Surg Oncol* 1987; **13:** 172–7.

14. Henderson DL, Hypertrophic surgical scar. In: *Atlas of Cutaneous Laser Surgery* (Apfelberg DB, ed.). New York: Raven Press, 1992:270–1.

15. Henderson DL, Post-thermal hypertrophic scar. In: *Atlas of Cutaneous Laser Surgery* (Apfelberg DB, ed.). New York: Raven Press, 1992:143–5.

16. Flores JT, Apfelberg DB, Maser MR et al, Trichoepithelioma: successful treatment with the argon laser. *Plast Reconstr Surg* 1984; **74:** 694–8.

17. Weston J, Apfelberg DB, Maser MR et al, Carbon dioxide laserabrasion for treatment of adenoma sebaceum in tuberous sclerosis. *Ann Plast Surg* 1985; **15:** 132–7.

18. Bellack GS, Shapshay SM, Management of facial angiofibromas in tuberous sclerosis: use of the carbon dioxide laser. *Otolaryngol Head Neck Surg* 1986; **94:** 34–40.

19. Becker DJ, Use of the carbon dioxide laser in

treating multiple cutaneous neurofibromas. *Ann Plast Surg* 1991; **26:** 582–6.

20. Rosio TJ, CO_2 laser treatment of homemade tattoo. In: *Atlas of Cutaneous Laser Surgery* (Apfelberg DB, ed.). New York: Raven Press, 1992:87–8.

21. Reid R, Muller S, Tattoo removal by CO_2 laser dermabrasion. *Plast Reconstr Surg* 1980; **65:** 717–28.

22. Sunde D, Apfelberg DB, Sergott T et al, Traumatic tattoo removal: comparison of four treatment methods in an animal model with correlation to clinical experience. *Lasers Surg Med* 1990; **10:** 158–64.

23. Baker SS, Muenzler WS, Small RG et al, Carbon dioxide laser blepharoplasty. *Ophthalmology* 1984; **91:** 238–44.

24. Morrow SM, Morrow LB, CO_2 laser blepharoplasty. A comparison with cold-steel surgery. *J Dermatol Surg Oncol* 1992; **18:** 307–13.

25. David LM, The laser approach to blepharoplasty. *J Dermatol Surg Oncol* 1988; **14:** 741–6.

26. Rosio TJ, Superficial vascular lasers: yellow light and 532 nm. In: *Surgical Dermatology: Advances in Current Practice* (Roenigk RK, Roenigk HH Jr, eds). London: Martin Dunitz, 1993:323–40.

27. Tan OT, Stafford TM, Murray S et al, Histologic comparison of the pulsed dye laser and copper vapor laser effects on pig skin. *Lasers Surg Med* 1990; **10:** 551–8.

28. McDaniel DH, Mordon S, Hexascan: a new robotized scanning laser handpiece. *Cutis* 1990; **45:** 300–5.

29. Scheibner A, Wheeland RG, Argon-pumped tunable dye laser therapy for facial port-wine stain hemangiomas in adults – a new technique using small spot size and minimal power. *J Dermatol Surg Oncol* 1989; **15:** 277–82.

30. Rosio TJ, Tunable dye laser treatment of spider angiomas. In: *Atlas of Cutaneous Laser Surgery* (Apfelberg DB, ed.). New York: Raven Press, 1992:378–9.

31. Neumann RA, Knobler RM, Venous lakes (Bean–Walsh) of the lips – treatment experience with the argon laser and 18 months follow-up. *Clin Exp Dermatol* 1990; **15:** 115–18.

32. Rosio TJ, Tunable dye laser plus diascopy for venous lake. In: *Atlas of Cutaneous Laser Surgery* (Apfelberg DB, ed.). New York: Raven Press, 1992:398–9.

33. Scheibner A, Kenny G, White W et al, A superior method of tattoo removal using the Q-switched ruby laser. *J Dermatol Surg Oncol* 1990; **16:** 1091–8.

34. Lowe NJ, Behr KL, Fitzpatrick R et al, Flash lamp pumped dye laser for rosacea-associated telangiectasia and erythema. *J Dermatol Surg Oncol* 1991; **17:** 522–5.

35. Rosio TJ, FEDL treatment of matte telangiectasias in collagen vascular disease and rosacea. In: *Atlas of Cutaneous Laser Surgery* (Apfelberg DB, ed.). New York: Raven Press, 1992:356–8.

36. Rosio TJ, Tunable dye laser treatment of large telangiectasias. In: *Atlas of Cutaneous Laser Surgery* (Apfelberg DB, ed.). New York: Raven Press, 1992:351–3.

37. Apfelberg DB, Smith T, Maser MR et al, Study of three laser systems for treatment of superficial varicosities of the lower extremity. *Lasers Surg Med* 1987; **7:** 219–23.

38. Goldman MP, Fitzpatrick RE, Pulsed-dye laser treatment of leg telangiectasia: with and without simultaneous sclerotherapy. *J Dermatol Surg Oncol* 1990; **16:** 338–44.

39. Garden JM, Bakus AD, Paller AS et al, Treatment of cutaneous hemangiomas by the flashlamp-pumped pulsed dye laser: prospective analysis. *J Pediatr* 1992; **120:** 555–60.

40. Goldberg DJ, Sciales CW, Pyogenic granuloma in children. Treatment with the flashlamp-pumped pulsed dye laser. *J Dermatol Surg Oncol* 1991; **17:** 960–2.

41. Glass T, Milgraum S, Flashlamp-pumped pulsed dye laser treatment for pyogenic granuloma. *Cutis* 1992; **49:** 351–3.

42. Ohshiro T, Maruyama Y, Nakajima H et al, Treatment of pigmentation of the lips and oral mucosa in Peutz–Jeghers syndrome using ruby and argon lasers. *Br J Plast Surg* 1980; **33:** 346–9.

43. Goldman L, Wilson RG, Radiation from a Q-switched ruby laser: effect of repeated impacts of power output of 10 megawatts on a tattoo of man, *J Invest Dermatol* 1965; **40:** 121–2.

58

Cosmetic cryosurgery

Rodney D Sinclair, Christopher Tzermias, Rodney Dawber

INTRODUCTION

Most cryosurgeons limit themselves to warts and solar keratoses; some also treat skin cancers. Many forget the diverse range of conditions, both pathological and cosmetic, amenable to treatment with liquid nitrogen. Cryosurgical treatments, when applied correctly, produce excellent cosmetic results, which fully justify a description of these techniques in a cosmetic surgery text.

As liquid nitrogen is freely available and cheap, and its use is relatively painless, it is often thought of as 'low-tech' and unable to compete with the newest lasers. On the contrary, cryosurgery is the equal of high-tech alternatives for therapeutic efficacy and aesthetic outcome for a wide range of conditions.

The following is a description of the specific cryosurgical techniques for treatment of a number of lesions seen by the cosmetic surgeon, and describes the steps to be taken to achieve good cosmetic results.[1,2]

TECHNIQUE AND TERMINOLOGY

While liquid nitrogen is not the only refrigerant available, it is the most commonly used, and the following descriptions are based on its use. The protocols presented are derived from experience gained with the Oxford cryosurgical unit, and, where available, descriptions from the medical literature are presented.

Liquid nitrogen can be applied by dipping a cotton bud into the flask (D), an open spray from a cryo-gun such as the Brymil Cryac (OS), or by use of a probe (P). Thermocouples, electrical impedance monitoring or ultrasound are not required for the treatment of these lesions, ensuring that the technique described is indeed 'low-tech' and accessible to anyone with a cryo-gun.[3]

The open spray technique consists of five steps (Figure 58.1).

1. The area to be treated is delineated by either marking pen (since ice blurs anatomical margins), a neoprene cone or adhesive putty (if there are vulnerable structures nearby), and the nozzle size or probe attachment for the cryo-gun is chosen: the 'A' nozzle for small areas and the 'D' for larger ones. Probes are especially useful when pressure on the lesion is required – for example, when treating vascular lesions.
2. The centre of the lesion is sprayed continuously from a distance of 1 cm from the skin until the field is frozen and confirmed to

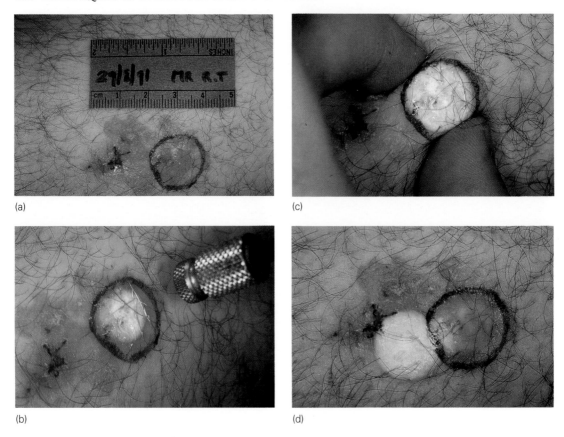

(a)

(b)

(c)

(d)

Figure 58.1 (a–d) Spot freeze technique demonstrated on a large patch of Bowen's disease requiring overlapping fields to obtain an even depth of freezing.

be so by palpatation. Large fields may be broken up into $2\,cm^2$ areas to ensure an even depth of freeze.

3. Time is added to the freeze according to the nature of the lesion being treated; that is, liquid nitrogen is sprayed into the centre of the lesion with the flow adjusted (by varied compressions of the trigger) to maintain the icefield as the predetermined size.

4. Freeze–thaw cycles (FTCs) are performed as necessary. To do this, the lesion is allowed to thaw over a few minutes, and then steps 2 and 3 are repeated. It is important to ensure that the lesion has thawed completely between cycles, and this is tested by palpatation.

The notation for treatment is

$$LN_2(OS),\ x\ seconds,\ y\ FTCs$$

where x is the number of seconds and y is the number of FTCs. This allows for reproducibility of treatment techniques and results by different operators, as well as audit of the outcome.

Table 58.1 Disturbances of pigmentation and melanocytic lesions

Lesion	Technique[a]	Time, No. of FTCs	Margin	Sessions and intervals	Response
Melasma	OS	Uniform ice formation, ×1	Feathering	4–6 weekly, according to response	Moderate
Idiopathic guttate hypomelanosis	OS	5 s, ×1	1 mm	4–6 weekly, according to response	Moderate to good
Tattoos	OS	30 s, ×2	1 mm	4–6 weekly, according to response	54% improved
Freckles	P	Uniform ice formation, ×1	Feathering	Usually only single treatment required	Variable
Solar lentigo	OS or P	5–10 s, ×1	Feathering	Usually only single treatment required	Good
Lentigo simplex	OS or P	Light, ×1	Feathering	Usually only single treatment required	Good

[a] See 'Technique and terminology' section.

Table 58.2 Vascular lesions and naevi

Lesion	Technique[a]	Time, No. of FTCs	Margin	Sessions and intervals	Response
AIDS-related Kaposi's sarcoma	OS	10–60 s, ×2	3 mm	3 at 3-weekly intervals	80% improved
Venous lake	P	10 s, ×1	1 mm	Usually only single treatment required	Excellent
Cherry angiomas	P	10 s, ×1	1 mm	Usually only single treatment required	Good
Angiokeratoma of Mibelli	P or OS	10 s, ×1	1 mm	3 at 2-monthly intervals	Good
Angiokeratoma of the scrotum	P or OS	5–10 s, ×1	1 mm	3 at 2-monthly intervals	Good
Spider naevus	P	10 s, ×1	1 mm	3 at 6-weekly intervals	Good
Capillary haemangioma	P	5–30 s, ×2	1 mm	2–4 at 8-weekly intervals	Excellent
Cavernous haemangioma	P	5–30 s, ×2	1 mm	2–4 at 8-weekly intervals	Excellent

[a] See 'Technique and terminology' section.

Variations on the open spray technique include the paintbrush (PB) method, where treatment is started at one side of the field and moves up and down across the field, and the spiral (Sp) method, where treatment begins in the centre of the field and is then rotated through ever-increasing circles.[4]

'Feathering' is a technique that may be

Table 58.3 Cysts, tumours and naevi

Lesion	Technique[a]	Time, No. of FTCs	Margin	Sessions and intervals	Response
Acne cyst	OS or D PB to peel	5–15 s, ×1	–	2–3 at monthly intervals	Good to excellent
Milia	P	Ice formation, ×1	1 mm	Usually only single treatment required	Good
Myxoid cyst	P or OS	30 s, ×2	1 mm	1–3 at 8-weekly intervals	86% improved
Syringoma	P	Ice formation, ×1	1 mm	2–3 at 1–2- monthly intervals	Good
Trichoepithelioma	P	Ice formation, ×1	1 mm	2–3 at 1–2- monthly intervals	Good
Trichillemmal cyst	OS	Ice formation, ×1	1 mm	2–3 at 1–2- monthly intervals	A minority respond
Steatocystoma multiplex	OS	Ice formation, ×1	1 mm	2–3 at 1–2- monthly intervals	A minority respond
Skin tag	OS or forceps	5–10 s, ×1	1 mm	Usually only single treatment required	Excellent
Hidrocystoma	OS or P	Ice formation, ×1	1 mm	2–3 at 1–2- monthly intervals	Small, good; large, minor
Dermatofibroma	OS or P	30 s, ×1	2 mm	1–3 at 1–2- monthly intervals	90% improved
Seborrhoeic keratosis	OS or D or PB	Ice formation, ×1	1 mm	Usually only single treatment required	Excellent
Sebaceous hyperplacia	OS or P	5–15 s, ×1	1 mm	Usually only single treatment required	Good
Chondrodermatitis nodularis helikis	OS or P	15 s, ×1	2 mm	2–3 at 1–2- monthly intervals	15–20% improved
Verrucous naevus	OS	5 s, ×1	1 mm	Up to 5 at 1–2- monthly intervals	Excellent
Hyperkeratosis naevoid of the nipple	OS	20 s, ×1	1 mm	Up to 5 at 1–2- monthly intervals	Excellent
Acrokeratosis verruciformis (Hopf)	OS	5 s, ×1	1 mm	Several at 6–8- weekly intervals	Excellent
Dermatosis papulosa nigrans	OS or P	Ice formation, ×1	Nil	Several at 6–8- weekly intervals	Excellent, but may depigment
Benign lichenoid keratosis	OS	5 s, ×1	1 mm	Several at 6–8- weekly intervals	Good
Andenoma sebaceum	OS	5–20 s, ×1	1 mm	3–6 at 3-weekly intervals	Satisfactory

[a] See 'Technique and terminology' section.

Table 58.4 Other conditions

Lesion	Technique[a]	Time, No. of FTCs	Margin	Sessions and intervals	Response
Keloid	OS or P	15–30 s, ×1	1 mm	5–10 at 4–8-weekly intervals	Variable
Acne scar	OS	Face 5 s, ×1 Back 5–15 s, ×1	1 mm	1–3 at 4–8-weekly intervals	Good to excellent
Rhinophyma	OS	30 s, ×2	Entire nose	4–6 at 8-weekly intervals	Satisfactory
Xanthelasma	OS	5 s, ×1	1 mm	2–3 at 4–8-weekly intervals	Satisfactory
Alopecia areata	D	2–5 s, ×2	Nil	4 at weekly intervals	Satisfactory
Porokeratosis plantaris discreta	OS	Ice formation, ×1	2 mm	2 at 2-weekly intervals	90.5% improved
Elastosis perforans serpiginosa	OS	10 s, ×1	1–2 mm	2 at weekly intervals	Excellent

[a] See 'Technique and terminology' section.

used for lesions where the freeze required for cure is of sufficient duration to induce permanent hypopigmentation. In order to prevent a sharp border between the ensuing area of pigmentation and loss of pigment, the border is sprayed to ice formation to produce mild hypopigmentation that diminishes the contrast between the treated and untreated areas. Sometimes the appearance of a hypopigmented treated patch on one cheek can be improved by spraying the other cheek to recreate symmetry.

If a lesion involves a single cosmetic unit, such as a solar keratosis on the nose, the best cosmetic outcome will be produced by lightly spraying the entire nose. Because any depigmentation so produced may be permanent, it is better to proceed cautiously when deliberately lightening the skin.

LESION SELECTION

Vast experience in the treatment of numerous and varied skin lesions by cryosurgery has been accumulated over the past 30 or so years since this treatment was popularized by Zacarian for skin neoplasms.[5,6] Much of this experience is summarized in Tables 58.1–58.4, while that pertaining to skin cancer can be found elsewhere.[7]

VASCULAR LESIONS

Spider naevi only require a light freeze. A 5 s single FTC is usually ample. Cryosurgery is a good alternative to fine-wire diathermy for people with pale complexions, especially for diffuse lesions with more than one feeding vessel (Figure 58.2). Diffuse telangiectasia, such as that associated with rosacea, can also be treated with good results, and is a substantially cheaper alternative to the use of a pulsed dye laser.

Cryosurgery is also useful for palliation of HIV-associated Kaposi's sarcoma. Small individual lesions (and a 3 mm margin) can be treated with a 15–30 s single FTC, with an 80% complete response.[8]

Cryoprobes are useful when treating venous

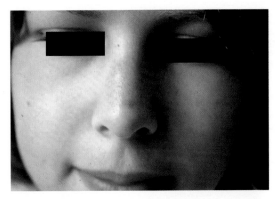

(a)

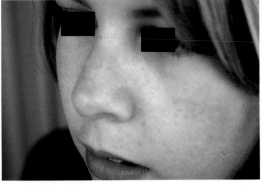

(b)

Figure 58.2 Spider naevus: (a) before and (b) after treatment.

ACNE

The first treatment to be advocated for acne was a solid carbon dioxide slush that acted as a peeling agent to reduce the oiliness of the skin and hastened the resolution of comedones and papules, as well as improving depressed pitted scars. This was superseded by cotton applicators dipped in liquid nitrogen, which has also been used for larger acne cysts. Better results and better control can be achieved with the open spray technique.[9] Small inflammatory papules require a 2–5 s single FTC, while the large cystic lesions of acne conglobata may require a 15–20 s single FTC, depending on their size.

Open spray liquid nitrogen has also been used as an alternative to dermabrasion for diffuse scarring.[10] The skin surface is divided into squares each about 4 cm on a side. Using the paintbrush technique, each segment is frozen for between 5 and 15 s, depending on the depth of the desired peel. Areas of hypertrophic scarring may require longer freezes because of the relative insensitivity of collagen to cold, while areas around the eyes, where the skin is thin, only require 5–10 s single FTCs. If more than one treatment is planned, one month is the suggested interval between sessions. Of the patients so treated, 95% were reported to have had good or excellent results,[10] which were similar to those achieved by superficial dermabrasion, with the advantage of their use in the presence of active acne.

SUN-DAMAGED SKIN AND FACIAL PEELING

Solar keratoses, solar lentigines, solar elastosis, sebaceous hyperplasia, colloid milium and the fine wrinkles of solar aging are all within the realms of unsightly sun-induced lesions amenable to cryosurgery. These lesions occur on highly visible sites, such as the face and hands, and may cause much distress. Cryosurgery is an excellent option for limited disease.

lakes, since they allow the operator to empty the lesion during treatment, which leads to lower tissue temperatures and higher cure rates. A single 10 s FTC is usually sufficient.

There is great variation in the size and depth of cavernus and capillary haemangiomas, and this is paralleled by the variation in freeze times required. For small thin lesions, a single 5 s freeze may suffice, while for larger lesions a 30 s double FTC will be required. Experience in the treatment of these lesions allows the operator to better judge the length of treatment required.

Many clinicians ignore sebaceous hyperplasia; however, a single 5 s FTC will often make these lesions disappear. The same applies to solar elastosis, solar lentigos and many solar keratoses.

For widespread changes, full-face cryo-peels can be used for effective depth-controlled removal of actinic keratoses, pigmented lesions and seborrhoeic keratoses.[10] Healing begins immediately, and is usually complete within 10 days. The skin is left smoother, pinker and tighter, and the results are equivalent to those of a chemical peel, but there is greater control of the depth of the icefield, so it can be adjusted to accommodate localized lesions.

SEBORRHOEIC KERATOSIS

Whether seborrhoeic keratoses are sun-related is still debated. Flat lesions can be effectively treated with a 5 s single FTC, but since keratin insulates the underlying epidermis from the cold, large hyperkeratotic lesions may still survive 30 s double FTCs. The main pitfalls of treatment are the induction of permanent alopecia if hair-bearing areas are treated, and the induction of hypopigmentation. It is for that reason that dermatosis papulosa nigra occurring on pigmented skin is best treated cautiously, and preferably with a test patch of a single lesion.

RHINOPHYMA

Cryosurgery has been used to treat rhinophyma;[11] however, in our hands it has proved to be less effective than dermabrasion or serial shaving. Thirty-second double FTCs are recommended, and can often be performed without anaesthesia or solely with EMLA cream. Multiple treatments are required, but are well tolerated. For mild cases, cryosurgery can still be considered as an inexpensive option with low risk and low morbidity that has some success.

TATTOOS

Good results have been seen after cryosurgery of tattoos in up to 50% of cases (Figure 58.3);[12] however, other modalities are now preferred, since a favourable outcome is more predictable. Nevertheless, for some patients desperate for treatment, there are no affordable alternatives.

KELOIDS

Many cryosurgeons disappointed by the apparent poor response of keloids to liquid nitrogen abandoned this form of treatment. Various techniques had been tried, including

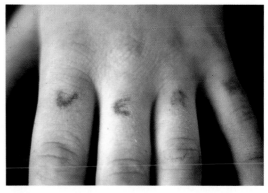

(a)

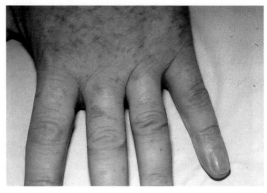

(b)

Figure 58.3 Home-made tattoo: (a) before and (b) after cryosurgery.

prophylactic and intralesional cryotherapy, without success. The poor response was attributed to the relative resistance of fibroblasts and collagen to cold.

More recently published work has suggested that previous treatment failure had been due to impatience, and that often a keloid that has not responded to two or three treatments at monthly intervals will begin to respond after the third or fourth. The protocol advocated suggests that a cryoprobe be used to induce a 30 s single FTC.[13] As there is no completely satisfactory alternative treatment for keloids, perhaps the time has come to revisit cryosurgery.

COMPLICATIONS

Inflammatory morbidity, inevitable side-effects and complications are difficult to separate with this modality of treatment.[14] Table 58.5 lists some of the well-known complications of cryosurgery. Some degree of pain is universal, but its intensity is extremely variable. Many cryosurgeons now use EMLA cream routinely – applied two hours before the treatment. Syncope can occur if the pain is severe, and many prefer to treat patients (particularly young men) lying down. During the freeze time, pain is felt as burning, and during the thaw phase, when pain is commonly worse than during the freeze, it is felt as throbbing. The periungual region and the temples are the most painful sites, and persistent headache is an occasional sequela after treatment of sites close to bone such as the forehead, temple or scalp.

Immediate haemorrhage, if it occurs, is often prolonged, but can usually ultimately be stopped with pressure alone. This can follow the taking of biopsies immediately prior to treatment, but can also occur if a pedunculated lesions is manipulated while frozen and cracks.

Oedema is the product of acute inflammation. Pronounced idiosyncratic oedema may occasionally occur after short freezes.

Table 58.5 Side-effects of cryosurgery
Immediate
• Pain
• Headache
• Haemorrhage
• Oedema and blister formation
• Syncope
Delayed
• Infection
• Haemorrhage
• Excessive formation of granulation tissue
Prolonged but usually temporary
• Hyperpigmentation
• Milia
• Hypertrophic scars
• Alteration of sensation
Prolonged and usually permanent
• Hypopigmentation
• Alopecia
• Atrophy
• Ectropion
• Notching of the eyelids, ear or vermillion border

Oedema is often more severe around the eyelids and lips. The oedema can be partly inhibited by a single application of a potent topical steroid immediately following treatment,[15] and if severe oedema is anticipated then systemic corticosteroids can be used.

Hypopigmentation is virtually universal following tumour doses of cryosurgery owing to the exquisite sensitivity of melanocytes to cold, and can occur unpredictably following lesser doses. In pigmented skin this will lead to an unacceptable cosmetic result; however, in fair-skinned people this is usually not a problem, and can be dealt with by feathering. Any such loss of pigmentation is permanent, but because the texture of the underlying skin is normal, it can be effectively disguised by cosmetics.

Alopecia will follow large doses of liquid nitrogen, and occasionally occurs at lower doses in an unpredictable fashion (Figure 58.4).[16] Like pigment loss, any hair loss is usually permanent, and so cryosurgical treatment of lesions in the scalp and beard areas is generally only considered for small lesions.

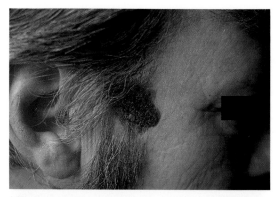

(a)

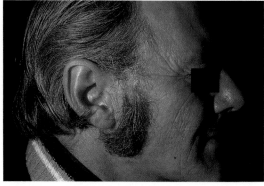

(b)

Figure 58.4 Demonstration of permanent alopecia following curative treatment of a seborrhoeic wart.

Scarring and wound contraction do not occur if the duration of the freeze after ice formation does not exceed 30 s, but it can occur with higher doses.[17] This is due to the relative resistance to cold of fibroblasts and collagen fibres, which leads to the preservation of the fibrous tissue network, which then acts as a scaffold upon which wound healing occurs. Cartilage is similarly cryoresistant, allowing lesions on the ears and nose to receive full 30 s double freezes of liquid nitrogen without distortion of the normal tissue contour.[18]

Sensory impairment following cryosurgery has been described in both patients and operators.[19] Touch, pain and cold sensation are all

Table 58.6 Contraindications to cryosurgery
• Agammaglobulinaemia
• Blood dyscrasias of unknown origin
• Cold intolerance
• Raynaud's disease
• Cold urticaria
• Cryoglobulinaemia
• Pyoderma gangrenosum
• Collagen and autoimmune disease

reduced, and may take as long as 18 months to recover. The extent of sensory impairment is more pronounced with longer freeze times. While this may be of advantage for repeat treatment of lesions or if analgesia is desired, patients must be warned of this complication if sensitive areas such as the fingertips are being treated.

Contra-indications to cryosurgery generally relate to intercurrent illnesses such as those listed in Table 58.6. Relative contra-indications arise with certain lesions, where the cosmetic result would be more favourable with different treatments, such as the beard areas or in patients with pigmented skin, or in sites where wound healing may be slow, such as the pretibial region. Cryosurgery can still be used on all these lesions, as long as the operator acknowledges that the cosmetic outcomes will be diminished.

CONCLUSIONS

As can be seen from the broad range of conditions listed in the tables, to distinguish between the use of cryosurgery for the treatment of disease and cosmetic usage is sometimes difficult. Many pathologies result in little functional impairment, but cause great psychological morbidity through their perceived unpleasant appearance. To dismiss these disorders as trivial or unworthy and of merely cosmetic significance is to deprive patients of balanced informed opinion, and may lead them towards others whose advice is influenced by self-interest.

For many of these conditions, there are few published data that specifically address how to perform the actual treatment. That is because experienced cryosurgeons will be able to judge the treatment required on the basis of the pathology of the lesion, its thickness and its site. For instance, a lesion on the lower leg of a person with venous insufficiency is likely to respond to shorter freeze times, and may have prolonged healing times. Even if all these treatments had been prospectively audited, more exact treatment protocols would be difficult to produce, since they would not allow for the many factors clinicians take into account when performing cryosurgery.

One reason why clinicians may get unsatisfactory outcomes is the use of inadequate treatment schedules. It is hoped that this description of the correct technique will ensure that others achieve results similar to those presented here. Cryosurgery is easy and can be learned quickly – but that is not the same as saying that no training is required. As Zacarian, the father of modern-day cryosurgery, said, 'A level of knowledge permitting an adequate understanding of the diagnosis and the pathophysiology of the condition to be treated must be a prerequisite. This is then to be combined with a degree in skill in dermatocryosurgical procedures to allow the selection of those methods necessary to carry out the treatment plan. These skills must be acquired. There are no short-cuts.'[6]

REFERENCES

1. Kuflik EG, Cryosurgery updated. Continuing medical education. *J Am Acad Dermatol* 1994; **31:** 925–44.

2. Sinclair RD, Dawber RPR, Cryosurgery of malignant and premalignant diseases of the skin: a simple approach. *Austr J Dermatol* 1995; **36:** 133–42.

3. Dawber RPR, Cold kills! *Clin Exp Dermatol* 1988; **13:** 137–50.

4. Colver GB, Dawber RPR, Malignant spots: spot freezes. In: *Surgical Gems in Dermatology*, Vol 2 (Robins P, ed.). New York/Tokyo: Igaku-Shoin, 1991:14–17.

5. Dawber RPR, Colver G, Jackson A, *Cutaneous Cryosurgery. Principles and Clinical Practice*, 2nd edn. London: Martin Dunitz, 1997:113.

6. Zacarian SA (ed), *Cryosurgery for Skin Cancer and Cutaneous Disorders*. St Louis, MO: Mosby Press, 1985.

7. Kuflik EG, Cage AA, *Cryosurgical Treatment for Skin Cancer*. New York/Tokyo: Igaku-Shoin, 1990:266.

8. Serfling U, Hood AF, Local therapies for Kaposi's sarcoma in patients with acquired immuno-deficiency syndrome. *Arch Dermatol* 1991; **127:** 1479–81.

9. Graham G, Cryosurgery for acne. In: *Cryosurgery for Skin Cancer and Cutaneous Disorders* (Zacarian SA, ed.). St Louis, MO: Mosby Press, 1985:59–76.

10. Chiearello SE, Full-face cryo (liquid nitrogen) peel. *J Dermatol Surg Oncol* 1992; **18:** 329–32.

11. Sonnex T, Dawber RPR, Rhinophyma treatment by liquid nitrogen cryosurgery. *Br J Dermatol* 1983; **109**(Suppl 24): 18.

12. Colver GB, Dawber RPR, Tattoo removal using a liquid nitrogen cryospray. *Clin Exp Dermatol* 1984; **9:** 364–6.

13. Zouboulis CC, Blume U, Buttner P et al, Outcome of cryosurgical treatment in patients with keloids and hypertrophic scars. *Arch Dermatol* 1993; **129:** 1146–51.

14. Dawber RPR, Cryosurgery: complications and contra-indications. *Clinics Dermatol* 1990; **8:** 96–100.

15. Hindson TC, Spiro J, Scott LV, Clobetasol propionate ointment reduces inflammation after cryosurgery. *Br J Dermatol* 1985; **112:** 599–602.

16. Burge SM, Dawber RPR, Hair follicle destruction and regeneration in guinea-pig skin after cutaneous freeze injury. *Cryobiology* 1990; **27:** 153–63.

17. Shepherd JP, Dawber RPR, Wound healing and scarring after cryosurgery. *Cryobiology* 1984; **21:** 157–69.

18. Burge SM, Shepherd JP, Dawber RPR, Effect of freezing the helix and rim or edge of the human and pig ear. *J Dermatol Surg Oncol* 1984; **10:** 816–19.

19. Sonnex TS, Jones RL, Wedell AG et al, Long-term effects of cryosurgery on cutaneous sensation. *Br Med J* 1985; **290:** 188–90.

59

Cosmetic denervation with botulinum (Botox) toxin

James E Fulton Jr

INTRODUCTION

When we heard Alstair Carruthers[1] make his presentation in 1992 at the American Society of Dermatologic Surgery in Scottsdale, Arizona, it was obvious that botulinum toxin (Botox) could help build our cosmetic dermatology practice. The infiltration of Botox into the muscles of facial expression results in weakening of the associated lines and expressions within 5–10 days. It is remarkable in its efficacy and safety, and the patients look refreshed for the next 3–6 months.

However, there were certain technical difficulties. The recommended directions suggested diluting 100 units with $1 \, cm^3$ of unpreserved saline and using it within 4–6 hours. This placed severe constraints on our cosmetic surgery practice as it is difficult to spread $1 \, cm^3$ over the muscles of facial expression in a cost-effective manner. We therefore began diluting the Botox to study methods for its more effective administration and storage.

We found that the Botox could be diluted and stored in the refrigerator and still retain clinical effectiveness and reduce the activity of the muscles of facial expression for 4–6 months.[2] This technique has become extremely important in promoting the cosmetic dermatology service we provide, and

results not only in satisfied patients, but also an acceptable income flow.

The relative and absolute contraindications for the use of Botox are shown in Table 59.1.

Table 59.1 Contraindications for the use of Botox
Relative contraindications
• Very thin patients (more lateral diffusion of Botox)
• Extensive use of anti-inflammatories (more bruising)
• Concerned about brow ptosis (skip the lower frontalis injections)
Absolute contraindications
• Pregnancy or breast feeding
• Neuromuscular diseases (myasthenia gravis)
• Allergic to human albumin or botulinum toxin

METHOD

Introduction

Patients are introduced to concept of Botox during their initial visit. They are told to stop taking aspirin and/or anti-inflammatories for at least two weeks before the series of injections. On the day of treatment they remove their make-up and sign the informed consent (Figure 59.1).

Patient:_____ Age:_____

To the Patient: You have the right to be informed about your skin condition and treatment so that you may make the decision whether or not to undergo the procedure after knowing the risks and hazards involved. This discosure is not meant to scare or alarm you; it is simply an effort to better inform you so that you may give or withhold your consent for the treatment program.

I have requested that _____ attempt to improve my facial expression lines with Botox®. This is the trademark for *botulinum* toxin. These injections have been used for more than a decade in children and adults to improve the problem of muscle spasm of the facial muscles. This toxin has also been useful to correct double vision due to muscular imbalance. Injection of minute amounts weakens the muscle and prevents frowning, crow's feet and expression lines. Although the results are usually dramatic, I have been informed that the practice of medicine is not an exact science and that no guarantees can be or have been made concerning expected results in my case.

Initial if true _____

The solution is injected with a small needle into the muscle. You see the benefits develop over the next five to seven days. Less frowning will be possible.

Side effects and complications have been minimal. Occasionally, slight swelling, and/or bruising may last for several days after the injections. Rarely, an adjacent muscle may be weakened for several weeks after an injection. I have been advised of the risks involved in such treatment, the expected benefits of such treatment, and alternative treatments, including no treatment at all.

Initial if true _____

I understand that several sessions may be needed to complete the injection series and that multiple sessions are planned.

Initial if true _____

I agree that this constitutes full disclosure, and that it supersedes any previous verbal or written disclosures. I certify that I have read, and fully understand, the above paragraphs, and that I have had sufficient opportunity for discussion and to ask questions.

Initial if true _____

First Procedure

_____   _____
Staff Signature   Patient Signature   Date

Second Procedure

_____   _____
Staff Signature   Patient Signature   Date

Third Procedure

_____   _____
Staff Signature   Patient Signature   Date

Figure 59.1 Botox injection informed consent.

Method of dilution

Our initial step was to determine how much the Botox could be diluted. The vial was diluted to 1 cm^3, 5 cm^3, 10 cm^3 and 20 cm^3 with unpreserved saline. The extents of denervation of the corrugator, frontalis and orbicularis oculi muscles were studied over the ensuring weeks.

Length of storage

Once we determined the most cost-effective dilution (10 cm^3/vial), we stored one of these reconstituted vials for 30 days in the refrigerator, and then compared its effectiveness with a freshly reconstituted vial by injecting these same muscles and again surveying the percent of denervation over the following weeks.

Method of injection

After surveying many injection methods, we found that the most effective way to denervate the muscle was to inject the toxin tangentially into the muscle (Figures 59.2 and 59.3). This was most easily accomplished with a 30-gauge, $\frac{1}{2}$-inch needle injected into the belly of the corrugator muscle. Similarly, a 30-gauge needle was used for denervating the latero-inferior aspect of the orbicularis oculi muscle at four different injection sites. A 1-inch, 30-gauge needle was injected tangentially into the frontalis muscles at several locations, starting a finger breadth or two above the eyebrow. The patient is told to raise both eyebrows and, usually, the third or fourth ridge is injected tangentially (Figure 59.4). The muscles were always tensed up during injections, and every attempt was made to inject directly into the apparent belly of muscle.

To reduce the sensation of injections and to reduce the bruising tendency, we rotated

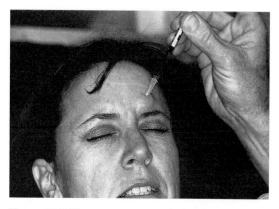

Figure 59.3 The corrugator muscle is injected tangentially into the mass of the muscle: the toxin is infused as the needle is withdrawn.

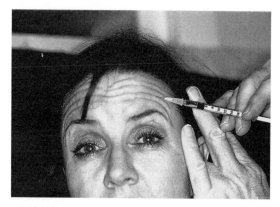

Figure 59.4 The frontalis muscle is injected tangentially with the toxin. The first mound above the eyebrow is not injected to avoid brow ptosis.

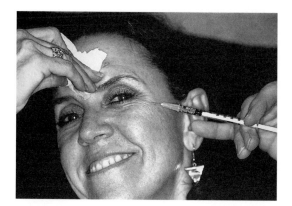

Figure 59.2 The method of injection of botulinum toxin. The muscle mounds between the linear depressions are injected with 0.1 cc (IU) of toxin.

ice compresses, injections and compression rapidly at each site. The sequence was to ice the left lateral orbicularis oculi; then, to move the ice to the right lateral orbicularis oculi and inject the left orbicularis with four 0.1 cm³ (4 units of Botox) injections. This was followed immediately with compression with a 4 × 4 gauze. We rotated around to the other orbital area and injected, while the ice was moved to the corrugator section of the forehead. Following icing, injection and compression of the corrugators, the left frontalis muscle was treated similarly before we

Table 59.2 Suggested guidelines

- Inject muscles with patient upright; do not let the patient lie down for 4 hours (so the Botox will not diffuse into the orbit)
- After the injections, exercise the muscles every 15 minutes for 1 hour (Botox attaches better to active muscles)
- Don't massage the muscles (may accelerate the diffusion to adjacent tissues)
- Inject the frontalis horizontally two or three centimetres above the brow (to reduce possible brow ptosis)

finished with the right frontalis muscle. Occasionally, other muscles of facial expression, such as the procerus, platsyma, levator labii superioris and depressor septi nasi, were also injected.

Guidelines for the administration of Botox are given in Table 59.2.

RESULTS

Clinical results

Our studies[2] indicated that we could dilute the Botox to the level of 1 unit per 0.1 cm^3 without losing efficacy (Figure 59.5). This dilution helped us to infiltrate the mass of the muscle more effectively, since we could easily see the distension of the muscle. At this dilution, there was ample fluid in each vial to infiltrate the muscles of five subjects. In comparing refrigerated with freshly reconstituted Botox, it became apparent that the length of storage of the reconstituted, unpreserved saline was not critical (Figure 59.6). Usually, we use a vial of Botox every 3 or 4 days.

The results on the last 1230 cases were impressive. Within 10 days, the facial lines began to soften. The results usually lasted for 4–6 months. The crow's feet were dramatically improved (Figure 59.7). The frontalis muscles were weakened and the forehead lines began to disappear (Figure 59.8). The corrugators proved to be the strongest muscles. They were the last ones to weaken and the first to return (Figure 59.9). They required the most frequent 'touch-ups'.

Side-effects

Difficulties with the injections have been minimal. Occasionally there was a non-responder that did not respond to repeat injections, and occasionally there was an injection that did not take and needed a 'touch-up' within 2–3 weeks after the initial injection. In 10% of the cases, a small bruise developed, especially in

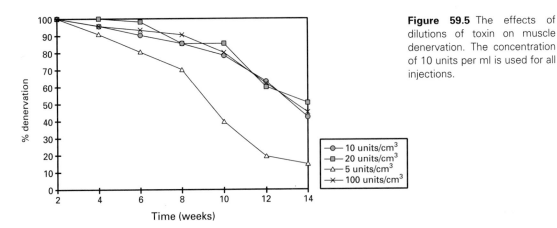

Figure 59.5 The effects of dilutions of toxin on muscle denervation. The concentration of 10 units per ml is used for all injections.

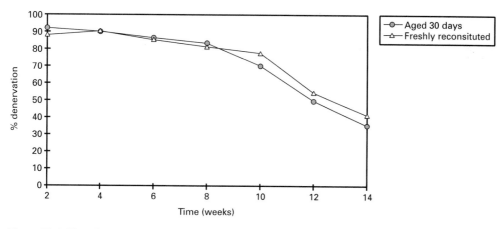

Figure 59.6 The effects of storage on the potency of toxin. Aging has no deleterious effects on muscle denervation.

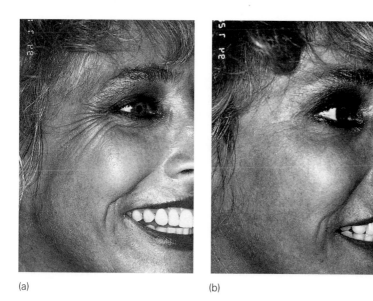

(a)

(b)

Figure 59.7 Denervation of the lateral orbicularis oculi diminishes crow's feet.

those patients on anti-inflammatories. Three percent of the cases complained about brow ptosis. Two cases developed eyelid ptosis, one case developed weakening of the zygomatic major muscle, and one patient developed diplopia. All of these side-effects resolved over 2–3 months, and have been minimal com-pared with the efficacy and patient satisfac-tion.

DISCUSSION

Following our initial dose-ranging studies, Botox became an effective tool in our

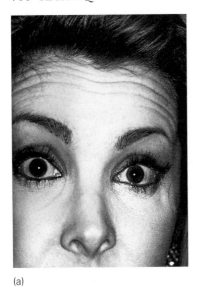 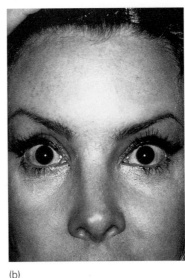

(a)   (b)

Figure **59.8** Denervation of the frontalis muscle reduces lines both at rest and during animation.

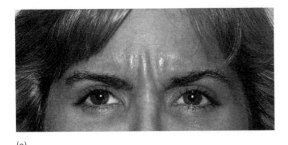 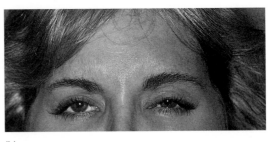

(a)   (b)

Figure 59.9 Denervation of the corrugator muscle reduces glabellar lines.

cosmetic dermatology practice. The benefits of Botox became a good motivating force for our patients. In 5–10 days after the injections, the muscles of facial expression began to relax. When combined with a skin care program, such as a glycolic acid/vitamin A conditioning lotion and a light glycolic acid peel, patients often felt and appeared 10 years younger, and even the resting lines softened. When the effects began to wear off, the patients immediately returned for a repeat injection. Occasionally, the benefits on a

glabellar crease would last beyond 4–6 months. These patients would no longer frown and had broken their habit pattern.

Botox injections are an almost ideal cosmetic procedure – you use it and get a benefit. If the patient does not like it, the skin returns to its previous condition, or, if they are satisfied, they return for repeat doses. The side-effects of severe bruising and migration of the Botox to a distant muscle or into the eye are rare and infrequent. This is especially true when the dose is diluted to a safe and effective level that denervates a muscle but does not leave excessive Botox around to migrate.

Routinely, we dilute with unpreserved saline to the level of 1 unit per 0.1 cm^3 and use the vial over 2–3 days. This allows us to fill 10 tuberculin syringes, and use approximately two tuberculin syringes or 20 units on each patient. This effectively denervates those muscles of expression for approximately 4–6 months. In some cases, expression returns more rapidly, but in others it lasts beyond 6 months. We have seen no evidence to indicate that the denervation becomes more permanent after multiple sessions.

Several investigators have complained that they are unable to achieve adequate denervation with these dilute doses of Botox. While observing their method of denervation, we found them injecting more perpendicularly to the muscle instead of tangentially into the bulk of the muscle mass. They were overcautious and often injected too superficially into the skin or too deeply below the periosteum. We have found no problem with injecting tangentially, since the lateral diffusion of this diluted Botox is insignificant.

REFERENCES

1. Carruthers J, Carruthers A, Treatment of glabellae frown lines with *C. botulinum* – An excitotoxin. *J Dermatol Surg Oncol* 1992; **18**: 17–21.
2. Garcia A, Fulton JE, Cosmetic denervation of the muscles of facial expression with *Botulinum* toxin. *Dermatol Surg* 1996; **22**: 39–43.

PART TEN

SIDE-EFFECTS AND SOCIAL ASPECTS OF COSMETOLOGY

60

Adverse cosmetic reactions

Smita Amin, Patricia G Engasser, Howard I Maibach

INTRODUCTION

The term 'cosmetic' is a familiar one, and its meaning has been expanded by an increase in the variety and complexity of substances used for cosmetic purposes. There are numerous ways to define and describe cosmetics. The Food, Drug and Cosmetic Act, which the US Food and Drug Administration (FDA) administers, defines cosmetics in the following manner:[1]

The term 'cosmetic' means [1] articles intended to be rubbed, poured, sprinkled, or sprayed on, introduced into, or otherwise applied to the human body or any part thereof for cleansing, beautifying, promoting attractiveness, or altering the appearance, and [2] articles intended for use as a component of any such articles: except the term shall not include soap.

Note two important aspects of this legal definition of cosmetics. First, in the United States, cosmetics in theory do not contain 'active drug' entities of any type, nor can they be promoted as altering any physiological state either in disease or health. Many countries do not recognize this legal distinction. The US

Modified version reprinted with permission from Toro JR et al, Cosmetic reactions. In: *Dermatotoxicology, 5th edn* (eds FN Marzulli, HI Maibach). Bristol, PA: Taylor & Francis, 1996:607–42.

FDA classifies products into cosmetics, over-the-counter (OTC) drugs and prescription drugs. By the US definition, antiperspirants are OTC drugs regulated by the FDA through the OTC drug monograph system, while deodorants are cosmetics. The second aspect of the US definition of cosmetics is the so-called soap exemption. 'Soap' in the classic sense, as made of natural ingredients, is the type of soap that is excepted by the definition above. However, if the soap product is made of detergent chemicals (synthetic surfactants), the product is regulated by the Consumer Product Safety Commission under the Federal Hazardous Substances Act, as a household product. If the soap contains a therapeutic ingredient for a medical condition, it is regulated either as a prescription or OTC drug.[2] Likewise, the classification of cosmetics is equally complex. The cosmetic industry itself divides the products into more general categories oriented as to their purpose as described in the definition.

Reactions to cosmetics constitute a small but significant portion of the cases of contact dermatitis seen by dermatologists in the United States. In a five-year study, the North American Contact Dermatitis Group (NACDG) found that 5.4% of 13 216 patients tested were identified as having reactions caused by cosmetics.[3]

This surely under-represents the true incidence, because most patients who experience reactions to newly purchased cosmetics seldom consult a physician and just stop using the suspected cosmetic. In addition, the NACDG reported that 59% of the reactions caused by cosmetics occurred on the face, including the periorbital area, and 79% were females. Half of the cases later proven to evoke reactions to cosmetics were initially unsuspected. Reactions to cosmetics can have a variety of presentations, including subjective and objective irritation, allergic contact dermatitis, contact urticaria, photosensitivity, pigmentation, and hair and nail changes.

IRRITANT DERMATITIS

Objective irritation

Skin irritation has been described by exclusion as localized inflammation not mediated by either sensitized lymphocytes or by antibodies – for example that develops by a process not involving the immune system. Skin irritation depends on endogenous and exogenous factors. Lammintausta et al[4] describe these factors in detail. Predictive testing in human beings and rabbits can reliably detect strong or moderate irritants as ingredients in cosmetics or the products themselves. This allows manufacturers to test thoroughly to eliminate these potential hazards before marketing. Mild irritants, however, are more difficult to detect. Individuals with fair, freckled skin may be easily irritated. This can, however, be misinterpreted by the inexperienced clinician; patients of all shades, including Blacks, may develop irritation to ingredients and combinations. Because the stratum corneum of the facial skin is penetrated easily, more irritant reactions occur, but are not always recognized clinically because of the complex biology of the human face. Many supposedly nonirritating moisturizers or emollient creams contain surfactants and emulsifiers that are mild irritants. These cosmetics are applied frequently to facial or inflamed skin, resulting in irritant reactions. In product use testing, reproducing an irritant reaction may be difficult, because penetrability of the stratum corneum varies with environmental conditions, and small panel testing may not account for the complexity and variance of the human genome. However, provocative-use testing may be performed at the original site of the reactions.

Application of some chemicals may directly destroy tissue, producing skin necrosis at the application site. Chemicals producing necrosis that results in formation of scar tissue are described as corrosive. Chemicals may disrupt cell functions and/or trigger the release, formation or activation of autocoids that produce local increases in blood flow, increase vascular permeability, attract white blood cells in the area or directly damage cells. The additive effects of the mediators result in local skin inflammation. A number of as yet poorly defined pathways involving different processes of mediator generation appear to exist. Although no agent has yet met all the criteria to establish it as a mediator of skin irritation, histamine, 5-hydroxytryptamine, prostaglandins, leukotrienes, kinins, complement, reactive oxygen species, and products of white blood cells have been implicated as mediators of some irritant reactions.[5] Chemicals that produce inflammation as a result of a single exposure are termed acute or primary irritants.

Some chemicals do not produce acute irritation from a single exposure, but may produce inflammation following repeated application to the same area of skin, i.e. cumulative irritation. Because of the possibility of skin contact during transport and use of many chemicals, regulatory agencies have mandated the screening of chemicals for the ability to produce skin corrosion and acute irritation. These studies are conducted in animals, using standardized protocols. However, the protocols specified by some agencies vary somewhat. It is not routinely appropriate to conduct screening studies for corrosion in humans, but acute irritation is sometimes evaluated in humans after animal studies have been completed. Tests for predicting irritation in both animals and humans have been widely utilized. Predictive irritation assays in animals include the modified Draize test, repeated-application patch tests, the guinea pig immersion test and the mouse ear test. Predictive human irritation assays include many forms of the single-application patch test, cumulative irritation assays, the chamber scarification test and the exaggerated exposure test. These predictive assays are reviewed in Marzulli and Maibach.[6] Sensitive bioengineering equipment used to evaluate pathophysiology of skin irritation includes transepidermal water loss, dielectric characteristics, skin impedance, conductance, resistance, blood flow velocity, skin pH, O_2 resistance and CO_2 effusion rate. The textbooks of Berardesca et al[7] and Elsner et al[8] describe these methods in detail.

Sensory or subjective irritation

Application of a cosmetic causing burning, stinging, or itching without detectable visible or microscopic changes is designated as subjective irritation. This reaction is common in certain susceptible individuals, occurring most frequently on the face. Some of the ingredients that cause this reaction are not generally considered irritants, and will not cause abnormal responses in nonsusceptible individuals. Materials that produce subjective irritation include dimethyl sulfoxide, some benzoyl peroxide preparations, salicylic acid, propylene glycol, amyldimethylaminobenzoic acid and 2-ethoxyethyl methoxycinnamate, which are ingredients of cosmetics and OTC drugs. Pyrethroids, a group of broad-spectrum insecticides, produce a similar condition that may lead to paraesthesia at the nasolabial folds, cheeks, periorbital areas and ears.[9]

Only a portion of the human population seems to develop nonpyrethroid subjective irritation. Frosch and Kligman[10] found that they needed to prescreen subjects to identify 'stingers' for conducting predictive assays. Only 20% of subjects exposed to 5% aqueous lactic acid in a hot, humid environment developed a stinging response. All stingers in their series reported a history of adverse reactions to facial cosmetics, soaps, etc. A similar screening procedure by Lammintausta et al[4] identified 18% of their subjects as stingers. Prior skin damage (e.g. sunburn, pretreatment with surfactants and tape stripping) increases the intensity of responses in stingers, and persons not normally experiencing a response report pain on exposure to lactic acid or other agents that produce subjective irritation.[11] Attempts to identify reactive subjects by association with other skin descriptors (e.g. atopy, skin type or skin dryness) have not yet been fruitful. However, Lammintausta et al[4] showed that stingers develop stronger reactions to materials causing nonimmunologic contact urticaria and increases in transepidermal water loss and blood flow following application of irritants via patches than nonstingers.[4]

The mechanisms by which materials produce subjective irritation have not been extensively investigated. Pyrethroids directly act on the axon by interfering with the gate channel mechanism and impulse firing.[12] It has been suggested that agents causing subjective irritation act via a similar mechanism, because no visible inflammation is present.

An animal model was developed to rate paraesthesia to pyrethroids, and may be useful for other agents.[9] Using this technique, it was possible to rank pyrethroids for their ability to produce paraesthesia. Lammintausta et al[4] and Berardesca et al[13] suggested that patients with subjective irritation have more responsive blood vessels.

As originally published, human subjective irritation assay volunteers were seated in the chamber (43°C and 80% relative humidity) until a profuse facial sweating was observed.[11] Sweat was removed from the nasolabial fold and cheek; then a 5% aqueous solution of lactic acid was briskly rubbed over the area. Those who reported stinging for 3–5 minutes within the first 15 minutes were designated as stingers and were used for subsequent tests. Lammintausta et al[4] reported a 15-minute treatment with a commercial facial sauna to produce facial sweating. This facial sauna technique is less stressful to both subjects and investigators, and produces similar results.

ALLERGIC CONTACT DERMATITIS

Although allergic contact dermatitis is the most frequently diagnosed reaction to cosmetics, it is clinically suspected initially in less than half the proven cases. Most cosmetics are complex mixtures containing perfumes, preservatives, stabilizers, lipids, alcohols, pigments, etc. Frequently, these components are responsible for cosmetic allergy.

Allergic contact dermatitis is cell-mediated. This type of skin response is often referred to as delayed contact hypersensitivity because of the relatively long period (about 24 hours) required for the development of the inflammation following exposure. Lymphocytes are responsible for producing delayed-type hypersensitivity (DTH) and for regulation of the immune system. Lymphocytes leaving the lymphoid organs are 'programmed' to recognize a specific chemical structure via a receptor molecule(s). If, during circulation through body tissues, a cell encounters the structure it is programmed to recognize, an immune response may be induced. To stimulate an immune response, a chemical must be presented to lymphocytes in an appropriate form.[14] Chemicals are usually haptens, which must conjugate with proteins in the skin or in other tissues in order to be recognized by the immune system. Haptens conjugate with proteins to form a number of different antigens that may stimulate an allergic response.[15] Hapten–protein conjugates are processed by macrophages or other cells expressing proteins on their surface. Although the exact nature of this process is not completely understood, it is known that physical contact between macrophages and T cells is required.[16] In the skin, keratinocytes produce interleukin-1, an important regulatory protein for induction of DTH.[17] Langerhans' cells express Ia antigen and may act as antigen-presenting cells.[18] Histologically, the DTH response has been described as a hyperproliferative epidermis with intracellular edema, spongiosis, intraepidermal vesiculation and mononuclear cell infiltrate by 24 hours. The dermis shows perivenous accumulation of lymphocytes, monocytes and edema. No reaction occurs if the local vascular supply is interrupted and the appearance of epidermal changes follows the invasion of monocytes. The histology of the response varies somewhat by species.

Many factors modulate development of DTH in experimental animals and humans. The method of skin exposure and rate of penetration influence the rate of sensitization. The effects of vehicle and occlusion are well documented.[19] Vehicle choice determines in part the absorption of the test material, and can influence sensitization rate, ability to elicit response at challenge and the irritation threshold. Application of haptens to irritated or tape-stripped skin, the dose per unit area, repeated applications to the same site,[20] increased numbers of exposures (this applies through 10–15 exposures only), an interval of 2–6 days between exposures[20] and treatment with adjuvant increase sensitization rates.[21,22] The development of DTH is under genetic control; not all individuals have the capability to respond to a given hapten. In addition, the status of the immune system determines if an immune response can be induced. For example, young animals may become tolerant to a hapten, and pregnancy may suppress expression of allergy.[20] The intrinsic biological variables controlling sensitization can be influenced only by selection of animals likely to be capable of mounting an immune response to the hapten. The extrinsic variables of dose, vehicle, route of exposure and adjuvant, can be manipulated to develop sensitive predictive assays.

Appropriate execution of predictive sensitization assays is critical. All too often, techniques are discredited when, in fact, the performance of the tests was inferior or study design (e.g. choice of dose) was inappropriate. A common error in choosing an animal assay is using Freund's complete adjuvant (FCA) when seeing dose–response relationships. The adjuvant provides such sensitivity that dose–effect relationships are muted. Although the dose must be high enough to ensure penetration, it must be below the irritation threshold at challenge to avoid misinterpretation of irritant inflammation as allergic. For instance, the quaternary ammonium compounds (e.g. benzalkonium chloride) rarely sensitize, but have been identified as allergens in some guinea pig assays. Knowing the irritation potential of compounds and choosing an appropriate experimental design will allow the investigator to design and execute these studies appropriately. John Draize developed the first practical animal assay to predict the proclivity of a chemical or a final product to produce allergic contact dermatitis. This test is widely used, and forms the basis for current testing. Modifications to this test include the Buhler method, Freud's adjuvant, the Freud's complete adjuvant test and the open epicutaneous test. If done properly, these tests will identify most of the contact allergens. Human testing supplements animal testing, but most sensitization studies have been done in humans. The Draize repeated-insult patch test is the standard assay to identify the propensity of a chemical to induce allergic contact dermatitis. Modifications to this test have been developed. A complete review of these assays can be found in reference 6. Patch testing of patients with suspected cosmetic contact dermatitis is discussed later in this chapter.

CONTACT URTICARIA SYNDROME

Contact urticaria has been defined as a wheal-and-flare response that develops within 39–60 minutes after exposure of the skin to certain agents.[23] Symptoms of immediate contact reactions can be classified according to their morphology and severity. Itching, tingling and burning with erythema is the weakest type of immediate contact reaction. Local wheal-and-flare with tingling and itching represents the prototype reaction of contact urticaria. Generalized urticaria after local contact is rare, but can occur from strong urticaria. Symptoms in other organs can appear with the skin symptoms in cases of immunologic contact urticaria syndrome. These include asthma, angioedema and anaphylaxis.

The strength of the reactions may vary greatly, and often the whole range of local symptoms – from slight erythema to strong edema and erythema – can be seen from the same substance if different concentrations are used in skin tests.[24] Not only the concentration but also the site of the skin contact affect the reaction. A certain concentration of contact urticant may produce strong edema and erythema on the skin of the back and face, but only erythema on the volar surfaces of the lower arms or legs. In some cases, contact urticaria can be demonstrated only on damaged or previously eczematous skin. Some agents (e.g. formaldehyde) produce urticaria on healthy skin following repeated but not single applications to the skin. Differentiation between nonspecific irritant reactions and contact urticaria may be difficult. Strong irritants, such as hydrochloric acid, lactic acid, cobalt chloride, formaldehyde and phenol, can cause a clear-cut immediate wheal if the concentration is high enough, but the reactions do not usually fade away within a few hours. Instead, they are followed by signs of irritation; erythema, scaling or crusting is seen 24 hours later. Some substances can only cause contact urticaria, for example benzoic acid and nicotinic acid esters. Diagnosis of immediate contact urticaria is based on a thorough history and skin testing with suspected substances. Skin tests for human diagnostic testing are summarized by von Krogh and Maibach.[23] Because of the risk of systemic reactions, such as anaphylaxis, human diagnostic tests should only be performed by experienced personnel with facilities for resuscitation on hand. Contact urticaria has been divided into two main types on the basis of proposed pathophysiological mechanisms: nonimmunologic and immunologic.[25] Recent reviews list agents suspected to cause each type of urticarial response.[26,27] Some common urticants are listed in Table 60.1. A flow sheet designed by von Krogh and Maibach[23] can be used to approach testing in suspected cases (Table 60.2).

Nonimmunologic contact urticaria

Nonimmunologic contact urticaria is the most common form, and occurs without previous exposure in most individuals. The reaction remains localized, and does not cause systemic symptoms or spread to become generalized urticaria. Typically, the strength of this type of contact urticaria reaction varies from sensory complaints of sting, itch or burn to an urticaria response, depending on the concentration, skin site and substance. The mechanism of nonimmunologic contact urticaria has not been completely delineated, but a direct influence on dermal vessel walls or a non-antibody-mediated release of histamine, prostaglandins, leukotrienes, substance P or other inflammatory mediators represents possible mechanisms. Lahti and Maibach[26] suggested that nonimmunologic urticaria produced by different agents may involve different combinations of mediators. Common nonimmunological urticants can be inhibited by oral acetylsalicylic acid and indomethacin[28,29] and by topical diclofenac and naproxen gel,[30] but not hydroxyzine, terfenadine[24,31] or capsaicin. This suggests that prostaglandins and leukotrienes may play a role in the inflammatory response.

The most-potent and best-studied substances producing nonimmunologic contact

urticaria are benzoic acid, cinnamic acid, cinnamic aldehyde and nicotinic acid esters. Under optimal conditions, more than half of a random sample of individuals show local edema and erythema reactions within 45 minutes of application of these substances if

---

Table 60.1 Some agents reported to cause urticaria in humans

Immunologic mechanisms
- Bacitracin
- Ethyl and methyl parabens
- Seafood (high-molecular-weight protein extracts)

Nonimmunologic mechanisms
- Cinnamic aldehyde
- Balsam of Peru
- Benzoic acid
- Ethyl aminobenzoate
- Dimethyl sulfoxide

Unknown mechanisms
- Epoxy resin
- Lettuce/endive
- Cassia oil
- Formaldehyde
- Ammonium persulfate
- Neomycin

Table 60.2 Test procedure for evaluation of immediate-type reactions in recommended order[a]

1. Open application
- Nonaffected normal skin:
  Negative

- Slightly affected (or previously affected) skin:
  Negative   Positive → positive diagnosis

2. Occlusive application (infrequently needed)
- Nonaffected normal skin:
  Negative

- Slightly affected (or previously affected) skin:
  Negative

3. Invasive (inhalant, prick, scratch, or intradermal injection)[b]

[a] Adapted from reference 23, with permission.
[b] When invasive methods are employed (especially scratch and inhalant testing), adequate controls are required.

the concentration is high enough. Benzoic acid and sodium benzoate are used as preservatives for cosmetics and other topical preparations at concentrations from 0.1% to 0.2%, and are capable of producing immediate contact reactions at the same concentrations.[32] Cinnamic aldehyde at a concentration of 0.01% may elicit an erythematous response associated with a burning or stinging feeling in the skin. Mouthwashes and chewing gums contain cinnamic aldehyde at concentrations high enough to produce a pleasant tingling sensation in the mouth and enhance the sale of the product. Higher concentrations produce lip swelling or typical contact urticaria in normal skin. Eugenol in the mixture may inhibit contact sensitization to cinnamic aldehyde and possibly nonimmunologic contact urticaria from this same substance. The mechanism of the putative quenching effect is not certain, but a competitive inhibition at the receptor level may be the explanation.[33] Provocative testing of patients suspected of nonimmunologic urticaria with individual ingredients such as benzoic acid, sorbic acid and sodium benzoate, common preservatives found in cosmetics, will frequently reproduce patients' symptoms.

Immunologic contact urticaria

Immunologic contact urticaria is an immediate Type I allergic reaction in people previously sensitized to the causative agent.[23] It is more prevalent in atopic patients than in nonatopic patients.[34] The molecules of a contact urticant react with specific immunoglobulin E (IgE) molecules attached to mast cell membranes. The cutaneous symptoms are elicited by vasoactive substances, such as histamine, released from mast cells. The role of histamine is conspicuous, but other mediators of inflammation, such as prostaglandins, leukotrienes and kinins, may influence the degree of response. Immunologic contact urticaria reaction can extend beyond the contact site, and generalized urticaria may be accompanied by other symptoms such as rhinitis, conjunctivitis, asthma and even anaphylactic shock. The term 'contact urticaria syndrome' was therefore suggested by Maibach and Johnson.[25] The name has generally been accepted for a symptom complex in which local urticaria occurs at the contact site, with symptoms in other parts of the skin or in target organs such as the nose and throat, lung, and gastrointestinal and cardiovascular systems. Anaphylactic reactions may result from substances that induce a strong hypersensitivity response or are easily absorbed from the skin.[35] Fortunately, the appearance of systemic symptoms is less common than the localized form, but it may be seen in cases of strong hypersensitivity or in a widespread exposure and abundant percutaneous absorption of an allergen.

Food substances are common causes of immunologic contact urticaria (Table 60.1). The orolaryngeal area is a site where immediate contact reactions are frequently provoked by food allergens, most often among atopic individuals. The actual antigens are proteins or protein complexes. As proof of immediate hypersensitivity, specific IgE antibodies against the causative agent can typically be found in the patient's serum using the RAST technique and skin test for immediate allergy. In addition, the prick test can demonstrate immediate allergy. The passive transfer test (Prausnitz–Kustner test) often gives a positive result. This is now performed in monkeys rather than humans.

ACNE AND COMEDONES

Acnegenesis and comedogenesis are distinct but often related types of adverse skin reactions to facial, hair and other products. Acnegenesis refers to the chemical irritation and inflammation of the follicular epithelium with resultant loose hyperkeratotic material within the follicle and inflammatory pustules and papules. Comedogenesis refers to the noninflammatory follicular response that leads to dense compact hyperkeratosis of the follicle. Mills and Berger[36] indicated that the time courses for the development of facial acne and comedones are different. While facial acne will appear in a matter of days, comedone formation in the human back and rabbit model takes longer to occur.

Classes of ingredients such as the lubricants isopropyl myristate and some analogs, lanolin and its derivatives, detergents, and D&C red dyes have been incriminated as acnegenic by the rabbit ear test.[37] Fulton[38] published a report about the comedogenicity and irritancy of commonly used cosmetics. Lists of comedogenic agents are not necessarily meaningful. Although they are important for pharmaceutical research and for the formulation of nonacnegenic products, they cannot alone predict the defects of the final product. The concentrations used in testing are often much greater than those in the final product. It is possible to use concentrations that are lower than the minimal acnegenic level. In addition, the vehicles in finished products can increase or decrease the acnegenic potential of individual compounds. In the final analysis, what is important is the testing of the finished product for its acnegenic and irritancy potential. When only inadequate data are available, an elimination regimen remains the only constructive approach to treat patients with suspected acne or comedones secondary to cosmetic use.

The rabbit ear assay is the major predictive animal model available. Kligman and Mills[39] developed the value of testing cosmetics and their ingredients by the rabbit ear assay. Several improvements to the model have been proposed.[40,41] However, the test is not standardized. The American Academy of Dermatology Invitational Symposium on Comedogenicity Panel suggested some guidelines for maximizing the usefulness of the rabbit ear model.[42]

Kligman and Mills[39] showed production of microcomedones in the backs of Black men after testing cosmetics with occlusion. One test for evaluating comedogenicity in humans is occlusive-patch application to the back followed by a cyanoacrylate follicular biopsy.[43] In this test the material previously positive in the rabbit ear assay is applied for four weeks under occlusion to the upper portion of the back of people with large follicles. This test needs refinement. However, if this occlusive patch test is negative, it provides additional assurance that the test material may be nonacnegenic.

Bronaugh and Maibach[44] reported that the rabbit ear test correlates well with pustule formation noted in use tests of cosmetics performed on women's faces. They noted that some cosmetics that produced papulopustules after 3–7 days of use on women's faces were strongly positive in the rabbit ear model. This may represent a manifestation of primary irritancy. Correlative studies with the rabbit pustulogenicity assay should be performed. The acute onset papulopustules are often described by the patient as a 'breakout'. The cause-and-effect relationship to cosmetics is strong, but is often missed by the dermatologist. Jackson and Robillard[45] proposed the ordinary clinical-usage test. This test, conducted for 4–6 weeks, may not provide reliable information on comedogenesis. However, follicular inflammation may be noted within 1–2 weeks of applications done twice a day to the face of people with acne-prone oily skin.

It is not known how long the applications need to be continued to observe true comedogenesis. Clinical observations should be done at least weekly for the first two weeks of using the product to detect follicle inflammation. The acute papulopustular form will be identified in short-term testing (days, in contradistinction to months). However, to conclusively incriminate cosmetics as a cause of comedonal acne, long-term testing using a single cosmetic on the faces of women will have to be conducted and the disease produced. Lines of cosmetics will ideally be manufactured that are screened with an appropriate rabbit ear test and then tested definitively on panels of acne-prone women for long term.

Wahlberg and Maibach[46] attempted to bridge the gap between the comedo identified in the rabbit ear assay and the more common acute papulopustule. They developed an animal model in which the rabbit's back is pierced with a needle and dosed topically. The resulting lesion closely resembles that seen in humans. Unfortunately, for several reasons, including reluctance to perform animal testing, identification of acnegenicity premarketing remains a weak link in the chain of dermatotoxicology.

PIGMENTATION

Hyperpigmentation of the face caused by contact dermatitis to ingredients in cosmetics occurs more frequently in dark-complexioned individuals.[47] An epidemic of facial pigmentation reported in Japanese women was attributed to 'coal tar' dyes, principally Sudan I, a contaminant of D&C red 31.[48,49] The following fragrance ingredients have also been implicated in causing pigmentation: benzyl salicylate, ylang-ylang oil, cananga oil, jasmin absolute, hydroxycitronellal, methoxycitronellal, sandalwood oil, benzyl alcohol, cinnamic alcohol, lavender oil, geraniol and geranium oil.[50] Histologic examination shows hydropic degeneration of the basal layer, pigment incontinence and little evidence of inflammation.[47] Mathias reported hyperpigmentation due to contact allergy to chromium hydroxide used as a dye in toilet soap.[51] Maibach[52] reported hyperpigmentation in a Black man sensitive to petrolatum. Dermatologists should search scrupulously for a causative agent in patients with hyperpigmentation. Eliminating the product results frequently in gradual fading of the pigment. Unfortunately, until a predictive assay is identified, most patients will be incorrectly identified as idiopathic.

Cosmetic chemicals have infrequently been associated with leukoderma. Nater and de Groot[53] and de Groot[54] listed chemicals associated with leukoderma. More recently, Taylor and colleagues[55] added seven more chemicals. Although Riley[56] reported that low concentrations of butylated hydroxyanisole (BHA) were toxic in culture guinea pig melanocytes, Gellin et al[57] could not induce depigmentation in guinea pigs or black mice by applying butylated hydroxyanisole. In addition, Maibach et al[58] were unable to produce depigmentation after a 60-day occlusive application of hydroxytoluene to darkly pigmented men. In 1984, the Cosmetic Ingredient Review Panel concluded that it is safe to use BHA in the present practices of use.

Hydroquinone has produced depigmentation in humans. Although it is a weak depigmenter at 2% concentration, it is a stronger depigmenter at higher concentrations and with different vehicles. Hydroquinone, used as a bleaching agent, has caused postinflammatory hyperpigmentation in South African Blacks. Findlay et al[59] from South Africa reported a long-term complication of the use of hydroquinone – deposits of ochronotic pigment in the skin along with colloid milia. Melanocytes, despite intense hydroquinone use, escaped destruction, the site of the injury shifted to the dermis, and the fibroblast and polymeric pigment adhered to thickened, abnormal collagen bundles. Similarly, an American Black woman developed this complication after intense use of a 2% hydroquinone cream.[60] Prolonged use of hydroquinone followed by sun exposure may lead to exogenous ochronosis with colloid milium production. In addition, a few cases of persistent hypopigmentation have incriminated topical hydroquinone in recent years.[61] Pyrocatechol has similar structure and effects to hydroquinone. The most frequent use of hydroquinone and pyrocatechol is in rinse-off type hair dyes and colors, in which the use concentration is 1% or less. In 1984, the Cosmetic Ingredient Review Panel declared hydroquinone and pyrocatechol safe for cosmetic use at 1% or less. The monobenzyl ether of hydroquinone is a potent depigmenting agent, and is not approved for cosmetic use in the United States. Its only approved use is as a therapeutic agent for patients with vitiligo. *p*-Hydroxyanisole is a potent depigmenting agent in black guinea pigs at concentrations near those used in cosmetics. However, it may cause depigmentation at distant sites from application in humans.

Angelini and co-workers[62] reported depigmentation of the lip margins from *p*-t-butylphenol in a lip liner. The *p*-t-butylphenol patch test site also depigmented, and the presence of *p*-t-butylphenol was confirmed by gas chromatography with mass spectroscopy. Most recently, Taylor and co-workers[55] reported four cases of chemical leukoderma associated with the application of semipermanent and permanent hair colors and rinses. They identified benzyl alcohol and *p*-phenylenediamine in three of the four cases. Depigmentation occurred at the hair color patch test sites in three of the four cases.

In addition, Mathias et al[63] reported perioral leukoderma in a patient who used a cinnamic aldehyde-containing toothpaste. Wilkenson and Wilkin[64] reported that azelaic acid is a weak depigmenter and its esters do not depigment pigmented guinea pig skin.

PHOTOSENSITIVITY

Contact photosensitivity results from ultraviolet (UV)-induced excitation of a chemical applied to the skin. Contact photosensitivity is divided into phototoxic and photoallergic reactions. Phototoxic reactions may be experienced by any individual, provided that the UV light contains the appropriate wavelengths to activate the compound and that the UV dose and the concentration of the photoreactive chemical are high enough. Clinically, it consists of erythema followed by hyperpigmentation and desquamation. Sunburn is the most common phototoxic reaction.

However, photoallergic reactions require a period of sensitization. The reactions are usually delayed, manifesting days to weeks or years after the UV exposure. The major problem with photoallergic reactions is that the patient may develop persistent light reaction for many years after the chemical has been removed. These patients tend to be exquisitely sensitive to the sun and usually have very low UVB and UVA minimal erythema doses. With the exception of the epidemic caused by halogenated salicylamides in soap in the 1960s, photosensitivity accounts for a small number of cosmetic adverse reactions. Maibach and colleagues[65] reported only 9 or 713 patients with photoallergic and photosensitive reactions. Musk ambrette, a fragrance in some aftershaves, has been reported as a major cause of cosmetic photosensitivity reactions.

Predictive testing in human skin is not always definitive. In the 1960s, identification of TCSA and related phenolic compounds was accomplished by photopatch testing clinically involved patients. Subsequently, Willis and Kligman[66] induced contact photoallergy to certain agents in normal human subjects using a modification of the maximization test, which was developed for evaluating the potential of chemicals to produce contact dermatitis.[67–69]

Kaidbey and Kligman[70] and Kaidbey[71] modified the photomaximization procedure. They were able to sensitize normal human volunteers readily to certain methylated coumarin derivatives (e.g. TCSA, 3,5-DBS, chlorpromazine and sodium omadine). A smaller number of positive induction responses was noted with TBS contaminated with 47% DBS, 4,5-DBS, Jadit and bithionol. Negative results were obtained with *p*-aminobenzoic acid (PABA) and musk ambrette, which have produced photoallergic contact dermatitis clinically. To date, there is no proven effective predictive testing model for photoallergic contact dermatitis in that most of the known photoallergens have been identified clinically and not in toxicologic assays. Furthermore, the refinement of risk assessment (not hazard identification) may be difficult; for example, sodium orridine is positive in the assay but not yet clinically, in spite of extensive use.

Photopatch testing

The criteria for separating allergic contact and allergic photocontact dermatitis utilizing patch-testing techniques are imprecise. General criteria and their interpretation are listed in Table 60.3. Often, the results are not 'all-or-none', as implied in the table. Frequently, there is a difference in response intensity, with either the contact or photocontact response being greater. All too infrequently, serial dilutions are performed with either the putative antigen or the amount of ultraviolet light employed. Until a significant number of patients are so studied, it will be unclear how many of them represent contact versus photocontact sensitization.

Wennersten et al[72] recommended that patients with suspected photocontact allergy be phototested prior to implementation of patch testing. The aim of this preliminary light testing is to detect any abnormal sensitivity to UVA and UVB wavebands. It is generally agreed that UVA sources are adequate and sufficient to elicit responses, an important convenience, since UVA does not produce erythema in normal fair-skinned subjects until a dose of 20–30 J/cm^2 is delivered. High doses of UVA such as 10–15 J/cm^2 for photopatch testing are unnecessary. Such doses increase the possibility of adverse reactions and increase the incidence of phototoxic reactions. Despite widespread use, there is little standardization in the UVA dosage used in photopatch testing. Doses range from 1 to 15 J/cm^2 at various centers.[73,74] The Scandinavian Photodermatitis Group was the first to formulate a protocol using 5 J/cm^2 of UVA in photosensitive patients: half their UVA minimal erythema dose (MED) for the procedure. However, most photoallergies will be defined with a far smaller dose (e.g. 1 J/cm^2). Duguid and co-workers[75] confirmed the adequacy of 5 J/cm^2 or less as a photoelicitation dose. Although some data on the dose of light required to elicit a response exist, it remains incomplete, and must be studied in context with the dose of antigen and the vehicle. Until the light and antigenic intensities are more fully defined, most physicians utilize a PUVA unit, a bank of UVA bulbs in a diagnostic unit, or a hot-quartz (Kromayer) unit, with an appropriate filter to remove any light with wavelengths below 320 nm (UVB). The effect of UV irradiation on photopatch test substances in vitro has been reported.[76] It appears that 5 J/cm^2 of UVA is almost always adequate.

It is also possible that some patients may require UVB to elicit photoallergic dermatitis.

Table 60.3 Patch and photopatch testing		
Contact test-site response	**Photocontact test-site response**	**Interpretation**
Positive	Positive	Allergic contact dermatitis
Negative	Positive	Photoallergic dermatitis
Negative	Negative	Not sensitized

However, since UVB testing is not done routinely, it may be some time before this is clarified. In addition, Epstein[77] observed that many patients are so sensitive to light that the dose delivered under an ordinary patch will elicit reactions. He provided details of testing the nonexposed site, utilizing a large light-impermeable black patch applied in a dimly lit room.

On request, many manufacturers provide patch-test kits of individual ingredients to photopatch test their products. A 'standard' series of sunscreen antigens has been proposed by the International Contact Dermatitis Research Group (ICDRG). Commercial sources of appropriately diluted sunscreen antigens are not presently available in the United States. In Europe, these test kits are commercially available. Sunscreen antigens are available in 2% concentrations, although the maximum nonirritating doses of putative antigens in a given vehicle have not been defined. Maibach et al[78] reported the test concentrations and vehicles for the dermatological testing of many cosmetic ingredients that may be in sunscreen formulations. We currently lack adequate virgin controls for the high concentrations used in contemporary formulations. When high concentrations are required to elicit allergic contact dermatitis, an impurity or a photoproduct may be the actual allergen.

The specific vehicle in which the allergens are dissolved or suspended is important.[79] The ICDRG list employs petrolatum as diluent. This vehicle appears to be adequate to elicit reactions in many patients. It is clear, however, that the bioavailability of the antigen may be too limited in some cases. Mathias and Maibach[80] required ethanol to demonstrate PABA sensitivity, and Schauder and Ippen[81] noted more pronounced test reactions to avobenzone in isopropyl myristate than petrolatum. This topic remains an area of investigation. Presumably each ingredient may require an optimal vehicle and concentration for eliciting a reaction.

Some patients develop dermatitis that appears allergic or photoallergic in a morphologic and historic sense, yet fails to demonstrate a positive patch or photopatch test, in spite of seemingly appropriate testing. Such false-negative reactions are more difficult to identify than false-positive reactions.[82] Table 60.4 provides the basic strategy employed in attempting to help these

---

Table 60.4 Strategy for identifying the cause when routine patch testing is negative

Intervention	Comment
Increase UVA dose	Avoid UVA erythema Use UVA control
Increase concentration of sunscreen	Upper limit of nonirritating dose not completely defined
Alter vehicle	Ethanol has been found to be effective
Test other components	Sunscreen manufacturers often helpful in providing test kits
Add suberythemogenic doses of UVB	
Perform provocative-use test on final formulation	
Consider 'compound' allergy	

patients. Unfortunately, in some patients, even these extensive work-ups fail to elicit the etiology of their reactions.

Many of the reported positive tests to date – and especially the cross-reaction studies – may well represent false-positives due to the excited skin syndrome. This state of skin hyperirritability often induced by a concomitant dermatitis is responsible for many nonreproducible patch tests. Bruynzeel and Maibach[83] detail strategies for minimizing such false-positives.

NAIL CHANGES

Paronychia, onycholysis, nail destruction, and discoloration are some of the most common cosmetic adverse reactions found in the nails. The physician should obtain a detailed description of nail grooming habits in patients who have paronychia, onycholysis, nail destruction or nail discoloration, because any of these problems may be caused by nail-cosmetic usage. Nail discoloration has been reported with the use of hydroquinone bleaching creams and hair dyes containing henna.[84,85]

HAIR CHANGES

Permanents and hair straighteners are intended to break the disulfide bonds that give hair keratin its strength. Improper usage or incomplete neutralization of these cosmetics causes hair breakage. Hair that has been damaged by previous applications of permanent waves, straighteners, oxidation-type dyes, bleaches, or excessive exposure to sunlight and chlorine is more susceptible to this damage. The dermatologist should always take a complete history in these cases, including a detailed account of the use of drugs, to detect any causes of telogen or anagen effluvium. Careful examination of the hair shafts is essential to detect any pre-existing abnormalities. Saving a sample of these hairs in the patient record may be invaluable should litigation against the beautician or supplier occur.[86]

INGREDIENT PATCH TESTING

The diagnosis and treatment of reactions to cosmetics has been facilitated by the Food and Drug Administration's (FDA) regulation requiring the ingredient labeling of all retailed cosmetics.[87] The European Community has also endorsed such labeling. The ingredients are listed in order of descending concentration. Because of the complexity of the composition of fragrances, their compositions are not given but are listed simply as 'fragrance'. The regulation was designed to aid the consumer in identifying ingredients at the time of purchase; therefore the list is often placed on the outer package, which may be discarded, rather than the container. Correspondence with the manufacturer or a trip to the cosmetic counter, however, can bring the needed information. This regulation, besides identifying ingredients, is helpful to dermatologists, because it mandated a uniform nomenclature for cosmetic ingredients. The *CTFA Ingredient Dictionary* (1993) published by the Cosmetic Toiletries and Fragrance Association is the source for the official names. This dictionary provides a brief description of the chemical, alternative names, and names of suppliers. Without this key reference book, the dermatologist is at a distinct disadvantage in advising patients in this area.

The standard screening patch-test tray includes some ingredients that are allergens found in cosmetics. Imidazolidinyl urea, diazolidinyl urea, thimerosal, formaldehyde and quaternium-15 are preservatives. Patch testing balsam of Peru screens for approximately 50% of the known allergic reactions to fragrance in the United States. Colophony and its constituents are used in the manufacture of eye cosmetics, transparent soap and dentifrice.[88] If a patient has a positive patch-test reaction to one of these chemicals, the clinician should consider allergic contact dermatitis to cosmetics as a possible diagnosis. We emphasize that cosmetic contact dermatitis can often be unsuspected. Any positive patch tests should be interpreted cautiously, because many cosmetics are mild irritants, and excited skin state may cause false-positive results. Ideally, a positive patch test should be confirmed with a repeat test several weeks later or with a provocative-use test. Reassessment of the patient's history and presenting findings and patch testing with the patient's cosmetics may establish the diagnosis.

Once a product or products has been implicated with patch testing, pinpointing the offending ingredient is an important part of the work-up so that the patient may be spared recurrent reactions. Cosmetic ingredient patch testing is complicated, because the proper concentration for closed patch testing is known only for a small percentage of these ingredients. Patch test concentrations and vehicles have been proposed for less than 450 of the nearly 2000 cosmetic ingredients listed.[78] The texts by Nater and de Groot[53] and by Cronin[89] are important sources for clinicians seeking information on ingredient patch testing.

Screening fragrance trays provide the most common fragrance allergens in the United States. Further information for patch testing fragrance ingredients is reviewed in several articles.[90,91] When the clinical history, appearance of the reaction, or patch-test results lead the clinician to conclude that a cosmetic has caused an adverse reaction, it is important to obtain the ingredients for patch testing. The Cosmetic, Toiletry, and Fragrance Association publishes a pamphlet called *Cosmetic Industry On Call.* This pamphlet lists the names of members of the industry who are willing to answer questions about their products. Physicians can contact these people to request specific ingredients for patch testing and information about patch-test concentrations. If the patient does or does not prove to have a

reaction due to the cosmetics, the manufacturer should be notified of the results. Manufacturers will not always send materials for patch testing, and the patient cannot be treated successfully and counseled on how to avoid recurrences. On occasion, 'fractionated' samples will be sent for patch testing. Because irritant concentrations of ingredients may be present in these samples, they are often not suitable to use for closed patch testing. Some manufacturers will supply individual ingredients in the concentration that they appear in the product. These are often unsatisfactory for patch testing, because the nonstandardized concentrations may be too low to provoke an allergic response or may be high enough to elicit irritation under occlusion.

COSMETIC PRODUCTS

Preservatives

After fragrances, preservatives are the next most common cause of cosmetic reactions.[3] The 10 most frequently used preservatives are listed in Table 60.5. A large number of specific studies have focused on individual preservatives as being identified as potential sensitizers and directly responsible for a number of adverse reactions.

Paraben esters (methyl, propyl, butyl and ethyl) are nontoxic and nonirritating preservatives that protect well against Gram-positive bacteria and fungi, but poorly against several Gram-negative bacteria, including pseudomonads.[92] Parabens, the most widely used preservatives in topical products, have long been known to be contact allergens at relatively high concentrations and at a low frequency.[93] However, their potential for being the causative agents in cosmetic adverse reactions has not diminished their use, and, in fact, it is on the increase. Although new parabens are available, it is unlikely that these will reduce paraben adverse reactions, since consumers tend to show a cross-reactivity to all parabens. Fortunately, parabens compared

Table 60.5 Preservative frequency of use (FDA data, June 1993 update)[a]	
Chemical name	**No. of products using chemical**
Methylparaben	6738
Propylparaben	5400
Propylene glycol	3922
Citric acid	2317
Imidazolidinyl urea	2312
Butylparaben	1669
Butylated hydroxyanisole (BHA)	1669
Butylated hydroxytoluene (BHT)	1610
Ethylparaben	1213
5-Choro-2-methyl-4-isothiazolin-3-one (methylchloroisothiazoline)	1042

[a] Adapted from Preservative frequency of use. *Cosmetics and Toiletries* 1993; **108**: 97–8.

with total use (tons × years) have a remarkable safety record. Although parabens may occasionally be sensitizers when applied to eczematous skin, cosmetics containing parabens infrequently cause clinical difficulties when they are applied to normal skin. Fisher[94] called this phenomenon the 'paraben paradox'. It is not known how often this phenomenon represents the excited skin state (due to high concentration of paraben in the patch-test mixture) rather than the paraben paradox.

Imidazolidinyl urea (Germall 115) has low toxicity and is nonirritating. It has a broad antimicrobial activity, especially when used in combination with parabens. Although formaldehyde is released on hydrolysis, the levels are too low to cause reactions in many formaldehyde-sensitive patients clinically or during patch testing. Diazolidinyl urea is a related preservative, the use of which is increasing.

Quaternium-15 is active against bacteria, but less active against yeast and molds. It is a formaldehyde releaser. A patient who has simultaneous positive patch test readings to quaternium-15 and formaldehyde should be studied carefully, since the patient may require special instructions. The patient may be allergic to both ingredients or sensitive only to formaldehyde reacting to its release by

this preservative in the occlusive patch test. In the latter situation, quaternium-15 may or may not be tolerated by the patient when present in cosmetics at a 0.2–0.3% concentration. A product use test should clarify the situation. A negative test relates to the product tested and not to all products, because of differences in bioavailability.

Formaldehyde as a preservative is used almost exclusively in wash-off products such as shampoos. Used in this manner, formaldehyde is seldom a cause of sensitization in the consumer, and is only infrequently problematic for the beautician.[95,96]

Bronopol (2-bromo-2-nitropropane-1,3-diol) has a broad spectrum of activity, most effectively against bacteria. It is a formaldehyde releaser, and may pose a problem for the formaldehyde-sensitive patient. In addition, this preservative may interact with amines or amides to produce nitrosamines or nitrosamides, which are suspected carcinogens. Patch testing with standard concentrations may produce marginal irritation responses. Positives are best retested, and if positive followed by a provocative-use test.

Kathon CG (5-chloro-2-methyl-4-isothiazolin-3-one and 2-methyl-4-isothiazolin-3-one) has developed great popularity as a preservative. It has been a preservative of choice for many formulators because of its broad applicability and ease of formulation. It is incorporated in many popular rinse-off products and some leave-on cosmetics under concentration restrictions. In spite of inducing sensitivity in guinea pigs at levels down to 25 ppm and elicitation levels down to 100 ppm and less, this preservative has infrequently produced sensitization from shampoo usage.[97] Kathon CG has been the subject of several adverse-reaction investigations. Depending on the study, it has shown significant rates of sensitization at concentrations from 2–5%.[98–100] Diagnostic testing should be performed at 100 ppm in water because 300 ppm in water induces active sensitization (B Bjorker, S Fregert, personal communication, 1984). Possibly 150–250 ppm might be more appropriate, but this requires additional study.

Preservation in the future

The cosmetic industry experiences two major challenges: the elimination of all animal testing and the development of preservative-free cosmetics. In recent years, strong socioeconomic pressure has focused interest and research on developing preservative-free products and preservation based upon natural extracts. Both of these approaches, while seemingly sound scientifically and from a marketing position, are fraught with problems. Natural preservatives are often complex mixtures, with many unknown chemicals. It is likely that some of these active materials may present sensitization rates equal to or greater than those of synthetic materials. The recently approved Sixth Amendment of the EC Cosmetic Directive has called for the elimination of all animal testing of personal care products and ingredients by 1998, unless alternative methods cannot be developed by then. While most new raw materials will be able to use new, alternative safety testing methods, preservatives will experience difficulty complying with existing requirements for chronic safety studies such as mutagenicity and teratogenicity, without relying on animals. Almost all regulatory agencies around the world currently require the use of in vivo methods to confirm the safety of biocidal ingredients. In vitro testing will most likely be used first as a prescreening test. At the present time, this may reduce the need for some animal testing. However, it is unlikely that all in vivo methods will be replaced by 1998. Before in vitro assays can replace animal testing, they should be validated against the known in vivo testing. This has the unfortunate drawback of increasing the safety testing cost, since the cost of acute in vitro testing is as high as acute in vivo testing.

Emulsifiers

Creams and lotions require the presence of an emulsifier to allow the combination of water and oil. Emulsifiers may act as mild irritants, especially if applied to slightly damaged skin. Pugliese[101] suggested that increased epidermal cell renewal or 'plumping' of the skin may be due to mild irritant effects of nonionic surfactants. Hannuksela et al[102] patch tested over 1200 eczematous patients with common emulsifiers.

One emulsifier, stearamidoethyl diethylamine phosphate, has been implicated in four cases of cosmetic contact dermatitis.[103] Irritant reactions are seen at the same concentration as allergic responses. When 5% triethanolamine stearate in petrolatum was tested, 9.5% of the patch tests showed irritant reactions. Even positive reactions to 1% triethanolamine in petrolatum should be confirmed by retesting and provocative-use testing.

Lanolin

Lanolin is a mixture of esters and polyesters of high-molecular-weight alcohols and fatty acids. This naturally occurring wax varies in its composition depending on its source. Adams and Maibach[3] reported in the NACDG study that lanolin and its derivatives remain among the ingredients that most commonly cause allergic contact dermatitis in cosmetics. Because of its superior emollient properties, lanolin is a popular ingredient for cosmetics.

Sulzberger et al[104] patch tested over 1000 patients suspected of having contact dermatitis, and 1% reacted to anhydrous lanolin. The allergen or allergens, which have not been identified, are found in the alcoholic fraction of lanolin. Patch testing is done most accurately using 30% wool alcohols in petrolatum. Similarly, Kligman[105] tested 943 healthy young women with hydrous lanolin and 30% wool wax alcohol. The results were interpreted as follows: no positive allergic patch tests were read, but irritant reactions to wool alcohols were common. Clark et al[106] estimated that the incidence of lanolin allergy in the general population is 5.5 per million. Lanolin is an important sensitizer when it is applied to eczematous skin eruptions, especially stasis dermatitis. However, cosmetics containing lanolin applied to normal skin are generally harmless. Cronin[89] reported only 26 cases of lanolin cosmetic dermatitis seen between 1966 and 1976 in women. In all of these cases, the lanolin-cosmetic dermatitis affected the face at some time during its course; almost half showed eyelid involvement. The history was of intermittent eruptions, often with swelling and edema.

Eye makeup preparations

Mascara, eyeliner, eye shadow, eyebrow pencil and powders are the most commonly used eye-area makeups. The upper-eyelid dermatitis syndrome is complex and often frustrating to the patient and dermatologist, because of chronicity and failure to respond to our well-intentioned assistance. Causes that we have documented are included in Table 60.6.

Although patients often consider this a reaction to eye makeup, the association is seldom proven. In the North American Contact Dermatitis Group study, 12% of the cosmetic reactions occurred on the eyelid, but only 4%

Table 60.6 Some causes of upper-eyelid dermatitis syndrome
• Irritant dermatitis
• Allergic contact dermatitis
• Photoallergic contact dermatitis
• Phototoxic dermatitis
• Contact urticaria
• Seborrheic dermatitis
• Rosacea diathesis
• Atopic dermatitis
• Psoriasis
• Collagen vascular diseases
• Conjunctivitis
• Blepharitis
• Dysmorphobia

of the reactions were attributed to eye makeup.[3] A workup of patients with eyelid dermatitis includes a careful history of all cosmetic usage, because facial, hair, and nail cosmetic reactions appear frequently on the eyelids.[107] Reactions to cosmetics on the eyelid are often the irritant type; and, to further complicate their diagnosis, they may be due to cumulative irritancy – the summation of several mild irritants (climatic, mechanical or chemical).

When the history does not clearly incriminate certain cosmetics, one should test with the screening patch-test trays as well as all cosmetics that may reach the eye area directly or indirectly. Occlusive patch tests with eyeliner or mascara may give an irritant reaction; thus weakly positive results should be interpreted cautiously. Waterproof mascara must be dried thoroughly for 20 minutes to volatilize hydrocarbon solvents before occluding – and even with this precaution, Epstein[108] noted some irritant reactions. Positive patch tests are repeated for confirmation, and individual ingredient patch testing should be carried out whenever possible. Patch testing cosmetics used in the eye area may occasionally give false-negative results when testing is done on the back or extremities.[107] A provocative-use test carried out in the antecubital fossa or the eyelid itself may ultimately prove the diagnosis.

In the United States, the pigments used in eye area cosmetics are restricted. No coal-tar derivatives may be incorporated. Only purified natural colors or inorganic pigments are used. Nickel contamination of iron oxide pigments has been implicated as a cause of allergic reaction to these cosmetics in the nickel-sensitive user.[109] Eye cosmetics are seldom fragranced, but other known allergens are used in these cosmetics. Almost all eye-area cosmetics are preserved with parabens combined with a second preservative such as phenylmercuric acetate, imidazolidinyl urea, quaternium-15 or potassium sorbate. The following antioxidants are sensitizers found in eye cosmetics: butylated hydroxytoluene, butylated hydroxyanisole,[110] propyl gallate,[111] di-t-butylhydroquinone,[112] colophony,[87] dihydroabietyl alcohol,[88,113] bismuth oxychloride[114] and lanolin.[115] Propylene glycol may act as an irritant or sensitizer. Soap emulsifiers, surfactants and solvents are all potential irritants used in these cosmetics.

Infected corneal ulcers due to abrasions from mascara resulted when the mascaras were not properly preserved.[116] These preservation problems appear to be solved, and reports of infected corneal ulcers have decreased. Patients should be urged to use their eye cosmetics hygienically and advised not to use eye cosmetics inside the lash line.

Hair preparations (non-coloring)

Permanents

Permanent waves are cosmetics that alter the disulfide bonds of hair keratin so that hair fiber configuration can be changed. The disulfide bonds of cystine are broken in the first step when the waving solution is applied to the hair wound around mandrels. In the second step, with neutralization, new disulfide bonds are formed by locking in the curl configuration of the hair.

The waving solutions contain reducing agents that can cause irritant reactions when allowed to run incautiously on the skin surrounding the scalp. Irritant reactions range from erythema to bullous dermatitis. Hair breakage and loss may result when permanent waves are used improperly – in too concentrated a form, for too long a time, or on hair previously damaged by dyes, straighteners or permanent waves. Old-fashioned hot waves occasionally caused chemical burns, which scarred the scalp, producing permanent alopecia, but modern permanents can cause breakage, which results in temporary loss.

In 1973, 'acid permanents' were introduced for beauty salon use.[117] Acid permanents are the most widely used permanent preparation today. These waving lotions, which contain anhydrous glyceryl monothioglycolate in acid form, are mixed at the time of application with a water-based ammonia solution to produce a neutral solution. The hair is covered with a plastic cap and placed under a hair dryer. Since the introduction of 'acid perms', irritant and allergic reactions have been noted to occur on the hands of hairdressers and the face, neck, scalp, and hair line of their customers from use of these permanents.[118,119] Patch testing can be carried out with 1.0% glyceryl thioglycolate (glyceryl monothioglycolate) in petrolatum or water (freshly prepared).

When clients are suspected of contact sensitization, glyceryl monothioglycolate (GMT) is one of the most likely sensitizers. Frosch et al[120] stated that sensitization seems to be much less frequent in clients than in hairdressers, due to less exposure; this was evident with ammonium persulfate (APS) (0% in clients versus 8% in hairdressers). Guerra et al[121] studied 261 hairdresser's clients. They reported the mean frequencies of sensitization as follows: *p*-phenylenediamine (PPD) 7%, *o*-nitro-*p*-phenylenediamine (ONPPD) 5%, GMT 3%, ammonium thioglycolate (AMT) 1% and APS 3%. Morrison and Storrs[122] indicated that the identification of GMT sensitization in a patient is of particular importance, since the clinical symptoms may continue for months even if the use of acid permanent waves is stopped. The allergen clings to the hair, and it is liberated in sufficient amounts during shampooing to maintain the dermatitis. This may elicit dermatitis on the face and neck, which may be confused with allergy or irritancy to shampoo. The operational definition for AMT has not been fulfilled. It is likely that most, if not all, patch-test reactions are irritant rather than allergic.

The 'cold waves' contain thioglycolic acid combined with ammonia or another alkali to raise the pH. The concentration of the thioglycolic acid and alkali can be varied to change the product's speed of action or to suit the type of hair to be waved, that is, hard to wave, normal, or easy to wave. The neutralizer contains hydrogen peroxide or sodium bromate. These permanents have been alleged to rarely cause allergic reactions. Ammonium thioglycolate can be patch tested as 1% or 2.5% in petrolatum.[87] Positives should be confirmed with serial dilution patch testing and provocative-use testing. Another type of permanent used primarily at home is the sulfite wave. Although the sulfite wave produces weaker curls and is slower, the odor is more pleasant. Neutralization is usually done with bromates.

Occasional allergic reactions have been alleged with these permanents. It is recommended to use 1% sodium bisulfite in water for patch testing.[123]

Straighteners

Straightening hair involves using a heated comb with petrolatum or a mixture of petrolatum, oils and waxes. The petrolatum or 'pressing oils' act as a heat-modifying conductor, which reduces friction when the comb travels down the hair fibers. Mechanical and heat damage can cause hair breakage. Over the years, the heated oils can injure the hair follicles, leading to scarring alopecia.

Chemical straighteners containing sodium hydroxide, 'lye', cleave the disulfide bonds of keratin thoroughly and straighten hair permanently. Experience and caution in applying these straighteners are important to avoid hair breakage and chemical burns. Similar products that contain guanidine carbonate mixed with calcium hydroxide are reputed to be milder. It is necessary to straighten new growth every several months. Care is taken not to 'double-process' the distal hair, which is already straightened. Some manufacturers advise against using permanent hair colors that require peroxide on chemically straightened hair to avoid damage.

Sulfite straighteners, chemically similar to sulfite permanents, are best suited to relaxing curly Caucasian hair. 'Soft Curls' have become a fashionable way of styling Black hair. Ammonium thioglycolate and a bromate or peroxide neutralizer are used to achieve restructuring of the hair.

Shampoos

When shampoos are used, they have generally a short contact time with the scalp, and are diluted and rinsed off quickly. These factors reduce their sensitizing potential. Consumers' complaints are commonly directed at their eye stinging and irritating qualities.[53] The importance of eye safety testing for these products became apparent 35 years ago when shampoos based on blends of cationic and nonionic detergents caused blindness in some users.

Modern shampoos are detergent-based, with a few containing small amounts of soap for conditioning. Anionic detergents and amphoteric detergents are occasional sensitizers.[124,125] Fatty acid amides used in shampoos as thickeners and foam stabilizers have caused allergic contact dermatitis in other products.[126] Formaldehyde or formaldehyde releasers may be used as preservatives in shampoos, but formaldehyde rarely causes contact dermatitis in hairdressers or consumers related to use of shampoos.[95,96] Other new preservatives used in shampoos include 5-chloro-2-methyl-4-isothiazoline-3-one and 2-methyl-4-isothiazoline-3-one. Individual ingredient patch testing is necessary to incriminate allergens in shampoos. They produce false-negative results because they are diluted in the final product.

Hair coloring preparations

Over 30 million Americans color their hair using five different types of dye:

- *Permanent hair dyes (type I)* are mixtures of colorless aromatic compounds that act as primary intermediates and couplers. The primary intermediates, *p*-phenylenediamine (PPD), toluene-2,5-diamine (*p*-toluenediamine) and *p*-aminophenol, are oxidized by hydrogen peroxide with couplers to form a variety of colors that blend to give the desired shade. These reactions take place inside the hair shaft, accounting for the fastness of these dyes. Permanent dyes are the most popular in the United States because of the variety of natural colors they can achieve.
- *Semipermanent hair dyes (type II)* contain low-molecular-weight *o*-nitro-*p*-phenylenediamine and anthraquinone dyes, which penetrate the hair cortex to some extent. Their color lasts through approximately five shampoos.
- *Temporary rinses (type III)* are mixtures of mild organic acids and certified dyes that coat the hair shaft. These shampoo off easily.
- *Vegetable dyes (type IV)* in the United States contain henna, which only colors hair red.
- *Metallic dyes (type V)* contain lead acetate and sulfur. When they are combed through the hair daily, they deposit insoluble lead oxides and sulfides that impart colors that range from yellow-brown to dark gray.

Types I and II contain 'coal tar' hair dyes, and in the United States they must bear a label warning about adverse reactions. Instructions for open patch testing are given. The law requires patch testing to be performed before each dye application. In practice, this is seldom carried out in homes or salons. 'Coal tar' dyes are added occasionally to temporary rinses; these rinses must also bear a warning label and patch-test instructions.

A persistent and significant number of reactions to hair dyes are seen by dermatologists each year. Seven percent of the reactions to cosmetics diagnosed by the North American Contact Dermatitis Group were caused by hair dyes.[3] Their severity ranges from mild erythema at the hairline and ears, to swelling of the eyelids and face, to an acute vesicular eruption in the scalp that requires prompt medical attention.

Most reactions to 'coal tar' dyes are reactions to PPD. Independent sensitization to toluene-2,5-diamine or 2-nitro-*p*-phenylenediamine dyes or resorcinol occurs rarely, but positive patch tests to toluene-2,5-diamine or 2-nitro-*p*-phenylenediamine dyes result generally from cross-sensitization to PPD.

One percent PPD in petrolatum is used in the standard closed patch test. Occasionally patients who have a +1 reaction to PPD do not have a significant reaction when they dye their hair, but stronger patch-test results should warn patients not to use these hair dyes. *p*-Phenylenediamine is a colorless compound. Patch-test material gradually darkens as PPD oxidizes, and it should be stored in dark containers and should be made fresh at least yearly.

The products of PPD's oxidation are not allergenic. Reiss and Fisher[127] studied the allergenicity of dyed hair. Twenty patients sensitive to PPD were tested to freshly dyed hair in closed patch tests, and all were negative. The findings of this study are particularly important to hairdressers sensitive to PPD, who may work with dyed hair all day. Occasional case reports have suggested that contact reactions occurred to another person's dyed hair.[128–131] We assume that the dyeing process must not have been carried out properly, and unoxidized products remained on the hair.

Patients sensitive to PPD should be warned about possible cross-reactions with local anesthetics (procaine and benzocaine), sulfonamides and *p*-aminobenzoic acid sunscreens. It is estimated that 25% of patients who are PPD-sensitive will react to semipermanent hair dyes. Patients who wish to try these as a substitute should do an open patch test with the dye first.

Several patients have been reported who experienced immediate hypersensitivity reactions to PPD, and this spectrum of reactions to hair dyes should now be considered as a diagnostic possibility in appropriate patients.[132] Some patients complain of scalp irritation after dyeing their hair, but we are unaware of published data on the potential of these dyes for irritation. Some hair-dye reactions occur most prominently in light-exposed areas, but the phototoxic and photoallergic potential of 'coal tar' dyes has not been investigated.

Henna has not been reported to cause allergic contact dermatitis when used as a hair dye, but a case has been reported from coloring the skin with henna.[133] Cronin[134] described a hairdresser who noted wheezing and coryza when she handled henna; this patient had a positive prick test to henna. Edwards and Edwards[135] reported a case of contact dermatitis due to lead acetate in the metallic dyes.

When hair is bleached, ammonium persulfate is added to hydrogen peroxide to obtain the lightest shades. Ammonium persulfate has several industrial uses, and it is known to cause irritant reactions commonly and allergic contact dermatitis occasionally.[92] Methods of testing for immediate hypersensitivity include rubbing a saturated solution of ammonium persulfate on intact skin, scratch tests or intracutaneous tests using a 1% aqueous solution of ammonium persulfate, and inhalation of 0.1 μg of ammonium persulfate powder. All of these methods can cause immediate hypersensitivity reactions, including urticaria, facial edema, asthma and syncope. Therefore they should be performed only when emergency treatment for anaphylaxis is available. These reactions are hista-mine-mediated, but it is not clear whether or not immunologic mechanisms are involved.[136] Hairdressers should be instructed that clients who develop hives, generalized itching, facial swelling or asthma when the hair is bleached should not have the process repeated using persulfate. Clients experiencing such reactions should receive immediate medical attention.

Facial makeup preparations

Eleven percent of the reactions to cosmetics in the NACDG study were attributed to facial makeup products, which include lipstick, rouge, makeup bases and facial powder.[3] Prior to 1960, allergic reactions to lipsticks were common: most were caused by D&C red 21 (eosin), an indelible dye used in long lasting, deeply colored lipsticks. The sensitizer in eosin proved to be a contaminant; improved methods of purification have reduced its sensitizing potential. Because eosin is strongly bound to keratin, patch tests are performed with 50% eosin in petrolatum.

Other dyes have occasionally been reported as sensitizers. Cronin[89] reported reactions to D&C red 36, D&C red 31, D&C red 19, D&C red 17, and D&C yellow 11. The latter is a potent sensitizer seldom used in lipsticks, but reported also as a sensitizing agent in eye cream[137] and rouge as well as lipstick.[138] D&C red 17 is not permitted in lipstick in the United States. D&C yellow 10, produced by the sulfonation of D&C yellow 11, is not a potent sensitizer.[139] Other sensitizers reported in lipsticks include castor oil acting as a pigment solvent,[140] the antioxidants propyl gallate and mono-t-butylhydroquinone,[111,141] the sunscreens phenyl salicylate and amyldimethylaminobenzoic acid,[142,143] lanolin[115] and fragrance.

Although reactions to lipstick are uncommon, dermatologists should consider this diagnosis even when the eruption has spread beyond the lips, because the sensitizing chemical may be present in cosmetics other than the lipstick. Each lipstick that the patient uses should be tested closed, and photopatch tests should be done, because some of the dyes used may be photoallergens.

Rouge or 'blush' is manufactured in various forms: powder, cream, liquid, stick and gel. It is designed to highlight the cheeks with color. The composition is not unique: powders are similar to face powder, and creams and liquids are similar to foundation. To achieve bright shades, organic colors are added to rouges, as they are to lipsticks. D&C yellow 11 caused allergic reactions to rouges as well as lipsticks.[138] Some women may use lipstick to color their cheeks in place of rouge, or rouge may be used all over the face to achieve a healthy glow. These practices need to be taken into account when evaluating patterns of contact dermatitis on the face.

Facial makeups or foundations are applied to the skin to give an appearance of uniform color and texture and to disguise blemishes or imperfections. They are produced in a variety of forms – emulsions of water and oil, oil-free lotions, anhydrous sticks, poured powders and pancake makeups – and the amount of coverage given is determined by the titanium dioxide (TiO_2) content. Because TiO_2 reflects light, some ordinary makeups achieve sun protection factor (SPF) values of 2 or even 4.[144] In recent years, sunscreen agents have been added to some foundations to increase these SPF values. When sunscreening claims are made for these cosmetics, the US government will consider these products as OTC drugs also. PABA derivatives, fragrances, emulsifiers, preservatives, propylene glycol and lanolin are chemicals with significant sensitizing potential used in these makeups. Synthetic esters, such as isopropyl myristate and lanolin derivatives, added to these makeups have been implicated as causes of acne by the rabbit ear test.[40]

Calnan[145] described a woman who had a positive patch test to her foundation on two occasions, and her facial eruption flared when she used this foundation. However, patch testing the individual ingredients of this foundation gave negative results. Calnan raised the possibility of compound allergy – the allergen is produced by a combination of more than one ingredient.

Sunscreens

Sunscreens can be classified into two major types: chemical and physical sunscreens.[146] Physical sunscreens such as titanium dioxide and zinc oxide reduce the amount of light penetrating the skin by creating a physical barrier that reflects, scatters or physically blocks the ultraviolet light reaching the skin surface. Chemical sunscreens, on the other hand, reduce the amount of light reaching the stratum corneum by absorbing the radiation. Examples of chemical sunscreens include *p*-aminobenzoic acid (PABA) and PABA derivatives such as Padimate O, cinnamates, benzophenones, salicylate derivatives and dibenzoylmethane derivatives.

Because chemical sunscreens are applied topically to the skin in relatively high concentrations (up to 26%), contact sensitization can occur. Similarly, because these chemicals absorb radiation, they have the potential to cause photosensitization. Both types of sensitization can occur not only with the various sunscreening agents but also with excipients such as emulsifiers, antioxidants and preservatives that are included in the various hydroalcoholic lotions, ointments, oil-in-water or water-in-oil emulsions. Despite extensive sunscreen use, there have been infrequent published reports of sunscreen-induced side-effects, including allergic/photoallergic reactions, but we have inadequate data to accurately predict the degree of hypersensitivity to sunscreening agents due to the lack of a well-developed adverse reaction reporting system.

Table 60.7 lists examples of the sunscreen formulations sold in the United States, together with the active ingredients and their sun protection factors (SPF), a measure of

Table 60.7 Selected sunscreen formulations available in the United States		
Trade name	**SPF**	**Active ingredients**
Four sunscreening ingredients		
Coppertone (Plough)	30	Padimate O, Parsol MCX, octyl salicylate, oxybenzone
Sundown (Johnson & Johnson)	30	Parsol MCX, octyl salicylate, oxybenzone, titanium dioxide
	20	Padimate O, Parsol MCX, octyl salicylate, oxybenzone
Cancer Garde (Eclipse Labs)	30	Padimate O, Parsol MCX, oxybenzone, titanium dioxide
T/I Screen (T/I Pharmaceuticals)	30+	Parsol MCX, octocrylene, octyl salicylate, oxybenzone
Block Out (Carter Products)	30	Parsol MCX, padimate O, octyl salicylate, oxybenzone
Supershade (Plough)	44	Parsol MCX, padimate O, homosalate, oxybenzone
Three sunscreening ingredients		
Solbar (Person and Covey)	50	Parsol MCX, octocrylene, oxybenzone
PreSun for Kids (Westwood)	39	Parsol MCX, octyl salicylate, oxybenzone
PreSun 29	29	Parsol MCX, octyl salicylate, oxybenzone
Bain de Soleil (Bain de Soleil)	30	Padimate O, Parsol MCX, oxybenzone
Ultrashade (Plough)	23	Padimate O, Parsol MCX, oxybenzone
Total Eclipse (Eclipse Labs)	15	Padimate O, octyl salicylate, oxybenzone
Sundown (Johnson & Johnson)	15	Padimate O, Parsol MCX, oxybenzone
Two sunscreening ingredients		
Supershade (Plough)	8, 15	Parsol MCX, oxybenzone
Coppertone (Plough)	4, 6, 8, 15	Padimate O, oxybenzone
Shade (Plough)	4, 6	Padimate O, oxybenzone
PreSun (Westwood)	8, 15	Padimate O, oxybenzone
Water Babies (Plough)	15	Parsol MCX, oxybenzone
Sundown (Johnson & Johnson)	4, 6, 8	Padimate O, oxybenzone
Block Out (Carter Products)	15	Padimate O, oxybenzone
Photoplex (Herbert Labs)	15	Padimate O, avobenzone
One sunscreening ingredient		
Coppertone (Plough)	2	Octyl salicylate
Bain de Soleil (Bain de Soleil)	2, 4	Padimate O
Eclipse (Eclipse Labs)	5	Padimate O
	10	Glyceryl PABA

sunscreen protection against sunburn. Most of the formulations that are combination sunscreens contain one or more UVB absorbers and a UVA absorber to provide much-needed protection against the damaging effects of UVA. Several sunscreens also include physical blockers such as titanium dioxide.

In general, as the SPF of the sunscreen formulation increases, the number of active ingredients increases to three or four, and in some cases the total amount of active sunscreens increases up to 26%. Not all formulations list the specific concentrations of the active ingredients, and it is possible that some may contain higher concentrations. As with many chemicals, increasing the concentrations of the active ingredients may increase the likelihood of sensitization.[147] The majority of sunscreens contain octyldimethyl PABA (Padimate O) as the main UVB absorber. The cinnamate derivative, octylmethoxycinnamate (Parsol MCX), is also used as a UVB absorber.

Most sunscreens with more than one ingredient contain oxybenzone as the additional ingredient. The absorption peak of this compound lies in the UVB region, and extends partially into the UVA. Other agents that absorb in the UVA region include sulisobenzone, dioxybenzone, menthylanthranilate and avobenzone. The latter chemical, which has an absorption maximum in the middle of the UVA region (358 nm), has been approved in the United States in two sunscreen formulations (Photoplex, Herbert Laboratories, Santa Ana, CA, and Coppertone, Sun and Shade) (Table 60.7). Representatives of all major sunscreen categories, including PABA derivatives, anthranilates, salicylates, cinnamates and benzophenones, that have caused allergic reactions are described next.

p-Aminobenzoic acid (PABA)

In 1975, Willis[148] suggested that the sensitization potential of *p*-aminobenzoic acid was minimal. Wennersten et al[149] reported that a total of 73 of 1883 (3.9%) subjects tested with 5% PABA in alcohol in the Scandinavian standard photopatch tray had either allergic or photoallergic responses to PABA. These subjects represent 73% of the total number of subjects with contact and photocontact sensitization to PABA. The use of PABA as a sunscreening agent in Europe and the United States has decreased significantly in recent years. PABA has been replaced by ester derivatives such as Padimate O that, unlike PABA, are not water-soluble and tend to remain on the surface layer, with less than 10% penetrating the corneum even after 24 hours.[150] These PABA esters appear to be less sensitizing than PABA; however, there are no data to substantiate this impression.

PABA derivatives

Sensitization to glyceryl PABA has been reported for the last 30 years.[151,152] Many of the cases of glyceryl PABA sensitization showed uniform strong reactions to benzocaine, suggesting that the sensitization may be due to the presence of impurities in the glyceryl PABA. This suggestion was first made by Fisher,[153] and has since been confirmed.[154] Benzocaine impurities (1–18%) occurred in many commercial sources of glyceryl PABA. Thus many of the early reports of contact allergy to glyceryl PABA may have falsely

implicated glyceryl PABA as the sensitizer. Thune[155] reported two cases of allergic/photoallergic reactions to glyceryl PABA in which there was no reaction to benzocaine, suggesting true allergy to the PABA derivative. However, no allergic responses were observed when these subjects were patched with glyceryl PABA that had been purified via high-pressure liquid chromatography.[156] This suggests the presence of an, as yet, unknown impurity or impurities other than benzocaine as the sensitization source. This shows the importance of utilizing purified raw materials in the manufacture of consumer products and the need for careful interpretation of patch test results.

Other PABA derivatives that have caused sensitization/photocontact sensitization include octyldimethyl PABA (Padimate O), amyldimethyl PABA (Padimate A), and ethyldihydroxy PABA. The number of case reports of sensitization/photocontact sensitization with Padimate O is less than that reported with PABA and glyceryl PABA, suggesting a lower sensitization potential with this derivative. This may be because Padimate O is not a true PABA ester, since it does not contain the NH_2 grouping present in glyceryl PABA, PABA and benzocaine.[157]

Although Padimate A was included as a safe and effective sunscreening agent,[146] this derivative can cause phototoxicity and may have accounted for the erythema response observed by Katz[158] 30 minutes after sun exposure. This compound is no longer used in sunscreens in the United States. In addition to benzocaine impurities in the glyceryl PABA raw materials, some PABA esters contain 0.2–4.5% PABA.[159] It is possible that PABA impurities may account for some of the reports of sensitization to the PABA derivatives.

Salicylates

There are two cases of contact allergy and two reports of photocontact allergy to homomenthyl salicylate in the literature[74,160] and no reports of sensitization to octyl salicylate, the major salicylate derivative in many sunscreens.

Cinnamates

Cinnamates are chemically related to or are found in balsam of Peru, balsam of Tolu, coca leaves, cinnamic acid, cinnamic aldehyde and cinnamon oil, ingredients used in perfumes, topical medications, cosmetics and flavoring. Thune[155] reported eight cases of sensitivity to cinnamates, two cases of photoallergy to 2-ethoxyethyl-*p*-cinnamate, and six subjects with contact allergy to other cinnamates such as amylcinnamaldehyde, amylcinnamic acid and cinnamon oil. Calnan[161] reported cross-sensitization among cinnamon derivatives.

Benzophenones

There have been reported cases of photocontact allergy[155,162] and contact allergy[163,164] to oxybenzone; and reports of contact allergy[3,165] and photocontact allergy to sulisobenzone.[74] Benzophenone-10 (Mexenone), a benzophenone derivative not used in sunscreens in the United States, can also cause contact and photocontact dermatitis.[166,167]

Dibenzoylmethanes

Dibenzoylmethane derivatives such as isopropyldibenzoylmethane (Eusolex 8020) and butyldibenzoylmethane (avobenzone) have been incorporated in European sunscreens as UVA absorbers since 1980. Instances of contact allergy/photoallergy to sunscreens and lipsticks containing dibenzoylmethanes or these derivatives have been reported, although the majority of reports have been associated with the isopropyl derivative.[168–170] As a result, manufacturers stopped incorporating Eusolex 8020 into their products.[171,172] Recently, the manufacturers of Eusolex 8020 have withdrawn it from the market.

There have been fewer reports of contact allergy/photoallergy to the butyldibenzoylmethane derivative, avobenzone. It is possible that some of these reactions to avobenzone may have been cross-reactions resulting from prior exposure to the isopropyl derivative.[169] Greater utilization of these compounds with appropriate testing should help clarify their relative sensitization potential.

Camphor derivatives

3-(4-Methylbenzylidene) camphor (Eusolex 6300) is a sunscreening agent used extensively in Europe, often in combination with Eusolex 8020, but it is not approved for use in the United States. There have been several reports of allergic and photoallergic reactions to sunscreens containing this agent.[172,173]

Miscellaneous

Other chemical sunscreens that have caused allergic reactions include diagalloyl trioleate,[174] the glycerol ester of *o*-amino-*m*-(2,3-dihydroxypropoxy)benzoic acid,[175] a dioxane derivative[176] and 2-phenyl-5-methylbenzol (witisol).[177] None of these ingredients are approved for use in sunscreens in the United States.

Titanium dioxide

Physical blockers such as titanium dioxide and zinc oxide have the advantage of not being sensitizers, but may be so occlusive that they can cause miliaria.[178] Kaminester[179] reported that the inclusion of titanium dioxide in a PABA sunscreen blocked the appearance of photoallergy. It is possible that the reflection and scattering of light by titanium dioxide reduced the amount of UV light that penetrated the skin and elicited photoallergy.

Excipients

Contact allergy can also be caused by excipients included in sunscreens. These chemicals include mineral oil, petrolatum, isopropyl esters, lanolin derivatives, aliphatic alcohols, triglycerides, fatty acids, waxes, propylene glycol, emulsifiers, thickeners, preservatives and fragrances. An extensive list of vehicle constituents in cosmetics that can cause allergic responses has been published.[53] de Groot[54] indicated that preservatives, fragrances and emulsifiers are the main classes of ingredients responsible for cosmetic allergy, with Kathon CG producing contact allergic reactions in 27.7% of subjects tested. Sunscreens available in the United States provide a complete list of ingredients, including the excipients. The listing of all ingredients in sunscreens should be encouraged so that consumers, especially those with known sensitivities to chemicals, are fully informed about the composition of the formulation prior to the purchase and application of the product to the skin.

Manicuring preparations

In the past, adverse reactions have been reported to numerous nail cosmetics that have subsequently been removed from the market because of reported hazards. Nail hardeners containing formaldehyde are in this category. In the United States, this type of hardener is permitted for use only on the free edge of the nail when the skin is protected from contact with the hardener. Some manufacturers sell products called 'hardeners', but they have merely increased the resin content of ordinary nail enamel. Nail enamels including base coats and top coats have a similar composition. The concentration of each of these chemicals depends on the quality to be achieved in the final product. The base coat will have increased amounts of resin to improve adhesion to the nail plate, but the top coat has increased nitrocellulose and plasticizers to enhance gloss and abrasion resistance.

Toluenesulfonamide/formaldehyde resin (TSFR) is responsible for contact dermatitis around the nails, but also at sites distant from the fingers – commonly the eyelids, around the mouth and chin, sides of the neck, on the genitalia, and, rarely, a generalized eruption. In contrast, free formaldehyde in nail hardeners causes mostly local reactions. Cronin[89] recommended 10% toluenesulfonamide/formaldehyde in petrolatum to perform a closed patch test. Norton[180] reported that

free-formaldehyde (FF) hardeners are the most common cause of nail cosmetic reaction, followed by methacrylate and cyanoacrylate resins, TSFR, acetone removers, and sodium and potassium hydroxide removers. Norton also reported onychomycosis, chromonychia, anonychia and pterigium inversum unguis secondary to FF nail hardeners. A small amount (0.1–0.5%) of free formaldehyde is in the resin.[145] Fisher[181] proposed that patients who are allergic to this resin may wear nail polish without problems if they allow it to dry thoroughly with their hands quietly at rest. Those who find this inconvenient can be advised to purchase certain 'hypoallergenic' brands of nail polish, which substitute alkyd or other resins. The patient should be asked to check the ingredient list for toluenesulfonamide/formaldehyde resin as a precaution. The durability and abrasion resistance of these other resins is said to be inferior to toluenesulfonamide/formaldehyde resin. Although onycholysis has been attributed to reactions to toluenesulfonamide/formaldehyde resin, no published data firmly support this.[182,183] A new nail enamel compound has been introduced by Almay and Revlon. The toluenesulfonamide/formaldehyde resin, the principal allergic sensitizer in nail enamels, has been replaced by glyceryl tribenzoate. In addition, these new enamels are toluene-free and replace dibutylphthalate by glyceryltriacetate. This new plasticizer, a polymer that prevents brittleness, provides longer wearability (Levy, personal communication, 1994). Another very recent innovation is quick-drying suspensions. Two recent patents employing acetone and halogenated hydrocarbons provide for a reduction in time of 50–70% over conventional nail enamel compositions without adversely affecting the other desirable properties of the coating. Environmentally safe nail enamels are a real challenge for the cosmetic industry. Water-based nail polish with adhesion, gloss and drying qualities will be developed.[184] A water- dilutable nail polish has been developed containing a mixture of polyurethanes, and vinyl and/or acrylic esters.[185,186]

Yellow pigmentation of the nail plate, darkest at the distal end, occurs commonly in women who wear colored nail polish. Samman[85] reproduced this staining with the following colors: D&C red 7, D&C red 34, D&C red 6 and FD&C yellow 5 lake. Nail enamel removers are mixtures of solvents such as acetone, amyl, butyl or ethyl acetate, to which fatty materials may be added.[187] These can be irritating to the skin and can strip the nail plate. Cuticle removers contain alkaline chemicals, frequently sodium or potassium hydroxide, to break the disulfide bonds of keratin. They should not be left on for prolonged periods or be used by people who are susceptible to paronychia. Cuticle removers are irritants.

'Sculptured nails' have become popular in recent years because they build an attractive artificial nail on the nail plate. They are prosthetic nails with a fresh acrylic mixture of methylmethacrylate monomer liquid and polymer powder. They are molded within a metabolized paperboard template on the natural nail surface to produce nails of the desired thickness and length. When hardened, the template is removed, the prosthesis filed and the surface is polished. Acrylate sculptured nails are of two varieties: methacrylate monomers, and polymers that polymerize in the presence of hydroquinone in ordinary light. Photobonded acrylate sculptured nails are based on acrylates that are photobonded. Allergic reactions to sculptured nails consist of paronychia, onychia, and severe and prolonged paresthesia. Fisher[188] reported that a patient developed a severe reaction to methyl methacrylate monomers resulting in permanent loss of all her fingernails. Fisher and Baran[189] reported that cyanoacrylates do not cross-react with other acrylates.

Unfortunately, irritant and allergic reactions to the liquid monomers, as well as secondary infections, may be painful and long-lasting. Paronychia, onycholysis, onychia,

and dermatitis of the finger and distant sites may occur. Fisher et al[190] reported allergic sensitization to the methyl methacrylate monomers in sculptured nails. In 1974, the FDA banned the use of methylmethacrylate in these cosmetics. However, analysis of 31 products sold between 1975 and 1981 revealed that this monomer was present in 9 of them.[191] Sensitization has also been reported to other monomers, and cross-reactions between acrylate monomers do occur.[188,192] Patch testing with 1.0–5.0% monomer in petrolatum or olive oil can help confirm the diagnosis of an allergic sensitization. Controls may be required if the patient responds to 5% and not to 1% of the monomer.

Preformed plastic nails may be designed to cover the nail plate or extended tips. Their prolonged use causes mechanical damage to the nail, and those covering the entire nail plate may cause injury by occlusion.[193] Sensitization to *p*-t-butylphenol formaldehyde resin in the nail adhesive and tricresylethyl phthalate in the artificial nail has been reported.[194] Nail mending and wrapping kits often help women grow the longer nails they desire, with few adverse reactions. A split nail can be repaired with cyanoacrylate glue with a negligible risk of sensitization. The repair is splinted with papers affixed by a nitrocellulose-containing glue. These papers, or in some cases linen or silk, are wrapped over the free edge of the nail to protect it from trauma. Use of more-sensitizing glues, of course, increases the risk of adverse reactions. The paper or cloth should not cover a large portion of the attached nail plate, to avoid complications of occlusion.

Oral hygiene products

Dentifrices and mouthwashes are incriminated infrequently as causing allergic contact reactions. This may be due to the short exposure time these products have with the skin and mucous membrane under ordinary use situations. If sensitization occurs inside the mouth, patch testing on the skin usually shows a positive reaction. Many of the products contain detergents and are unsuitable for closed patch testing. To avoid irritant reactions, one should test open in the antecubital fossa and confirm positive results with tests in controls. To help patients avoid further reactions, ingredient patch testing should be done. Fisher[195] reviewed concentrations for patch testing ingredients found in toothpastes and mouthwashes. If the physician suspects allergic contact dermatitis and negative patch tests on the skin do not reflect mucosal sensitivity, ingredients may be incorporated in Orabase (Squibb). This material can be held against the inside of the lip for 24 hours, and then examined for erythema. Reports of allergic sensitization to toothpastes in the last decade have primarily involved flavoring agents.[196] Cinnamic aldehyde has been the most frequent offender, because it was introduced in a relatively high concentration in toothpaste sold in several countries.[197–199] A case of contact dermatitis to cinnamic aldehyde resulted in depigmentation about the vermilion border.[63]

Personal cleanliness products

The action of bacteria upon sterile apocrine secretions produces a characteristic odor. Lipophilic diphtheroids produce unique axillary odors.[200] Although deodorants are considered cosmetics, antiperspirants are regulated as over-the-counter (OTC) drugs as well as cosmetics. Many of these products have been reformulated in the last decade because of government regulations.[201] Hexachlorophene was banned because of its neurotoxicity and halogenated salicylanilides because of their photoallergic nature. Chlorofluorocarbon propellants were removed from aerosols because of their role in depleting the stratosphere of ozone. The chlorofluorocarbons have been replaced by hydrocarbon propellants – isobutane, butane and propane – which are flammable. The FDA OTC Antiperspirant Review Panel recommended the removal of zirconium-containing chemicals from aerosol antiperspirants because of the potential for formation of granuloma in the lung. Sodium zirconium acetate salts had caused granulomatous lesions in the skin of the axilla.

Simple deodorants reduce the number of bacteria in the axilla. Most deodorants contain triclosan as an active ingredient. Triclosan is an antimicrobial agent used in soaps and shampoos. Draize testing showed a low-sensitizing potential for this chemical.[202] Allergic contact dermatitis to this chemical has been reported, but this requires confirmation.[87] We recommend a patch test with 1–2% triclosan in petrolatum in suspected cases. The OTC Review Panel published a list of aluminium and aluminium–zirconium chemicals permitted in antiperspirants. These chemicals are not regarded as sensitizers. Irritant reactions to aluminium salts in antiperspirants are common because of the environmental heat, moisture, and the friction and inflammation caused by shaving in the axilla. Allergic reactions are due to the other chemicals in antiperspirants – most frequently the fragrance ingredients. Similarly, feminine hygiene sprays are primarily fragrance products that cause irritant reactions when sprayed too close.

Baby products

These products are marketed primarily to use on the skin and scalps of infants. Some experimental data suggest that infants are less easily sensitized than adults. However, Epstein[203] reported that 44% of infants under one year of age could be sensitized to pentadecylcatechol, but that 87% of children over three years of age were sensitized in the same experiment. In clinical practice, allergic contact dermatitis is diagnosed infrequently in young children.[204] Patch testing with ingredients in standard concentrations may result in a higher incidence of irritant reactions in young children.[205,206] Because the diaper area is a frequent site of irritant contact dermatitis, careful attention should be paid to the products used there.

Generally, baby products are fragranced. Baby oil, talc and corn starch have simple compositions with little sensitizing potential beside that of the fragrances. Baby lotions or creams may contain fragrance, preservatives, lanolin or propylene glycol, which are common sensitizers.[114] Propylene glycol, present in these lotions and the moistened towelettes marketed for cleansing the diaper area, is a common irritant. In the treatment of infants with diaper rash, it is important to examine the ingredients of the cosmetics used on the diaper area.

Bath preparations

Adverse reactions to bubble bath reported to the FDA include skin eruptions, irritation of the genitourinary tract, eye irritation, and respiratory disorders.[207–209] The genitourinary tract reactions in children have been the most serious; many children have been subjected to extensive urologic workups before the cause was established. The skin eruptions are assumed usually to be irritant reactions due to the detergent content of these cosmetics.

Other skin care preparations

Depilatories

Most depilatories today contain mercaptans such as calcium thioglycolate 2.5–4.0% in conjunction with an alkali to bring the pH to between 10 and 12.5.[187] The keratin of the cortex is more vulnerable before it emerges from the follicle, and depilatories attack it there, leaving a soft rather than a sharp end. For this reason, the use of depilatories in place of shaving can prevent pseudofolliculitis barbae in some Black men. Powdered facial depilatories, produced for beard removal, contain barium or strontium sulfide because these chemicals are quicker acting.

Unfortunately, they cause more irritation and produce an unpleasant odor. In order to use the less malodorous thioglycolate depilatories for coarser-beard removal, hair accelerators such as thiourea, melamine or sodium metasilicate are added. Depilatories cannot be patch tested directly, and these thioglycolates are seldom sensitizers.

Epilating waxes

Epilating waxes are usually warmed to soften, and they harden and enmesh the hair after application. When the wax is pulled off, the hair is removed by the root. Some modified waxes do not have to be warmed, and can be applied with a backing material. These cosmetics may contain beeswax, rosin (colophony), fragrance or rarely benzocaine as potential sensitizers.[187] The problems usually seen with these epilating cosmetics are due to mechanical irritation.

COSMETIC INTOLERANCE SYNDROME

Fisher[210] coined the term 'status cosmeticus' for the condition in which a patient is no longer able to tolerate the use of many or any cosmetic on the face. Patients complain of itching, stinging, burning or discomfort. This group seriously challenges our diagnostic skills as well as our ability to be empathetic, because the severity of patients' symptoms does not match objective signs of disease. Most of these patients have only subjective symptoms, but some may have mild inflammation. The cosmetic intolerance syndrome is not a single entity, but rather a symptom complex due to multiple factors – exogenous and endogenous.[65] Therefore these patients need a thorough history, physical examination and workup. Some patients have occult allergic contact dermatitis, allergic photocontact dermatitis or contact urticarial reactions. Therefore the causal agents are documented by careful clinical review and patch testing.

People who have a seborrheic or rosacea diathesis with or without inflammation seem to have flared this condition by overusing cleansing creams and emollients. Both of these conditions may be accompanied by facial erythema or scaling. Some patients require anti-inflammatory therapy, as do atopic patients who develop this state. Some chemicals can produce itching or stinging or both in patients with 'status cosmeticus'; therefore, whenever possible, these chemicals should be avoided by these patients.

When the offending agent cannot be found, prolonged elimination of cosmetics seems to help some women, who after 6–12 months or more are able to gradually return to the use of other cosmetics (Table 60.8). Additions of skin care products should be made one at a time, and no more frequently than every two weeks. The final program should be simple and limited in the number and frequency of cosmetics used. Goldenberg and Safrin[211] suggested that stinging effects of cosmetics irritants may be neutralized by 'anti-irritants'. They proposed three possible mechanisms of action of anti-irritants: to complex the irritant, to block the reactive sites in the skin, and to prevent physical contact with the skin.

Table 60.8 Management of patients who are intolerant to cosmetic usage

1. Examine every cosmetic and skin care agent

2. Patch and photopatch test to rule out occult allergic and photoallergic contact dermatitis, or contact urticaria

3. Limit skin care to
   - water washing without soap or detergent
   - lip cosmetics
   - eye cosmetics (if the eyelids are not symptomatic)
   - face powder
   - glycerol and rose water as moisturizer (only if needed)
   - 6–12 months of avoidance of other skin care agents and cosmetics

4. Watch for and test, if necessary, depression and other neuropsychiatric aspects

OCCUPATIONAL DERMATITIS: HAIRDRESSERS

Cosmeticians may perform a variety of personal care tasks, including hair grooming, manicuring and applying makeup. It is primarily the hair-care tasks that account for the high rate of occupational hand dermatitis. Cronin[212] noted that beauticians frequently develop a dry, scaling dermatitis over the metacarpophalangeal joints. Novice beauticians and those in training are required to shampoo many customers each day, and the resulting irritation is frequently the initial cause of hand dermatitis. These hairdressers have a good chance of improving as they learn to protect and lubricate their hands. However, patients with atopic eczema may have a particularly difficult time with hand dermatitis as hairdressers, although we do believe they should not be barred from this career. Young atopic patients who are contemplating career choices should be appraised of the occupational hazards of hairdressing.

When beauticians with hand dermatitis are patch tested at different centers, the percentage of reactions varies. PPD is usually the leading offender when allergy is present.[213] Frosch and co-workers[120] reported that the major contact sensitizer of hairdressers in Europe was GMT. Sensitization is at least as frequent to PPD; in some countries (Germany, UK, Spain) sensitization frequencies were high. This has to be emphasized in comparison with the relatively low frequencies to AMT. The recently introduced acid permanent waves pose a higher risk of sensitization to hairdressers than the alkaline permanent waves that have been used since the early 1940s. The low figures for GMT sensitization in some centers may be explained by lower usage in salons or by more careful handling.

There is still a strong prejudice against the use of gloves in this occupation. In Denmark, most hairdressers wear gloves when dyeing and permanent waving. In Germany, most protect their hands only against hair dyes. In Italy, only

12.5% of 240 hairdressers wear gloves for permanent waving, whereas 51% wear them for hair dyeing.[214] A relatively low sensitization to GMT was found in Italy because of its infrequent usage. Guerra et al[214] demonstrated that vinyl gloves may not always suppress the reaction to GMT in sensitized individuals. They found that three of eight patients patch-tested with GMT through vinyl gloves were positive after three days. Better plastic materials must be looked for, if GMT continues to be used in European salons. Furthermore, it must be kept in mind that wearing gloves over a prolonged time poses its own risks. The primary goal in the prevention of occupational dermatitis must be reduction of exposure to highly sensitized agents. Guerra et al[214] reported GMT was the number-one sensitizer. After the series described by Storrs,[119] the German CDRG reported sensitization to GMT in 38% of 87 patients in 1989, and in 31% of a second series of 178 patients.[215] Holness and Nethercott[216] found 23.5% of 34 patients positive to GMT. GMT sensitization may become increasingly frequent if no further action is taken. Hairdressers need to be instructed to handle this type of permanent wave with caution. Direct skin contact should be avoided. Gloves and improved handling technique may lead to a decrease in the frequency of sensitization, which may, in comparison with hair dyes, be acceptable to this occupational group.

Rietschel et al[217] and other investigators have shown that allergens can penetrate gloves. Fisher[218] reported that polyethylene laminate gloves (4-H glove, Safety 4 Company, Denmark) protect allergic patients from epoxy resin and acrylic monomers. McClain and Storrs,[219] in a placebo-controlled double-blind patch-test study, reported that the 4-H glove was effective in preventing allergic contact dermatitis in GMT-sensitized volunteers, protecting four of four patients after an 8-hour exposure and two of three after 48 hours. Reference 220 provides extensive documentation about protective gloves. Frosch et al[120] found PPD to be the second most common sensitizer – very close to GMT. However, sensitization figures for PPD derivatives were considerably lower, ranging from 37%. In the Italian study, the figures were similar for PPD but higher for the derivatives. Frosch and colleagues[120] were unable to conclude that ONPPD had the lowest sensitization risk. They stated that pyrogallol and resorcinol are the least frequent sensitizers in the hairdressers' series.

Nickel, preservatives such as (chloro)-methylisothiazolinone and formaldehyde, surface-active agents such as cocamidopropylbetaine, and hydrolyzed animal proteins, as well as perfume ingredients, may also be responsible for dermatitis in hairdressers. To work-up hairdressers with hand eczema, we use the standard hairdressers screening series. This series includes resorcinol, *p*-toluenediamine sulfate, glyceryl monothioglycolate, ammonium thioglycolate, ammonium persulphate, *p*-aminodiphenylamine hydrochloride, pyrogallol and *o*-nitro-*p*-phenylenediamine. At the same session, we apply 1.0% glyceryl thioglycolate in petrolatum, and pieces of the hairdresser's protective glove applied on both sides.

Hairdressers who are nickel-sensitive also have a serious challenge. There is evidence that permanent solutions may leach nickel out of metal objects.[221] Fastidious care in the selection of stainless-steel tools and use of dimethylglyoxime for testing pins, clips, and other paraphernalia allows some patients to continine in this career. Tomb and co-workers[222] reported a young hairdresser who developed acute periorbital eczema and marked edema of eyelids, lip erosions and eczema of her fingertips to two instant glues used to attach false hair. A patch test to ethyl cyanoacrylate adhesive was strongly positive. Hairdressers with allergic contact dermatitis need to be told that protective gloves may not provide an absolute barrier to allergens.[119]

Ingredient labeling of retailed cosmetics in the United States has greatly aided dermatologists in caring for patients with contact dermatitis. There is no regulation requiring similar labeling for cosmetics used in beauty salons.

REFERENCES

1. Code of Federal Regulations. 1986. 21201(i) paragraph 40.

2. Jackson EM, Cosmetics: substantiating safety. In: *Dermatoxicology*, 4th edn (Marzulli N, Maibach HI, eds). New York: Hemisphere, 1991.

3. Adams RM, Maibach HI, A five-year study of cosmetic reactions. *J Am Acad Dermatol* 1985; **13:** 1062–9.

4. Lammintausta K, Maibach HI, Wilson D, Mechanisms of subjective (sensory) irritation: propensity of nonimmunologic contact urticaria and objective irritation in stingers. *Derm Beruf Unwelt* 1988; **36:** 45–9.

5. Prottey C, The molecular basis of skin irritation. In: *Cosmetic Science*, Vol I (Breuer MM, ed.). London: Academic Press, 1978:275–349.

6. Marzulli FN, Maibach HI (eds) *Dermatoxicology*, 4th edn. New York: Hemisphere, 1991.

7. Berardesca E, Elsner P, Maibach HI, *Bioengineering of the Skin: Cutaneous Blood Flow and Erythema.* Boca Raton, FL: CRC Press, 1994.

8. Elsner P, Berardesca E, Maibach HI, *Bioengineering of the Skin: Water and the Stratum Corneum.* Boca Raton, FL: CRC Press, 1994.

9. Cagen SZ, Malloy LA, Parker CM et al, Pyrethroid mediated skin sensory stimulation characterized by a new behavioral paradigm. *Toxicol Appl Pharmacol* 1984; **76:** 270–9.

10. Frosch PJ, Kligman AM, A method for appraising the stinging capacity of topically applied substances. *J Soc Cosmet Chem* 1977; **28:** 197–207.

11. Frosch PJ, Kligman AM, The chamber scarification test for assessing irritancy of topically applied substances. In: *Cutaneous Toxicity* (Drill VA, Lazar P, eds). New York: Academic Press, 1977:127–44.

12. Vivjeberg HP, VandenBercken J, Frequency dependent effects of the pyrethroid insecticide decamethrin in frog myelinated nerve fibers. *Eur J Pharmacol* 1979; **58:** 501–4.

13. Berardesca E, Cespa M, Farinelli N et al, In vivo transcutaneous penetration of nicotinates and sensitive skin. *Contact Dermatitis* 1991; **25:** 35–8.

14. Landsteiner K, Jacobs J, Studies on the sensitization of animals with simple chemical compounds. II. *J Exp Med* 1935; **64:** 625–9.

15. Polak L, Polak A, Frey JR, The development of contact sensitivity to DNFB in guinea pigs genetically differing in their response to DNP–skin protein conjugate. *Int Arch Allergy Appl Immunol* 1974; **46:** 417–26.

16. Unanue ER, Antigen-presenting function of the macrophage. *Annu Rev Immunol* 1984; **2:** 395–428.

17. Cunningham-Rundles S, Cell-mediated immunity. In: *Immunodermatology* (Safai B, Good RA, eds). New York: Plenum, 1981:133.

18. Lever WF, Schaumburg-Lever G, *Histopathology of the Skin*, 6th edn. Philadelphia: Lippincott, 1983.

19. Magnusson B, Kligman AM, *Allergic Contact Dermatitis in the Guinea Pig.* Springfield, IL: Charles C Thomas, 1970.

20. Magnusson B, Kligman AM, The identification of contact allergens by animals assay. The guinea pig maximization test. *J Invest Dermatol* 1969; **52:** 268–76.

21. Maguire HC, Mechanism of intensification by Freund's complete adjuvant of the acquisition of delayed hypersensitivity in the guinea pig. *Immunol Commun* 1973; **1:** 239–46.

22. Maguire HC, Alteration in the acquisition of delayed hypersensitivity with adjuvant in the guinea pig. *Monogr Allergy* 1974; **8:** 13–26.

23. von Krogh G, Maibach HI, The contact urticaria syndrome. *Semin Dermatol* 1982; **1:** 59–66.

24. Lahti A, Nonimmunologic contact urticaria. *Acta Derm Venereol (Stockh) Suppl* 1980; **60**(91): 1–49.

25. Maibach HI, Johnson HL, Contact urticaria syndrome. Contact urticaria to diethyltoluamide (immediate-type hypersensitivity). *Arch Dermatol* 1975; **111:** 726–30.

26. Lahti A, Maibach HI, Species specificity of nonimmunologic contact urticaria: guinea pig, rat and mouse. *J Am Acad Dermatol* 1985; **13:** 66–9.

27. Harvell J, Bason M, Maibach HI, Contact urticaria and its mechanisms. *Food Chem Toxicol* 1994; **32:** 103–12.

28. Lahti A, Oikarinen A, Viinikka L et al, Prostaglandins in contact urticaria induced by benzoic acid. *Acta Derm Venereol (Stockh)* 1983; **63:** 425–7.

29. Lahti A, McDonald DM, Tammi R, Maibach HI, Pharmacological studies on nonimmunologic contact urticaria in guinea pigs. *Arch Dermatol Res* 1986; **279:** 44–9.

30. Johansson J, Lahti A, Topical non-steroidal anti-inflammatory drugs inhibit non-immunologic immediate contact reactions. *Contact Dermatitis* 1988; **19:** 161–5.

31. Lahti A, Terfenadine does not inhibit non-immunologic contact urticaria. *Contact Dermatitis* 1987; **16:** 220–3.

32. Marzulli FN, Maibach HI, The use of graded concentration in studying skin sensitizers: experimental contact sensitization in man. *Food Cosmet Toxicol* 1974; **12:** 219–27.

33. Guin JD, Meyer BN, Drake RD, Haffley P, The effect of quenching agents on contact urticaria caused by cinnamic aldehyde. *J Am Acad Dermatol* 1984; **10:** 45–51.

34. Fisher AA, Management of facial irritation due to cosmetics in patients with 'status cosmeticus' (cosmetic intolerance). *Cutis* 1990; **46:** 291–3.

35. Lahti A, Maibach HI, Immediate contact reaction: contact urticaria syndrome. *Semin Dermatol* 1987; **6:** 313–20.

36. Mills OH, Berger RS, Defining the susceptibility of acne prone and sensitive skin populations to extrinsic factors. *Dermatol Clin* 1991; **9:** 93–8.

37. Fulton JE, Pay SR, Fulton JE, Comedogenicity of current therapeutic products, cosmetics and ingredients in the rabbit ear. *J Am Acad Dermatol* 1984; **10:** 96–105.

38. Fulton JE, Comedogenicity and irritancy of commonly used ingredients in skin care products. *J Soc Cosmet Chem* 1989; **40:** 321–33.

39. Kligman AM, Mills OH, Acne cosmetica. *Arch Dermatol* 1972; **106:** 843–50.

40. Kligman AM, Kwong T, An improved rabbit ear model for assessing comedogenic substances. *Br J Dermatol* 1979; **100:** 699–702.

41. Tucker SB, Flannigan SA, Dunbar M Jr, Drotman RB, Development of an objective comedogenicity assay. *Arch Dermatol* 1986; **122:** 660–702.

42. American Academy of Dermatology, American Academy of Dermatology invitational symposium of comedogenicity. *J Am Acad Dermatol* 1989; **20:** 272–7.

43. Mills OH Jr, Kligman AM, A human model for assessing comedogenic substances. *Arch Dermatol* 1982; **118:** 903–5.

44. Bronaugh RL, Maibach HI, Primary irritant, allergic contact, phototoxic, and photoallergic reactions to cosmetics and tests to identify problem products. In: *Principles of Cosmetics for the Dermatologist* (Frost P, Horwitz SN, eds). St Louis, MO: CV Mosby, 1982.

45. Jackson EM, Robillard NF, The controlled use test in a cosmetic product safety substantiation program. *J Toxico-Cutan Ocular Toxicol* 1982; **1:** 117–32.

46. Wahlberg JE, Maibach HI, Sterile cutaneous pustules: a manifestation of primary irritancy? Identification of contact pustulogens. *J Invest Dermatol* 1981; **76:** 381–3.

47. Rorsman H, Riehl's melanosis. *Int J Dermatol* 1982; **21:** 75–8.

48. Sugai T, Takahashi Y, Takagi T, Pigmented cosmetic dermatitis and coal tar dyes. *Contact Dermatitis* 1977; **3:** 249–56.

49. Kozuka T, Tashiro M, Sano S et al, Pigmented contact dermatitis from azo dyes. I. Cross-sensitivity in humans. *Contact Dermatitis* 1980; **6:** 330–6.

50. Nakayama H, Harada R, Toda M, Pigmented cosmetic dermatitis. *Int J Dermatol* 1976; **15:** 673–5.

51. Mathias CG, Pigmented cosmetic dermatitis from contact allergy to a toilet soap containing chromium. *Contact Dermatitis* 1982; **8:** 29–31.

52. Maibach HI, Chronic dermatitis and hyperpigmentation from petrolatum. *Contact Dermatitis* 1978; **4:** 62.

53. Nater JP, de Groot AC, *Unwanted Effects of Cosmetics and Drugs Used in Dermatology*, 2nd edn. New York: Elsevier, 1985.

54. de Groot AC, Adverse reactions to cosmetics. Thesis, State University of Groningen, 1988.

55. Taylor JS, Maibach HI, Fisher AA, Bergfeld WF, Contact leukoderma associated with the use of hair colors. *Cutis* 1993; **52:** 273–80.

56. Riley PA, Acquired hypomelanosis. *Br J Dermatol* 1971; **84:** 290–3.

57. Gellin GA, Maibach HI, Misiaszxek MH et al, Detection of environmental depigmenting substances. *Contact Dermatitis* 1979; **5:** 201–13.

58. Maibach HI, Gellin G, Ring M, Is the antioxidant butylated hydroxytoluene depigmenting agent in man? *Contact Dermatitis* 1975; **1:** 295–6.

59. Findlay GH, Mornson JGL, Simson IW, Exogenous ochronosis and pigmented colloid millium from hydroquinone bleaching creams. *Br J Dermatol* 1975; **93**: 613–22.

60. Cullison D, Abele DC, O'Quinn JL, Localized exogenous ochronosis. *J Am Acad Dermatol* 1983; **8**: 882–9.

61. Fisher AA, Current contact news. Hydroquinone uses and abnormal reactions. *Cutis* 1983; **31**: 240–4, 250.

62. Angelini E, Marinaro C, Carrozzo AM et al, Allergic contact dermatitis of the lip margins from *para*-tertiary-butylphenol in a lip liner. *Contact Dermatitis* 1993; **28**: 146–8.

63. Mathias CG, Maibach HI, Conant MA, Perioral leukoderma simulating vitiligo from use of a toothpaste containing cinnamic aldehyde. *Arch Dermatol* 1980; **116**: 1172–3.

64. Wilkenson MG, Wilkin JK, Azelic acid esters do not depigment pigmented guinea pigs. *Arch Dermatol* 1990; **126**: 252–3.

65. Maibach HI, Engasser P, Management of cosmetic intolerance syndrome. *Clinics Dermatol* 1988; **6**: 102–7.

66. Willis I, Kligman AM, The mechanism of photoallergic contact dermatitis. *J Invest Dermatol* 1968; **51**: 378–84.

67. Kligman AM, The identification of contact allergens by human assay. I. A critique of standard methods. *J Invest Dermatol* 1966; **47**: 369–74.

68. Kligman AM, The identification of contact allergens by human assay. II. Factors influencing the induction and measurement of allergic contact dermatitis. *J Invest Dermatol* 1966; **47**: 375–92.

69. Kligman AM, The identification of contact allergens by human assay. III. The maximization test. A procedure for screening and rating contact sensitizers. *J Invest Dermatol* 1966; **47**: 393–409.

70. Kaidbey KH, Kligman AM, Photo-maximization test for identifying photoallergic contact sensitizers. *Contact Dermatitis* 1980; **6**: 161–9.

71. Kaidbey KH, The evaluation of photoallergic contact sensitizers in humans. In: *Dermatotoxicology*, 2nd edn (Marzulli FN, Maibach HI, eds). Washington, DC: Hemisphere, 1983:405–14.

72. Wennersten G, Thune P, Jansen CT, Brodhagen H, Photocontact dermatitis: Current status with emphasis on allergic contact photosensitivity (CPS) occurrence, allergens and practical phototesting. *Semin Dermatol* 1986; **5**: 277–89.

73. Holzle E, Neumann N, Hansen B et al, Photopatch testing: the 5-year experience of the German, Austrian and Swiss Photopatch Test Group. *J Am Acad Dermatol* 1991; **25**: 59–68.

74. Menz J, Muller S, Connoly SM, Photopatch testing: a 6-year experience. *J Am Acad Dermatol* 1988; **18**: 1044–7.

75. Duguid C, O'Sullivan D, Murphy GM, Determination of threshold UV-A elicitation dose on photopatch testing. *Contact Dermatitis* 1993; **29**: 192–4.

76. Bruze M, Regert S, Luggren B, Effects of ultraviolet irradiation of photopatch test substances in vitro. *Photodermatology* 1985; **2**: 32–7.

77. Epstein S, Masked photopatch tests. *Contact Dermatitis* 1963; **41**: 369.

78. Maibach HI, Akerson JM, Marzulli FN et al, Test concentrations and vehicles for dermatological testing of cosmetic ingredients. *Contact Dermatitis* 1980; **6**: 369–404.

79. Fisher T, Maibach HI, Patch testing in allergic contact dermatitis: an update. *Semin Dermatol* 1986; **5**: 214–24.

80. Mathias CG, Maibach HI, Dermatoxicology monographs. I. Cutaneous irritation: factors influencing the response to irritants. *Clin Toxocil* 1978; **13**: 333–46.

81. Schauder S, Ippen H, Photoallergic and allergic contact eczema caused by dibenzoylmethane compounds and other sunscreening agents. *Der Hautarzt* 1988; **39**: 435–40.

82. Rycroft RJG, False reactions to non-standard patch test. *Semin Dermatol* 1986; **5**: 225–30.

83. Bruynzeel DP, Maibach HI, Excited skin syndrome (angry back). *Arch Dermatol* 1986; **122**: 323–8.

84. Fitzpatrick TB, Arndt KA, El Mofty AM, Pathak MA, Hydroquinone and psoralens in the therapy of hypermelanosis and vitiligo. *Arch Dermatol* 1966; **93**: 589–600.

85. Samman PD, Nail disorders caused by external influences. *J Soc Cosmet Chem* 1977; **28**: 351–6.

86. Whitmore CW, Maibach HI, *Courtroom Medicine: The Skin.* New York: Matthew Bender, 1984.

87. Food, Drug, and Cosmetic Products Warning Statements. *Federal Register* 1975; **40**: 8912.

88. Rapaport MJ, Sensitization to abitol. *Contact Dermatitis* 1980; **6:** 137.

89. Cronin E, *Contact Dermatitis.* New York: Churchill Livingstone, 1980.

90. Larsen WG, Maibach HI, Fragrance contact allergy. *Semin Dermatol* 1982; **1:** 85–90.

91. Fisher AA, Patch testing with perfume ingredients. *Contact Dermatitis* 1975; **1:** 166–8.

92. White IR, Catchpole HE, Rycroft RJG, Rashes among persulfate workers. *Contact Dermatitis* 1982; **8:** 168–72.

93. Schubert H, Baumbach N, Prater E, et al, Patch testing with parabens. *Contact Dermatitis* 1990; **23:** 245–6.

94. Fisher AA, Cosmetic dermatitis. II. Reaction to some commonly used preservatives. *Cutis* 1980; **26:** 136–7, 141–2, 147–8.

95. Lynde CW, Mitchell JC, Patch test results in 66 hairdressers 1973–81. *Contact Dermatitis* 1982; **8:** 302–7.

96. Bruynzeel DP, van Ketel WG, de Haan P, Formaldehyde contact sensitivity and the use of shampoos. *Contact Dermatitis* 1984; **10:** 179–80.

97. Chan PK, Baldwin RC, Parsons RD et al, Kathon biocide: manifestations of delayed contact dermatitis in guinea pigs is dependent on the concentration of induction and challenge. *J Invest Dermatol* 1983; **81:** 409–11.

98. Pascher F, Hunziker N, Sensitization to Kathon CG in Switzerland. *Contact Dermatitis* 1989; **20:** 115–19.

99. Hjorth N, Roed-Peterson J, Patch testing to Kathon CG. *Contact Dermatitis* 1986; **14:** 155–7.

100. Shuster S, Shapiro J, Measurement of risk of sensitization and its application to Kathon. *Contact Dermatitis* 1987; **17:** 299–302.

101. Pugliese PT, Cell renewal – an overview. *Cosmet Toiletries* 1983; **98:** 61–5.

102. Hannuksela M, Kousa M, Pirila V, Contact sensitivity to emulsifiers. *Contact Dermatitis* 1976; **2:** 201–4.

103. Taylor JS, Jordan WP, Maibach HI, Allergic contact dermatitis from stearamidoethyl diethylamine phosphate: a cosmetic emulsifier. *Contact Dermatitis* 1984; **10:** 74–6.

104. Sulzberger MB, Warshaw T, Hermann F, Studies of hypersensitivity to lanolin. *J Invest Dermatol* 1953; **20:** 33–43.

105. Kligman AM, Lanolin allergy crisis or comedy. *Contact Dermatitis* 1983; **9:** 99.

106. Clark EW, Blondeel A, Cronin E et al, Lanolin of reduced sensitizing potential. *Contact Dermatitis* 1981; **7:** 80–3.

107. Sher MA, Contact dermatitis of the eyelids. *S Afr Med J* 1979; **55:** 511–13.

108. Epstein E, Misleading mascara patch tests. *Arch Dermatol* 1965; **91:** 615–16.

109. van Ketel WG, Liem DH, Eyelid dermatitis from nickel contaminated cosmetics. *Contact Dermatitis* 1981; **7:** 217.

110. Turner TW, Dermatitis from butylated hydroxyanisol. *Contact Dermatitis* 1977; **3:** 282.

111. Cronin E, Lipstick dermatitis due to propyl gallate. *Contact Dermatitis* 1980; **6:** 213–14.

112. Calnan CD, Ditertibarybutylhydroquinone in eyeshadow. *Contact Dermatitis Newsl* 1973; **13:** 368.

113. Dooms-Goossens A, Degreef H, Luytens E, Dihydroabietyl alcohol (Abitol), a sensitizer in mascara. *Contact Dermatitis* 1979; **5:** 350–3.

114. Eiermann HJ, Larsen W, Maibach HI, Taylor JS, Prospective study of cosmetic reactions: 1977–1980. *J Am Acad Dermatol* 1982; **6:** 909–17.

115. Schorr WF, Lip gloss and gloss-type cosmetics. *Contact Dermatitis Newsl* 1973; **14:** 408.

116. Wilson LA, Reid FR, Wood TO, *Pseudomonas* corneal ulcer. The causative role of contaminated eye cosmetics. *Arch Ophthalmol* 1979; **97:** 1640–1.

117. Brauer EW, Cosmetics for the dermatologist. In: *Clinical Dermatology*, Vol 4 (Dennis DJ, McGuire J, eds). Philadelphia: Harper & Row, 1984.

118. Rapaport M, Irritant contact dermatitis to glyceryl monothioglycolate. *J Am Acad Dermatol* 1983; **9:** 739–42.

119. Storrs FJ, Permanent wave contact dermatitis: contact allergy to glyceryl monothioglycolate. *J Am Acad Dermatol* 1984; **11:** 74–85.

120. Frosch DB, Camarasa JG, Dooms-Goossens A et al, Allergic reactions to a hairdressers' series: results from 9 European centers. *Contact Dermatitis* 1993; **28:** 180–3.

121. Guerra L, Bardazzi F, Tosti A, Contact dermatitis in hairdressers' clients. *Contact Dermatitis* 1992; **26:** 108–11.

122. Morrison LH, Storrs FJ, Persistence of an allergen in hair after glyceryl monothioglycolate-containing permanent wave solutions. *J Am Acad Dermatol* 1988; **19:** 52–9.

123. Schorr WF, Multiple injuries from permanents. Presented at Cosmetic Symposium, American

Academy of Dermatology, 3 December 1983, Chicago, IL.

124. Sylvest B, Hjorth N, Magnusson B, Lauryl ether sulfate dermatitis in Denmark. *Contact Dermatitis* 1975; **1**: 359–62.

125. van Haute N, Dooms-Goossens A, A shampoo dermatitis due to cocobetaine and sodium lauryl ether sulphate. *Contact Dermatitis* 1983; **9**: 169.

126. Hindson C, Lawlor F, Coconut diethanolamine in a hydraulic mining oil. *Contact Dermatitis* 1983; **9**: 168.

127. Reiss F, Fisher AA, Is hair dyed with para-phenylenediamine allergenic. Arch. 73. Mitchell, JC. Allergic contact dermatitis from *para*-phenylenediamine presenting as nummular eczema. *Contact Dermatitis Newsl* 1972; **11**: 270.

128. Foussereau J, Reuter G, Petitjean J, Is hair dyed with PPD-like dyes allergenic? *Contact Dermatitis* 1980; **6**: 143.

129. Hindson C, *o*-Nitro-*para*phenylenediamine in hair dye – an unusual dental hazard. *Contact Dermatitis* 1975; **1**: 333.

130. Cronin E, Dermatitis from wife's dyed hair. *Contact Dermatitis Newsl* 1973; **13**: 363.

131. Warin AP, Contact dermatitis to partner's hair dye. *Clin Exp Dermatol* 1976; **1**: 283–4.

132. Engasser PG, Maibach HI, Cosmetics and dermatology: hair dye toxicology. In: *Recent Advances in Dermatology*, Vol 6 (Rook AJ, Maibach HI, eds). New York: Churchill Livingstone, 1985:127.

133. Pasricha IS, Gupta R, Panjwani S, Contact dermatitis to henna (*Lawsonia*). *Contact Dermatitis* 1980; **6**: 288–9.

134. Cronin E, Immediate-type hypersensitivity to henna. *Contact Dermatitis* 1979; **5**: 198–9.

135. Edwards EK Jr, Edwards EK, Allergic contact dermatitis to lead acetate in a hair dye. *Cutis* 1982; **30**: 629–30.

136. Fisher AA, Dooms-Goossens A, Persulfate hair bleach reactions. Cutaneous and respiratory manifestations. *Arch Dermatol* 1976; **112**: 1407–9.

137. Calnan CD, Quinazoline yellow dermatitis D&C Yellow 11 in an eye cream. *Contact Dermatitis* 1981; **7**: 271.

138. Calnan CD, Quinazoline yellow SS in cosmetics. *Contact Dermatitis* 1976; **2**: 160–6.

139. Sato Y, Kutsuna H, Kobayashi T, Mitsui T, D&C nos. 10 and 11: chemical composition analysis

and delayed contact hypersensitivity testing in the guinea pig. *Contact Dermatitis* 1984; **10**: 30–8.

140. Sai S, Lipstick dermatitis caused by ricinoleic acid. *Contact Dermatitis* 1983; **9**: 524.

141. van Joost T, Liem DH, Stolz E, Allergic contact dermatitis to monotertiary-butylhydroquinone in lip gloss. *Contact Dermatitis* 1984; **10**: 189–90.

142. Calnan CD, Cronin E, Rycroft RJG, Allergy to phenyl salicylate. *Contact Dermatitis* 1981; **7**: 208–11.

143. Calnan CD, Amyldimethylamino benzoic acid causing lipstick dermatitis. *Contact Dermatitis* 1980; **6**: 233.

144. Lanzet M, Modern formulations of coloring agents: facial and eye. In: *Principles of Cosmetics for the Dermatologist* (Frost P, Horwitz SN, eds). St Louis, MO: CV Mosby, 1982:133.

145. Calnan CD, Compound allergy to a cosmetic. *Contact Dermatitis* 1975; **1**: 123.

146. Food and Drug Administration, Sunscreen drug products for over-the-counter human drugs: proposed safety, effective and labeling conditions. *Federal Register* 1978; **43**: 38 206.

147. Thompson G, Maibach H, Epstein J, Allergic contact dermatitis from sunscreen preparations complicating photodermatitis. *Arch Dermatol* 1977; **113**: 1252–3.

148. Willis I, Photosensitivity. *Int J Dermatol* 1975; **14**: 326–37.

149. Wennersten G, Thune P, Brodthagen H et al, The Scandinavian multicenter photopatch study: preliminary results. *Contact Dermatitis* 1984; **10**: 305–9.

150. Weller P, Eireman S, Photocontact allergy to octyl-dimethyl PABA. *Aust J Dermatol* 1984; **25**: 73–6.

151. Caro I, Contact allergy/photoallergy to glyceryl PABA and benzocaine. *Contact Dermatitis* 1978; **4**: 381–2.

152. Marmelzat J, Rapaport MJ, Photodermatitis with PABA. *Contact Dermatitis* 1980; **6**: 230–1.

153. Fisher AA, Sunscreen dermatitis due to glyceryl PABA: significance of cross-reactions to this PABA ester. *Cutis* 1976; **18**: 495–6, 500.

154. Hjorth N, Wilkinson D, Magnusson B et al, Glyceryl *p*-aminobenzoate patch testing in benzocaine-sensitive subjects. *Contact Dermatitis* 1978; **4**: 46–8.

155. Thune P, Contact and photocontact allergy to sunscreens. *Photodermatology* 1984; **1**: 5–9.

156. Bruze M, Gruvberger B, Thune P, Contact and photocontact allergy to glyceryl *para*-aminobenzoate. *Photodermatology* 1988; **5**: 162–5.

157. Fisher AA, Dermatitis due to benzocaine present in sunscreens containing glyceryl PABA (Escalol 106). *Contact Dermatitis* 1977; **3**: 170–1.

158. Katz SI, Relative effectiveness of selected sunscreens. *Arch Dermatol* 1970; **101**: 466–8.

159. Bruze M, Fregert S, Gruvberger B, Occurrence of *para*- aminobenzoic acid and benzocaine as contaminants in sunscreen agents of *para*-aminobenzoic acid type. *Photodermatology* 1984; **1**: 277–85.

160. Rietschel RL, Lewis CW, Contact dermatitis to homomenthyl salicylate. *Arch Dermatol* 1978; **114**: 442–3.

161. Calnan CD, Cinnamon dermatitis from an ointment. *Contact Dermatitis* 1976; **2**: 167–70.

162. Knobler E, Almeida L, Ruzkowski AM et al, Photoallergy to benzophenone. *Arch Dermatol* 1989; **125**: 801–4.

163. Camarasa JG, Serra-Baldrich E, Allergic contact dermatitis to sunscreens. *Contact Dermatitis* 1986; **15**: 253–4.

164. Fowler JF, Allergic cheilitis due to benzophenone-3. Presented to the Patch Test Clinic Symposium at the American Academy of Dermatology Annual Meeting 1987, San Antonio, TX.

165. Ramsay DL, Cohen H, Baer RL, Allergic reaction to benzophenone. *Arch Dermatol* 1972; **105**: 906–8.

165. Bury JN, Photoallergies from benzophenones and β-carotene in sunscreens. *Contact Dermatitis* 1980; **6**: 211–39.

167. De Groot AC, Weyland JW, Contact allergy to butyl methoxydibenzoylmethane. *Contact Dermatitis* 1987; **16**: 278.

168. English JSC, White IR, Allergic contact dermatitis from isopropyl dibenzoylmethane. *Contact Dermatitis* 1986; **15**: 94.

169. Schauder S, Ippen H, Photoallergic and allergic contact dermatitis from dibenzoylmethanes. *Photodermatology* 1986; **3**: 140–7.

170. De Groot AC, van der Walle HB, Jagtman BA, Weyland JW, Contact allergy to 4-isopropyl-dibenzoylmethane and 3-(4-methylbenzylidene)camphor in sunscreen Eusolex 8021. *Contact Dermatitis* 1987; **16**: 249–54.

171. Roberts DL, Contact allergy to Eusolex 8021. *Contact Dermatitis* 1988; **8**: 302.

172. Alomar A, Cerda MT, Contact allergy to Eusolex 8021. *Contact Dermatitis* 1989; **20**: 74–5.

173. Hunloh W, Goerz G, Contact dermatitis from Eusolex 6300. *Contact Dermatitis* 1983; **9**: 333–4.

174. Sams WM, Contact photodermatitis. *Arch Dermatol* 1956; **73**: 142–8.

175. van Ketel WG, Allergic contact dermatitis from an aminobenzoic acid compound used in sunscreens. *Contact Dermatitis* 1977; **3**: 283.

176. Fagerlund V-L, Kalimo K, Jansen C, Valonsuoja-aineet fotokontaktiallergian aiheuttajina. *Duodecim* 1983; **99**: 146–53.

177. Mork N-J, Austad J, Contact dermatitis from witisol, a sunscreen agent. *Contact Dermatitis* 1984; **10**: 122–3.

178. Fisher AA, *Contact Dermatitis*, 2nd edn. Philadelphia: Lea & Febiger.

179. Kaminester LH, Allergic reaction to sunscreen products. *Arch Dermatol* 1981; **117**: 66.

180. Norton LA, Common and uncommon reactions to formaldehyde-containing nail hardeners. *Semin Dermatol* 1991; **10**: 29–33.

181. Fisher AA, Suppression of reactions to certain cosmetics. *Cutis* 1977; **20**: 170, 176, 182–7.

182. Paltzik RL, Enscoe I, Onycholysis secondary to toluene sulfonamide formaldehyde resin used in a nail hardener mimicking onychomycosis. *Cutis* 1980; **25**: 647–8.

183. Brauer EW, Onycholysis secondary to toluene sulfonamide formaldehyde resin used in a nail hardener mimicking onychomycosis. *Cutis* 1980; **26**: 588.

184. Mitchell L, Schlossman ML, Wimmer E, Advances in nail enamel technology. *J Soc Cosmet Chem* 1992; **43**: 331–7.

185. Yamazaki K, Tanaka M, Development of a new w/o emulsion-type nail enamel. In: *Preprints 16th IFSCC Congress, 1990*, Vol 1: 464–95.

186. So D, *US Patent* 4,903,840; 1990.

187. Wilkinson JB, Moore RJ, *Harry's Cosmetology*. New York: Chemical Publishing, 1982.

188. Fisher AA, Cross reactions between methyl methacrylate monomer and acrylic monomers presently used in acrylic nail preparations. *Contact Dermatitis* 1980; **6**: 345–7.

189. Fisher AA, Baran R, Adverse reactions to acrylate sculpture nails with particular reference to

prolonged paresthesia. *Am J Contact Dermatitis* 1991; **2**: 38–42.

190. Fisher AA, Franks A, Glick H, Allergic sensitization of the skin and nails to acrylic plastic nails. *J Allergy* 1957; **28**: 84–8.

191. Fuller M, Analysis of paint-on artificial nails. *J Soc Cosmet Chem* 1982; **33**: 51–3.

192. Marks JF, Bishop ME, Willis WF, Allergic contact dermatitis to sculptured nails. *Arch Dermatol* 1979; **115**: 100.

193. Baran R, Pathology induced by the application of cosmetics to the nail. In: *Principles of Cosmetics for the Dermatologist* (Frost P, Horwitz SN, eds). St Louis, MO: CV Mosby, 1982.

194. Burrows D, Rycroft RJG, Contact dermatitis from PTBP resin and tricresyl ethyl phthalate in a plastic nail adhesive. *Contact Dermatitis* 1981; **7**: 336–7.

195. Fisher AA, Patch tests for allergic reactions to dentifrices and mouthwashes. *Cutis* 1970; **6**: 554–61.

196. Andersen KE, Contact allergy to toothpaste flavors. *Contact Dermatitis* 1978; **4**: 195–8.

197. Drake TE, Maibach HI, Allergic contact dermatitis and stomatitis caused by a cinnamic aldehyde-flavored toothpaste. *Arch Dermatol* 1976; **112**: 202–3.

198. Magnusson B, Wilkinson DS, Cinnamic aldehyde in toothpaste. 1. Clinical aspects and patch tests. *Contact Dermatitis* 1975; **1**: 70–6.

199. Kirton V, Wilkinson DS, Sensitivity to cinnamic aldehyde in a toothpaste. 2. Further studies. *Contact Dermatitis* 1975; **1**: 77–80.

200. Labows JN, McGinley KZJ, Kligman AM, Axillary odor: current status. In: *Principles of Cosmetics for the Dermatologist* (Frost P, Horwitz SN, eds). St Louis, MO: CV Mosby, 1982:89.

201. Jass HE, Rationale of formulations of deodorants and antiperspirants. In: *Principles of Cosmetics for the Dermatologist* (Frost P, Horwitz SN, eds). St Louis, MO: CV Mosby, 1982:98.

202. Marzulli FN, Maibach HI, Antimicrobials: experimental contact sensitization in man. *J Soc Cosmet Chem* 1973; **24**: 399–421.

203. Epstein WL, Contact-type delayed hypersensitivity in infants and children: Induction of rhus sensitivity. *Pediatrics* 1961; **27**: 51–3.

204. Hjorth N, Contact dermatitis in children. *Acta Derm Venereol (Stockh)* 1981; **95**: 36–9.

205. Marcussen PV, Primary irritant patch-test reactions in children. *Arch Dermatol* 1963; **87**: 378–82.

206. Epstein E, Contact dermatitis in neonates and infants. In: *Neonatal Skin* (Maibach HI, Boisits EK, eds). New York: Marcel Dekker, 1982:223.

207. Simmons RJ, Acute vulvovaginitis caused by soap products. *Obstet Gynecol* 1955; **6**: 447–8.

208. Bass HN, Bubble bath as an irritant to the urinary tract of children. *Clin Pediatr* 1968; **7**: 174.

209. Roberts HJ, Bubble bath cystitis and cosmetic vulvitis neglected hazards. *J Fla Med Assoc* 1973; **60**(8): 31–5.

210. Fisher AA, Current contact news (cosmetic actions and reactions: therapeutic, irritant, and allergic). *Cutis* 1980; **26**: 22–4, 29–30, 32.

211. Goldenberg RL, Safrin L, Reduction to topical irritation. *J Soc Cosmet Chem* 1977; **28**: 667–701.

212. Cronin E, Dermatitis of the hands in beauticians. In: *Occupational and Industrial Dermatology* (Maibach HI, Gellin GA, eds). New York: Year Book Medical Publishers, 1982:215.

213. Wahlberg JE, Nickel allergy and atopy in hairdressers. *Contact Dermatitis* 1975; **1**: 161–5.

214. Guerra L, Tosti A, Bardazzi F et al, Contact dermatitis in hairdressers: the Italian experience. *Contact Dermatitis* 1992; **26**: 101–7.

215. Frosch PJ, Aktuelle Kontaktallergerne. *Hautarzt* 1989; **41**(Suppl 10): 129–33.

216. Holness DL, Nethercott JR, Dermatitis in hairdressers. In: *Dermatology Clinics*, Vol 8 (Adams RM, Nethercott JR, eds). Philadelphia: Saunders, 1990:119–26.

217. Rietschel HL, Huggins L, Levy N et al, In vivo and in vitro testing of gloves for protection against UV-curable acrylate resin systems. *Contact Dermatitis* 1984; **11**: 279–82.

218. Fisher AA, 'Hypoallergenic' surgical gloves for special situations. *Cutis* 1975; **15**: 797.

219. McClain DC, Storrs FJ, *Am J Contact Dermatitis* 1992; **3**: 201–5.

220. Mellström GA, Wahlberg JE, Maibach HI (eds), *Protective Gloves for Occupational Use*. Boca Raton, FL: CRC Press, 1994.

221. Dahlquist I, Fregert S, Gruyberger B, Release of nickel from plated utensils on permanent wave liquids. *Contact Dermatitis* 1979; **5**: 52–3.

222. Tomb RR, Lepoittevin J, Durepaire F et al, Ectopic contact dermatitis from ethyl cyanoacrylate instant adhesives. *Contact Dermatitis* 1993; **28**: 206–8.

61

Social, psychological and psychiatric aspects of cosmetic use

John A Cotterill

INTRODUCTION

The skin is an organ of communication, and from earliest times we have modified the appearance of this organ in three main ways: by scarification, tattooing and body painting. Modern cosmetics, as used in the Western world, can be regarded as but one extension of body painting. From the anthropological point of view, it is interesting that body painting often becomes much more widely practised at times of love or during preparations for war. However, these observations cannot necessarily be extrapolated to Western civilization.

THE COSMETIC INDUSTRY AND BODY IMAGE CREATION

Concepts about what is desirable in body image terms vary enormously, not only as a function of time, but also geographically. With regard to time, there is no doubt that Miss World in 1997 is a much different woman than her first predecessor in 1912. The modern Miss World is much taller, with a slimmer waist and hips and with smaller breasts than her forerunner 85 years ago. Indeed, the 1980s and 1990s have been dominated in Western female society by a complete aversion to adipose tissue. The cosmetic industry, in its advertisements, has constantly stressed to women that young skin is what is desirable. Ideally, this skin must be odour-free, wrinkle-free, grease-free and spot-free. In short, it should be like a baby's skin. Plenty of hair on the scalp is desirable, but facial hair or hair under the arms, on the arms, on the breasts, chest, abdomen or legs is frowned upon. The sophisticated woman in the 1980s began to have the lateral margins of her pubic hair shaved. In addition, any visit to a pharmacy or supermarket in these present times will demonstrate the inordinate number of products labelled, for instance, 'baby' oil, 'baby' talc or 'baby' shampoo. These particular products are not targetted at babies – who are not well-known for their shopping abilities – but at women, who are being asked by the advertising industry to become completely infantile in their skin care. Indeed, one large skin-care organization, Johnson & Johnson, exhorts women to 'be a Johnson's baby', harnessing this infantile aspect of skin care to their advertising campaign. The success of this type of propaganda is soon appreciated by any dermatologist in his clinic when women patients, one after the other, will say, 'and I was only using baby oil or baby talc, or baby shampoo, on my skin so I don't understand what has gone wrong'. These women are really saying to the dermatologist that they thought they were treating their skin in an appropriate way, but in fact are all victims of the society in which they find themselves and being completely infantile in their skin care.

In short, the woman of the 1980s and 1990s is expected to deny virtually all her secondary sex characteristics in her quest for a more youthful and perfect, baby-like skin. This is a very unhealthy target for women to aim at, and it is not surprising to the writer that so many young girls and women nowadays develop anorexia nervosa – a condition par excellence of body image disturbance in which infantile body habitus becomes all important, dominated by an extreme fear of weight gain.

The pendulum is continually swinging, and it is now becoming more fashionable in the 1990s to have larger breasts and larger lips. There are those women in the vanguard of media manipulation, such as models, who are obliged to follow the current trends and are generating a good standard of living for practitioners working in the area of increasing breast and lip size. The degree of swing in the pendulum is being counterbalanced to some extent by concern about the possible development of breast cancer following some types of breast augmentation procedures.

THE COSMETIC INDUSTRY AND ITS ADVERSE EFFECT ON DOCTOR/PATIENT RELATIONSHIPS IN MEDICINE

The majority of women, even in the 1990s, know little of skin anatomy or physiology, and all their information on their skin usually comes from women's magazines, beauticians or the cosmetic industry's advertising campaigns. Thus one reads that 'the skin needs to breathe' and that 'the pores must be unblocked'. At the same time, the skin must be repeatedly 'cleansed' and 'moisturized' to keep it healthy. There is a bewildering array of topical creams, all claiming to make the skin younger in one way or another. With the possible exception of retinoic acid used topically, I have seen no convincing scientific data to substantiate any of the claims for youthful skin that are made by the cosmetic industry for their products in their advertisements. From the point of view of continuing to stimulate the market, the cosmetic industry seems quite happy to continue its paternalistic role, treating women as children as far as responsible and accurate information about the skin and its care is concerned. It is lamentable that the cosmetic industry often treats the enquiring dermatologist in the same way, although this must change with recent EC legislation requiring cosmetic houses to verify advertising claims with scientific data.

Whilst exhorting women to quest further and further after a more youthful skin, at the same time the cosmetic industry encourages women to become tanned, and usually equates a tanned skin with health. The fact is that ultraviolet light is a major aging factor as far as the skin is concerned, can significantly depress not only skin immunological responses but also systemic immunological processes, and can produce a whole host of other skin problems varying from 'Majorca' acne (acne aestivale), to solar keratoses and frank skin malignancy such as rodent ulcers, squamous carcinoma and malignant melanoma. The cosmetic industry is failing to put these sort of data in front of their potential clients, and at the same time continues to be infantile in the content of the data it presents to women in their magazine advertisements. It is therefore not surprising that the data presented to women by the media make it extremely difficult for doctors, and for dermatologists in particular, to have a reasonable and adult conversation with the 'sophisticated woman' patient of the 1990s about her skin. Whilst the writer accepts that the medical profession, and dermatologists in particular, probably have much more to do in educating people about their skin and its care, and about the prevention of skin malignancy, and malignant melanoma in particular, the advertising and cosmetic industries are showing few signs of responsibility in this area, and the incidence of malignant melanoma continues to double each 10 years in the UK and other countries in northern Europe.

BODY IMAGE: SELF-PERCEPTION AND SELF-ESTEEM

The skin is a vital part of the perception of an individual's concept of his or her body image. The most important skin body areas involved include the face, eyes, mouth and nose, hair and scalp, breasts in females and the genital area in males. Body odour is also important in body image, and is largely cutaneous in origin. Positive body image leads to a high self-esteem and confidence, which is usually reflected with success within the society in which the individual finds him or herself.

Indeed, there are several studies to show that people with a more attractive appearance do have numerous advantages over those perceived as less attractive.[1] Thus individuals without acne have a better chance of gaining employment than those with acne.[2] Moreover, outwardly attractive geriatric patients are looked after far better than those perceived as non-attractive by their carers.[3] In order to attain these advantages, cosmetics can be used to reinforce an individual's body image. Indeed, Ryan[4] has postulated that 'everyone seeks to attain the status of a confident nude', and cosmetics may have a place in this quest.

With regard to self-perception, the more attractive one is, the more highly one may think of oneself – so an improvement in attractiveness following the use of cosmetics could lead to an increase in self-esteem. Graham and Jouhar[5] found that an increased use of colour in facial make-up was related to high sensitivity towards the body and fears of

a negative evaluation of one's appearance by others.

Cosmetics can be used, however, not only to influence self-perception, but also to modify perception of the self by others and thus to possibly influence interpersonal relationships.

Detailed studies by Graham and Jouhar[5] showed that people related more favourably in terms of appearance and personality after using cosmetic treatments compared with when they related without cosmetic treatments. Facial make-up seemed to enhance the evaluation of the more outgoing aspects of personality (sociable, confident), and hair care seemed to enhance the evaluation of the softer, more general aspects of personality (caring, sensitive).

Graham and Jouhar[5] examined how attractive a standard range of cosmetics commonly used by women was thought to be by both men and women. The study was rated for both daytime and night-time social situations. The cosmetic rated most attractive by men used by women was perfume, for both night and daytime. Mascara gained the highest rating by women when rated for use at night and during the day. All cosmetics tended to be rated as more attractive at night than during the day.

Finally, the importance of cosmetics in general health care, both in physical disease and in patients with psychological or psychiatric problems, is becoming more appreciated. Cosmetic camouflage may be used for patients with birthmarks such as port wine stains and in patients with burns, severe acne scarring or other forms of scarring and vitiligo. Attention to appearance, and the use of cosmetics in particular, may have a place in the management of patients recovering from depressive illness.[6] The importance of an elderly patient looking good has already been alluded to. Kligman and Graham[7] described the positive effects accruing from a professional makeover of the skin in elderly women. The effect of the makeover on self-perception was compared with that of a control group, and was found to have a striking beneficial effect on the psychological status, with positive short-term effects on appearance, socializing, good feeling, self-image, outlook and social attitudes. The benefits were found to be greater from those perceived as unattractive than for those already perceived as attractive. The makeover consisted of the application of skin products to cleanse and tone the skin, and these were followed with appropriate foundation lotions, a blusher, rouge, eyebrow liner, eyeshadow and various shades of mascara for the eyelashes and, finally, lipstick. Kligman and Graham[7] described the transformation attainable by a skilled artist as 'usually spectacular'.

PERSONALITY AND COSMETICS

Some individuals have a very vulnerable personality as far as body image perception, self-esteem and confidence are concerned. Even the smallest blemish can produce disparate misery in these anxious, mirror-checking, narcissistic, beauty-conscious, highly demanding, obsessional individuals who set themselves unrealistically high standards, not only in how they should look, but also in their anxieties about how other people see them. Women with such personality traits often become beauticians and attract other women with similar personality characteristics. On the other hand, there are patients who have gross acne pustulation of the face who seem quite indifferent to it. Most individuals lie somewhere between these two extremes. The great variability in personality from person to person explains why the tiniest lesion on the nose causes disproportionate anxiety in some vulnerable individuals, whereas it may not be perceived at all by others.

DERMATOLOGICAL PATHOMIMICRY: MILLARD'S SYNDROME

Patients with Millard's syndrome[8] learn to reproduce their original skin problem or attempt to mimic it. The payoff for this behaviour is usually to gain some sort of 'emotional strokes' and possibly sympathy from close family or friends. It is not unusual to see unhappy women presenting repeatedly with a cosmetic dermatitis. These women know that they are allergic to fragrance or to various preservatives in their cosmetics or to dyestuffs in their hair tint, but continue to use these products on an intermittent basis, usually to manipulate their partners.

SELF-ANOINTERS: COSMETIC HABITUATION

There is a sizeable group of patients, almost all females, who are unable to get through life without putting a wide range of cosmetics of one sort or another on their skin, and their face in particular. In short, these women are habituated to cosmetics, and may develop a contact dermatitis. Patch testing in these women usually pinpoints the source of their allergic problems, but because of their obsession with anointing their skin they are unable to give up this behaviour. It is not unusual for such women to bring 30 or 40 different types of cosmetic for patch testing purposes, and as part of every shopping expedition they buy more creams or moisturisers.

DERMATITIS SIMULATA[9]

Some females attempt to mislead the dermatologists by applying dyestuffs to their skin. This may be part of the picture of artefact dermatitis, and has also been observed in children who are victims of Munchausen's syndrome by proxy (Meadow's syndrome).[10] The abusing mothers attempt to mimic skin disease in their children as part of their general onslaught on the child.

This type of behaviour may also be seen in people seeking compensation. For instance, I recently had a woman patient who was suing a bus company following a slip on some oil three or four years previously. She claimed that her skin had become tattooed by the oil. In reality, when I saw her it was quite easy to remove some black pigment from the involved area of the face. However, she had deceived her two previous examining doctors with this simulated skin problem.

THE WITCHCRAFT SYNDROME[11]

In this syndrome an acute social urticaria was produced in many women clients at a hairdressers by the hairdresser's daughter, who was angry at her father, who was in turn angry with her for becoming pregnant out of wedlock. The daughter had found that she could apply histamine-releasing agents to her clients' facial skin using the palms of her hands. Presumably the thickened skin on the palms of her hands prevented her developing skin problems, whereas her clients all developed a very acute urticaria.

DYSMORPHOPHOBIA (BODY DYSMORPHIC DISORDER, DERMATOLOGICAL NON-DISEASE)

Dysmorphophobia is a term used to describe patients who complain about some form of physical disability that is apparent only to themselves and not to any other observer. This condition is basically a disturbance of perception of cutaneous body image. Rich symptomatology is apparent in important body image areas, including the face, scalp, breasts and genital area. The presenting symptoms referable to the face include a complaint of burning, excessive redness and excessive grease, excessive facial hair, unusually large pores and scarring. None of these changes perceived by the patients can be perceived by the examining doctor. These patients are ill, but have no organic dermatological problems, and the term 'dermatological non-disease' has been used to describe this group of largely female patients.[12] The commonest psychiatric illness present is depression, and women with facial symptomatology are usually severely depressed.[13] A proportion of these women are depressed enough to consider suicide, and a recent study showed that 24% made a suicide attempt.[14] It is vital, therefore, that the practising dermatologist recognizes this common and important group of patients.

Symptoms referable to the scalp include excessive hair loss and a burning sensation that is unremitting, morning noon and night. A premorbid obsessional personality is reasonably common in this group of individuals, who often score quite highly on depression inventories if they are performed.

A whole range of psychiatric illness may be present in this group, including personality disorders, schizophrenia and, in the elderly, dementia. Emotional and marital problems are also well represented.

PATIENTS WITH MINIMAL SKIN DISEASE

There is a small group of patients with minimal acne who plague their family doctors and dermatologists for therapy, usually demanding treatment with 13-*cis*-retinoic acid. The suspicion is that this group of patients contains individuals with very vulnerable personalities, which means that the tiniest pimple can induce such a lowering of self-esteem and confidence that depression results. Suicide is one possible sequel in this group. MacDonald Hull et al[15] have shown that these patients respond well to treatment with 13-*cis*-retinoic acid. Unfortunately, this drug is very expensive, and there are those who feel that in the prevailing economic climate it is not right and proper to prescribe this expensive drug for these patients. However, MacDonald Hull et al[15] were able to show that patients were able to return to society and to gainful employment after treatment, and the risk of suicide was obviated.

PSYCHOLOGICAL CONSEQUENCES OF HAVING A PORT WINE STAIN[16]

Patients with port wine stains do not score abnormally on standard depression and anxiety inventories, but there is no doubt that their port wine stain, especially if it is in a visible area, has a very significant effect on the quality of their lives. It is apparent that it is unusual for men with extensive port wine stains to marry, although women with this condition often do so. Many women with facial port wine stains have never been seen without cosmetic camouflage by their husbands. I have seen two adult patients in the last year who have tried to commit suicide because of their port wine stain. Considerable difficulties can be encountered in attempts to socialize with other members of society and in achieving gainful employment. One of my patients nearly died of thyrotoxicosis because she refused to have surgery in case her cosmetic camouflage became compromised during the anaesthetic or surgical procedure. Another patient took exception to an appointment being sent to her in an envelope that bore the hospital logo on the postmark because she had never told her husband that she had a port wine stain and felt he must have realized some treatment was under way when the envelope arrived at her home. She wrote a long letter stating that in future all appointments should be sent in a plain envelope.

Cosmetic camouflage in this group of patients can have a very positive effect on the quality of their lives, although successful laser therapy also seems to help their self-esteem to a disproportionately high degree. Indeed, one problem with laser therapy is that patients' expectations are often far higher than the final results achieved. The satisfactory end point is a port wine stain that can be covered by conventional cosmetics rather than by heavy-duty masking camouflage. A smooth skin surface is also important to the adult female with a port wine stain, so laser ablation of the vascular blebs that so often complicate a port wine stain in later life enables the affected person to apply cosmetics, and cosmetic camouflage in particular, much more evenly and acceptably.

The most realistic aim of laser therapy is to try and reach that happy state of affairs where the patient is able to apply ordinary cosmetics rather than cosmetic camouflage to their facial skin in the laser-treated area, giving a presentable appearance without any undue problems. Perfect removal of a port wine stain following laser therapy is rarely achieved.

CONCLUSIONS

Just as the heart or kidney may be subject to failure, so may the skin. The skin is an organ of communication, and for many people feeling good can only occur with a self-perception of looking good. Moreover, relationships with other people may depend very much on the physical appearance of the skin.

The cosmetic industry works very hard extolling women to quest after an ever more youthful-looking skin. Indeed, the end point of this desire is a baby-like skin, coupled with a denial of secondary sex characteristics.

In the elderly and those with dermatological stigmata such as port wine stains, vitiligo or scarring, the use of cosmetics can lead to very significant elevation of self-esteem, confidence and reversal of depression. In addition, relationships with others, and with carers in particular, may become more optimal, particularly in the elderly, in this situation.

Some dermatologists will be afraid to cross the Iron Curtain that exists between the world of pure dermatology and skin disease and the world of cosmetics. A common language needs to be developed between these two worlds, which at present are poles apart. Dermatologists do realize that patients want to look and thus feel good, and should not be afraid to use cosmetics in appropriate circumstances. Both the medical profession and the cosmetic industry should discuss together ways of educating people, and women in particular, about their skin and its care. It seems pointless that an industry should on the one hand exhort women to an ever more youthful skin, whilst encouraging them to photo-age their skin with sunbathing on the other hand.

The move by the cosmetic industry to include photoprotective agents in some – albeit a minority – of their products is surely a move in the right direction for the next millennium.

REFERENCES

1. Adams GR, Huston TL, Social perception of middle-aged persons varying in physical attractiveness. *Dev Psychol* 1975; **11:** 657–8.
2. Cunliffe WJ, Acne and unemployment. *Br J Dermatol* 1986; **115:** 386.
3. Connor CL, Walsh RP, Litzelman DK, Alvarez MG, Evaluation of job applicants: the effects of age versus success. *J Gerontol* 1978; **33:** 246–52.
4. Ryan TJ, The confident nude – or – whither dermatology? *Dermatol Pract* 1987; **5:** 8–18.
5. Graham JA, Jouhar AJ, The importance of cosmetics in the psychology of appearance. *Int J Dermatol* 1983; **22:** 153–6.
6. Red Cross Report – Basic skin care and cosmetics for the chronically ill, the mentally disturbed and the aged infirm – A service of the British Red Cross Society. *J Dermatol Surg Oncol* 1981; **7:** 455–99.
7. Kigman AL, Graham JA, The psychology of cutaneous ageing. In: *Ageing and the Skin* (Balin, AK, Kligman AM, eds). New York: Raven Press, 1989:347–55.
8. Millard LG, Dermatological pathomimicry (a form of patient maladjustment). *Lancet* 1984; **ii:** 969–71.
9. King CM, Chalmers RJG, Another aspect of contrived disease: 'dermatitis simulata'. *Cutis* 1984; **34:** 463–4.
10. Meadows R, Munchausen's syndrome by proxy. *Arch Dis Child* 1982; **57:** 92–8.
11. Bandman HJ, Wahl B, Contact urticaria artefacta (witchcraft syndrome). *Cont Derm* 1982; **8:** 145–6.
12. Cotterill JA, Dermatological non-disease: a common and potentially fatal disturbance of cutaneous body image. *Br J Dermatol* 1981; **104:** 611–18.
13. Hardy GE, Cotterill JA, A study of depression and obsessionality in dysmorphophobic and psoriatic patients. *Br J Psych* 1982; **140:** 19–20.
14. Veale D, Boocock A, Gournay K et al, Body dysmorphic disorder. A survey of 50 cases. *Br J Psych* 1996; **169:** 169–201.
15. MacDonald Hull S, Cunliffe WJ, Hughes BR, Treatment of the depressed and dysmorphophobic acne patient. *Clin Exp Dermatol* 1991; **16:** 210–11.
16. Lanigan SW, Cotterill JA, Psychological disabilities amongst patients with port wine stains. *Br J Dermatol* 1989; **121:** 209–15.

Index

Page numbers in *italic* refer to illustrations.

Abrasives, 50, 159, 168
Absorbant deodorants, 173
Absorbents, 50
Absorption, percutaneous *see*
    Percutaneous absorption
Acetone, 163, 352–3
N-Acetyl-4-*S*-
    cysteaminylphenol, 403
Acid permanent waves, 726–7,
    738
Acid rinse, dry hair, 180–1
Acne, 127, 433–44, 715–17
  adjunctive treatments, 436
  astringents, 163
  ceramides, 102
  CO_2 laser resurfacing, 596–7,
    597
  collagen injections, 619
  cosmetics, 441–4
  cryosurgery, 694, 695, 696
  dermabrasion, 596–7, *597*,
    602, *602*, 610
  facial make-up, 730
  gender variations, 496
  make-up, 436
  menopausal women, 490, 493
  minimal, 751
  prophylaxis, 443–4
  self-esteem, 749, 751
  skin cleaning, 117, 433–5
  and the sun, 437–8
  surgery, 438–41
  systemic treatment, 140–1,
    443–4

  toners, 163
  topical treatment, 79, 140,
    442–3, 588–9
  treatment tolerance, 437
Acnegenesis, 304, 441–2
Acoustic spectrometry, 272,
    277
Acrokeratosis verruciformis,
    694
Actinic cheilitis, 662, *664*, 665,
    686–7
Actinic damage *see* Solar
    elastosis; Solar keratoses;
    Solar lentigo; Solar
    urticaria; Sun damage;
    Sunscreens
Actinic dermatitis, 327
Adapalene, 442
Additives, 50
  hand and body lotions, 290
  nail varnishes, 216–17
Adenoma sebaceum,
    cryosurgery, 694
Adipose tissue
  body image, 747
  gender variations, 19
  liposculpturing, 553–67
  syringe fat transfer, 569–84
Adnexal tumours, 670, 687
Adolescents
  puberty, 496–7
  skin cleansers, 508
  sunscreens, 510–11
Adrenocortical disease, 383–4

Adsorbent deodorants, 173
Adverse reactions *see* Toxicity
Advertising influences, 747–8
Aerosol propellants, 736
Aftershave products, 42, 498,
    718
Aging of skin, 455–67
  body image, 749–50
  ceramide levels, 102–3
  electrical stimulation, 645,
    646–9, *646–8*, 651–4,
    654
  gender variations, 17–21, 23,
    25, 27–9, 496
  inflammatory reactions,
    469–85
  intrinsic, 456
  mechanical properties, 20–1,
    541
  menopause, 28–9, 487–93
  normal skin, 125–6
  rejuvenation surgery,
    569–84, 613–22
  transepidermal water loss,
    530–1
  UV protection, 123
  see also Photoaging
AIDS-related Kaposi's sarcoma,
    693, 695
Albinism, 328
Alcohols
  adverse reactions, 717, 725
  thermal sensory analysis,
    551

Allergic contact dermatitis, 346–7, 712–13
  artificial nails, 236, 240, 735
  children, 736–7
  delayed type-hypersensitivity, 712
  fragrances, 41–2, 45–7
  hairdressers, 739
  lanolin, 725
  nail polish, 224–6
  oral hygiene, 735–6
  patch testing, 722
  and photocontact dermatitis, 719
  photopatch testing, 719
  race differences, 519–20
  shampoos, 727
  transepidermal water loss, 533
  triclosan, 736
  vitamin E, 78
  vulvar skin, 339–40
Allergic contact urticaria, 43
Allergic reactions
  collagen injections, 614, 616, 617–18, 619, 620, 621
  deodorants, 736
  facial make-up, 729, 730
  fragrances, 41–7
  hair preparations, 726–9, 738–9
  immunologic contact urticaria, 715
  preservatives, 723, 726
  sunscreens, 730, 732–4
Alopecia
  androgenetic, 489, *489*, *490*, 493, 633
  cryosurgery, 695, 698–9, *699*
  phototrichograms, 545, 546
  surgical treatments, 633
  α-Hydroxy acids (AHAs), 145
  and electrical stimulation, 654
  exfoliation, 168, 585–6
  face masks/scrubs, 158, 159, 160, 161
  menopausal women, 492–3
  percutaneous absorption, 91–2
  photoaging, 463
Aluminium salts, deodorants, 174–5, 446, 736

Aminexil, hair care, 501
Ammonium persulphate, 729
Ammonium thioglycolate (AMT), 726, 727, 738
Amphoteric surfactants, 137, 507
Amyl dimethyl PABA (Padimate A), 732
α-Amylcinnamic alcohol, allergic contact dermatitis, 41, 42
Anaesthesia
  dermabrasion, 599
  laser resurfacing, 663
  and *p*-phenylenediamine, 728–9
  reduction liposculpturing, 557–8
  rhinophyma, 668
  syringe fat transfer, 575–6
Androgenetic alopecia, 489, *489*, *490*, 493, 633
Androgens
  acne, 127, 140–1
  hair growth, 30, 381–6, 387–8
  menopausal women, 488–91, 492, 493
  sweat secretion, 496
Angiokeratomas, cryosurgery, 693
Angiomas
  cryosurgery, 693, 695
  laser treatments, 674, 678–9, 683
Animal origin, ingredients of, 56
Animal testing
  acnegenesis, 716
  comedogenesis, 716
  corrosivity, 62, 710–11
  Draize assay, 33, 37, 64, 178, 713
  electrical stimulation, 653
  percutaneous absorption, 62, 63, 64, 81
  regulation, 49, 60–4, 67–73, 724
  sensitization assays, 712–13
  subjective irritation, 711
Anionic surfactants, 114, 115–16, 137, 507
Ankle flare, 376

Anti-aging bio-activators, 492
Anti-androgenic topical products, 493
Antibiotics
  acne, 140, 437, 443
  hyperpigmentation, 399, 400
  and nail discolouration, 226
Anticorrosives, 50
Antidandruff agents, 50, 141–2, 186, 194–5, 198–9
Antifoaming agents, 50
Anti-inflammatory agents, photoaging, 464
Antimicrobials, 50
  acne, 140, 434
  deodorants, 172, 173–4, 445–6, 502, 736
  hand and body lotions, 290
  oily skin cleansers, 117
  shaving products, 498
Antioxidants, 50
  adverse reactions, 726, 729
  infrared radiation, 314
  α-lipoic acid, 79
  in moisturizers, 122, 370
  photoaging, 464, 470, 472–5, 476–8, *479*, 483–4
Antiperspirants, 50, 174–5, 736
  idiopathic hyperhidrosis, 446
  men, 501–2
  regulation, 709
Antiseptics
  children's cleansers, 508
  foaming solutions for acne, 434
  idiopathic hyperhidrosis, 446
Antistatic agents, 50
Antiwrinkle products, laser profilometry, 3–5, 8–9
Arachidonic acid (AA), premature aging, 476–7, *481*
Argon lasers, 680, 686
Argyria, 399, 401
Artecoll, 620–1
Artefact dermatitis, 750
Asiatic pills, 399, 401
Astringents, 155, 161–3, 167
Athlete's foot, 502
Atopic dermatitis
  ceramides, 102
  children, 511
  dry skin of, 128, 145

transepidermal water loss,
367–8, 531
Atopic dermatitis (AD),
367–72
Atopic eczema
and autosomal dominant
ichthyosis, 360
children, 508
hairdressers, 738
Autologen, 620
Autologous collagen, 619–20
Autonomic function, 26
Autosomal dominant
ichthyosis (ADI), 359–61
Avobenzone, 732, 733
Awls, syringe liposculpturing,
555
Azelaic acid (AA), 140, 403–4,
718

Babies
adult use of products for,
747–8
adverse reactions, 736–7
cleansers, 508
diaper dermatitis, 508–9
dry skin, 511
powders, 509
safety aspects, 506, 511–12
shampoos, 506–8
skin permeability, 505–6
sunscreens, 510
transepidermal water loss,
530
Bacteria
atopic dermatitis, 367, 370
body odour, 736
diaper dermatitis, 509
fluorescent, 35–6, 146
nails, 229
vulvar skin, 334–6, 340
Bacterial vaginosis, 336
Baker's phenol, 585, 586
Baldness, 427, 501
cryosurgery, 695, 698–9, *699*
surgical treatments, 633–42
Ballistometry, elasticity
measurement, 271
Balsam of Peru, 42, 43, 46, 47,
721–2
Barber's itch, 498
Barrier condition,
moisturizers, 121–2

Barrier creams, testing, 525–6
Barrier function, stratum
corneum, 104, 107–9,
351–2, 356, 529, 532
Basal cell carcinoma
camouflage make-up, *419*
surgical scars, 606, *607*
Bath preparations
adverse reactions, 737
atopic dermatitis, 370
moisturizing efficacy, 259,
261
Beards
depilatories, 737
imitation, 425, *426*
shaving, 435, 497–9
Beauticians, dermatitis, 738
Becker's naevus, 395, *395*, 405
Benzocaine impurities,
sunscreens, 732
Benzoic acid, contact urticaria,
714–15
Benzophenones, sunscreens,
320–1, 733
Benzoyl peroxide, 140, 141
in cosmetics, 442
percutaneous absorption, 79
side-effects, 437, 443
Benzyl alcohol, 717
Benzyl salicylate, 41, 46, 717
Bergamot oil, 43, 396
Berlocque dermatitis, 43, 396,
402
Binders, 50
'Bindi' depigmentation, 401
Biocides, hand and body
lotions, 290
see also Antimicrobials
Bioengineering techniques,
128–37
cutaneous microcirculation,
23–5, 523–7
limitations, 527
moisturizer efficacy, 250–82,
296–8
transepidermal water loss,
529–34
Biological additives, 50
Biopsies, skin surface *see* Skin
surface biopsies
BIOSPEC imager, 135
Biotechnologically-derived
ingredients, 55, 57

Bismuth oxychloride, 726
Bleaching
agents, 50, 717
damaged hair care, 179–80,
181, 182–3
dyschromias, 404
hair, 201, 386, 729
Blepharoplasty, laser, 671–4,
672
Blood flow
gender variations, 23–5
non-invasive assessment,
523–8
race variations, 519
testing skin cleansers, 118
Blood vessel problems *see*
Telangiectases; Vascular
problems
Blushers, 730
Body contouring, syringe fat
transfer, 571
see also Liposculpturing
Body dysmorphic disorder, 751
Body hair, 201–4
Body image, 343–4, 747–8,
749–50, 751
Body lotions, 285–307
efficacy, 292–9
function, 285–6
ingredients, 287–90
leading US brands, 286
physical structure, 290–2
toxicology, 300–5
Body masks, 160
Body odour
deodorants, 171–6, 501–2, 736
idiopathic hyperhidrosis,
445–6
vulvar skin microbiology, 336
Botanicals, 50
Botulinum toxin (Botox),
701–7
clinical results, 704, *704*
consent to treatment, 701,
702
contraindications, 701
dilution, 701, 702, 704,
706–7
hyperhidrosis, 453
injection, 703–4, *703*, 707
photoaging, 464
side-effects, 704–5, 706–7
storage, 702–3, 704, *705*

Bovine cornea tests, 146
Bowen's disease, *692*
Breasts, syringe fat transfer, 571, *583*
Bromocriptine, hirsutism, 389
Bronopol, 723
Bubble bath, 737
Buffering agents, 50
Burns, depigmentation, 394
Butylated hydroxyanisole (BHA), 717, 726
Butylated hydroxytoluene, 726
p-t-butylphenol, 718, 735

Café-au-lait
    hyperpigmentation, 405, *680*, 682, 685
Caffeine, percutaneous absorption, 89–90
Camouflage make-up, 417–32
    baldness, 427, 501
    body image, 749
    brushes, 427
    children, 425
    clinical considerations, 418–19
    colour correctors, 426–7
    contouring, 427
    cover creams, 421–3, *422, 423*
    dyschromias, 409–10
    eyelid incision eyes, 427
    face cleansing, 421, *421*
    financial factors, 420–1
    indications, 417, *418, 419*
    materials checklist, 420
    mature patients, 427
    men, 425–6, *426*
    patient instruction, 431
    patient interviews, 420
    physical considerations, 421
    procedure, 423–5
    prostheses, 427–31
    psychological consequences, 752
    storage kit, 419
    telangiectases, 375, 378
Camphor, sunscreens, 733
Cananga oil, 717
Candida albicans
    diaper dermatitis, 509
    nail plate, 229
    phototoxicity assays, 36

vulvar skin, 334
Cannulas, syringe liposculpturing, 553–4, *554*, 555–6, *555*
Capacitance measurement, 131, 253, 254–61, 274, 275, 296–7
Capillary microscopy, 524
Carbon dioxide laser, 592–3, 596–7, *597*, 661, 662, 680
    actinic cheilitis, 686–7
    adnexal tumours, 670
    photoaging, 686–7
    rhinophyma, 596, *598*, 666–9, *667*, 687
    tattoo removal, 412, 670–1, *671*, 686
    thickened scars, 669, 687
    tuberous sclerosis, *668*
    xanthelasma, 666, 687
Carcinogens
    percutaneous absorption, 80–1, 88
    tars, 186–7
Carotenoderma, 399–400
Castor oil, 729
Cationic polymers, hair care, 183
Cationic surfactants, 114, 137, 182–3, 507
Cell culture assays, 33–5, 146
Celluloses
    dry hair care, 183
    nail varnish, 214
Ceramides, 99–112, *100, 106*
    atopic dermatitis, 369
    barrier function, 104, 351–2, 356, 532
    barrier repair, 107–9
    biosynthesis, 107–8, *107*
    desquamation, 104–7
    gender variations, 19–20
    in irritant dermatitis, 351–2, 354–6, *354*
    linoleic acid, 144
    major classes, 99–101, 351
    racial differences, 102–3, 515
    variations in levels of, 101–4
Cerulodermas, 391, 392, 397–400
Cheilitis
    with isotretinoin treatment, 437

laser treatment, 662, *664*, 665, 686–7
Chelating agents, 51
Chemabrasion
    cryo-peels compared, 697
    dyschromias, 405, 588, 593
    and electrical stimulation, 654
    facial peels, 585–94
    menopausal women, 493
    photoaging, 463
Chemical Abstract Service (CAS), 49, 52
Chemical peeling *see* Chemabrasion
Chemoscarification, telangiectases, 375
Cherry angiomas, cryosurgery, 693
Chewing gums, contact urticaria, 715
Chicken pox scars, 606, *606*
Children, 505–13
    adult use of products for, 747–8
    adverse reactions, 511–12, 736–7
    bubble bath, 737
    camouflage make-up, 425
    haemangiomas, 684
    laser therapies, 675, 684
    puberty, 496–7
    safety, 506
    shampoos, 506–8
    skin cleansers, 508
    skin permeability, 505–6
    skin protection, 508–11
    transepidermal water loss, 530
Chloasma, 685
Chlorofluorocarbons, 736
Chloroxine, 226
Chlorpromazine
    hyperpigmentation, 399, 400
Chondrodermatitis nodularis helikis, 694
Chorioallantoic membrane system (CAM), 34, 36
Chromium hydroxide, 717
Cigarette smoke, aging effects, 470, 475, *475–6*, 493
Cimetidine, hirsutism, 388–9

Cinnamic acid
contact urticaria, 714–15
sunscreens, 320, 321, 526, 731, 733
Cinnamic alcohol, 41, 42, 717
Cinnamic aldehyde
allergic contact dermatitis, 41, 42, 736
contact urticaria, 43, 714–15
depigmentation, 718
Clay-based masks, 156, 160–1, 169
Cleansers, 114–19
bend of elbow washing test, 6
children, 508
dry skin, 115–16
mixed skin, 116
normal skin, 137–8
oily skin, 116–17
testing, 117–19
see also Masks
Climatic influence
ceramide levels, 103–4, *105*
cosmetic skin parameters, 1–15
skin and gender, 25, 29
Clofazimine
hyperpigmentation, 399
Clothing, sun protection, 461, 510
Clove bud oil, 47
Coal tars
hair care, 142, 186–7, 198, 728
percutaneous absorption, 80–1
pigmentation, 717
Coefficient-of-friction devices, 272
Cohesography, 272
Cold stress, gender variations, 25
Collagen
age variation, 2, 496
Artecoll, 620, 621
autologen, 620
autologous, 619–20
electrical stimulation, 653, 654
facial chemical peels, 586, 591
Fibrel, 617
gender variations, 17, 28–9, 496

hygroscopic properties, 143, 248
in menopause, 488, 490, 492
Zyderm, 613
Zyplast, 613
Collagenase, 478, 480, *480–1*
Collodion baby, 361
Colophony, 721–2, 726
Colorants, 51, 216, 729–30, 735
Colorimetry, 28, 524, 539
Colour of skin
cover cream matching, 422–3
measurement, 28, 524, 539
and photoaging, 458–9, 462
self-tanning products, 151–4
see also Pigmentation
Comedogenesis, 304, 441–2, 715–17
Comedones, acne surgery, 438–41, *438–41*
Conductance measurement
moisturizer efficacy, 131, 252–3, 254–61, 275, 296–7
racial differences, 518–19
Congenital adrenal hyperplasia (CAH), 383–4, 386, 388
Consumer testing, 86–7, 147, 298
Contact dermatitis, 710–12
artificial nails, 236, 240
emulsifiers, 724
eye make-up, 725–6
facial make-up, 729–30
fragrances, 41–7, 396
hairdressers, 727, 729, 738–40
incidence, 709–10
lanolin, 725
moisturizers, 300
nail cosmetics, 224–6, 242, 502, 734
oral hygiene products, 735–6
patch testing, 722
photopatch testing, 719
race differences, 515, 519–20
role of lipids in, 351–7
sensitive skin, 343–9
transepidermal water loss, 532–3
triclosan, 736
vitamin E, 78
in vitro toxicity assays, 36

vulvar skin, 337–40
Contact thermometry, 524
Contact urticaria
fragrances, 43
moisturizers, 304
nail varnish, 226
vulvar skin, 337
witchcraft syndrome, 751
Contact urticaria syndrome (CUS), 337, 347, 713–15
Contraceptives, vaginal, 338–9
Corneal ulcers, 726
Corneocytes
facial masks, 156, *157*
skin surface biopsies, 130–1, *130*
transepidermal water loss, 530
Corneometers, 5, 8, 131, 253, 257, 274, 296–7
Corona phlebectatica paraplantaris, 376
Corrosivity, testing, 62, 710–11
Corticosteroids
dyschromias, 404
hirsutism, 388
pathological dry skin, 145
pseudofolliculitis, 499
seborrheic dermatitis, 142
vulvar allergic contact dermatitis, 339
Cosmetic Industries in the European Union (COLIPA), 63, 72–3
Cosmetic industry
body image, 747–8, 752
doctor/patient relationships, 748–9
patient education, 752–3
Cosmetic intolerance syndrome (CIS), 344, 345, 348, 737–8
Cosmetic Toiletries and Fragrance Association, 721, 722
Coumarins
contact dermatitis, 41, 42–3
photosensitivity, 718
Couperose, 373, 374–5
Crenotherapy, telangiectases, 375
Critical surface tension (CST), 281

Crow's feet
  botulinum toxin, 704, *705*
  collagen injections, 614, 615,
    616
  electrical stimulation, 651
Cryoanaesthesia, 558, *558*
  dermabrasion, 599
  syringe fat transfer, 575, 576
Cryosurgery, 691–700
  complications, 698–9
  contraindications, 699
  dyschromias, 404–5, 407–8,
    693, 698
  feathering, 693, 695
  freeze-thaw cycles, 692
  lesion selection, 693–8
  paintbrush method, 693
  spot freeze technique, 691–2,
    692
  telangiectases, 375, 695, *696*
Cushing's disease, 384
Cutaneous absorption *see*
    Percutaneous absorption
Cutaneous blood flow *see*
    Blood flow
Cutaneous virilism, 385–6
Cuticles, 223–4, 227–8, 735
Cyanoacrylate, 735
Cyproterone acetate (CPA), 387
Cysts, cryosurgery, 694, 696
Cytokines
  photoaging, 458
  premature aging, 471, 478,
    479, 480, *481*

Dandruff, 193–200
  antidandruff agents, 50,
    141–2, 186, 194–5, 198–9
  clinical features, 193, *193,
    194*
  etiology, 194
  incidence, 193
  pathology, 193–4
  shampoos, 195–8
Decubitus ulcers, 653
Delayed type-hypersensitivity
    (DTH), 712
Denaturants, 51
Denervation, botulinum toxin,
    701–7
Dentifrices, 735–6
Deodorants, 51, 171–6, 445–6,
    501–2, 709, 736

Depilatories, 51, 499, 502, 737
Depression, 749, 751
Dermabrasion, 595–611
  anaesthesia, 599
  complications, 608–9
  contraindications, 610
  dressings, 600–2, *601*
  dyspigmentation risk, 411
  and electrical stimulation,
    654
  equipment, 595–6, *596*
  indications, 602–4
  laser resurfacing, 592–3,
    596–7, *597, 598*, 662–5
  patient selection, 597–8
  photoaging, 463, 607–8,
    608–10
  preoperative work-up, 598–9
  scar revision, 605–6, *606–7*
  tattoo removal, 412–13, *603*
  technique, 599–600, *600*
Dermatitis simulata, 750–1
Dermatofibroma, cryosurgery,
    694
Dermatologic non-disease,
    343–4, 348, 751
Dermatological bars, acne, 434
Dermatosis papulosa nigrans,
    694, 697
Desogestrel, hirsutism, 388
Desquamation
  effect of ceramides, 104–7
  moisturizer efficacy, 267
  skin surface biopsies, 130–1
Detergents
  atopic dermatitis, 370
  bubble bath, 737
  shampoos, 177–8, 184–5, 727
Diagalloyl trioleate, 733
2,4–diaminoansole (DAA), 81
Diaper dermatitis, 508–9, 737
Diazolidinyl urea, 721–2, 723
Dibenzoylmethanes,
    sunscreens, 321, 733
Digital image processing, 266
Dihydroabietyl alcohol, 726
Dihydroxyacetone (DHA),
    151–4
  decolouring test, 5–6, 11–13,
    12, 13
5,6–Dihydroxyindole (DHI),
    500
Diluents, nail varnish, 215–16

Dimethyl sulphoxide (DMSO),
    96
DIN parameters, laser
    profilometry, 3–5, *4*, 8–9,
    10
Dioxane, percutaneous
    absorption, 80
Diseased skin, absorption,
    77–8
DNA
  hygroscopic properties, 143,
    248
  photoaging, 458, 459, 460,
    462, 464
Doctor/patient relationships,
    748–9
Draize assay, 33, 37, 64, 178,
    713
Drugs
  cosmetics distinguished, 86,
    113
  drug-induced
    hyperpigmentation,
    399–400
  Japanese regulation, 66
  US regulation, 65, 709
Dry eyes, isotretinoin, 437
Dry hair, 178–83, 190–1,
    507–8, 511
Dry skin, 128
  acquired, 128
  atopic dermatitis, 368–70
  care of, 143–6
  children, 511
  cleansers, 115–16
  constitutional, 128
  elderly people, 530–1
  see also Ichthyosis;
    Moisturizers
D-Squames, 267, 298
  antidandruff efficacy, 199
  facial masks, 156, *157*
Dyes
  facial make-up, 729–30
  hair, 51, 407, 500, 717–18,
    728–9
Dyschromias, 391–415
  cellular-level
    photothermolysis,
    679–82
  ceruloderma, 391, 392,
    397–400
  chemabrasion, 405, 588, 593

classification, 391–2
cryosurgery, 404–5, 407–8, 693, 698
etiology, 400–1
laser treatments, 405–6, 411, 679–82, 685–6
leucoderma, 391, 392–5, 717, 718
management, 401–11, 588
melanoderma, 391, 392, 395–7
racial variations, 394, 401, 402, 404, 517, 520
risk after surgery, 411
Dysmorphophobia, 343–4, 751

Earth-based masks, 156, 160–1, 169
Econazole shampoo, 195–6
Eczema
   and autosomal dominant ichthyosis, 360
   children, 508
   hairdressers, 738, 739
   transepidermal water loss, 531
EINECS inventory, 52
Elastase, 478, 480, *480*
Elasticity
   after electrostimulation, 652
   measurement, 268–71, 297–8, 540–1
Elastin
   hygroscopic properties, 143, 248
   menopausal women, 492
Elastosis perforans serpiginosa, 695
Electrical measurement, skin hydration, 5, 131–2, 133, 251–61, 274–8, 518–19
Electrical stimulation of skin (ESS), 643–55
   electrorhytidopuncture, 643–4, *645*, 646, 650
   patient selection, 645
   procedure, 646
   research into, 653
   results, 646–9, 651–3
   role in treatment of aging, 653–4
   side-effects, 650
   Simonin's apparatus, 643

Top Derm, 643, 644, *645*, 646, 650
Electrical treatments
   couperose, 374–5
   idiopathic hyperhidrosis, 447–53, *448*, *450–2*
   menopausal women, 493
   see also Electrical stimulation of skin
Electrocautery, leg telangiectases, 379
Electrodermal asymmetry, 25
Electrodermal responses, 25
Electrolysis, hair removal, 202–3, 386, 502
Electromagnetic spectrum, 309, *309*
   see also Infrared radiation; Ultraviolet radiation
Electrorhytidopuncture, 643–4, *645*, 646, 650
Elimination programmes, 343
Ellipsometry, 281
Emollients, 51, 249, 250, 287–8, 368–70
Emulsifiers, 289, 724
Emulsions
   acne, 435
   moisturizers, 119–20, 144, 258–9, 290–2, 369–70
Endoscopic surgery, idiopathic hyperhidrosis, 446–7
Eosin, 729
Ephelides *see* Freckles
Epidermabrasion, 168
Epidermis, *100*
Epilating wax, 201, 386, 502, 737
Epithelioma adenoides cysticum, 602, *604*
Erbium-YAG laser, 661, 662
Erythema, and percutaneous absorption, 81
Essential fatty acids (EFAs)
   dry skin, 144, 145
   moisturizers, 288
Estrogen *see* Oestrogen
Ethnic cosmetics, 515–21
   see also Racial differences
Eugenol
   allergic contact dermatitis, 41, 42
   contact urticaria, 715

European Centre for Validation of Alternative Methods (ECVAM), 61–3, 64, 71
European List of Notified Chemical Substances (ELINCS), 49, 52
European Union (EU), cosmetic regulation, 49–64, 65, 67–73, 85, 86, 721, 724
Evaporimeters, 133, *133*, 279
Excipients, 733–4
Exfoliation, 167–8, 585–93
   masks, 158, 159, 161
Expert sensory panels, 298
Extensometry, 268
Eye creams, 210
Eye irritancy
   animal testing, 62, 63, 64, 178
   baby care products, 506, 507
   isotretinoin, 437
   moisturizers, 305
   shampoos, 178, 506, 507, 727
Eye make-up, 205–12, 725–6
Eyebrows
   pencils, 209–10, 425–6, 430–1, *431*
   reconstruction, 430–1, *431*
   recreation, 429–30, *429–30*
   ventilated, 430
Eyelashes
   false, 428–9, *428*
   mascaras, 205, 206–7, 725, 726, 749
Eyelid dermatitis, 725
Eyelid incision lines, 427
Eyeliners, 208–9, 210
Eye-shadows, 207–8
Eytex, 145–6

Facial chemical peel, 585–94
Facial hair, 201–4, *203*, 435, 497–9
Facial make-up
   adverse reactions, 729–30
   body image, 749–50
Facial masks, 156–61, 168–9, 436
Facial recontouring, syringe fat transfer, 571–9

Facial scrubs, 156, 158, 159–60, 168

Facial telangiectases, 373–5
see also Port wine stains

Fat
autologous collagen, 619–20
gender variations, 19
liposculpturing, 553–67
syringe transfer, 569–84

Fatty acid amides, shampoos, 727

Feet, sweating, 445–53, 501–2

Fibrel, 617–19, *617–19*

Fibroblasts
electrical stimulation, 653
infrared damage, 310
TCA chemical peels, *590*, 591–2

Fick's law, skin hydration, 246–7

Film formers, 51, 214

Film modifiers, nail varnish, 214

Filmogenic compounds, 144, 249, 250

Fine-needle sclerotherapy, 375, 378, *378*

Finger nails *see* Nails

Fluorescent bacteria, 35–6, 146

5–Fluorouracil cream, 586–7

Flutamide, hirsutism, 388

Foam
antifoaming agents, 50
antiseptic solutions for acne, 434

Folliculitis, 498

Food allergens, 715

Formaldehyde
adverse reactions, 721–2, 723, 727, 734
nail varnishes, 214, 217–18, 225–6, 241–2, 734

Foundations, adverse reactions, 730

Fourier-transform infrared (FTIR) spectroscopy, 131, 132, *132*, 278

Fragile skin, 128

Fragrances
baby products, 737
deodorant, 171–2, 445
idiopathic hyperhidrosis, 445
moisturizers, 289–90, 303

patch testing, 722
pigmentation, 717
regulation, 51–3, 58–9, 721
sensitivity to, 41–7, 303, 396

Freckles, 396
imitation, 425
removal, 402, 404, 405, 685, 693

Free radicals
menopausal women, 492
premature aging, 470, 471–2, 477, 480, *481*

Fresheners, 155, 161–3, 167

Freund's complete adjuvant (FCA), 713

Frown lines, botulinum toxin, 703–4, *703*, 706, *706*

Furfuracea *see* Dandruff

Furocoumarins, 42, 43, 526

Gardnerella vaginalis, 336

Gel nails, 237–8

Gels
acne, 434–5
hydroalcoholic, 189

Gender variations in skin, 17–32, 495–6
anatomical characteristics, 17–19
biochemical composition, 19–20
cutaneous microvasculature, 23–5
exogenous triggers, 21–3
functional differences, 21
hormonal influence, 19–20, 21, 23, 28–30
mechanical properties, 20–1
pilosebaceous unit, 29–30
sensory functions, 25–6
skin colour, 27–8
structural characteristics, 17–19

Genitals
virilization, 386
vulva, 331–42

Genodermatoses, laser treatments, 670, 687

Geraniol, 41, 42, 717

Geranium oil, 717

Gloves, hairdressers, 738–9

Glucose utilization, toxicity assay, 34, 35

Glycerides, moisturizers, 288

Glycerol (glycerin), moisturizers, 143, 248, 257–8, 259, 288–9, 295

Glyceryl monothioglycolate (GMT), 726–7, 738, 739

Glyceryl PABA, 732

Glyceryl tribenzoate, 734

Glycolic acid
exfoliation, 168, 585–6
face masks, 159, 160, 161
menopausal women, 492–3

Glycosaminoglycans, 120, 143, 248, 458

Gonadal dysgenesis, 384

Gonadotrophin-releasing hormone agonists, 388

Gore-tex, 621–2, 623–32

Grafts
fat, 569–84
hair, 634–7, 639–40
melanocytes, 410–11

Greasy hair, 141–2, 183–8

Greasy skin *see* Oily skin

Haemangiomas, 375
cryosurgery, 693, 696
laser therapy, 684
see also Naevi; Port wine stains

Hair, 177–91
adverse reactions to products, 717–18, 721, 723, 724, 726–9
body image, 747
camouflage make-up, 427
colouring products, 499–500, 717–18, 728–9
conditioners, 190–1
cryosurgery, 695, 698–9, *699*
dry, 178–83, 190–1
dyes, 51, 407, 500, 717–18, 728–9
gender variations, 20, 29–30
greasy, 183–8
hirsutism, 30, 203–4, *203*, 381–9, 489, 687–8
masks, 160
men, 497–501, 502
menopausal women, 489, *489*, *490*, 493
methylolated compounds, 190

permanent waving, 188–9, 721, 726–7, 738–9
phototrichograms, 545–7
pomades, 191, 443–4
punch autograft, 640
removal, 201–4, 386–7, 497–9, 502, 687–8, 737
rotational scalp flaps, 640–1
scalp reduction, 637–9, *638*, 640, *640*, 641
setting lotions, 190
sprays, 190
straighteners, 189–90, 721, 727
strip grafting, 639
thickeners, 500–1
transplants, 634–7, *634–7*, *640*, 641
see also Shampoos
Hairdressers, 727, 729, 738–40
Hairpieces, 501, 633
Hamamelis virginiana, 162
Hand lotions, 285–307
  efficacy, 292–9
  function, 285–6
  ingredients, 287–90
  leading US brands, 286
  physical structure, 290–2
  toxicology, 300–5
Hands
  idiopathic hyperhidrosis, 445–53
  occupational dermatitis, 738–40
  syringe fat transfer, 571
Haptens, 712–13
Hats, sun protection, 461, 510
Heat stress, 25
Heel pad thickness, 19
Henna, 729
Hen's egg tests, 146
Herpes
  antiherpetic medication, 339, 610
  and dermabrasion, 610
  postherpetic neuralgia, 551
Hexachlorophene, 736
Hidrocystoma, cryosurgery, 694
Highley Hand Wash protocol, 295
Hirsutism, 30, 203–4, *203*, 381–9, 489, 687–8

HIV-related Kaposi's sarcoma, 693, 695
Hormone replacement therapy, 28–9, 490–1
Hormones
  acne, 127, 140–1, 443
  gender variations, 19–20, 21, 23, 28–30
  hirsutism, 30, 381–6, 387–9
  menopause, 487–91, 492, 493
  photoaging, 464
Human testing *see* In vivo human testing
Humectants, 51, 120, 142–4, 248, 250, 288–9
Humidity *see* Climatic influence, cosmetic skin parameters
Hydration, 246–7
  children's skin, 511
  cosmetic efficacy, 86, 533–4
  gender variations, 20–1, 28
  measurement, 5, 8, 129, 131–5, 253, 257, 296–7
  racial differences, 515, 516, 518–19
  relation with TEWL, 247, 529, 530, 531–3, *532*
  see also Moisturizers
Hydrocolloid masks, 169
Hydrocortisone, dyschromias, 404
Hydroquinone
  adverse reactions, 721, 726, 729
  depigmentation, 401–3, 717–18, 721
  percutaneous absorption, 76–7, *76*, *77*
  photoaging, 464
Hydroxy acids, 145
  and electrical stimulation, 654
  exfoliation, 168, 585–6
  face masks/scrubs, 158, 159, 160, 161
  menopausal women, 492–3
  percutaneous absorption, 91–2
  photoaging, 463
  see also Lactic acid; Salicylic acid

p-Hydroxyanisole, 718
Hydroxycitronellal, 41, 42, 717
21–Hydroxylase deficiency, 384
Hydroxytoluene, 717, 726
Hygiene products
  adverse reactions, 736
  body odour, 171, 172, 173–5, 445–6, 736
  dry skin, 142
  female hygiene sprays, 338, 339
  men, 501
  normal skin, 137–8
  oily skin, 139–40
  oral, 715, 718, 735–6
Hygrometers, 131, 253, 257
Hylan Gel, 621
Hyperandrogenism, 385–6, 488–90, 491
Hyperhidrosis, idiopathic, 445–54
Hyperprolactinaemia, 384

Ichthyosis, 128, 359–65
  ceramide levels, 101–2
  hydrating products, 145
Idiopathic guttate hypomelanosis (IGH), 393–4, *394*, 407–8, 410, 693
Idiopathic hyperhidrosis, 445–54
Imidazolidinyl urea, 721–2, 723, 726
Immediate pigmentation darkening (IPD), 539
Immune system
  aging of skin, 470–2, 478, 480
  delayed type-hypersensitivity, 712
Immunologic contact urticaria, 715
Impedance, moisturizer efficacy, 252, 254–61, 269, 273–6
In vitro testing
  percutaneous absorption, 75, 77
  predicting irritancy, 33–40
  replacing animal testing, 60–4, 724

In vivo human testing, 146–7
  comedogenicity, 716–17
  confocal microscopy, 280
  contact urticaria syndrome,
    714, 715
  irritants, 710–12
  lipid peroxidation, 472–5
  lipid role in irritation, 353–6
  photosensitivity, 718
In vivo testing, animals *see*
    Animal testing
Indentometry, elasticity
    measurement, 271
Infants *see* Babies; Children
Inflammatory reactions,
    modulation, 469–85
Infrared radiation, 309–15
Infrared spectroscopy, 131,
    132, *132*, 277, 278
Infrared thermography, 524
Insulin, hirsutism and, 385–6
International Fragrance
    Association (IFRA), 41
  Code of Practice, 52, 58–9
  restricted materials, 42, 44–5,
    52
International Nomenclature
    Cosmetic Ingredient
    (INCI) names, 49, 50
Inventory of Fragrance
    Ingredients, 51–3
Iontophoresis, 447–53, *448,
    450–2*
Iron oxide, sun blocks, 321
Irritancy and irritation
  agents of, 710–11
  animal testing, 62, 63, 64
  anti-irritants, 738
  astringents, 163
  bend of elbow washing test,
    6, 11, *11*
  blood flow assessment, 526–7
  children's toiletry, 506,
    507–8, 511–12, 736–7
  corrosives, 62, 710–11
  deodorants, 736
  eye make-up, 725
  face masks, 160
  gender variations, 21–3
  hair preparations, 726–7, 729
  moisturizers, 122, 300–5
  nail cosmetics, 215–16,
    217–18, 224–8, 237, 238,
    ⁻40, 241–2, 502, 735

objective, 346, 710–11
patch testing, 722
primary irritants, 710
racial differences, 515–16,
    517–18, *517, 518,* 519–20
self-tanning products, 153
'sensitive skin', 343–9
sensory (subjective), 302,
    344–6, 711–12
shampoos, 178, 507–8
skin cleansers, 118–19
testing protection from,
    525–6
thermal sensory analysis,
    549–52
transepidermal water loss,
    532–3
in vitro tests, 33–40, 145–6
in vivo human testing, 146–7
vulvar skin, 334
Irritant contact dermatitis,
    710–12
  baby products, 508
  causes, 345
  racial differences, 515
  role of lipids in, 351–7, 532
  vulvar skin, 337–40
Isoeugenol, 41, 42, 46
Isopropyldibenzoylmethane,
    733
Isotretinoin
  acne treatment, 140, 437,
    442, 443, 751
  and dermabrasion, 609
  photoaging, 463

Japan, cosmetic regulations,
    66–7
Jasmine absolute, 47, 717
Juri procedure, scalp flaps,
    640–1

Kaposi's sarcoma, 693, 695
Kathon CG, 723–4
Keloids, 608–10, 669, 687, 695,
    697–8
Kenacid blue assay, 34, 35, 36
Keratinocytes
  ceramides, 108–9
  delayed type-hypersensitivity,
    712
  dry skin, 119, 121–2
  infrared radiation, 310–11
  racial differences, 516, 517

Keratolytic substances, 144–5
Ketoconazole
  hirsutism, 388
  shampoo, 195, 196–8
Khellin photochemotherapy,
    406
Kligman regression protocol,
    292–4

Labelling information
    systems, 49–50, 59, 65, 66,
    67, 721
  hand and body lotions, 287,
    299
Lactic acid
  irritancy, 711–12
  masks, 160, 161
  moisturizing efficacy, 143,
    248, 258
Lamellar ichthyosis, ceramides,
    101–2
Lanolin, 144, 181, 288, 292,
    293
  adverse reactions, 724–5,
    726, 729
Laser Doppler flowmetry
    (LDF), 23, 523–4
  barrier creams, 525
  limitations, 527
  photoaging treatment, 525
  skin irritation, 526–7
Laser profilometry, 129
  cosmetic skin parameters,
    3–5, 8–9
  mask efficacy, 159
  moisturizer efficacy, 266
Laser treatments, 657–89
  actinic cheilitis, 662, *664,*
    665, 686–7
  adnexal tumours, 670, 687
  blepharoplasty, 671–4, *672*
  cellular-level
    photothermolysis,
    679–82
  deep-pigment lasers, 661
  definitions, 657
  dyschromias, 405–6, 411,
    679–82, 685–6
  and electrical stimulation,
    654
  genodermatoses, 670, 687
  hair removal, 386–7, 687–8
  menopausal women, 493
  procedures, 661

relative indications, 658, 659

resurfacing, 592–3, 596–7, *597*, *598*, 661, 662–5

rhinophyma, 596, *598*, 666–9, *667*, 687

scalp reduction, 669–70

scars, 592–3, 596–7, 665–6, 669, 687

superficial-pigment lasers, 661, 680

tattoo removal, 412, 670–1, *671*, 681–2, *681*, 686

techniques, 659–82

telangiectases, 375, 379, 674, 675, *676*, *677*, 683–4, 752

training, 658

tuberous sclerosis, *668*

vascular problems, 674–9, 683–5

whole-tissue surgical lasers, 661

xanthelasma, 666, 687

Lavender oil, 717

Legs

syringe fat transfer, 571

telangiectases, 376–80, *376*, *377*, *378*, 684

transepidermal water loss, 531

Lentigos, 396, 403, 405, 588, 685, 693

Leucocytes

delayed type-hypersensitivity, 712

polymorphonuclear, 471, 478, 480

premature aging, 480–3

Leucoderma, 391, 392–5, 717, 718

Levarometry, 270

Lichen amyloidosis, 398–9

Lichenoid keratosis, cryosurgery, 694

Linoleic acid, 144, 145, 249

Lipids

cleanser formulation, 114, 115, 118

moisturizer formulation, 119, 122

premature aging, 471, 472–5, 477–8, 696

quantification, 539–40

role in irritant dermatitis, 351–7, 532

shaving, 497

stratum corneum, 99, *106*, 107–8

surfactant action, 137

see also Ceramides; Sebum

Lipofilling *see* Syringe fat transfer

α-lipoic acid, 79

Lipometer, 136

Liposculpturing, 553–67

anaesthesia, 557–8, *558*

approaches, 558–9

complications, 563

dressings, 561

electrolyte balance, 561

equipment, 553–6

fluid balance, 561

goals, 556

patient marking, 557, *558*

patient positioning, 559, *559*

preoperative preparation, 556–7

technical considerations, 561–2

technique, 560–1

warnings, 562

Liposomes, 143–4, 248, 259, 261

Lips

augmentation, 620, 621, 622, 626, 629–31, *629–31*

cheilitis, 437, 662, *664*, 665, 686–7

laser resurfacing, *664*, 665

Lipsticks, 729–30, 733

Liquid nitrogen cryotherapy, 404–5, 407–8, 691–700

Liquid soaps, acne, 434–5

'Liver spots', 404

Lotions

aftershave, 498

baby products, 737

emulsifiers, 724

hair care, 142, 187

see also Hand lotions

Lubricants *see* Emollients

Lupus erythematosus, 327

Lymphocytes

delayed type-hypersensitivity, 712

premature aging, 480–3

transformation test, 36

Lymphokine assays, 36

Macromolecules, humectants, 143, 248

Macrophage migration inhibition test, 36

Macular amyloidosis, 399

Magnetic resonance imaging (MRI)

skin hydration, 134–5, *134*, 278

stratum corneum imaging, 280

Malassezia genus, 194–5, 395, 403

Mascaras, 205, 206–7, 725, 726, 749

Masks, 155, 156–61, 168–9, 436

Matting, telangiectases, 376–7

Medroxyprogesterone acetate (MPA), 388

Melanins

pigmentation, 391, 405

Q-switched laser treatments, 682

racial differences, 516–17

sun protective effect, 462

Melanocytes

dyschromias, 391–8, 403–5, 408, 410–11, 685, 717

racial differences, 516–17

Melanoderma, 391, 392, 395–7, 398

Melasma, 396–7, *397*

chemabrasion, 588

cryosurgery, 693

depigmentation agents, 401–2, 403, 404

laser therapy, 406

Men, 495–502

beauty products, 502

body image, 749

camouflage make-up, 425–6, *426*

depilatories, 499, 502

hair care, 499–501

port wine stains, 752

shaving with acne, 435

shaving products, 497–9

washing products, 501

see also Gender variations in skin

Menopause, 28–9, 487–94
Menstruation
  menstrual pads, 339
  vulvar skin microbiology,
    335–6
Mercurials, dyschromias, 404
Metabolic activity, skin, 88
Metal content, hair, 20
Methyl methacrylate (PMMA),
  620–1, 735
Methylcoumarins, 42, 718
Micropigmentation tattooing,
  409, *409*
Microrelief *see* Skin surface
  relief
Microtox system, 34, 35–6
Microvasculature *see*
  Vasculature
Milia, cryosurgery, 694
Millard's syndrome, 750
Mimicry, skin disorders, 750–1
Mineral oils
  atopic dermatitis, 369, 370
  moisturizers, 288
Mineral origin, ingredients of,
  56
Minocycline
  acne, 437, 443
  hyperpigmentation, 399, 400
  and nail discolouration, 226
Minoxidil
  hair care, 500–1, 633
  menopausal women, 493
Mixed skin, cleansers, 116
Moisture accumulation test
  (MAT), 133
Moisture-retaining effects
  climatic influence, 7–8, *7*, *9*
  stratum corneum, 99
Moisturizers, 119–23, 245–83
  action of, 247–50, 285–7
  atopic dermatitis, 368–70
  barrier condition, 121–2
  cleansers and, 115–16
  definitions, 245–6
  efficacy assessment, 86,
    250–82, 292–9, 369, 525
  excessive cell renewal, 121
  ingredients, 250, 287–90
  menopausal women, 491–2
  normal skin, 139
  physical structure, 290–2
  skin hydration, 246–7

skin surface extensibility,
  120, *120*
toxicology, 300–5
UV protection, 122–3
variable forms, 250
water-holding substances,
  142–4, 247
Monobenzyl ether of
  hydroquinone (MBEH),
  402–3, 718
Monomethyl ether of
  hydroquinone (MMEH),
  403
Mouthwashes, 715, 735–6
MTT dye uptake and
  reduction assay, 33, 34–5,
  36
Mud packs, 156, 160–1, 169
Muller's phlebectomy, 378–9,
  378–9
Muscle denervation,
  botulinum toxin, 701–7
Musk ambrette
  contact dermatitis, 41, 42
  photosensitivity, 718
Myxoid cysts, cryosurgery, 694

Naevi
  Becker's naevus, 395, *395*,
    405
  classification, 373
  cryosurgery, 405, 693, 694,
    695, *696*
  dermabrasion, 602, *603*
  laser therapy, 405–6, 685
  see also Port wine stains
Naevus flammeus *see* Port wine
  stains
Naevus of Ota, 397–8, *398*,
  405–6, 685
Nail lacquers, drug delivery,
  96–7
Nails, 213–44
  anatomy, 219–20, *219*
  artificial, 228, 233–7, *234–6*,
    239–40, *239*, 735
  care, 220–4
  decoration, 220–1, *220*, *221*
  discolouration, 226, 721, 735
  function, 220
  gel, 237–8
  hardeners, 217–18, 241–2,
    734

instrument damage, 228–30
mending, 240–1, *240*, 735
onycholysis, 228, 235, 237,
  241–2, 721, 734
onychoschizia, 221, *222*
paronychia, 721, 735
physico-chemical properties,
  96
pterygium inversum, 242,
  242
reactions to cosmetics,
  224–8, 237, 238, 240,
  241–2, 502, 721, 734–5
sanitary practices, 229–30
texture, 221
transungual drug therapy,
  95–7
varnishes, 213–18, 223,
  224–7, 734–5
wrapping, 241, *241*, 735
Nappies, dermatitis, 508–9
Narcissus absolute, 46–7
Nasolabial furrows
  collagen injections, 614, 615,
    616, 618–19, 620
  Gore-tex, 622, 623–6, *623–8*
Natural moisturizing factors
  (NMF), 142–3, 247, 248
Neuropathies, diagnosis, 551
Neutral red dye uptake assay,
  33–4, 36, 146
Newborns
  cleansers, 508
  skin permeability, 505–6
  transepidermal water loss,
    530
Nickel, adverse reactions, 726,
  739
Nicotinic acid esters, 714–15
Nitrocellulose, nail varnish,
  214
N-Nitrosodiethanolamine
  (NDELA), 80
Nonimmunologic contact
  urticaria, 714–15
Nonionic surfactants, 114, 137,
  507
Normal skin, 125–6
  care of, 137–9
  cleansers, 116
  stratum corneum lipids, *106*
Nova Dermal Phase Meter,
  296

Nuclear magnetic resonance (NMR) spectroscopy, 131, 134–5, *134*, 278, 280

Oakmoss absolute, 41, 42, 46
Occlusive agents, 119–20, 142, 144, 250, 258–9, 287–8, 370
Occupational dermatitis, 727, 729, 738–40
Occupational dyschromias, 398, 400
Octyl dimethyl PABA, 731, 732
Octyl methoxycinnamate, 731
Ocular irritancy *see* Eye irritancy
Odour *see* Body odour
OECD, testing guidelines, 71–2
Oestrogen
    cutaneous microvasculature, 23, 28
    menopausal women, 487–8, 490–1, 492, 493
    stratum corneum hydration, 21, 28
Oil-in-water emulsions, 120, 144, 258–9, 290, 291, 369–70, 435
Oils rich in PUFA, 144, 145
Oily skin, 2–4
    care of, 139–43
    cleansers, 114, 116–17
    complex type, 127, 139–42
    simple type, 127, 139
Onycholysis, 228, *228*, 229, 721
    with artificial nails, 235, *235*, 237
    due to formaldehyde, 241–2, 734
Onychoschizia, 221, *222*
Opacifiers, 51
Optical techniques
    blood flow measurement, 523–5
    skin properties, 281
    skin surface relief, 538–9
Oral care agents, 51, 715, 718, 735–6
Organic solvents, irritation, 352–5
Ovarian hormones, menopause, 488
Ovaries

polycystic ovary syndrome, 382–3, 385, 386, 387, 389
    tumours, 383
Oxidation *see* Antioxidants
Oxidizing agents, 51
Oxybenzone, 731–2
Oxygen pressure, transcutaneous, 23, 24, 25, 524–5

Package labelling systems, 49–50, 59, 65, 66, 67, 721
    hand and body lotions, 287, 299
Pain sensation, 25
p-Aminobenzoic acid (PABA), 319, 320, 718, 730, 731, 732, 733
Parabens, 722–3, 726
Paraesthesia, pyrethoids, 711
Paraffin, 249, 259, 261
Paronychia, 721, 735
Patch testing, 146–7, 713, 721–2
    artificial nails, 236, 240, 735
    children, 506, 736–7
    cosmetic habituation, 750
    eye make-up, 725
    facial make-up, 730
    hair preparations, 726, 727–8
    nail hardeners, 242, 734
    oral hygiene products, 736
    percutaneous absorption, 81–2
    photosensitivity, 719–21
    racial differences, 516
Patient/doctor relationships, 748–9
Peeling
    chemical *see* Chemabrasion
    cryosurgery, 697
Pentadecylcatechol, 736
Percutaneous absorption, 75–94
    cosmetic efficacy, 86–7, 89–92
    diseased skin, 77–8
    dynamics, 92–3
    measuring methods, 75–7
    product development, 79
    racial differences, 516
    regulation, 62, 63, 64, 85, 86
    safety and efficacy, 87
    skin viability, 77

toxicity, 62, 63, 64, 79–82, 87–9
    vitamins, 78–9, 90–1
Perfumes *see* Fragrances
Permanent waves, 190–1, 721, 726–7, 738–9
Persistent light reaction, 327
Personal cleanliness *see* Hygiene products
Personality, 749, 750
Perspiration *see* Sweat
Petrolatum
    hair straighteners, 727
    moisturizers, 249, 259, 261, 288, 292, *293*, 295, *295*
    photosensitivity, 720
pH
    cleansers, 115, 138, 434
    exfoliants, 168
    shampoos, 507
    vulvar skin, 332
Pharmacokinetics, 88–9
    caffeine, 89–90
    α-hydroxy acids, 91–2
    sunscreens, 90
    vitamins, 91
Phenols
    depigmentation, 718
    facial peels, 585, 586
    photosensitivity, 718
Phenothiazine
    hyperpigmentation, 399, 400
Phenylalanine, dyschromias, 407
p-phenylenediamine (PPDA, PPD), 81–2, 728–9, 738, 739
Phlebectomy, Muller's, 378–9, *378–9*
Phosphobacterium phosphoreum, 35–6, 146
Phospholipase A_2, 476, *476*, *481*
Photo-acoustic spectroscopy (PAS), 277
Photoaging, 126, 456–65
    α-hydroxy acids, 463
    anti-inflammatory agents, 464
    antioxidants, 464
    clinical signs, 459–60
    clinical study methods, 464–5

Photoaging – *cont.*
cryosurgery, 696
    dermabrasion, 607–8, *608–10*
    electrical stimulation of skin,
        645, 646–9
    facial peels, 463
    histologic changes of, 460
    inflammatory reactions,
        469–70, 472–8, 480,
        483–4
    laser therapy, 662, *664*, 665,
        686–7
    pathogenesis, 457–9
    prevention, 460–2
    retinoids, 462–3, 525
    surgical procedures, 463–4
    topical hormones, 464
Photoallergy reaction, 325,
    718–20, 730, 732–3
Photochemotherapy
    dyschromias, 400, 406–7
    and photoaging, 459
Photodermatitis, 42, 324, 325,
    346–7
Photography, studying
    photoaging, 464, 465
Photopatch testing, 719–21
Photopulse plethysmography
    (PPG), 523
Photosensitivity, 326–8,
    718–21, 730, 732–3
Photothermolysis
    cellular-level, 679–82
    vascular, 674–9
Phototoxic contact dermatitis,
    43, 396
Phototoxic protection factor
    (PPF), 318
Phototoxicity, 323, 324–5,
    718
    animal testing, 62, 63, 64
    fragrances, 42
    moisturizers, 304–5
    sunscreens, 732
    in vitro assays, 36
Phototrichograms, 545–7
Phytophotodermatitis, 324
Pigmentation, 391–415
    adverse reactions, 717–18
    artefact dermatitis, 750–1
    cellular-level
        photothermolysis,
        679–82

ceruloderma, 391, 392,
    397–400
classifying disorders of,
    391–2
cryosurgery for disorders of,
    693
dyspigmentation risk after
    surgery, 411
etiology of disorders, 400–1
following cryosurgery, 698
gender variations, 27–8
hair repigmentation, 500
leucoderma, 391, 392–5, 717,
    718
managing dyschromias,
    401–11, 588, 679–82,
    685–6
measurement, 28, 524, 539
measuring regeneration, 5–6
melanoderma, 391, 392,
    395–7
and photoaging, 458–9, 462
problems with dermabrasion,
    610
racial variations in disorders,
    394, 401, 402, 404, 517,
    520
testing cleansers, 118
Pigment-darkening protection
    factor, 319
Pilosebaceous unit
    gender variations, 29–30
    greasy hair, 184
Pityriasis alba, 394–5
Pityriasis capitis *see* Dandruff
Pityriasis versicolor, 395, *395*,
    403, 404
Pityrosporum yeasts, 127, 128,
    141, 194–5, 197, 436
Plants
    botanicals, 50
    ingredients from, 56–7
Plasticizers, nail varnish,
    214–15, 734
Plucking hair, 201–2, 386
Poikiloderma of Civatte, 683
Poison ivy, 339
Poison oak, 339
Polarized light, testing
    cleansers, 118, *118*
Polycystic ovary syndrome
    (PCO), 382–3, 385, 386,
    387, 389

Polymethyl methacrylate
    (PMMA), 620–1
Polymorphonuclear leucocytes
    (PMN), 471, 478, 480
Polymorphous light eruption
    (PLME), 326
Polyols, moisturizers, 143, 248,
    257–8, 259, 288–9, 295,
    296
    see also Glycerol; Propylene
        glycol
Polyunsaturated fatty acids
    (PUFA), 144, 145
Pomades, 191, 443–4
Porokeratosis plantaris
    discreta, 695
Porphyrias, 326
Port wine stains, 375
    camouflage make-up, *418*
    laser therapy, 375, 675, *676*,
        752
    psychological consequences,
        752
Post-dermabrasion
    hyperpigmentation, 400
Postherpetic neuralgia, 551
Post-inflammatory
    hypermelanosis, 397,
    397
    depigmenting agents, 401–2,
        404
    with dermabrasion, 610
    facial peels, 588, 593
    laser therapy, 406, 685
Post-inflammatory
    hypomelanosis, 394, *394*
Post-traumatic
    depigmentation, 394,
    410–11
Potassium permanganate,
    337–8
Powders
    baby, 509
    facial make-up, 730
Pregnancy, hirsuties in, 383
Preservatives, 51
    adverse reactions, 722–4,
        726, 727–8
    contact urticaria, 715
    moisturizers, 289–90, 300
Pressure sensitivity, 25
Progestogens, menopausal
    women, 488, 491, 493

Progressive disseminated essential telangiectasia, 375, *375*

Propellants, 51, 736

Propionibacterium acnes, 127
azelaic acid, 140
benzoyl peroxide, 79, 140
liquid soaps, 434
skin cleansers, 117
topical antibiotics, 140

Propyl gallate, 726, 729

Propylene glycol, 143, 145, 248, 726, 737

Prostheses, camouflage therapy, 427–31

Protease activity, premature aging, 471, 478, 480, *480–1*, 484

Protein derivatives, hair care, 181–2

Pseudofolliculitis, 498–9, *499*, 737

Pseudomonas infections, nails, 229

Psoralen photochemotherapy
dyschromias, 400, 406
and photoaging, 459

Psoralens, 324–5, 526

Psoriasis
ceramide levels, 101–2
transepidermal water loss, 531

Psychiatric illness, 751

Psychology of cosmetic use, 747–53

Pterygium inversum, 242, *242*

Puberty, 496–7
see also Adolescents

PUVA lentigines, 396, 400

PUVA therapy, 400, 406, 459

Pyogenic granulomas, 685

Pyrethroids, 711

Pyrimidine (thymidine) dimers, photoaging, 458, 462, 464, 477, *478*

Pyrithione zinc (PTZ) shampoo, 195–6

Pyrocatechol, 717–18

Pyrrolidone carboxylic acid (PCA), moisturizing effect, 142, 247, 248, 257, 258, 261

Q-switched lasers, 661, 680–2

dyschromias, 405–6, 412, 681–2, *681*, 685, 686

hirsutism, 687–8

Quaternary ammonium compounds, 141, 182

Quaternium-15, 721–2, 723, 726

Quaternized protein hydrolysates, 183

Rabbit ear assay, acnegenesis, 716–17

Racial differences, 515–21
ceramides, 102–3, 515
dyschromias, 394, 401, 402, 404, 517, 520, 717
face masks, 160
hair growth, 204
photoaging, 458–9
senile xerosis, 102–3
stratum corneum, 102–3, 515–16, 517
*Ra*DIN parameter, 4–5, *4*, *10*

Radiolabelling, percutaneous absorption, 76–7, 81

Reducing agents, 51

Reduction liposculpturing, 553–67

Regulation of cosmetic products, 49–73, 85–6
animal testing, 49, 60–4, 67–73, 724
IFRA-restricted fragrance materials, 42, 44–5, 52
Japan, 66–7
labelling, 49–50, 59, 65, 66, 67, 721
USA, 64–6, 113, 162, 215–16, 709, 721

Relief analysis *see* Skin surface relief

Reodorants, 172

Repetitive irritant test (RIT), 525–6

Research Institute of Fragrance Materials (RIFM), 41

Retinoids
acne treatment, 140, 437, 442–3, 751
and dermabrasion, 609
dyschromias, 404

and electrical stimulation, 654
irritant potential, 527
menopausal women, 492–3
photoaging, 462–3, 525
pseudofolliculitis, 499

Rhinophyma
cryosurgery, 695, 697
laser treatments, 596, *598*, 666–9, *667*, 687

Riehl's melanosis, 398

Rinsing products, 435

Rosacea, 373–4, 683, 695, 737–8

Rouge, 730

Rubber masks, 169

*Rz*DIN parameter, 4, *4*, 5, *10*

Safety
astringents, 163
children's toiletry, 506, 507–8, 511–12
face masks, 160
moisturizers, 300–5
percutaneous absorption, 62, 63, 64, 79–82, 85–9, 93
regulation of cosmetics, 44–5, 49–73, 85, 709, 724
shampoos, 178
skin cleansers, 118–19
tars, 186–7
toluene, 215–16, 217–18
in vitro tests, 33–40, 145–6
in vivo human testing, 146–7
see also Toxicity

Salicylic acid
acne, 436
hair care, 198
masks, 160, 161
sensitivity to, 41, 46, 717
sunscreens, 320, 731, 732–3

Sandalwood oil, 41, 46–7, 717

Scalp
dysmorphophobia, 751
seborrhoea of, 127–8, 183–8, 193

Scalp flaps, hair loss, 640–1

Scalp reduction
hair loss, 637–9, *638*, 640, *640*, 641
laser treatments, 669–70

Scanners, vascular
photothermolysis, 676–7
Scars
cryosurgery, 695, 696, 697–8
dermabrasion, 595–610
electrical stimulation of skin,
643, 645, 646, *649–51*,
653
Fibrel, 617–19, *618–19*
laser treatments, 592–3,
596–7, 665–6, *665*, 669,
687
Sclerotherapy, telangiectases,
375, 378, *378*
Scratch-resistance test, 272
Scrubs, 156, 158, 159–60, 168
Seasonal influences
ceramide levels, 103–4, *105*
cosmetic skin parameters,
1–15
hair distribution, 29
thermoregulatory response,
25
Sebaceous hyperplasia,
cryosurgery, 694, 696, 697
Seborrhoeic dermatitis, 127–8
astringents/toners, 163
cosmetic intolerance
syndrome, 737–8
dandruff and, 193, 194, *194*
greasy hair, 127–8, 183–8
selenium disulphide, 186
treatment, 141, 195, 196,
197–8
Seborrhoeic keratosis,
cryosurgery, 694, 697
Sebum
acne, 117, 140–1, 433, 443
atopic dermatitis, 368
gender variations, 21, 29,
496
hair care, 177–8, 180–1, 184–8
measurement, 135–7
menopausal women, 489–90
quantification, 539–40
skin cleansers, 116–17
Sebum excretion rate (SER),
135, 136
Sebumeter, 136
Sebutape, 136–7
Selenium sulphide, 186,
196–7
Self-esteem, 749–50

Self-tanning products, 151–4,
462
Senile skin, 128
Senile xerosis, ceramide levels,
102–3
Sensitive skin syndrome,
343–9, 549, 551–2
Sensitization, 302–4, 712–13
Sensory functions
cryosurgery, 699
gender variations, 25–6
thermal, 25, 549–52
Sensory (subjective) irritation,
302, 344–6, 711–12
Shampoos, 177–8
adverse reactions, 378, 723,
724, 727–8
babies, 506–8, 511
children, 506–8
dandruff, 195–8
efficacy, 178
greasy hair, 141–2, 184–8
irritant potential, 526–7
men, 499
normal hair, 138
Shaving
and acne, 435
hair removal, 201, 386
products for men, 497–9
Silicon Microphysiometer, 34,
35
Silicones
dry hair care, 183
injectable, 622
moisturizers, 249, 288
Silver pigmentation, 399, 401
Skin critical surface tension
(CST), 281
Skin equivalents, 34, 35
Skin surface biopsies (SSBs),
129–31, *130*, 137
moisturizer efficacy, 267
pigmentation disorders, 392
Skin surface hygrometers, 131,
253, 257, 296
Skin surface relief, 129, *129*,
130, 537–9
after electrostimulation,
652
climatic influence, 3–5, 8–9
mask efficacy, 159
moisturizer efficacy, 265–6
studying photoaging, 464–5

Skin surface water loss
(SSWL), 532–3
Skin tags, cryosurgery, 694
Skinfeel SDA, 298
Skintex, 34, 36, 37, 146
Smoke, aging effects, 470, 475,
475–6, 493
Soaps
acne, 433–4
adverse reactions, 717, 726
anionic surfactants, 114, 115,
137
atopic dermatitis, 370
children, 508
men, 501
normal skin, 137–8
oily skin, 139–40
regulation, 709
shampoos, 178
shaving, 497, 498
Social aspects of cosmetic use,
747–53
Social customs, dyschromia
and, 401
Sodium benzoate, 715
Sodium bicarbonate,
deodorant, 173
Sodium dodecyl sulphate
(SDS), 355–6
Sodium hydroxide
barrier cream efficacy, 525
hair straightening, 727
Sodium lauryl sulphate (SLS)
blood flow assessment, 525,
526–7
gender variations, 22–3
race differences in irritant
reactions, *517*, 518,
518
transepidermal water loss,
532–3
Soft-tissue augmentation,
613–22
Artecoll, 620–1
autologen, 620
autologous collagen, 619–20
Fibrel, 617–19, *617–19*
Gore-tex, 621–2, 623–32
Hylan Gel, 621
injectable silicone, 622
syringe fat transfer, 569–84
Zyderm/Zyplast, 613–16,
613–17

Solar elastosis, 460, 696
Solar keratoses
    dermabrasion, 602, *604*, 608,
        609
    facial chemical peels, 587–8,
        587–8
    sunscreen protection, 323
Solar lentigo, 396, *396*, 405,
    693, 696
Solar urticaria, 326–7
Solvents, 51
    irritation, 352–5
    nail varnish, 215
Sorption/desorption test
    (SDT), 133, 257, 531
Spearmint oil, 47
Spider angiomas
    cryosurgery, 693, 695, *696*
    laser treatments, 674, 678,
        683
Spironolactone, 387–8
Squamometry
    antidandruff efficacy, 199
    facial masks, 156, *157*
    moisturizer efficacy, 267,
        298
    Staphylococcus spp
    atopic dermatitis, 367, 370
    diaper dermatitis, 509
    nails, 229
    vulvar skin, 334, 335, 336,
        340
Starches, dry hair care, 183
Static electricity, 50
Status cosmeticus, 343, 348,
    737
Steam treatment, acne, 444
Stearamidoethyl diethylamine
    phosphate, 724
Steatocystoma multiplex, 694
Steroids
    dyschromias, 404
    hirsutism, 388
    iatrogenic dyschromia, 400
    pathological dry skin, 145
    pseudofolliculitis, 499
    seborrheic dermatitis, 142
    vulvar allergic contact
        dermatitis, 339
Stingers, 711–12
Stinging test, 147, 506
Stratum corneum
    acne, 102

atopic dermatitis, 102, 369
barrier function, 104, 107–9,
    351–2, 356, 529, 532
ceramides, 19–20, 99–109,
    100, 106, 107
DHA decolouring test, 5–6,
    11–13
gender variations, 19–21, 28
ichthyosis, 101–2
imaging techniques, 280
inflammatory reactions, 471
irritation prevention, 302
lipid role in irritant
    dermatitis, 351–6
psoriasis, 101–2
racial differences, 102–3,
    515–16, 517
senile xerosis, 102–3
skin surface biopsies, 129–31,
    130
winter xerosis, 103–4, *105*
X-linked recessive ichthyosis,
    362
see also Hydration;
    Transepidermal water
    loss
Streptococci
    diaper dermatitis, 509
    vulvar skin, 335–6
Strip grafting, hair loss, 639
Subjective (sensory) irritation,
    302, 344–6, 711–12
Suction chamber, elasticity,
    270, 297
Suicide, 751, 752
Sulphur compounds
    acne, 436
    blood flow assessment, 525,
        526–7
    dandruff, 196–7, 198
    gendered irritant reactions,
        22–3
    hair preparations, 185–6,
        727, 729
    hair removal, 202, 499, 737
    racial differences in
        reactions to, *517*, 518,
        518
    SDS irritation, 355–6
    transepidermal water loss,
        532–3
Sun damage
    acne patients, 437–8, 444

CO_2 laser resurfacing, 592,
    593
dyschromias, 396, *396*, 404,
    405
face masks, 159–60
facial chemical peels, 586–8,
    587–8
hair, 179, *179*
protection from *see*
    Sunscreens
racial differences, 516
see also Photoaging
Sun protection factors (SPFs),
    318
climatic influence, 13, *14*
foundations, 730
moisturizers, 123
of suntans, 462
US formulations, 730–1
Sunscreens, 138–9, 317–29
    active ingredients, 319–21
    adverse reactions, 720, 729,
        730–4
    against actinic keratoses, 323
    blood flow assessment, 526
    children, 509–11
    coumarins, 42
    drug photosensitive skin
        reactions, 323–4
    excipients, 733–4
    facial make-up, 730
    history, 317–18
    infrared radiation, 311–15
    menopausal women, 492
    normal skin, 322
    percutaneous absorption, 90
    photoallergy reaction, 325
    photoinstability, 321
    photosensitivity, 326–8, 720
    phototoxicity reaction, 323–5
    physical blockers, 313–14,
        321, 462, 730, 733
    preventing photoaging,
        461–2, 484
    in self-tanning products, 153
    skin colour measurement,
        539
    substantivity, 319
    systemic agents, 321–2
    US formulations, 730–1
    UVA protection, 318–19,
        320–1, 323–5, 461–2,
        463, 539

Suntan products
  children, 510
  DHA decolouring test, 5–6,
    11–13, *12, 13*
  self-tanning, 151–4, 462
Suntans, and photoaging, 462
Surfactants, 51, 137
  bend of elbow washing test, 6
  in cleansers, 114–16
  dry skin, 142
  hair care, 141, 182–3
  for normal skin products, 138
  percutaneous absorption,
    92–3
  shampoos, 141, 183, 188,
    506–7
  transepidermal water loss,
    532
Sweat
  antiperspirants, 50, 174–5,
    446, 501–2, 709, 736
  atopic dermatitis, 367–8
  deodorants, 51, 171–6,
    445–6, 501–2, 736
  gender variations, 496
  idiopathic hyperhidrosis,
    445–54
  men, 496, 501–2
Sympathetic surgery,
    idiopathic hyperhidrosis,
    446–7
Syndets
  children, 508
  dry skin, 142
  normal skin, 138
  oily skin, 139
Syringe fat transfer, 569–84
  adipose tissue washing, 577–8
  anaesthesia, 575–6
  complications, 580–1
  delayed harvesting, 579
  extraction technique, 577
  facial recontouring, 571–9
  history, 569–70
  implant conservation,
    579–80
  indications, 571
  instruments, 576–7
  postoperative course, 579,
    580
  reinjection, 578, *578*
  remodelling, 578–9
  results, 581–2, *581–3*

Syringe liposculpturing,
    553–67
Syringoma, cryosurgery, 694
Systemic toxicity, 87–9

Tactile Sensor, 298
Tags, cryosurgery, 694
Talc, 509, 737
Tannic acid, dermabrasion,
    412–13
Tans and tanning
  children, 510
  DHA decolouring test, 5–6,
    11–13, *12, 13*
  photoaging, 462
  self-tanning products, 151–4,
    462
Tars
  hair care, 141–2, 186–7, 198,
    728
  percutaneous absorption,
    80–1
  pigmentation, 717
Tattoos and tattooing
  camouflage make-up, 426–7,
    501
  covering dyschromias, 408–9
  cryosurgery, 693, 697, *697*
  dermabrasion, 412–13, *603*
  laser removal, 412, 670–1,
    671, 681–2, *681*, 686
Tazarotene, 442–3
Teenagers *see* Adolescents
Telangiectases, 373–80
  cryosurgery, 375, 695, *696*
  laser treatments, 674, 675,
    676, 677, 683–4
  see also Naevi; Port wine
    stains
Temperature effects *see*
    Climatic influence,
    cosmetic skin parameters
Testosterone
  acne, 127, 141
  hair growth, 30, 381–2, 383,
    384, 385, 387–8
  menopausal women, 488, 492
Tetracyclines
  acne, 437, 443
  hyperpigmentation, 399, 400
  and nail discolouration, 226
Tetrahymena thermophila assay,
    34, 36

Tewameters, 279
Thermal sensation
  analysis, 549–52
  gender variations, 25
Thermometry, 524
Thermoregulatory response,
    25
Thickness of skin
  gender variations, 17, 18, 19
  measurement, 541–3
Thiersch grafts, 410, *410*
Thimerosal, 721–2
Thioglycolates
  hair removal, 202, 499, 737
  permanent waves, 726–7,
    738, 739
Thixotropic behaviour, 216
Thymidine (pyrimidine)
  dimers, photoaging, 458,
    462, 464, 477, *478*
Titanium dioxide
  acne, 443
  adverse reactions, 730, 733
  sun block, 313–14, 321, 462,
    730, 733
Toe nails *see* Nails
Toluene
  hair preparations, 728
  nail varnish, 214, 215–16,
    217–18, 225–6, 734
Toners, 155, 161–3, 167
Tonometry, elasticity
  measurement, 270
Toothpaste, 718, 735–6
Top Derm, 643, 644, *645*, 646,
    650
Torque meters, skin hydration,
    133–4, 269, 297
Torsion recovery,
    measurement, 540–1
Total protein assays, 34, 35, 36,
    145–6
Toupees, 501, 633
Toxicity, 709–46
  acnegenesis, 715–17
  animal testing, 60–4, 67–73,
    724
  astringents, 163
  bath preparations, 737
  blood flow assessment, 526–7
  children's toiletry, 506,
    507–8, 511–12, 736–7
  comedogenesis, 715–17

cosmetic intolerance
    syndrome, 737–8
depilatories, 737
emulsifiers, 724
epilating waxes, 737
eye make-up, 725–6
face masks, 160
facial make-up, 729–30
hair preparations, 721, 723,
    724, 726–9
hygiene products, 736
incidence, 709–10
lanolin, 724–5
moisturizers, 300–5
nail cosmetics, 215–18,
    224–8, 237, 238, 240,
    241–2, 502, 721, 734–5
occupational dermatitis,
    738–40
oral care agents, 715, 718,
    735–6
patch testing, 721–2
percutaneous absorption, 62,
    63, 64, 79–82, 87–9
photosensitivity, 718–21, 730
pigmentation, 717–18
preservatives, 722–4, 726
regulation, 55, 57–8, 60–7,
    709
shampoos, 178, 507–8, 723,
    724, 727–8
sunscreens, 730–4
tars, 186–7
in vitro assays, 33–40, 145–6
in vivo human testing, 146–7
see also Allergic contact
    dermatitis; Contact
    urticaria; Irritant contact
    dermatitis
Transcutaneous oxygen
    pressure, 524–5
gender variations, 23, 24, 25
Transepidermal water loss
    (TEWL), 529–34
atopic dermatitis, 367–8, 531
children, 530
cosmetic efficacy testing,
    533–4
dry skin, 128, 531
elderly people, 530–1
face masks, 168–9
gender variation, 21, 22–3,
    28

hydrating products, 121–2,
    142, 144
and hydration, 247, 529, 530,
    531–3, *532*
lipid role in irritation, 352,
    353, 355–6
measurement, 131, 133, 251,
    252, 254, 255, 279, 5230
principal factors, 128
racial differences, 517–19,
    517–18
skin cleansers, 116, 118
vulvar skin, 332–4
Transmission protection
    factor, 319
Transplants
hair, 634–7, *634–7, 640*, 641
melanocytes, 410–11
Transungual drug therapy,
    95–7
Traumatic wounds
dermabrasion, 605, 606,
    607
electrical stimulation, *650*,
    653
Tretinoin
acne treatment, 140, 437,
    442, 443, 751
and dermabrasion, 609
dyschromias, 404
and electrical stimulation,
    654
menopausal women, 492–3
photoaging, 462–3, 525
Trichilemmal cyst, cryosurgery,
    694
Trichloroacetic acid (TCA),
    405, 585, 586–92
Trichoepithelioma,
    cryosurgery, 694
Triclocarban, 174
Triclosan, 174, 736
Triethanolamine stearate, 724
Triglycerides, moisturizers,
    288
Tuberous sclerosis, laser
    resurfacing, *668*
Twistometer, 540–1

Ultrasound, 280, 541–3
Ultraviolet radiation, 309
absorbers, 51
acne patients, 437, 444

face masks for photodamage,
    159, 160
immediate pigmentation
    darkening, 539
and infrared, 311
lipid role in irritation, 356
moisturizers, 122–3
photochemotherapy, 400,
    406, 459
photoreactions, 304–5
photosensitivity, 718, 719–20
protection *see* Sunscreens
vitamin E absorption, 91
see also Photoaging
Urea, 143, 145, 248, 258, 259,
    369
adverse reactions, 721–2,
    723, 726
[³H]Uridine uptake assay, 33,
    34, 35
Urticaria *see* Contact urticaria;
    Contact urticaria
    syndrome
USA
cosmetic regulations, 64–6,
    113, 162, 215–16, 709,
    721
hand/body lotions, 286, 299
sunscreen ingredients, 320
Usage tests, 86–7, 147, 298
UV radiation *see* Ultraviolet
    radiation
UVA erythema protection
    factor (APF), 319

Vaginal contraceptives, 338–9
Vascular problems
cryosurgery, 693, 695–6
laser treatments, 674–9,
    683–5
see also Telangiectases
Vasculature
gender variations, 23–5
non-invasive assessment,
    523–8
race differences, 519
testing skin cleansers, 118
Venous lakes, cryosurgery, 693,
    695–6
Venous telangiectases of legs,
    376–80, *376, 377, 378*
Verrucous naevus, cryosurgery,
    694

Viability of skin, percutaneous absorption, 77
Vinyl masks, 169
Virilization
    hirsutism, 383, 384, 385, 386
    menopause, 488–90
Viscoelasticity
    after electrostimulation, 652
    measurement, 268–71, 297–8, 540–1
Viscosity controlling agents, 51
Viscosity modifiers, nail varnish, 216
Vitamin A
    cleansers, 115–16
    hair care, 181
    moisturizers, 116, 120, 121
    percutaneous absorption, 90, 91
    see also Tretinoin
Vitamin B
    hair care, 181
    percutaneous absorption, 90, 91
Vitamin C
    lipid peroxidation, 472, *473*
    percutaneous absorption, 90, 91
    sunscreens, 526
Vitamin D, children, 510
Vitamin E
    hair care, 181
    percutaneous absorption, 78–9, 91
    premature aging, 472, *473*, 478, *479*
Vitiligo, 392–3, *393*, 400
    management, 402, 406, 407, *409*, 410, *410–11*, *418*, 588, 718
Vulva and vulvar skin, 331–42

Washing test, bend of elbow, 6, 11, *11*
Water content
    moisturizers, 119–21, 257, 287
    nails, 96
    see also Emulsions; Hydration
Water-soluble polymers, moisturizers, 289
Wax masks, 168–9
Waxes, filmogenic properties, 249
Waxing, hair removal, 201, 386, 502, 737
Weathering, hair, 179, *179*
Wigs, 501, 633
Winter xerosis, 103–4, *105*
Wipes, 508
Witch hazel, 162
Witchcraft syndrome, 751
Women
    body image, 343–4, 747–8, 749–50, 751
    cosmetic habituation, 750
    dermatitis simulata, 750–1
    doctor/patient relationships, 748–9
    hirsutism, 30, 203–4, *203*, 381–9
    Millard's syndrome, 750
    port wine stains, 752
    skin care education, 752–3
    see also Gender variations in skin
Wood's lamp, 392
Wrinkles
    Artecoll implants, 621
    botulinum toxin, 704, *705–6*
    cryosurgery, 696
    dermabrasion, 608, *609*
    electrical stimulation of skin, 643, 644, 645, 646–9, *646–8*, 651–4, *654*

enzyme activity, 480
    facial chemical peels, 588
    gender variations, 496
    hormonal influence, 21, 28–9
    hormone replacement therapy, 491
    laser resurfacing, 662, 663, *664*
    photoaging, 460, 462–4
    skin surface relief, 3–5, 8–9, 129, 538–9
    syringe fat transfer, 573
    Zyderm injections, 614, 615
    Zyplast injections, 614, 615, *616*

Xanthelasma
    cryosurgery, 695
    laser treatment, 666, 687
Xeroderma pigmentosum (XP), 327–8, 459
Xerosis, 145
    hydrating products, 144–5
    with isotretinoin, 437
    skin surface biopsies, 130, *130*
    stratum corneum ceramide levels, 102–4, *105*
Xerosis vulgaris, 128
X-linked recessive ichthyosis (XRI), 361–2

Ylang-Ylang oil, 46–7, 717

Zinc oxide, sun blocks, 321, 733
Zinc pyridine thione, 141
Zirconium salts, 736
Zovirax cream, 339, 610
Zyderm, 613–16, *613–17*
Zyplast, 613–16